PHYSICAL DIAGNOSIS SECRETS

SALVATORE MANGIONE, MD

Clinical Associate Professor of Medicine
Center for Research in Medical Education and Health Care
Director, Physical Diagnosis Curriculum
Jefferson Medical College of Thomas Jefferson University
Philadelphia, Pennsylvania

HANLEY & BELFUS, INC./ Philadelphia

Publisher: HANLEY & BELFUS, INC.
Medical Publishers
210 South 13th Street
Philadelphia, PA 19107
(215) 546-7293; 800-962-1892
FAX (215) 790-9330
Web site: http://www.hanleyandbelfus.com

Note *to the reader*: Although the information in this book has been carefully reviewed for correctness of dosage and indications, neither the authors nor the editors nor the publisher can accept any legal responsibility for any errors or omissions that may be made. Neither the publisher nor the editors make any warranty, expressed or implied, with respect to the material contained herein. Before prescribing any drug, the reader must review the manufacturer's current product information (package inserts) for accepted indications, absolute dosage recommendations, and other information pertinent to the safe and effective use of the product described.

Library of Congress Cataloging-in-Publication Data

Physical diagnosis secrets / edited by Salvatore Mangione.
     p.   cm. — (The Secrets Series®)
Includes bibliographical references and index.
ISBN 1-56053-164-9 (alk. paper)
  1. Physical diagnosis—Miscellanea. I. Mangione, Salvatore,
1954–   . II. Series.
  [DNLM: 1. Physical Examination examination questions.
2. Diagnostic Techniques and Procedures examination questions.
3. Signs and Symptoms examination questions.   WB 18.2 P578 2000]
RC76.P524   2000
616.07'54'076—dc21
DNLM/DLC
for Library of Congress   98-43417
                                        CIP

PHYSICAL DIAGNOSIS SECRETS   ISBN 1-56053-164-9

Last digit is the print number: 9 8 7 6 5 4 3 2 1

To my dog, who made it all possible.

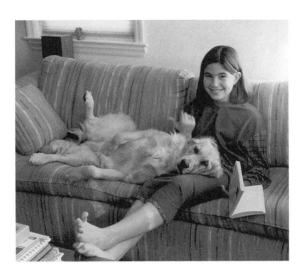

And to my editor, Bill Lamsback, for his North-American tolerance of my South-European procrastination.

To be able to explore is, in my opinion, a large part of the Art
Hippocrates, *Epidemics III*

It was six men of Indostan, to learning much inclined,
who went to see the elephant (Though all of them were blind),
that each by observation, might satisfy his mind.

The first approached the elephant, and, happening to fall,
against his broad and sturdy side, at once began to bawl:
"God bless me! But the elephant, is nothing but a wall!"

The second, feeling of the tusk, cried: "Ho! what have we here,
so very round and smooth and sharp? To me tis mighty clear,
this wonder of an elephant, is very like a spear!"

The third approached the animal, and, happening to take,
the squirming trunk within his hands, "I see," quoth he,
the elephant is very like a snake!"

The fourth reached out his eager hand, and felt about the knee:
"What most this wondrous beast is like, is mighty plain," quoth he;
"Tis clear enough the elephant is very like a tree."

The fifth, who chanced to touch the ear, Said; "E'en the blindest man
can tell what this resembles most; Deny the fact who can,
This marvel of an elephant, is very like a fan!"

The sixth no sooner had begun, about the beast to grope,
than, seizing on the swinging tail, that fell within his scope,
"I see," quoth he, "the elephant is very like a rope!"

And so these men of Indostan, disputed loud and long,
each in his own opinion, exceeding stiff and strong,
Though each was partly in the right, and all were in the wrong!

So, oft in theologic wars, the disputants, I ween,
tread in utter ignorance, of what each other mean,
and prate about the elephant, not one of them has seen!

John Godfrey Saxe (1816–1887)

CONTENTS

CONTRIBUTORS

Sylvia R. Beck, MD
Assistant Professor, Department of Ophthalmology, Medical College of Pennsylvania; Clinical Instructor, Wills Eye Hospital, Philadelphia, Pennsylvania

Dale Berg, MD
University of Minnesota Medical School and Harvard Medical School, Minneapolis, Minnesota

Carol Fleischman, MD
Assistant Professor, Department of Internal Medicine, Medical College of Pennsylvania, Hahnemann School of Medicine, Philadelphia, Pennsylvania

Debra Grossman, MD, MPH
Clinical Assistant Professor of Dermatology, University of Pennsylvania School of Medicine; Bucks Dermatology and Laser Center, Langhorne, Pennsylvania

Cynthia Guzzo, MD
Director of Worldwide OTC, Merck Research Laboratories, Blue Bell, Pennsylvania; Adjunct Clinical Associate Professor, Department of Dermatology, University of Pennsylvania School of Medicine, Philadelphia, Pennsylvania

Bruce I. Hoffman, MD
Associate Professor, Department of Medicine, Medical College of Pennsylvania, Hahnemann University School of Medicine, Philadelphia, Pennsylvania

Salvatore Mangione, MD
Clinical Associate Professor of Medicine, Center for Research in Medical Education and Health Care, Director of Physical Diagnosis Curriculum, Jefferson Medical College of Thomas Jefferson University, Philadelphia, Pennsylvania

Cameron Quanbeck, MD
Department of Psychiatry, UCLA Neuropsychiatric Institute, Los Angeles, California

Loren A. Rolak, MD
Director, The Marshfield Clinic Multiple Sclerosis Center, Marshfield, Wisconsin; Clinical Associate Professor of Neurology, University of Wisconsin, Madison, Wisconsin

Ira Strassman, MD
Assistant Professor, Department of Pediatrics, Jefferson Medical College of Thomas Jefferson University, Philadelphia, Pennsylvania

Richard Tipperman, MD
Clinical Associate Professor, Wills Eye Hospital, Philadelphia, Pennsylvania; Active Staff, Graduate Hospital, Medical College of Pennsylvania, Parkview Hospital, Philadelphia, Pennsylvania; Holy Redeemer Hospital, Meadowbrook, Pennsylvania; Lankenau Hospital, Wynnewood, Pennsylvania

Janice Wood, MD
Assistant Professor, Department of Medicine, Loyola University Medical Center, Maywood, Illinois; Loyola University Hospital, Chicago, Illinois

Katherine Worzala, MD
University of Minnesota School of Medicine, Minneapolis, Minnesota

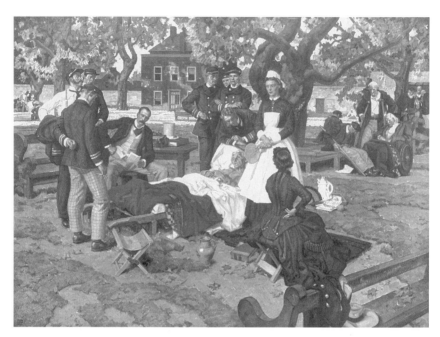

Osler at Old Blockley (Philadelphia General Hospital), by Dean Cornwell. (Reproduced by permission of Wyeth-Ayerst Laboratories.)

PREFACE

Physical diagnosis occupies an uncertain position at the turn of the millennium. There has been recent interest in validating, refining, and sometimes discarding traditional methods and signs. A physical diagnosis interest group has arisen within the general internal medicine community, the *American College of Physicians* has sponsored an update course on physical diagnosis, and the *Journal of the American Medical Association* has initiated a series of articles on the "rational clinical examination." Perhaps most important, physicians in practice rate history-taking and physical examination as their most valuable skills. On the other hand, a distressing literature documents the lack of competence in physical diagnosis among primary care residents and even physicians-in-practice, few training programs provide structured teaching in these skills, and attending "rounds" too often avoid the bedside.

At times physical diagnosis reminds us of the lowly troglodyte in the Gary Larson cartoon at the end of this book, holding in his hand a stone wheel while fellow troglodytes drive a Cadillac and poke fun at him.

Still, there are plenty of reasons to promote the teaching of physical examination. Among these are cost-effectiveness, the possibility of making inexpensive serial observations, the early detection of critical findings, the intelligent and well-guided selection of costly diagnostic technology, and the therapeutic value of the physical contact between physician and patient. In times when the "fun" seems to have abandoned the practice of medicine, physical diagnosis and other bedside skills can restore the satisfaction and intellectual pleasure of making a diagnosis using only our own wits and senses.

In our age of high technology it is also important that we identify which areas of physical examination retain value for 21st century medicine and which need to be abandoned. The *Conventional Teaching Watch* sections of this book, based on general consensus or literature validation, represent our attempt at separating the wheat from the chaff. A ranking of this sort is essential to guide a more intelligent learning of physical diagnosis.

In reviewing the various maneuvers and findings which, over the centuries, created physical examination, we made a deliberate attempt at presenting some information about the men and women behind the eponyms (and for this we relied on the great little book by B.G. Firkin and J.A. Whitworth, *The Dictionary of Medical Eponyms*). We believe that learning about the character and personality of these physicians might shed some light on why physical diagnosis enjoyed so many contributions in the last century and so few in our own. The great bedside diagnosticians of the last century were passionately interested in everything human. Most, if not all of them, were humanists, lovers of the arts and literature, travelers and historians, poets and painters, curious of any field that could enrich the human spirit. William Osler, the pinnacle of 19th century bedside medicine, believed so strongly in the value of a liberal education that he provided his medical students with a list of ten books (ranging from Plutarch and Montaigne to Marcus Aurelius and Shakespeare) to read for half an hour before going to sleep.

As Bernard Lown puts it, today's physicians "seem at times more interested in laying on tools than laying on hands." Rejuvenating physical diagnosis might therefore need a revival of the time-honored link between the art and the science of medicine. We agree with William Osler that medicine is "an art of probabilities and a science of uncertainties," and that these two aspects are inseparable, very much like those Siamese twins for whom trying to separate one from the other would only kill them both. Rekindling interest in the bedside and in the humanistic aspect of medicine may therefore represent two facets of the same challenge. We also agree with Socrates that one of the most effective ways to teach is to question. We hope that *Physical Diagnosis Secrets*, in following this tradition and that of the proven and time-tested Secrets Series®, will serve as a valuable and an engaging resource for learning and for truly appreciating the art and the science of physical diagnosis.

Salvatore Mangione, M.D.

THE FAR SIDE
By GARY LARSON

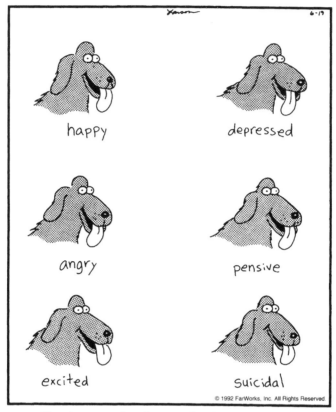

How to recognize the moods of an Irish setter

1. GENERAL APPEARANCE, FACIES, AND BODY HABITUS

Salvatore Mangione, M.D.

I knew you came from Afghanistan. From long habit, the train of thought ran so swiftly through my mind that I arrived at the conclusion without being conscious of immediate steps. There were such steps, however. The train of reasoning ran: "Here is a gentleman of a medical type, but with the air of a military man. Clearly, an army doctor then. He has just come from the tropics, for his face is dark, and that is not the natural tint of his skin, for his wrists are fair. He has undergone hardship and sickness, as his haggard face says clearly. His left arm has been injured. He holds it in a stiff and unnatural manner. Where in the tropics could an English army doctor have seen much hardship and got his arm wounded? Clearly in Afghanistan." The whole train of thought did not occupy a second. I then remarked that you came from Afghanistan and you were astonished.

Arthur Conan Doyle, *A Study in Scarlet*, 1887

TOPICS COVERED IN THIS CHAPTER

Posture
State of hydration
State of nutrition
Body habitus and body proportions
Facies
Apparent age

Apparent race and sex
Alertness and state of consciousness
Degree of illness, whether acute or chronic
Degree of comfort
State of mind and mood
Gait

CONVENTIONAL TEACHING WATCH

Assessment of general appearance is the most fun (and Sherlockian) of all aspects of the physical examination. It is also the most challenging. Nonetheless, astute bedside observation can be extremely helpful and often provides a diagnosis even before the patient is interviewed or examined.

FINDING/MANEUVER		CONVENTIONAL TEACHING REVISITED
Posture	⇑	Valuable information can be obtained by astutely evaluating the patient's posture.
State of hydration	⇑	Another essential aspect of bedside exam, particularly in selective cases
State of nutrition	⇑	Assessment of malnourishment (and its adverse impact on infections and wound healing) or obesity is an important aspect of exam.
Body habitus and body proportions	⇑	Pay attention to distribution of body fat, which may serve as important prognostic indicator because of its association with chronic diseases.
Facies	⇑	Plethora of names, many time-honored.
Degree of illness	⇑	Medical equivalent of infamous observation, "Patient does not look good."
Gait	⇑	As for facies, long list of terms has been gathered over time, and all are quite helpful in reaching a diagnosis.

1. What is the value of carefully examining the general appearance of the patient?

The Sherlockian value of making a diagnosis even before interviewing or touching the patient. General appearance literally can be assessed while the patient is walking down the street. The art of attentive and knowledgeable observation is a time-honored hallmark of the medical profession, and its process was beautifully articulated by Sir Arthur Conan Doyle (himself a physician and former student of the charismatic bedside diagnostician, Joseph Bell) in describing the first encounter between Holmes and Watson. The Sherlockian process requires practice and knowledge and is quite challenging. But it is also the most valuable, rewarding, and fun aspect of bedside diagnosis. It is best learned by having the luck to work with a physician who is skilled at it.

2. Which aspects of the patient should be assessed during a careful and attentive evaluation?

- Posture
- State of hydration
- State of nutrition
- Body habitus and body proportions
- Facies
- Apparent age
- Apparent race and sex
- Alertness and state of consciousness
- Degree of illness, whether acute or chronic
- Degree of comfort
- State of mind and mood
- Gait

Often the untrained eye is able to detect whether a patient "looks weird." But this awareness remains subliminal and never leads to a more cogent insight. The trained eye, on the other hand, is able not only to detect weirdness but also to recognize the reasons behind it. A mental database search then attaches a medical label. As Holmes says, the entire process takes only a few milliseconds, yet it requires a series of intermediate intuitive steps.

POSTURE

3. What information can be obtained from observing the patient's posture?

Valuable information. In **abdominal pain**, for example, the patient's posture is usually so typical that it may help to localize the site of pain:

- Patients with **pancreatitis** usually lie in a fetal position—on the side with knees and legs bent over.
- Patients with **renal or perirenal abscesses** bend toward the side of the lesion.
- Patients with **peritonitis** usually are quite still to avoid any movement that may worsen the pain.
- Patients with **intestinal obstruction** are usually restless.
- Patients who lie supine with one knee flexed and the hip externally rotated usually are said to have the **psoas sign**, which may reflect either a local abnormality around the iliopsoas muscle (such as an inflamed appendix, inflamed terminal ileum due to Crohn's disease, or inflamed diverticulum) or inflammation of the muscle itself. In the olden days the psoas sign indicated a tuberculotic abscess, usually originating in the spine and spreading downward along the muscle. Abscesses of this kind were referred to as "cold abscesses" because they were characterized by no heat or other signs of inflammation. Now the most common cause of iliopsoas muscle involvement is not tuberculosis but intramuscular bleeding due to anticoagulation.

Patients with a large **pericardial effusion** (particularly those in tamponade) usually sit up in bed and lean forward with a posture often described as "the praying Muslim posture." Neck veins are greatly distended.

4. What is the posture of patients with dyspnea?

Quite varied, and still a very valuable source of information. Orthopnea, paroxysmal nocturnal dyspnea, platypnea and orthodeoxia, trepopnea, respiratory alternans, and abdominal paradox provide clues for determining not only the severity of dyspnea but also its etiology. For a detailed description of these respiratory postures, refer to chapter 13.

STATE OF HYDRATION

5. What is hypovolemia?

Hypovolemia is characterized by volume depletion and dehydration:

- **Volume depletion** is a loss of extracellular salt through either kidneys (diuresis) or gastrointestinal tract (hemorrhage, vomiting, diarrhea). Because of circulatory instability, volume depletion usually is associated with an increase in the serum urea nitrogen-to-creatinine ratio, which provides a valuable biochemical marker.
- **Dehydration** is a loss of intracellular water. It eventually causes cellular desiccation and an increase in serum sodium and plasma osmolality (two useful biochemical markers).

6. Is there any reason to consider volume depletion and dehydration as separate processes?

The major reason is management. **Volume depletion** requires rapid infusion of normal saline to correct a situation of hemodynamic instability, whereas **dehydration** is usually not as dramatic and responds to a less aggressive infusion of 5% dextrose in water.

7. What is the value of physical examination in assessing patients with hypovolemia?

The two goals of the examination are (1) to determine whether hypovolemia is present and (2) to confirm its degree.

8. How do you determine whether hypovolemia is present?

By performing the **tilt test**, which measures postural changes in heart rate and blood pressure. The test is conducted as follows:

1. Ask the patient to lie in a supine position.
2. Wait at least 2 minutes.
3. Measure heart rate and blood pressure while the patient is supine.
4. Ask the patient to stand.
5. Wait 1 minute.
6. Measure heart rate and blood pressure while the patient is standing.

Heart rate should be measured by counting over a 30-second period and multiplying by two. This method is more accurate than counting over a 15-second period and multiplying by four.

9. Why is it important to have the patient supine for at least 2 minutes before asking him or her to stand?

This approach increases the sensitivity of the test. A period of two minutes in the supine position is necessary to cause maximal leg pooling of blood upon subsequent standing. The pooling, in turn, causes maximal drop in cardiac output and maximal increment in heart rate. Within 1–2 minutes after standing, about 7–8 ml/kg of blood shift to the lower body, thereby decreasing intrathoracic volume, stroke volume, and cardiac output and at the same time increasing circulating catecholamines and systemic vascular resistance.

10. Is there any benefit in asking the patient to lie supine longer than 2 minutes before assuming a standing position?

No. Keeping the patient supine longer than 2 minutes does not add much to the sensitivity of the test.

11. Is sitting equivalent to standing?

Not at all. In fact, sitting has been shown to reduce significantly the degree of leg pooling and thus the sensitivity of the tilt test.

12. What is the normal response to the tilt test?

Going from supine to standing, a normal patient usually exhibits the following signs:

- **Heart rate** increases by 10.9 ± 2 beats/min and usually stabilizes after 45–60 seconds.

• **Systolic blood pressure** decreases only slightly (by 3.5 ± 2 mmHg) and also stabilizes within 1–2 minutes.

• **Diastolic blood pressure** increases by 5.2 ± 2.4 mmHg and stabilizes within 1–2 minutes. As patients become older, however, the postural increase in heart rate becomes smaller.

13. What are the findings of a tilt test in hypovolemia?

1. The most helpful finding is a **postural increase in heart rate of at least 30 beats/min** (which has a sensitivity of 97% and a specificity of 96% for blood loss > 630 ml). This finding (as well as severe postural dizziness; see below) may last 12–72 hours if intravenous fluids are not administered.

2. The second most helpful finding is **postural dizziness so severe that it is impossible to complete the test**. Severe dizziness has the same sensitivity and specificity as tachycardia. Conversely, mild postural dizziness has no proven diagnostic value.

3. **Hypotension of any degree while standing** has little diagnostic value. In fact, a drop in systolic blood pressure ≥ 20 mmHg upon assuming a standing position may be seen in 10% of normovolemic people below the age of 65 and 11–30% of normal people above the age of 65. It has a sensitivity of only 9% for blood losses of 450–630 ml.

4. **Supine hypotension** (systolic blood pressure < 95 mmHg) and **tachycardia** (> 100 beats/min) may be absent, even in patients with blood losses greater than 1 liter. Thus, although quite specific for hypovolemia when present, supine hypotension and tachycardia have low sensitivity. Paradoxically, patients with blood loss may even have bradycardia (usually as a result of vagal reflex).

Most studies have been conducted in patients with blood loss. Bedside maneuvers for the assessment of hypovolemia due to vomiting, diarrhea, or decreased oral intake have not been studied as extensively.

14. What is the significance of an abnormal tilt test?

An abnormal tilt test usually reflects volume loss. However, it also may reflect either an inability of the heart to increase output (usually because of failure) or a series of neurogenic disorders (such as use of certain antihypertensive agents, various forms of autonomic neuropathies, prolonged bed rest, and even the weightlessness of space travel).

15. What is poor skin turgor?

Poor skin turgor is another bedside indicator of hypovolemia and is indicated by the loss of skin elasticity (see also chapter 21). The physiology behind this test is based on the extreme change in elastin characteristics as a result of change in moisture. Thus, a loss of elasticity (which may be caused by as little as 3.4% loss in wet weight) may prolong the recoil time of the skin by 40 times. As a result, the skin exhibits "tenting" after being pinched by the examiner's thumb and forefinger. Conversely, the skin of a normal person quickly returns to its original position. Older patients tend to have less elastic skin. Thus, this test may be useful in children but has no real diagnostic value in adults. In all patients the standard remains a set of basic laboratory tests: serum electrolytes, urea nitrogen, and creatinine.

16. What is the capillary refill time?

It is another bedside maneuver to assess volume status (see also chapter 21). The patient's hand is placed at the same level as the heart, and the distal phalanx of the middle finger is compressed for 5 seconds and then released. The time necessary for the phalanx to regain its normal color is the capillary refill time. At normal room temperature (21° Celsius) the upper limits of normal are as follows:

• 2 seconds for children and adult men
• 3 seconds for adult women
• 4 seconds for the elderly

Interobserver agreement has been well studied and found to be quite good. In adults this test has little sensitivity but high specificity (11% and 89%, respectively).

17. What other bedside findings can give an estimate of volume status?
- Dry mucous membranes
- Dry axillae
- Sunken eyes
- Longitudinal tongue furrows

Interobserver agreement for some of these findings (axillary sweat) has been studied in a group of acutely ill elderly patients and found to be moderate (80% agreement).

STATE OF NUTRITION

18. What information should be obtained about the patient's state of nutrition?
First determine whether the patient is well nourished or malnourished. Then determine whether the patient is overweight and, if so, to what degree. The distribution of obesity also should be determined.

19. What is the clinical value of assessing the body distribution of obesity?
Quite high. In fact, the location of obesity correlates strongly with its effects on health. Obesity may be central (that is, involving primarily the trunk) or peripheral (that is, involving primarily the extremities).

Central obesity is characterized by a bihumeral diameter that is greater than bitrochanteric diameter. In such patients subcutaneous fat has a descending distribution and is concentrated primarily in the upper half of the body (neck, cheeks, shoulder, chest, and upper abdomen).

Peripheral obesity is characterized by a bitrochanteric diameter that is greater than the bihumeral diameter. In such patients subcutaneous fat has an ascending distribution and is concentrated primarily in the lower half of the body (lower abdomen, pelvic girdle, buttocks, and thighs).

Men tend to have primarily central obesity, whereas women usually have peripheral obesity. Central obesity also carries a much worse prognosis because of its higher association with hypertension, diabetes, atherosclerotic cardiovascular diseases, and other chronic conditions (see below).

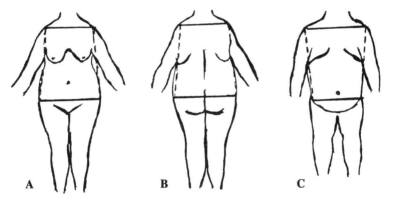

Peripheral (*A* and *B*) and central (*C*) obesity.

20. What is the BMI?
BMI is the acronym for body mass index, the federal government's standard for body weight. BMI is calculated as a ratio between weight and height and provides a better measurement of body fat than the traditional height and weight charts. According to the old standards, men were considered overweight if they had a BMI of 27.3 or higher. The cut-off for women was even higher (27.8). On the basis of the recently revised guidelines, anyone with a BMI of 25 or higher is considered abnormal. Because of these new definitions, more than one-half of all Americans aged 20–74 are overweight, whereas one-fifth are considered obese. (See p 7.)

21. How do you measure the BMI?

The best way is to use a BMI chart (see table on facing page): one simply locates height (inches) and weight (pounds) and finds the corresponding BMI at the intersection of the two. The BMI also can be determined by calculating in kilograms and dividing it by the height in meters squared (BMI = kg/m^2). The following formula is a shortcut:

1. Multiply weight (in pounds) by 703.
2. Multiply height (in inches) by height (in inches).
3. Divide the answer in step 1 by the answer in step 2.

22. Are there any exceptions to the BMI?

Yes. Although the BMI is a better predictor of disease risk than body weight alone, certain people should not use the BMI to determine their risk. For example, because of their larger muscle mass, competitive athletes and body builders may have an index that is excessively high. Similarly, women who are pregnant or lactating also may not be able to use it. Finally, the BMI should not be used in growing children or frail and sedentary elderly people.

23. Why is the BMI important?

A high BMI is associated with an increased risk for serious medical problems:

- Hypertension
- Cardiovascular disease
- Dyslipidemia
- Adult-onset diabetes mellitus (type II)
- Sleep apnea
- Osteoarthritis
- Female infertility
- Various other conditions:
  Idiopathic intracranial hypertension
  Lower extremity venous stasis disease
  Gastroesophageal reflux
  Urinary stress incontinence

Prevention of further weight gain is imperative, and weight reduction is crucial to preserve health. The same value of BMI carries a worse prognosis in the presence of comorbid conditions.

24. What is a comorbid condition?

Any condition associated with obesity that worsens as the degree of obesity increases and, conversely, improves as obesity is successfully treated. Risk of disease based only on BMI increases whenever the patient has one or more comorbid conditions.

25. How do you identify malnutrition?

Primarily through history and physical examination and by using a technique known as the Subjective Global Assessment (SGA) of nutritional status. Patients fall into one of three major classes:

1. Class A (well-nourished)
2. Class B (moderately malnourished)
3. Class C (severely malnourished)

26. What are the physical examination components of the SGA?

Detecting loss of subcutaneous fat, loss of muscle, and shift of intravenous fluid. They are recorded as normal (0), mild (1+), moderate (2+), or severe (3+):

1. The best locations for assessment of **subcutaneous fat loss** are the triceps region of the arms, midaxillary line at the costal margin, interosseous and palmar areas of the hand, and deltoid regions of the shoulder. Loss of subcutaneous fat appears as a lack of fullness; skin fits loosely over the deeper tissues.

2. **Muscle wasting** usually is best assessed by palpation (although inspection at a distance also may help). The best locations for assessment of muscle wasting are the quadriceps femoris and deltoids. Shoulders of malnourished patients appear "squared off" as a result of both muscle wasting and subcutaneous fat loss.

3. **Loss of fluid from the intravascular to extravascular space** refers primarily to ankle or sacral edema and ascites. Edema is best assessed by palpation—that is, by pressing over the ankles or sacral area. Fluid displaced from the subcutaneous tissues as a result of compression is

Body Mass Index

HEIGHT \ WEIGHT	100	105	110	115	120	125	130	135	140	145	150	155	160	165	170	175	180	185	190	195	200	205	210	215	220	225	230	235	240	245	250
5'0"	20	21	21	22	23	24	25	26	27	28	29	30	31	32	33	34	35	36	37	38	39	40	41	42	43	44	45	46	47	48	49
5'1"	19	20	21	22	23	24	25	26	26	27	28	29	30	31	32	33	34	35	36	37	38	39	40	41	42	43	43	44	45	46	47
5'2"	18	19	20	21	22	23	24	25	26	27	27	28	29	30	31	32	33	34	35	36	37	37	38	39	40	41	42	43	44	45	46
5'3"	18	19	19	20	21	22	23	24	25	26	27	27	28	29	30	31	32	33	34	35	35	36	37	38	39	40	41	42	43	43	44
5'4"	17	18	19	20	21	21	22	23	24	25	26	27	27	28	29	30	31	32	33	33	34	35	36	37	38	39	39	40	41	42	43
5'5"	17	17	18	19	20	21	22	22	23	24	25	26	27	27	28	29	30	31	32	32	33	34	35	36	37	37	38	39	40	41	42
5'6"	16	17	18	19	19	20	21	22	23	23	24	25	26	27	27	28	29	30	31	31	32	33	34	35	36	36	37	38	39	40	40
5'7"	16	16	17	18	19	20	20	21	22	23	23	24	25	26	27	27	28	29	30	31	31	32	33	34	34	35	36	37	38	38	39
5'8"	15	16	17	17	18	19	20	21	21	22	23	24	24	25	26	27	27	28	29	30	30	31	32	33	33	34	35	36	36	37	38
5'9"	15	16	16	17	18	18	19	20	21	21	22	23	24	24	25	26	27	27	28	29	30	30	31	32	32	33	34	35	35	36	37
5'10"	14	15	16	17	17	18	19	19	20	21	22	22	23	24	24	25	26	27	27	28	29	29	30	31	32	32	33	34	34	35	36
5'11"	14	15	15	16	17	17	18	19	20	20	21	22	22	23	24	24	25	26	27	27	28	29	29	30	31	31	32	33	33	34	35
6'0"	14	14	15	16	16	17	18	18	19	20	20	21	22	22	23	24	24	25	26	26	27	28	28	29	30	31	31	32	33	33	34
6'1"	13	14	15	15	16	16	17	18	18	19	20	20	21	22	22	23	24	24	25	26	26	27	28	28	29	30	30	31	32	32	33
6'2"	13	13	14	15	15	16	17	17	18	19	19	20	21	21	22	22	23	24	24	25	26	26	27	28	28	29	30	30	31	31	32
6'3"	12	13	14	14	15	16	16	17	18	18	19	19	20	21	21	22	23	23	24	24	25	26	26	27	27	28	29	29	30	31	31
6'4"	12	13	13	14	15	15	16	16	17	18	18	19	19	20	21	21	22	23	23	24	24	25	26	26	27	27	28	29	29	30	30

BMI Category	Health Risk Based Solely On BMI	Risk Adjusted for the Presence of Comorbid Conditions and/or Risk Factors
19-24	Minimal	Low
25-26	Low	Moderate
27-29	Moderate	High
30-34	High	Very High
35-39	Very High	Extremely High
40+	Extremely High	Extremely High

its hallmark. Such displacement is clinically manifested by a persistent depression of the compressed area (pitting), which lasts more than 5 seconds.

Once gathered, these physical features are combined subjectively with other clinical findings and an SGA is generated. There is no clearcut weighting recommendation for combining these features, even though the following variables are usually given high clinical importance:

- Weight loss of more than 10%
- Loss of subcutaneous tissue
- Poor dietary intake
- Muscle wasting

For example, patients with all three physical signs of malnutrition plus a weight loss of at least 10% usually are classified as severely malnourished (class C). The SGA technique is not highly sensitive for the diagnosis of malnutrition, but it is quite specific.

27. Why should one bother to assess for malnutrition?

Malnutrition is an important risk factor for the development of major complications such as infection or poor wound healing.

FACIES

28. Define facies.

Facies is Latin for face and refers to peculiar and unusual facial features that often are pathognomonic of a particular disease. The physician with a trained eye can quickly recognize these features and make a diagnosis simply by walking in the waiting room.

29. Which disease processes are associated with a typical facies?

Quite a few. The following list is not exhaustive:

1. **Facies antonina** is one of the facial expressions of leprosy. It is characterized by alteration in the eyelids and anterior segment of the eye.

2. **Facies leonina**, another facial expression of advanced lepromatous leprosy, is characterized by prominent ridges and furrows on the forehead and cheeks. It also is called leontiasis because of the lion-like appearance of affected patients.

3. **Rhinophyma** is a typical facial feature immortalized by Ghirlandaio in his Louvre painting of an old man and popularized (albeit involuntarily) by W.C. Fields.

4. **Adenoid facies** is the long, open-mouthed, and dumb-looking face of children with adenoid hypertrophy. It often is associated with a pinched nose and narrow nares. The mouth is always open because upper airway congestion has made patients obligatory mouth breathers. Adenoid facies also is typical of recurrent upper respiratory tract allergies. Its diagnostic features are (1) Dennie's lines, which are horizontal creases under both lower lids (first described by the American physician Charles Dennie); (2) a nasal pleat, which is the horizontal crease just above the tip of the nose produced by the recurrent upward wiping of nasal secretions; and (3) allergic shiners, which are bilateral shadows under the eyes produced by chronic venous congestion. Incidentally, upward wiping of nasal secretions with either the palm or dorsum of the hand is so common that often it is called the "allergic salute." The facies of a child with upper respiratory allergies or hypertrophied adenoids is so typical that an astute physician often can make the diagnosis just by walking into the patient's room.

5. **Facies bovina** is the cowlike face of Greig's syndrome, characterized by ocular hypertelorism (i.e., extreme width between the eyes) due to an enlarged sphenoid bone. It often is associated with other congenital deformities, such as osteogenesis imperfecta, Sprengel deformity (congenital elevation of the scapulae), and mental retardation. (See also question 30.)

6. **Elfin facies** is characterized by a short and upturned nose, widely spaced eyes, full cheeks, wide mouth with patulous lips, deep husky voice, and a friendly personality. It is often associated with hypercalcemia, supravalvar aortic stenosis, and mental retardation.

7. **Cherubic facies** is the characteristic childlike facies of cherubism, a familial fibrous dysplasia of the jaws characterized by enlargement in childhood and regression in adulthood. A cherubic facies also is seen in some forms of glycogenosis.

8. **Corvisart's facies** is characteristic of patients with aortic regurgitation or heart failure. It is puffy, purplish, and cyanotic with swollen eyelids and shiny eyes. It was first described by the French physician Jean Nicolas Corvisart, one of Laennec's teachers and the main advocate for use of percussion in bedside diagnosis.

9. **Aortic facies** is another face of patients with aortic regurgitation. Its hallmark is a pale and sallow complexion.

10. **De Musset's facies** is the bobbing motion of the head, synchronous with each heartbeat. It typically is seen in patients with severe aortic regurgitation but is neither sensitive nor specific for the disease. In fact, it also has been reported in patients with a large stroke volume (hyperkinetic heart syndrome) and even in patients with massive left pleural effusion. A variant of De Musset's sign is seen in tricuspid regurgitation: the systolic bobbing motion of the head tends to be more lateral as a result of the regurgitant column of blood rising along the superior vena cava. (See also questions 31 and 32.)

11. **Mitral facies** is the face of mitral stenosis, characterized by pink and slightly cyanotic cheeks. This form of cyanosis affects primarily the periphery of the body (i.e., acrocyanosis), such as the tip of the nose, cheeks, hands, and feet. It is due to peripheral desaturation caused by low and fixed cardiac output. When patients with mitral stenosis develop right-sided heart failure and tricuspid regurgitation as a result of longstanding pulmonary hypertension, the overall skin color becomes sallow and often overtly icteric. This appearance contrasts quite well with the persistently cyanotic cheeks.

12. **Hippocratic facies** is a tense and dramatic expression of the face with sunken eyes, sharp nose, hollow cheeks and temples, open mouth, dry and cracked lips, cold and drawn ears, and leaden complexion. It was first described by Hippocrates and typically is observed in impending death as a result of severe and prolonged illness.

13. **Hound-dog facies** is the facial appearance of cutis laxa and is characterized by loose facial skin hanging in folds (much like a hound dog). Cutis laxa or dermatochalasis, a congenital disease characterized by degeneration of elastic fibers, causes the excessive amount of skin hanging in folds. Vascular anomalies also may be present, together with pulmonary emphysema and diverticula of the alimentary tract or bladder.

14. **Hurloid facies** is the coarse and gargoyle-like facial appearance of mucopolysaccharidoses and mucolipidoses. Hurler's syndrome (described in 1919 by the German pediatrician Gertrud Hurler) is due to a deficiency of a-L-iduronidase. The result is accumulation of an abnormal intracellular material and severe abnormality in the development of skeletal cartilage and bone. Patients with Hurler's syndrome have dwarfism, kyphosis, deformed limbs, limitation of joint motion, spadelike hands, corneal clouding, hepatosplenomegaly, mental retardation, and gargoyle-like facies.

15. **Potter's facies** is characteristic of bilateral renal agenesis (Potter's disease) and other severe renal malformations. It is characterized by ocular hypertelorism with prominent epicanthic folds, low-set ears, receding chin, and flattening of the nose.

16. **Facies of chronic renal failure** is similar to myxedema, except that the facial edema is due to accumulation not of connective tissue but of water as a result of hypoproteinemia.

17. **Facies scaphoidea** is a dish-like or hollowed facial malformation (from the Greek *scaphos* = boat-shaped, hollowed). It is characterized by protuberant forehead, depressed nose and maxilla, and prominence of the chin.

18. **Battle's sign** is the classic sign of trauma, more specifically of a basilar skull fracture with bleeding into the middle fossa. The name typically is given to a bruise located over the mastoid process, although at times the same name has been applied to blood behind the eardrum or a bruise behind the mastoid. Battle's sign may occur on the ipsilateral or contralateral side of the skull fracture and may take as long as 3–12 days to develop. The sign is not highly sensitive (2–8%) but has a high predictive value (almost 100%).

19. **Raccoon eyes** are bruises over the ocular orbits associated with external trauma to the eyes, skull fracture, and intracranial bleeding. A form of raccoon eyes also may be seen with amyloidosis; the bleeding is due to capillary fragility and usually is precipitated by a Valsalva

maneuver and its resulting increase in central venous pressure or by a simple proctoscopy, which also may lead to Valsalva's maneuver and therefore to a capillary leak.

20. **Scleroderma facies** is characterized by a sharp nose and shiny, tightly drawn skin. As a result, wrinkles may even disappear. Most patients have hyperpigmentation, associated at times with areas of vitiligo and a few telangiectasias. The opening of the mouth is often quite narrow.

21. **Facies of lupus erythematosus** is characterized by a classic malar, butterfly-like rash, often involving the bridge of the nose.

22. **Smoker's face** is becoming an increasingly familiar entity because tobacco remains a prevalent addiction among teenagers. Smokers tend to look much older than their stated age. They have coarse facial features and wrinkled, grayish, atrophic skin. Comparing pictures of smokers and nonsmokers may be a great way to discourage smoking among teens (especially girls)—even better than quoting the latest cancer statistics.

23. **Hutchinson's facies** is the peculiar facial expression produced by drooping eyelids and motionless eyes of ophthalmoplegia.

24. **Myasthenic facies** is the facial expression of myasthenia gravis, characterized by drooping of the eyelids (ptosis) and corners of the mouth. Weakness of facial muscles may lead to paucity of expressivity and an apathetic look.

25. **Myopathic facies** may be seen in various congenital myopathies and in many ways is similar to myasthenic facies. Patients have protrusion of the lips, drooping of the lids, and general relaxation of the facial muscles due to muscular weakness.

26. **Parkinson's facies** is the expressionless or masklike facies of Parkinson's disease. It has a fixed and apathetic look.

27. **Tetanus facies** classically is characterized by *risus sardonicus* (Latin for sardonic grin). The patient's mouth is open with the lips tightened transversally to resemble the expression of Batman's menace, the Joker.

28. **Graves' facies** is associated with Graves' disease and characterized by exophthalmos and lid lag. The face typically is anxious-looking.

29. **Myxedematous facies** is a puffy face with a sallow color (due not to jaundice but to accumulation of carotene) and dry, rough skin. The hair is coarse and the eyes boggy. The lateral third of the eyebrows is typically missing.

30. **Acromegalic facies** is characterized by thickening of the facial bones, prominence of the mandible and supraciliary areas, a thick nose, and large lips. Acromegaly (from the Greek *akron* = extremity and *megalos* = large) is characterized by progressive enlargement of the peripheral parts of the body, such as head, face, hands, and feet.

31. **Cushing's facies** is a typical moon facies: round, mildly plethoric, and a bit oily. Some patients have acne and alopecia combined with an increase in facial hair. They also may have a buffalo hump, buccal fat pads, striae, and central obesity.

30. Who was Greig?

David Greig (1864–1936) was a Scottish surgeon and quite an interesting character. A graduate of Edinburgh University, he served in the army first in India and then in South Africa, where he participated in the Boer War. On returning to Scotland he became supervisor at the Baldwin Institute for Mentally Retarded Children and curator of the Museum of the Royal College of Surgeons. Both appointments fostered a peculiar fascination with skulls (either normal or abnormal) that lasted for the rest of his life and gave him a shot at fame. He was so enamored with skulls that he was rumored to have hoarded as many as 300 in his private collection. He wrote extensively about skull deformities and even published a paper describing the skull characteristics of Sir Walter Scott. An avid reader, Greig was interested in both music and literature and published a collection of his own poetry ("The Rhymes of D.R.I.").

31. What is Lincoln's sign?

Lincoln's sign is one of the varieties of De Musset's sign. The term refers to a picture of Abe Lincoln taken during the Civil War that shows the president quietly sitting with his legs crossed.

The tip of Lincoln's raised foot is fuzzy and indistinct. Because nineteenth-century photography required long exposure times, it has been speculated that Lincoln may have had aortic regurgitation, probably due to Marfan's syndrome, and that the fuzziness of his foot could have been caused by its bobbing with each heartbeat.

32. Who was De Musset?

Alfred De Musset was French, he was a poet, and he lived in the nineteenth century. Thus, he had all of the major risk factors for acquiring syphilis, which he compliantly did. The eponymous sign was noticed first by De Musset's brother, Paul, during breakfast with their mother in 1842. When informed of this peculiar motion, Alfred simply put his forefinger and thumb to his front and calmly stopped the bobbing. Paul subsequently reported the event in his biography of his famous brother. Incidentally, De Musset is probably best known for being the lover of Georges Sand and for being dumped by her in favor of Frédéric Chopin (showing that she preferred pulmonary tuberculosis to syphilitic aortitis).

APPARENT AGE

33. What conditions make you look older than your stated age?

Other than a job in academic medicine, the most common reason for looking older than your stated age is cigarette smoking (see question 29). Chronic exposure to sunlight (especially ultraviolet light) also makes you look older by accelerating skin aging and wrinkling (actinic face). Progeria is a pathologic acceleration of the aging process, affecting children and leading to premature senescence and death within a few years.

34. Which conditions make you look younger than your stated age?

Not many, unfortunately. Good genes, of course, always help. Yet a few conditions tend to give a youthful look to the patient, including hypogonadism and other endocrine disorders of developmental arrest or retardation. Panhypopituitarism also has been associated with a youthful look, although patients usually have a sallow complexion and many fine wrinkles. Finally, anorexia nervosa and even use of immunosuppressive agents in organ-transplant patients have been associated with a persistent adolescent-like appearance. Being mildly underweight also conveys an impression of youth and health, but this effect is probably more cultural, based on our ever-increasing obsession with thinness. A few years ago, in fact, when "consumption" from tuberculosis was still a major killer, being overweight was considered a sign of health. This is still the case in many parts of the world, where people's main concern is not how to lose weight but how to put food on the table at least once a day.

35. What is a toxic-looking patient?

A patient who is anxious, flushed, sweaty, and febrile with tachycardia and evidence of respiratory distress (usually rapid and shallow breathing). Such patients need immediate attention. The underlying cause is usually sepsis, but it also may be poisoning (such as salicylate intoxication), thyroid storm, psychotic crisis, or heat stroke.

GAIT

36. How much information can be gathered through assessment of gait?

It depends on the disease, of course. Yet by inspecting the way that the patient walks into the office or climbs onto the examination table it is often possible to make a diagnosis of neurologic or musculoskeletal disorders. Because the primary care physician is often the first person to evaluate patients with such disorders, it is important to be fully familiar with at least some characteristics of the various gaits.

37. What is the difference between stance and gait?

Stance is the position assumed by a standing person (the French derivative of the Italian *stanza*).

Gait is the walking style of the individual (from Old Norse *gata* = path). Each of us has a peculiar way of walking that often can be recognized from a distance. One may conclude that a gait tells a lot not only about neuromuscular physiology and pathology but also about character and even occupation. Contrast, for example, Henry Fonda's understated and elegant walk with John Wayne's flamboyant and macho gait.

38. What neurologic structures participate in the control of stance and gait?

- **Basal ganglia:** responsible for automatic movements, including the swinging of arms opposite to the legs during walking.
- **Locomotor region of the midbrain:** responsible for initiating walking.
- **Cerebellum:** responsible for maintaining proper posture and balance; also controls the major characteristics of movement, such as trajectory, velocity, and acceleration.
- **Spinal cord:** responsible for coordination of movement and for conveying proprioceptive and sensory input from joints and muscles to the higher centers for feedback and autoregulation.

39. What are the characteristics of a normal gait?

The body is erect, the head is straight, and the arms hang loosely on each side, moving automatically in a direction opposite to the movement of the legs. The feet are slightly everted, almost in line with each other, and the internal malleoli come close to touching while walking. Steps are usually small and equal.

40. What are the physiologic components of gait?

1. **Antigravity support:** provided by reflexes located in the spinal cord and brainstem; antigravity reflexes are responsible for maintaining full extension of hips, knees, and neck.

2. **Stepping:** a basic pattern of movement based on sensory input from soles and body (including inclination forward and from side to side) and integrated at the midbrain level.

3. **Equilibrium:** responsible for maintaining balance and center of gravity during shifting of weight from one foot to the other.

4. **Propulsion:** involves leaning forward and slightly to one side, permitting the body to fall a certain distance before being checked by leg support.

41. What historical information should be gathered to help interpret an abnormal gait?

- Worsening of the gait disturbance at night (because of darkness)
- Association with vertigo or light-headedness
- Association with pain, numbness, or tingling in the limbs
- Presence of muscle weakness
- Presence of bladder or bowel dysfunction
- Presence of stiffness in the limbs
- Problems initiating or terminating walking

42. How should one examine a patient with a gait abnormality?

By closely evaluating:

- How the patient gets up from a chair (useful, for example, in Parkinson's disease or limb girdle dystrophy)
- How the patient initiates walking (also useful in Parkinson's disease)
- How the patient walks at a slow pace
- How the patient walks at a fast pace
- How the patient turns
- How the patient walks on toes (toe-walking cannot be done by patients with Parkinson's disease, sensory ataxia, spastic hemiplegia, or paresis of the soleus or gastrocnemius muscle)
- How the patient walks on heels (heel-walking unmasks patients with motor ataxia, spastic paraplegia, or foot drop)

- How the patient walks a straight line in tandem (i.e., heel to toe): useful in all gait disorders
- How the patient walks with eyes first open and then closed (patients with sensory ataxia do much worse with eyes closed, whereas patients with motor ataxia or cerebellar ataxia do poorly either way)
- How the patient stands erect with eyes first open and then closed

This evaluation should be carried out by looking at the patient from the front, back, and side.

43. What is an antalgic gait?

It is a gait resulting from pain on weightbearing, which may be caused by hyperesthesia (from neurologic diseases) or, more simply, by painful lesions on the bottom of the foot. The stance phase is typically shortened on the affected side. Similarly, the foot is gently lowered to the ground on the affected side and lifted almost immediately.

44. What is a cerebellar gait?

It is the unsteady and staggering gait of cerebellar ataxia. It is totally irregular in rate, range, and direction and often accompanied by a tendency to fall to either one side or the other, forward or backward. Stance is widened, but often not enough to prevent staggering. Titubation while standing worsens considerably when patients are asked to close their feet together and usually leads to swaying and even falling. Opening or closing the eyes while standing neither improves nor worsens balance, in strong contrast to sensory ataxia (see below). Walks are highly cautious. Steps vary in length and often are accompanied by swaying to one side or the other to the point that patients often look for something to lean on, whether a cane, bed rail, or sometimes even the wall. Cerebellar gait is due to compromise of the cerebellum (the organ normally responsible for proper balance and posture) and resembles very much the walk of alcohol intoxication. Other signs of cerebellar disease (such as limb ataxia and nystagmus) are usually present.

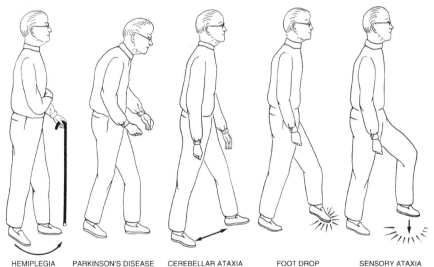

HEMIPLEGIA   PARKINSON'S DISEASE   CEREBELLAR ATAXIA   FOOT DROP   SENSORY ATAXIA

Common types of gait abnormalities. (From Swartz MH: Textbook of Physical Diagnosis, 3rd ed. Philadelphia, W.B. Saunders, 1997, with permission.)

45. What is a sensory ataxia gait?

It is the gait of patients who have lost sensory and proprioceptive sensation in their lower extremities. When tertiary syphilis was epidemic, a gait of this sort was almost pathognomonic of tabes dorsalis. Patients with sensory ataxia are unaware of the position of their limbs in space.

They walk, therefore, by taking steps that are higher than necessary while carefully watching the ground. They also walk with a wide gait (as in cerebellar ataxia). Yet only patients with sensory ataxia (or peroneal nerve palsy) typically slap their foot to the ground (they do so to increase their peripheral input). Patients with sensory ataxia also keep their legs widely apart while standing. But in contrast to patients with cerebellar ataxia, usually they can stand straight if their eyes are open. It is only with eyes closed that they sway and even fall (because of the loss of compensatory visual input). This is also why they have great difficulty in walking at night.

46. What is a (high) steppage gait?

It is the peculiar walk of patients with lower motor neuron disease and can be seen with various forms of peripheral neuropathy, spinal muscular atrophy, and peroneal neuropathy (see below). It is characterized by the foot drop. The ankle cannot be dorsiflexed during walking. Thus, the foot is raised high so that the drooping toes can clear the ground. The foot is then brought down suddenly in a flapping manner. Because the toe of the lifted foot tends to point toward the ground, the patient may still stumble and fall. A patient with a foot drop also wears and tears the soles of the shoes asymmetrically. This observation may be a quick and Sherlockian way to make a diagnosis. If the proximal (girdle) muscles are affected, the patient's gait has a waddling quality (see anserine gait, below).

47. What is a Charcot-Marie-Tooth (CMT) gait?

It is much like a high-steppage gait. In earlier forms of CMT, the high-steppage gait can be spotted easily by having the patient run. The drooping toes require high elevation of the knees to clear the ground. CMT is a progressive and hereditary degeneration on the peripheral nerves and roots (peroneal nerve paralysis) that leads to a slowly progressive wasting of the distal muscles of the extremities. CMT involves feet and legs initially and hands and arms later. It rarely involves muscles more central than the elbows or above the mid-third of the thighs. **Pes cavus** (an exaggeration of the normal foot arch due to involvement of the extensor and everter muscles of the foot) is often the first sign of the disease. The foot becomes plantarflexed, inverted, and adducted, producing a typical equinovarus deformity. Calluses are common as well as perforating ulcers. Later all muscles below the middle third of the thigh also may atrophy, causing the patient's lower extremities to resemble a "stork leg." Deficits may involve touch and pain sensation (usually in feet earlier and hands later) as well as proprioception. Deep tendon reflexes of the involved limbs are usually absent.

48. Who were Charcot, Marie, and Tooth?

Jean M. Charcot (1825–1893) is a legend in French medicine. His contributions to the field of neurology include the first description of amyotrophic lateral sclerosis, the characterization of multiple sclerosis as a separate entity (while observing the disease in his housemaid), and several studies in hysteria and hypnotism. A talented artist and animal lover who refused animal experimentation, Charcot was also an excellent teacher (his students included Sigmund Freud and Josef Babinski) and a charismatic clinician.

Pierre Marie (1853–1940) was a French physician who started as a law student. Trained by Charcot, he eventually succeeded his famous mentor at the Saltpetriere Hospital. He contributed widely to neurology, particularly in the area of aphasia. He also was responsible for one of the first descriptions of acromegaly.

Henry Tooth (1856–1925) was a British physician and army surgeon during the Boer War. He kept an interest in military medicine and during World War I worked with honor both in Malta and on the Italian front. Tooth was well liked by both students and colleagues. He was also a good musician who played regularly in an orchestra and an excellent spare-time carpenter. He described CMT disease in his Cambridge M.D. thesis in the same year (1886) as Charcot and Marie.

49. What is a parkinsonian gait?

It is the frozen gait of patients with Parkinson's disease. It is characterized by a series of very small steps, at first barely clearing the ground. The walk is quite slow and has no associated automatic movement (such as the swing of the arms). Patients find it particularly difficult to get started. This difficulty is present not only in getting up from a chair but also in starting to walk after standing still. Other characteristics include festination (acceleration of the rate of movement after the walk has finally begun) and propulsion (the tendency to fall forward and the reason for festination). In the standing position the head of the patient is bent downward, the thoracic spine is bent forward, the arms are moderately flexed at the elbows, and the legs are slightly flexed at hips and knees. During walking the trunk is bent farther forward, the arms are either immobile at the side or carried ahead of the body (typically they do not swing), and the legs remain bent at the hips, knees, and ankles. Falls are quite common, because patients fail to make compensatory flexion or extension movements of the trunk in an attempt to maintain balance.

50. What is apraxic gait?

It is the gait of patients with frontal lobe disease or normopressure hydrocephalus. A milder form may be seen as a result of aging. Apraxic gait is characterized by forward flexion of the upper trunk and flexion of arms and knees. The automatic arm swing is much decreased. Feet are wide apart and shuffled (hence the term "magnetic gait," as if the feet were glued to the ground). The cause of apraxic gait is not muscle weakness but inability to perform properly the various motor functions. Thus, sensory capacity and deep tendon reflexes are usually normal, although the plantar reflex may be of the Babinski type.

51. What is the gait of spastic paraplegia?

It is the gait of patients with spinal cord disease who have a combination of spasticity and weakness in the lower extremities. Their walk requires much effort and is characterized by short steps with slow and stiff movements. The legs are extended at the hips and knees and adducted at the hips. In contrast to a parkinsonian gait, the toes always stay on the ground. As a result, one leg must swing across the other instead of straight forward, thereby producing a typical criss-cross motion ("scissor gait"). Because the feet often scrape along the floor, the soles of the shoes become worn along the toes. To compensate for the stiff movement of the legs, the patient may move the trunk from side to side.

52. What is a gait of spastic hemiplegia (circumduction gait)?

It is the typical walk of patients who have suffered an internal capsule hemispheric stroke (hemiplegic gait). On the affected side, patients have (1) upper extremity adduction and flexion at all levels (elbow, wrist, and fingers) and (2) lower extremity extension at all levels (hip, knee, and ankle). The foot is internally rotated. Spastic hemiplegic patients have great difficulty in flexing the involved hip and knee and dorsiflexing the ankle. As a result, they do not drag the foot limply behind them but swing it on the affected side in a half circle (circumduction). The upper body tilts to the opposite side (in compensation for the semicircular movement of the leg), and the walk is difficult and slow.

53. What is an anserine gait?

It is the duck-like waddle (from the Latin *anserinus* = goose) of patients with girdle muscular dystrophy and progressive muscular atrophy. Patients walk with short steps and tilt the body from side to side in a characteristic sway. The legs are spread wide apart, and the shoulders are sloped slightly forward. When standing, they have an exaggerated lumbar lordosis and a protuberant abdomen. Getting up from a chair is also quite typical (not to mention difficult). First, patients bend forward, placing both hands on the knees. Then they push themselves up by sliding their hands up the thighs (Gower's maneuver).

54. What is a malingering gait?

It is a gait of either hysterical disorders or malingering patients seeking medicolegal compensation. This gait is characterized by any kind of movements of arms and legs that follow no physiologic pattern. Despite these theatrical movements, patients are quite capable of maintaining their balance and usually never allow themselves to fall. No objective signs of neurologic deficit are found on exam.

BIBLIOGRAPHY

1. Detsky AS, Smalley PS, Chang J: Is this patient malnourished? JAMA 271:54–58, 1994.
2. McGee S, Abernethy WB, Simel DL: Is this patient hypovolemic? JAMA 281:1022–1029, 1999.
3. Sapira JD: The Art and Science of Bedside Diagnosis. Baltimore, Urban & Schwarzenberg, 1990.
4. Willis JL, Schneiderman H, Algranati PS: Physical Diagnosis. Baltimore, Williams & Wilkins, 1994.

2. VITAL SIGNS

Salvatore Mangione, M.D.

Immediately below a completely compressed artery (with obliteration of the lumen) no sounds are heard. As soon as the first drop of blood escapes from under the site of pressure, we hear a clapping sound very distinctly. This sound is heard when the compressed artery is released and even before the appearance of pulsation in the peripheral branches.

N.S. Korotkoff: On methods of studying blood pressure.
Bull Imperial Acad Med St. Petersburg 4:365, 1905

Humanity has but three great enemies: Fever, Famine, and War. Of these by far the greatest, by far the most terrible is fever.

Sir William Osler, JAMA 26:999, 1896

A quartan fever kills old men and heals young.—Italian proverb

TOPICS COVERED IN THIS CHAPTER

Pulse and heart rate
  Normal heart rate
  Tachycardia and bradycardia
  Pulsus alternans
Respiratory rate and rhythm
Temperature
  Definition of fever
  Significance of fever
  Methods of measurement
  Common fever patterns
    Factitious
    Relapsing
    Pel-Ebstein
    Remittent
    Intermittent
    Charcot's
    Hectic
    Continued (sustained)
    Malarial
    Ephemeral
    Epimastical
    Exanthematous
    Exhaustion
    Miliary
    Polyleptic
    Undulant
    Essential
  Temperature-pulse dissociation
  Extreme pyrexia
  Inappropriately low fever
  Hypothermia

Blood pressure
  Methods of measurement (direct vs. indirect)
  History of the sphygmomanometer
  When, where, and how blood pressure should be measured
  Definition of hypertension
  Over- or underestimates of blood pressure
  Accuracy in blood pressure measurement
  Osler's sign
  Pseudohypertension
  Pseudohypotension
  Differences between palpatory and auscultatory determination of blood pressure
  Calibration of an aneroid sphygmomanometer
  Pulse pressure
    Increased
    Decreased
  Branham's sign
  Pulsus paradoxus
  Reversed pulsus paradoxus
  Trousseau's sign
  Rumpel-Leede sign
  Hill's sign
  Severe hypertension
  Malignant hypertension

CONVENTIONAL TEACHING WATCH

Assessment of vital signs is the initial, still essential part of bedside examination. Unfortunately, it is often relegated to nonphysicians, sometimes even to technicians. Yet, as the phrase implies, vital signs provide a wealth of crucial information, some of which may require special skills and knowledge.

FINDING/MANEUVER		CONVENTIONAL TEACHING REVISITED
Vital statistics	⇔	Valuable, but probably not as crucial as vital signs.
Pulse and heart rate	⇑	Even in absence of electrocardiogram, quite a bit can be learned from peripheral pulse.
Respiratory rate and rhythm	⇑	As above
Temperature	⇑	If you don't take a temperature, you can't find a fever.
Fever patterns	⇓	Fever has fascinated mankind for thousands of years. Not surprisingly, a smorgasbord of various terms has been generated. Many of these "fevers," albeit interesting, belong more to the history (and folklore) than to the science of medicine.
Temperature/pulse dissociation	⇔	Useful finding with relatively narrow differential diagnosis.
Hypothermia	⇑	Very important; normal mercury thermometers may miss it.
Blood pressure	⇑	Essential vital sign. Physicians need to know not only how, when, and where to measure it, but also the limitations of the test, both under- and overestimates.
Osler's sign	⇔	Helpful for detection of pseudohypertension, but probably not as much as traditionally thought.
Pseudohypotension	⇔	Not uncommon problem in patients in shock; intraarterial recording provides diagnosis.
Pulse pressure	⇑	Useful finding with important differential diagnosis, both increased and decreased.
Branham's sign	⇔	Useful maneuver to identify arteriovenous fistula.
Pulsus paradoxus	⇑	Very important; physicians need to know how to detect it.
Trousseau's sign	⇔	Time-honored sign of (latent) tetany.
Rumpel-Leede sign	⇓	Part of the folklore and history of bedside diagnosis.
Hill's sign	⇓	Neither sensitive nor specific for aortic regurgitation.

1. What are the vital statistics?
Weight and height, both important measurements. In contrast to vital signs, vital statistics tend to be more stable over time. Thus, they provide less crucial clinical information.

2. What are the vital signs?
They are crucial (hence vital) measurements that should be obtained in every important patient interaction. They consist of heart rate, respiratory rate, temperature, and blood pressure.

PULSE

3. What is a normal heart rate?
60–100 beats per minute (bpm). A rate below 60 bpm is considered **bradycardia**, and a rate above 100 bpm is considered **tachycardia**.

4. Which characteristics of the pulse should be assessed?

Regularity and, if the pulse is irregular, whether the irregularity itself is regular or irregular. For example, a regular tachycardia usually suggests a diagnosis of sinus tachycardia, atrioventricular reentry tachycardia, or ventricular tachycardia. Conversely, an irregularly irregular tachycardia is almost always due to atrial fibrillation. The flutter is a regularly irregular tachycardia due to variable atrioventricular block. A regularly irregular pulse also can be felt in patients with second-degree heart block, in whom skipped beats occur at regular intervals.

5. What is pulsus alternans?

A pulse that is regular in rate and rhythm but alternates between a weaker and a fuller volume. Pulsus alternans is typical of congestive heart failure and may or may not be associated with electrical alternans (an alternation on the electrocardiogram [EKG] of tall and small QRS complexes, still within the range of a regular heart rate).

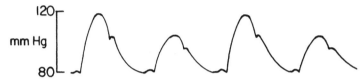

Pulsus alternans. Note that every other beat has a lower systolic pressure. (Adapted from Abrams J: Prim Cardiol, 1982.)

RESPIRATORY RATE AND RHYTHM

6. What kind of information can be gathered through the assessment of rate, rhythm, and depth of respiration?

Much valuable information. Intelligent observation of these respiratory parameters may generate an entire alphabet soup of terminology, often conducive to specific diagnoses. For a more detailed description of these terms and disease processes, see chapter 13.

TEMPERATURE

7. Define fever.

Fever is a bodily temperature above 98.6°F (37°C). Many normal people, however, reach higher levels because of exercise or exposure. Thus, a true fever should be considered an oral temperature greater than 100.2°F (37.9°C).

8. What is the difference between rectal and oral temperature?

Rectal temperature is a little higher than oral temperature. The difference is usually 1°F (0.55°C) but may be even greater in mouth breathers or patients who are tachypneic (independently of whether they breathe through the mouth). In such patients the difference in temperatures usually averages 1.67°F (0.93°C), but it may be even greater with faster respiratory rates. Recent ingestion of either cold or hot substances (including smoking a cigarette) may be responsible for falsely low or falsely high oral temperatures.

9. What about axillary temperatures?

They are highly inaccurate and should be avoided.

10. How long does it take for a thermometer to equilibrate when it is placed under the patient's tongue?

Approximately 3 minutes with the old mercury thermometers and approximately 1 minute with the newest models.

11. What is the clinical significance of fever?

It usually indicates the presence of infection. Fever, however, also may be present in inflammatory processes (e.g., several autoimmune diseases), cancers, drug reactions, environmental exposures (e.g., heat stroke), and certain dysmetabolic and endocrine disorders (e.g., Graves' disease, Addisonian crisis).

12. What is factitious fever?

It is a self-induced, artificial fever (from the Latin *factitius* = made by art). Techniques to create fever vary, depending on patients' imagination and skills. The most commonly used method is to ingest and hold hot liquids in the mouth immediately before a temperature check. Factitious fever often (but not always) can be counteracted by rectal temperature checks, which also may act as a deterrent or punishment, or by measuring the temperature of the urine immediately after voiding. Urinary temperature, however, is a little lower than oral temperature.

13. What is relapsing fever?

Relapsing fever is characterized by a number of febrile attacks that last about 6 days and are separated by afebrile intervals of about the same length. A relapsing fever is usually the result of an infectious process (such as brucellosis, malaria, borreliosis, or tuberculosis), but it also may be due to Hodgkin's disease or familial Mediterranean fever.

14. What is Pel-Ebstein fever?

Pel-Ebstein fever is seen in 16% of patients with Hodgkin's disease. It is characterized by febrile episodes lasting for hours or days, followed by afebrile periods of days and sometimes even weeks. It is, therefore, a form of relapsing fever. It was described in the nineteenth century by the Dutch Pieter Pel and the German Wilhelm Ebstein. Ebstein had interests far beyond medicine, ranging from arts and literature to history. He even wrote a few books about the diseases of famous Germans, such as Luther and Schopenhauer, and a medical reinterpretation of the Bible.

15. What is remittent fever?

Fever that abates every day but still does not completely resolve.

16. What is intermittent fever?

Fever that resolves completely every day.

17. What is Charcot's intermittent fever?

A special intermittent fever, usually accompanied by chills, right upper quadrant pain, and jaundice. It is due to stones that intermittently obstruct the common duct.

18. What is hectic fever?

Fever characterized by a daily afternoon spike (from the Greek *hektikos* = habitual) and often accompanied by facial flushing. It usually is seen in active tuberculosis and is a form of intermittent fever with much wider temperature excursions.

19. What is continued or sustained fever?

Fever of some duration with no intermissions or marked remissions in temperature. It is typical of either gram-negative sepsis or central nervous system damage.

20. What is malarial fever?

Malarial fevers vary considerably, depending on the organism involved. Typical fevers include the following:

1. **Quotidian fever** (from the Latin *quotidianus* = daily) is a fever with daily paroxysms. It usually is caused by double tertian malaria, which is infection by two distinct groups of *Plasmodium vivax* that sporulate alternately every 48 hours. It also may be caused by the most pernicious form of malarial parasite, *P. falciparum*, in combination with *P. vivax*. Finally, it may

be seen in infections by two distinct *P. falciparum* generations that mature on different days. This fever occurs twice a day. Double quotidian fever is *not* a malarial fever but a daily two-spike fever seen in as many as one-half of all cases of gonococcal endocarditis.

2. **Tertian fever** (from the Latin *tertianus* = third) is a fever that recurs every third day, counting the day of an episode as the first day. As a result, it occurs every 48 hours. Tertian fever is typical of *P. vivax*.

3. **Quartan fever** (from the Latin *quartanus* = fourth) is a fever that recurs every 72 hours (or every fourth day, counting the day of an episode as the first day). It is due to *P. malariae*. A double quartan fever is due to infection with two independent groups of quartan parasites; the febrile paroxysms occur on two successive days followed by one day without fever.

4. **Malignant tertian fever** is typical of *P. falciparum* (falciparum fever). It also is called aestivoautumnal fever and Roman fever (because it was a common ailment in the Roman countryside not too many decades ago). It is characterized by 48-hour paroxysms of a severe form of malaria, accompanied by acute cerebral, renal, or gastrointestinal manifestations. These manifestations are usually due to clumping of the infected red blood cells, which causes secondary capillary obstruction.

21. What is ephemeral fever?
A febrile episode lasting no more than a day or two.

22. What is epimastical fever?
Epimastical fever (from the Greek *epakmastikos* = coming to a height) increases steadily until it reaches its acme and then declines by either crisis or lysis (crisis indicates a sudden drop, whereas lysis indicates a more gradual improvement).

23. What is exanthematous fever?
Fever associated with an exanthem.

24. What is fatigue (exhaustion) fever?
Elevation of body temperature after excessive and continued muscular exertion. It may last for up to several days.

25. What is miliary fever?
An infectious fever characterized by profuse sweating and production of **sudamina** (minute vesicles caused by retention of fluid in a sweat follicle). It was commonly described in the past during severe epidemics.

26. What is monoleptic fever?
Continued fever that has only one paroxysm.

27. What is polyleptic fever?
Fever occurring in two or more paroxysms, as typically is seen in malaria (from the Greek *poly* = multiple and *lepsis* = paroxysm).

28. What is undulant fever?
Undulant fever refers to the wavy appearance of the long temperature curve typically seen in brucellosis.

29. What is essential fever?
Fever of unknown etiology. It is defined as a temperature of at least 100.4°F (38°C) for 3 weeks or longer without an identifiable cause. In adults fever of unknown origin (FUO) is most commonly due to infection, either closed-space (abscess) or disseminated (malaria, tuberculosis, HIV, endocarditis, fungemia). Less common causes include (1) cancer (particularly lymphomas, hypernephromas, hepatomas, and hepatic metastasis of extrahepatic tumors); (2) autoimmune

diseases (collagen vascular diseases and vasculitis); and (3) drug reactions. Patients with iatrogenic fever due to drugs often have a temperature/pulse dissociation (see below), look quite well despite their high fever, and have other signs of allergic reactions, such as skin rash or eosinophilia.

30. What is temperature/pulse dissociation?

A rise in temperature that is not matched by an equivalent rise in heart rate. Normally, each degree of increase in temperature is accompanied by a 10-bpm increase in heart rate. The increase in heart rate, however, may not occur. The differential diagnosis of this dissociation is usually infectious (e.g., salmonellosis, typhoid fever, brucellosis, legionellosis, mycoplasma pneumonia, meningitis with an increase in intracranial pressure). But it also may be iatrogenic (as in drug fever) or due simply to the use of digitalis or beta blockers.

31. What are the causes of extreme pyrexia?

Very high temperatures (> 105°F or 40.6°C) are usually due to disorders of the thermoregulatory centers of the nervous system (central fever), including heat stroke, cerebrovascular accidents, or a major anoxic brain injury following cardiac arrest. Malignant hyperthermia and neuroleptic malignant syndrome are other important causes of very high fevers of central origin (often leading to temperatures > 106°F or 41.2°C). Fevers of this degree usually are not caused by an infectious process. The exception is an infection of the central nervous system, such as meningitis or encephalitis.

32. What are the causes of an inappropriately low fever?

Fevers lower than expected can be seen in patients with chronic renal failure (especially if they are uremic) and patients receiving antipyretics (such as acetaminophen) and nonsteroidal antiinflammatory agents. Cardiocirculatory collapse is another important reason for an inappropriate rise in body temperature.

33. What is hypothermia? What are its causes?

Hypothermia is a body temperature below 98.6°F (37°C). Yet, given the normal fluctuations in temperature, true hypothermia is considered any body temperature below 95°F (35°C). Moderate hypothermia is defined as a body temperature of 73.4–89.6°F (23–32°C), whereas profound hypothermia is defined as a temperature of 53.6–68°F (12–20° C). Temperatures of this degree are missed by routine thermometers; they require a thermistor.

Depending on the setting, the most common cause of hypothermia is either overwhelming sepsis or environmental exposure. Other causes include cerebrovascular accidents, endocrine disorders (hypoglycemia, hypothyroidism, panhypopituitarism, adrenal insufficiency), and intoxication (drugs and alcohol). Patients who feel hypothermic to touch are often simply peripherally vasoconstricted.

BLOOD PRESSURE

34. How is blood pressure measured?

It depends. In practice the standard of measurement is the **indirect** method, which relies on a blood pressure cuff (sphygmomanometer) and may be either palpatory or auscultatory. The gold standard, however, remains **direct** measurement based on intraarterial determination via a rigid-walled catheter.

35. Why is it important to measure blood pressure accurately?

Unrecognized hypertension may lead to cardiovascular disease and decrease life expectancy. Hypertension is a common medical problem, affecting as many as 1 of 5 North American adults. It is easily treatable but often clinically silent, at least in its initial phases. Thus, only regular and accurate blood pressure measurements can detect it in time to initiate effective therapy. There is another reason to be accurate. Erroneous overestimates of blood pressure may cause a normal person to be labeled hypertensive with significant economic, medical, and psychological repercussions. Thus, correct and frequent ambulatory measurements of blood pressure are an important part of every physician's armamentarium.

36. What does sphygmomanometer mean?

It is Greek for measurement of a weak pulse (*sphygmos* = pulse, *manos* = scanty, and *metron* = measurement).

37. Who invented the sphygmomanometer?

Like many successes in history, the sphygmomanometer enjoys the privilege of many fathers (failures are almost always orphans). In this case the proud parents were the French Pierre Potain, the Italian Scipione Riva-Rocci, the Russian Nicolai Korotkoff, and the American Harvey Cushing. Cushing did not participate in the ideation of the device but was instrumental in its diffusion to North America. Incidentally, the mercury sphygmomanometer just celebrated its 100th anniversary; it was invented in 1896.

38. Who made the first direct measurement of blood pressure? How?

The first direct measurement of arterial pressure was made in England in 1733. The English botanist and chemist Stephen Hales (1677–1761) decided to sacrifice his horse to find out whether in fact "blood pressure" existed. In his backyard he cannulated the carotid artery of the poor animal and then measured the height of the column of blood extending from the carotid into a glass tube. This measurement was carried out from the time of cannulation until the horse's death. Based on his observations, Hales concluded that the animal indeed had something that he called "blood pressure" and suggested that this pressure varies between arteries and veins, between dilations and contractions of the heart, and between large and small animals. He published his observations under the title "Haemasticks" and then went on to bigger and better things, such as telling housewives that putting an inverted teacup in their pies would prevent the crust from becoming soggy.

39. Who was Potain? What contribution did he make to the measurement of blood pressure?

The French physician Pierre Potain first described the gallop rhythms and later inspired the figure of the great Parisian diagnostician in Proust's *Remembrance of Things Past*. Potain was one of the several giants produced by nineteenth century French medicine. He was also an interesting man. As an intern he survived a rendezvous with cholera, which he contracted during the 1849 epidemic. He then survived an even more dangerous rendezvous with the Prussians, whom he faced during the 1870 war, fighting as a simple foot soldier. Potain became one of Trousseau's protégés (see below), a great promoter of cardiac auscultation, and a compassionate teacher. He was famous for answering his own questions if an examinee failed to provide the answers in time. His unique contribution to blood pressure measurement was a contraption made of a compressible bulb filled with air. It was attached by a rubber tube to an aneroid manometer. The bulb then was pressed on the arterial pulse until the pulse disappeared. The manometric recording at the time of the disappearance of the pulse reflected the patient's systolic blood pressure.

40. Who first thought of the mercury sphygmomanometer?

Scipione Riva-Rocci, one of Potain's students. Riva-Rocci first trained and worked under Forlanini on the idea of a therapeutic pneumothorax for the control of pulmonary tuberculosis. While studying air-filling of the pleural cavity at controlled pressures, he became interested in a noninvasive measurement of blood pressure. In 1896, at the age of 33, Riva-Rocci came up with the idea of a mercury sphygmomanometer—a device attached to a manometer in which the varying pressures were shown by differences of elevation in a column of mercury instead of a revolving pointer, as in Potain's aneroid (or dial) manometer. This idea was quite good for medicine, but it may have been fatal for Riva-Rocci, who years later died of a chronic neurologic condition probably contracted in the laboratory. Riva-Rocci made several improvements in Potain's instrument:

1. He proposed the use of the brachial instead of the radial artery (which made measurements easier and more accurate).

2. He proposed the use of a wrap-around inflatable rubber cuff that made Potain's over-readings much less common. (Later Von Recklinghausen increased the width of the cuff from 5 to 13 cm.)

3. He proposed guidelines for the correct use of the instrument to avoid errors.

4. He proposed an instrument so simple and easy to carry that it made blood pressure measurement feasible even at the bedside. Indeed, the success of his device is proved by the fact that, with only minor modifications, it is still much the same tool 100 years later.

Riva-Rocci also had good insights into the "white-coat" effect of blood pressure measurement, which he first described.

41. How did Riva-Rocci's device reach the United States?

Despite such achievements, Riva-Rocci's sphygmomanometer may have remained an Italian secret were it not for Harvey Cushing's visit to Pavia in 1901. Cushing spent several days with Riva-Rocci at the Ospedale di San Matteo, made a drawing of the instrument, received one as a gift, and brought everything back to Johns Hopkins. The rest is history.

42. Who perfected the indirect measurement of blood pressure?

The problem with both Potain's and Riva-Rocci's sphygmomanometers was that they provided a reading only of systolic pressure (by releasing the arterial pulse after its obliteration). The Russian physician Nicolai Sergeyevich Korotkoff came to the rescue. Korotkoff actually stumbled onto his discovery of auscultatory pressure, as often happens in medical breakthroughs. A surgeon in the czar's army, he had just completed a tour of duty during the Russian-Japanese War of 1904 and, at the age of 30, was working in St. Petersburg on an animal model of postsurgical arteriovenous fistulas. One day Korotkoff was listening over a dog's artery before releasing a tourniquet. Suddenly he heard loud sounds. Intrigued, he noted that the sounds correlated with systole and diastole and reported his observations in 1905. Korotkoff suggested that listening for the appearance and disappearance of pulse sounds may serve as a signal for maximal and minimal blood pressures. The article, written in Russian, did not create much noise in Europe, but it created a tremendous noise in Russia, winning Korotkoff an enviable reputation as a madman. Only after the article finally reached Germany (and from there England) did the auscultatory method of Korotkoff replace the pulse obliteration method of Riva-Rocci and Potain. Modern measurement of systolic and diastolic blood pressure was finally born. Korotkoff was arrested during the Russian Revolution and died in 1920.

43. What is the proper technique for indirect measurement of blood pressure?

The American Heart Association has published guidelines for indirect auscultatory measurement:

Technique for Measuring Blood Pressure

The intent and purpose of the measurement should be explained to the patient in a reassuring manner and every effort should be made to put the patient at ease. (Include a 5-minute rest before the first measurement.) The sequential steps for measuring the blood pressure in the upper extremity, as for routine screening and monitoring purposes, should include the following:

1. Have paper and pen at hand for immediate recording of the pressure.

2. Seat the patient in a quiet, calm environment [with feet flat on the floor, back against the chair] with his or her bared arm resting on a standard table or other support so that the midpoint of the upper arm is at the level of the heart.

3. Estimate by inspection or measure with a tape the circumference of the bare upper arm at the midpoint between the acromium and olecranon process and select an appropriately sized cuff. The bladder inside the cuff should encircle 80% of the arm in adults and 100% of the arm in children less than 13 years old. If in doubt, use a larger cuff. If the available cuff is too small, this should be noted.

Table continued on facing page

Technique for Measuring Blood Pressure (Continued)

4. Palpate the brachial artery and place the cuff so that the midline of the bladder is over the arterial pulsation; then wrap and secure the cuff snugly around the patient's bare arm. Avoid rolling up the sleeve in such a manner that it forms a tight tourniquet around the upper arm. Loose application of the cuff results in overestimation of the pressure. The lower edge of the cuff should be 1 in (2 cm) above the antecubital fossa where the head of the stethoscope is to be placed.

5. Place the manometer so that the center of the mercury column or aneroid dial is at eye level [except for tilted-column floor models] and easily visible to the observer and the tubing from the cuff is unobstructed.

6. Inflate the cuff rapidly to 70 mmHg, and increase by 10 mmHg increments while palpating the radial pulse. Note the level of pressure at which the pulse disappears and subsequently reappears during deflation. This procedure, the palpatory method, provides a necessary preliminary approximation of the systolic blood pressure to ensure an adequate level of inflation when the actual, auscultatory measurement is made. The palpatory method is particularly useful to avoid underinflation of the cuff in patients with an auscultatory gap and overinflation in those with very low blood pressure.

7. Place the earpieces of the stethoscope into the ear canals, angled forward to fit snugly. Switch the stethoscope head to the low-frequency position (bell). The setting can be confirmed by listening as the stethoscope head (i.e., the bell orifice) is tapped gently.

8. Place the head of the stethoscope over the brachial artery pulsation, just above and medial to the antecubital fossa but below the edge of the cuff, and hold it firmly [but not too tightly] in place, making sure that the head makes contact with the skin around its entire circumference. Wedging the head of the stethoscope under the edge of the cuff may free one hand but results in considerable extraneous noise [and is nearly impossible with the bell in any event].

9. Inflate the bladder rapidly and steadily to a pressure 20–30 mmHg above the level previously determined by palpation; then partially unscrew (open) the valve and deflate the bladder at 2 mm[Hg]/sec while listening for the appearance of the Korotkoff sounds.

10. As the pressure in the bladder falls, note the level of the pressure on the manometer at the first appearance of repetitive sounds (Phase I) and at the muffling of these sounds (Phase IV) and when they disappear (Phase V). During the period that the Korotkoff sounds are audible, the rate of deflation should be no more than 2 mm per pulse beat, thereby compensating for both rapid and slow heart rates.

11. After the Korotkoff sound is heard, the cuff should be deflated slowly for at least another 10 mmHg to ensure that no further sounds are audible and then rapidly and completely deflated. The patient should be allowed to rest for at least 30 seconds.

12. The systolic (Phase I) and diastolic (Phase V) pressures should be recorded immediately, rounded off (upward) to the nearest 2 mmHg. In children and when sounds are heard nearly to a level of 0 mmHg, the Phase IV pressure also should be recorded (example: 108/65/56 mmHg). All values should be recorded together with the name of the patient, the date and time of the measurement, the arm on which the measurement was made, the patient's position, and the cuff size (when a nonstandard size is used).

13. The measurement should be repeated after at least 30 seconds, and the two readings should be averaged. In clinical situations, additional measurements can be made in the same or opposite arm, in the same or an alternative position.

44. When should blood pressure be measured?

It should be measured in every significant patient interaction, whether ambulatory or hospital-based. At each exam you should obtain two or more readings from the same arm with the patient supine or seated. The average value should be recorded in the chart. If the readings differ by more than 5 mmHg diastolic, you should take additional readings until a stable pressure is reached. Measure blood pressure in both arms at the first visit, and use the arm with the higher pressure thereafter (the arm with the lower pressure is abnormal).

45. Where should blood pressure be measured?

It should be measured at least once in both upper extremities. A difference in systolic blood pressure between the two arms > 10–15 mmHg is considered significant. This measurement requires two independent observers, working simultaneously on the two arms and then switching sides. You also should measure blood pressure in the lower extremities if clinically indicated (see below).

46. How is hypertension defined?

With great difficulty. In fact, there are no real cutoff points in blood pressure values below which the risk for cardiovascular disease is minimal and above which disease definitely develops. Even mild hypertension should receive strong consideration, and systolic hypertension should not be disregarded.

Classification of Blood Pressure for Adults Aged 18 Years and Older

CATEGORY	SYSTOLIC (mmHg)	DIASTOLIC (mmHg)
Normal	< 130	< 85
High normal	130–139	85–89
Hypertension*		
Stage 1 (mild)	140–159	90–99
Stage 2 (moderate)	160–179	100–109
Stage 3 (severe)	180–209	110–119
Stage 4 (very severe)	≥ 210	≥ 120

• Based on the average of two or more readings taken at each of two or more visits after an initial screening. Adapted from the Fifth Report of the Joint National Committee on Detection, Evaluation, and Treatment of High Blood Pressure. (Adapted from Reeves RA: Does this patient have hypertension? How to measure blood pressure JAMA 273:1211–1217, 1995.)

General consensus defines hypertension as the blood pressure level above which the risk for cardiovascular disease increases significantly. This threshold is set at about (or above) 140/90 mmHg. Treatable hypertension is the blood pressure level above which treatment has been found to be more beneficial than harmful. This threshold is set at a blood pressure that is consistently:

• ≥ 160 mmHg systolic (tested only in the elderly) with or without diastolic elevation *or*
• ≥ 90 mmHg diastolic (tested in young and elderly patients)

Blood pressure is quite variable and often decreases with observation. Thus, it is important to monitor patients over time before labeling them hypertensive (see below).

47. Which factors can overestimate or underestimate the true blood pressure value?

Several factors can either increase or decrease blood pressure during routine ambulatory measurements. Familiarity with these factors is important.

Factors Affecting the Immediate Accuracy of Office Blood Pressure

FACTOR	MAGNITUDE (SBP/DBP, mmHg)
Increases Recorded Blood Pressure	
Examinee	
Soft Korotkoff sounds	DBP
Missed auscultatory gap	DBP (rare, huge)
Pseudohypertension	2 to 98/3 to 49
"White coat" reaction	
To physician	11 to 28/3 to 15
To nonphysician	1 to 12/2 to 7
Paretic arm (due to stroke)	2/5
Pain, anxiety	May be large
Acute smoking	6/5
Acute caffeine	11/5
Acute ethanol ingestion	8/8

Table continued on facing page

Factors Affecting the Immediate Accuracy of Office Blood Pressure (Continued)

FACTOR	MAGNITUDE (SBP/DBP, mmHg)
Increases Recorded Blood Pressure *(Continued)*	
Examinee *(cont.)*	
Distended bladder	15/10
Talking, signing	7/8
Setting, equipment	
Environmental noise	DBP
Leaky bulb valve	≥ 2 DBP
Blocked manometer vents	2 to 10
Cold hands or stethoscope	Not stated
Examiner	
Expectation bias	Probably < 10
Impaired hearing	DBP
Examination	
Cuff too narrow	–8 to +10/2 to 8
Cuff not centered	4/3
Cuff over clothing	5 to 50
Elbow too low	6
Cuff too loose	Not stated
Too short rest period	Varied estimates
Back unsupported	6 to 10
Arm unsupported	1 to 7/5 to 11
Too slow deflation	–1 to +2/5 to 6
Too fast deflation	DBP only
Parallax error	2 to 4
Using phase IV (adult)	6 DBP
Too rapid remeasure	1/1
Cold season (vs. warm)	6/3 to 10
Decreases Blood Pressure	
Examinee	
Soft Korotkoff sounds	SBP
Recent meal	–1 to 1/1 to 4
Missed auscultatory gap	10 to 50 SBP
High stroke volume	Phase V can = 0
Habituation	0 to 7/2 to 12
Shock (additional pseudohypotension)	33 SBP
Setting, equipment	
Noisy environs	SBP
Faulty aneroid device	Can be > 10
Low mercury level	Varies
Leaky bulb	≥ 2 SBP
Examiner	
Reading to next lowest 5 or 10 mmHg or expectation bias	Probably ≤ 10
Impaired hearing	SBP only
Examination	
Left vs. right arm	1/1
Resting for too long (25 min)	10/0
Elbow too high	5/5
Too rapid deflation	SBP only
Excessive bell pressure	≥ 9 DBP
Parallax error (aneroid)	2 to 4

SBP = systolic blood pressure, DBP = diastolic blood pressure. (Adapted from Reeves RA: Does this patient have hypertension? How to measure blood pressure. JAMA 273:1211–1217, 1995.)

The following factors have no effect on blood pressure measurement: menstrual phase, chronic caffeine ingestion, phenylephrine nasal spray, cuff self-inflation, discordance in sex or race of examinee and examiner, thin shirtsleeve under cuff, bell vs. diaphragm, cuff inflation per se, hour of day (during work hours), and room temperature.

48. What are the most common reasons for variations in blood pressure?

They usually are related to the patient, equipment, or examiner. Patients show tremendous blood pressure variability over time. With two or more measurements at each visit, the standard deviation between visits is 5–12 mmHg systolic and 6–8 mmHg diastolic. This between-visits variability is greater than within-visit fluctuations; thus, more visits are necessary to ensure diagnostic precision. The interval between visits, however, should take into account both blood pressure level and clinical status. The Joint National Committee recommends repeat measurements within 1 month for blood pressure initially in the range of 160–179 mmHg systolic or 100–109 mmHg diastolic (stage 2), within 2 months for stage 1, within 1 week for stage 3, and immediate evaluation for stage 4. In addition, arrhythmias (particularly atrial fibrillation) also may cause beat-to-beat variations in cardiac output and thus increase interobserver variation in blood pressure measurements. Averaging several readings may help to overcome this problem.

Finally, although interobserver agreement is usually high for blood pressure measurement, examiners may be responsible for errors. In fact, differences among examiners of 10/8 mmHg are quite common. Of interest, auscultatory automatic monitors had fewer discrepancies than a control group of experienced clinicians.

49. How accurate is blood pressure measurement by sphygmomanometer?

Accurate with some limitations. Blood pressure values recorded with the indirect auscultatory method correlate quite well with simultaneous intraarterial direct recordings ($r = 0.94$–0.98). But the Korotkoff phase I sounds do not appear until 4–15 mmHg below the direct systolic blood pressure, whereas Korotkoff phase V sounds disappear above the true diastolic value (by 3–6 mmHg). Thus, there are still minor discrepancies between the two methods.

Physicians also may be responsible for some inaccuracies. For example, despite previously agreeing to use three readings for diagnosis, a group of British general practitioners diagnosed hypertension after only one blood pressure measurement in 58% of patients. Similarly, 37% of German ambulatory physicians and British hospital-based clinicians record Korotkoff phase IV (muffling) rather than the more accurate phase V as the signal for diastolic blood pressure. The most common technical error, however, is usually failure to use a sufficiently large cuff. In one survey, only 25% of primary care physicians had a large cuff available in their office. Finally, aneroid instruments (used by 34% of practitioners) often go out of calibration, usually downward. One survey found that 30% of office sphygmomanometers were in fact off by 10 mmHg or more; they need to be periodically recalibrated.

Finally, in some patients the blood pressure in a physician's office is considerably and consistently higher than the daytime ambulatory value. This phenomenon is called the "white coat" effect and is seen in as many as 10–40% of untreated and borderline hypertensive patients. Even treated patients often show blood pressure differences that are greater than 20/10 mmHg. This phenomenon tends to be greater in female patients than in male patients and responds more to the white coat of doctors than to the white coat of nurses.

50. What is Osler's maneuver? How is it carried out?

Osler's maneuver is a bedside test for the detection of pseudohypertension. This relatively uncommon condition is seen in less than 2% of otherwise healthy elderly people. Osler's maneuver is carried out by inflating the blood pressure cuff to the point of obliteration of the radial pulse and then feeling the radial artery. If the examiner is still able to palpate the artery, the maneuver is said to be positive (positive Osler's sign). In this case the artery remains palpable as a firm tube. If a cuff is not available, the examiner can obliterate the radial pulse by compressing the brachial artery with his or her other thumb.

51. What is the significance of a positive Osler's sign?

A positive Osler's sign (palpability of an artery in the absence of its pulse) is a sign of arteriosclerosis. Its presence, therefore, suggests that both systolic and diastolic blood pressures may be overestimated because a stiff arterial wall is more difficult to compress.

52. How useful is Osler's sign?

Probably not as much as traditionally taught. For example, in 65 geriatric patients classified as either Osler-positive or Osler-negative by unanimous consensus among three observers, there was moderate intraobserver consistency ($\kappa = 0.49$) with another group of six physicians and only modest interobserver agreement ($\kappa = 0.37$). Definitive confirmation of pseudohypertension requires an intraarterial measurement of blood pressure.

53. What is pseudohypotension?

It is a condition seen in shock. The high peripheral vascular resistance of patients in shock tightens their arteries to the point that generation of Korotkoff sounds is severely impaired. As a result, the sounds are too weakened to allow effective measurement of either systolic or diastolic blood pressure and may lead to a gross underestimate. Thus, a high peripheral vascular resistance (as seen in shock) is an important cause of pseudohypotension.

Pearl. *Both pseudohypertension and pseudohypotension can be counteracted by direct intraarterial recording of blood pressure.*

54. Is there any difference in systolic blood pressure as determined by palpation and auscultation?

Yes, but not a lot. Palpated systolic blood pressure is about 7 mmHg lower than the auscultatory value. Thus, physicians who have a hearing impairment may still do quite well by relying on the palpatory method for both systolic and diastolic pressures.

55. How do you calibrate an aneroid sphygmomanometer?

It should be calibrated against a mercury unit by using a y-connector and tubing so that the cuff can be connected to both sphygmomanometers. Alternative methods include the following:

1. Connect the aneroid bulb/dial unit to the cuff of the mercury sphygmomanometer (which is attached to it). Close the valve, and wrap the cuff to avoid its unrolling.

2. Slowly inflate the cuff until the mercury column rises to about 90 mmHg. Compare the readings in the two instruments by holding the aneroid dial near the mercury column.

3. Obtain repeat readings at high and low pressure values (e.g., 210 mmHg, 180 mmHg, 50 mmHg).

56. What is pulse pressure?

It is the difference between systolic and diastolic blood pressure. Thus, in a patient with systolic blood pressure of 120 mmHg and diastolic blood pressure of 80 mmHg, the pulse pressure is 40 mmHg.

57. What is an abnormally widened pulse pressure? What are the causes?

An abnormally widened pulse pressure is greater than 50% of the systolic blood pressure. For example, in a patient with systolic blood pressure of 140 mmHg and diastolic blood pressure of 60 mmHg, the pulse pressure is 80. The most common cause is hyperkinetic heart syndrome, a hemodynamic state characterized by high stroke volume and low peripheral vascular resistances. It may be seen in the following conditions:

- Aortic regurgitation
- Patent ductus arteriosus (PDA)
- Exercise
- Fever
- Anemia
- Arteriovenous fistulas
- Beriberi
- Paget's disease
- Cirrhosis
- Pregnancy
- Thyrotoxicosis
- Severe exfoliative dermatitis

Many of these conditions are characterized by arteriovenous (AV) fistulas. The fistulas may be either large and single, as in PDA, or small and multiple, as in Paget's disease (the fistulas are in the bone), pregnancy (the entire placenta functions as a big AV fistula), exfoliative dermatitis (the fistulas are in the skin), and cirrhosis (the fistulas are both hepatic and extrahepatic). The shunt from these fistulas is responsible for the high output and hyperdynamic state.

58. What is the significance of a widened pulse pressure in only one extremity?

It indicates the presence of an AV fistula in that extremity. Branham's sign helps to confirm this suspicion.

59. What is Branham's sign?

It is the typical bradycardia seen after compression (or excision) of a large AV fistula. Slowing of the heart rate is caused by inhibition of the Bainbridge reflex, which operates continuously in patients with large fistulas. The Bainbridge reflex is a compensatory increase in heart rate caused by a rise in right atrial pressure, which is commonly seen in patients with AV fistulas because of the large shunts. Compensatory tachycardia is due to stretching of the right atrium and is caused by inhibition of vagal influence and activation of sympathetic acceleratory mechanisms. The Bainbridge reflex is also the mechanism for the supraventricular tachyarrhythmias of patients with acute pulmonary embolism.

60. How do you test for Branham's sign?

By inflating a blood pressure cuff over the suspected limb. The heart rate slows down, only to reaccelerate upon cuff deflation (and secondary reopening of the AV fistula).

61. Who were Branham and Bainbridge?

Henry Branham was a nineteenth-century American surgeon.

Francis Bainbridge (1874–1921) was an English physiologist whose most important contribution was in the field of exercise. He was a small, quiet man and an unimpressive lecturer.

62. What is an abnormally narrowed pulse pressure? What are the causes?

A pulse pressure is considered abnormally narrowed if it is less than 25% of the systolic value. For example, a patient with systolic blood pressure of 100 mmHg and diastolic blood pressure of 90 mmHg has a pulse pressure of 10. The most common cause is a drop in left ventricular stroke volume, as in patients with obstruction to left ventricular filling or left ventricular emptying (i.e., tamponade, constrictive pericarditis, or aortic stenosis). It also may be seen in extreme tachycardia, in which the filling time for the ventricle is severely reduced. Finally, it may be seen in shock as a result of increased peripheral vascular resistance.

63. What is pulsus paradoxus?

It is an exaggeration of the normal respiratory variation in systolic pressure. With inspiration the systolic blood pressure decreases, and with expiration it increases. These changes are physiologic but may become detectable at the bedside, even by simply palpating the peripheral pulse. Thus, with inspiration the pulse becomes weaker, whereas with expiration it becomes stronger. To detect an inspiratory weakening of the pulse the decrease in systolic blood pressure must be at least 20 mmHg. An easier and more sensitive way to detect smaller variations is to measure the blood pressure. In this case, an abnormal pulsus paradoxus is defined as an inspiratory drop in systolic blood pressure greater than 10 mmHg.

64. Why is it paradoxical?

Because the changes in pulse volume are independent of the changes in pulse rate. This paradox goes back to the original patient described by Kussmaul in 1873. The man had such a decrease in systolic pressure during inspiration that his peripheral pulse completely disappeared. The paradox to Kussmaul was that the patient maintained a heartbeat despite losing his pulse.

This paradox was also the reason for the Latin term, *pulsus respiratione intermittens* (intermittent pulse as a result of respiration). Pulsus paradoxus was described first by Lower in the 17th century. Lower had no sphygmomanometer (it had not been invented yet) and therefore relied only on the peripheral pulse. Hence the name pulsus. This term is now outdated, considering that the pulsus is detected primarily by measuring inspiratory changes in systolic blood pressure, not by feeling the peripheral pulse. Lower's initial observation was largely ignored until it was rediscovered by Kussmaul two centuries later.

65. Describe the pathophysiology of pulsus paradoxus.

It is an exaggeration of the normal drop in systolic blood pressure (and therefore in the fullness of the arterial pulse) during inspiration.

Inspiration causes a decrease in intrathoracic pressure and hence an increase in venous return to the right ventricle. It also causes a decrease in left ventricular venous return (because of the pooling of blood in the inflated lungs and a left shift in the ventricular septum). The smaller, end-diastolic left ventricular volume results, in turn, in a lower stroke volume and, thus, in a lower systolic blood pressure. If this drop is severe enough (> 20 mmHg), it results in a palpable weakening in peripheral pulse.

Exhalation, on the other hand, leads to an increase in left ventricular filling (because of the squeezing of blood from the deflating lungs and the right shift in the ventricular septum). This increase in ventricular filling leads, in turn, to an increased left ventricular stroke volume and increased systolic blood pressure. If severe enough, it may lead to an increase in pulse volume.

All of these respiratory variations are physiologic. But in certain pathologic states they may become large enough to cause more profound and detectable changes in blood pressure and pulse volume.

66. What are the most common causes of pulsus paradoxus?

The most common cause is pericardial tamponade. Almost 100% of patients with tamponade, in fact, have pulsus paradoxus. This percentage is lower (70%) in more chronic cases but approaches 100% in acute cases with rapid fluid accumulation. Pulsus paradoxus also occurs in 30–45% of patients with constrictive pericarditis, but the condition must have an exudative component and not be completely "dry."

The other major cause of pulsus paradoxus is obstructive lung disease, particularly status asthmaticus. Lung hyperinflation leads to an excessive inspiratory pooling of blood and therefore to a drop in systolic blood pressure. Pulsus paradoxus, for example, has been reported in as many as 80% of patients with asthma, correlating well with the degree of reduction in FEV_1. In such patients pulsus paradoxus is usually not highly sensitive but quite specific for an $FEV_1 < 0.5$–0.7 L. Pulsus paradoxus also has been reported (albeit not consistently) in pulmonary embolism, shock, right ventricular infarction, right ventricular failure, and severe congestive heart failure.

Pulsus paradoxus may be absent (false negative) when either pericardial stiffness poses an asymmetric obstacle to the filling of the two ventricles or respiratory changes to ventricular filling occur differently or not at all. Examples of such situations include (1) stiff left ventricular wall (as a result of hypertrophy), (2) severe left ventricular failure, (3) atrial septal defect, (4) aortic regurgitation, (5) severe tamponade with shock, and (6) loculated pericardial fluid.

67. What is reversed pulsus paradoxus?

It is an increase in systolic blood pressure that coincides with inspiration rather than expiration and is typical of hypertrophic obstructive cardiomyopathy (also called idiopathic hypertrophic subaortic stenosis). Reversed pulsus paradoxus also may be seen in patients with left ventricular failure and positive-pressure ventilation. In both cases either the ventricle is too stiff to fill adequately, or positive pressure ventilation reverses the respiratory changes in intrathoracic pressure.

68. How is pulsus paradoxus measured?

By standing at the bedside in such a way that you can monitor at the same time the patient's respiratory movements and the column of mercury in the sphygmomanometer. Fully inflate the blood pressure cuff until you achieve auscultatory silence. Then start deflating the cuff slowly, at the same time paying attention to chest and abdominal wall expansions. As soon as you hear the first Korotkoff sounds, stop deflating the cuff and record the pressure reading. You will notice that sounds can be heard only in exhalation. Start deflating the cuff again slowly, until you hear Korotkoff sounds in both inspiration and expiration. Record the second blood pressure reading. The difference between the two recordings, expressed in mmHg, is the pulsus paradoxus.

69. What is Trousseau's sign?

There are actually two Trousseau's signs:

1. **Thrombophlebitis** associated with a visceral carcinoma, which may be either superficial or deep and often has a migratory characteristic. This sign (often called Trousseau's syndrome) has been reported in association with cancers of the stomach, pancreas, lung, breast, and prostate.

2. **Carpal spasm** in patients with overt tetany, which also is associated with extension of the foot (carpopedal spasm), extension of the body, and opisthotonos. The spasm of the hand involves wrist flexors and finger extensors. The fingers are flexed at the metacarpophalangeal joints but extended at the phalangeal joints; the thumb is flexed and adducted into the palm. This hand so typically resembles the hand of a physician making a vaginal examination that often it is called obstetrician's hand (*main d'accoucheur* in Trousseau's original description).

70. What are the causes of obstetrician's hand?

Any cause predisposing to tetany, such as hypocalcemia, hypomagnesemia, hypophosphatemia, or alkalemia.

71. How can one trigger carpal spasm in patients with latent tetany?

By occluding the arterial pulse for 5 minutes with a blood pressure cuff. This test has a sensitivity of 66% in hypocalcemia with a false-positive rate of 4%. Therefore, it does not eliminate the need for blood testing. Another sign of muscular hyperexcitability is Chvostek's sign (facial twitching triggered by mechanical stimulation of cranial nerve VII). The test usually is carried out by tapping the bone anterior to the ear, which corresponds to the exit point of cranial nerve VII. In latent tetany Chvostek's sign has high false-positive rates: 19–74% in children and 4–29% in adults. It has a sensitivity of 27%.

72. Who was Trousseau?

Armand Trousseau (1801–1867) was one of the great leaders of nineteenth-century Parisian medicine. Among his "firsts" were the performance of tracheostomy (in France), use of thoracentesis, and creation of the term aphasia. Trousseau was a superb clinician and a much beloved teacher. He trained, among others, Lasegue, Brown-Sequard, and Da Costa. Sadly, in the last part of his life he diagnosed himself with gastric carcinoma by recognizing the same migratory superficial thrombophlebitis that he previously had described in patients with occult malignancy.

73. What is the Rumpel-Leede sign?

It is a test of capillary fragility, carried out by increasing venous pressure in the forearm with a blood pressure cuff and then inspecting the skin for petechial eruptions. The test is named after the two physicians who first described it: the German Theodore Rumpel and the American Carl Leede. It is, however, often called the Hess test after Alfred Hess (1875–1933), the American physician who had noticed this phenomenon while treating children with scurvy.

74. What is Hill's sign?

It is a sign of severe aortic regurgitation (see chapter 11) and consists of a systolic blood pressure at the thigh that is 20 mmHg higher than the systolic blood pressure at the arm. The systolic blood pressure of the lower extremities is often higher than the systolic blood pressure in the upper extremities (by as much as 10–15 mmHg). This normal difference, however, is present only with indirect recording. By direct intraarterial measurement, there is no discrepancy between upper and lower extremity pressures. Hill's sign is an exaggeration of the normal difference and indicates a high stroke volume. Thus, it is not specific to aortic regurgitation but also may be encountered in other hyperdynamic states (see above). It is also not particularly sensitive for aortic regurgitation (it is negative in moderate aortic regurgitation). If present, however, it usually confirms a diagnosis of severe aortic regurgitation.

75. What is the mechanism of Hill's sign?

The mechanism is not entirely clear. According to one theory, a high stroke volume generates a summation between the regular pulse wave of the aortic pressure and a rebound wave originating from the periphery. Because of the characteristics of the rebound wave, however, this summation takes place only in the lower extremities.

76. What causes systolic blood pressure to be lower in the lower extremities than in the upper extremities?

It depends on the age of the patient. In elderly patients the most common cause is atherosclerotic obstruction (or dissection) of the aorta. In younger patients the cause is usually coarctation of the aorta. Patients with these conditions may have systolic blood pressures that are at least 6 mmHg less in the lower extremities than in the upper extremities.

77. How do you measure the blood pressure in the lower extremities?

By placing the cuff over the thigh and palpating or auscultating over the popliteal artery.

78. Who was Hill?

Sir Leonard Hill (1866–1952) was an English physiologist who modified the original Riva-Rocci mercury sphygmomanometer by using a pressure gauge. In 1923 he won the Nobel Prize for physiology for his discovery of heat production and muscle metabolism.

79. What is severe hypertension?

Systolic blood pressure $\geq$ 180 mmHg or diastolic blood pressure $\geq$ 100 mmHg.

80. What is malignant hypertension?

A form of hypertension associated with one or more of the following manifestations of end-organ damage: rapid deterioration of renal function, retinal hemorrhages or optic nerve involvement, left ventricular failure, myocardial ischemia, or cerebrovascular accidents. The syndrome may occur independently of the level of hypertension. Thus, patients with very high blood pressure may not develop malignant hypertension, whereas patients with pressures as low as 180/120 mmHg may present with it.

BIBLIOGRAPHY

1. Beard K, Bulpitt C, Mascie-Taylor H, et al: Management of elderly patients with sustained hypertension. BMJ 304:412–416, 1992.
2. Blank SG, West JE, Muller FB, et al: Wideband external pulse recording during cuff deflation: A new technique for evaluation of the arterial pressure pulse and measurement of blood pressure. Circulation 77:1297–1305, 1988.
3. Collins R, Peto R, MacMahon S, et al: Blood pressure, stroke, and coronary heart disease. Part II: Short-term reductions in blood pressure: Overview of randomized drug trials in their epidemiological context. Lancet 335:827–838, 1990.

4. Joint National Committee: The Fifth Report of the Joint National Committee on Detection, Evaluation, and Treatment of High Blood Pressure (JNC V). Arch Intern Med 153:154–183, 1993.
5. McKay DW, Campbell NR, Parab LS, et al: Clinical assessment of blood pressure. J Hum Hypertens 4:639–645, 1990.
6. Neufeld PD, Johnson DL: Observer error in blood pressure measurement. Can Med Assoc J 135:633–637, 1986.
7. Reeves RA: A review of the stability of ambulatory blood pressure: Implications for diagnosis of hypertension. Clin Invest Med 14:251–255, 1991.
8. Smith TD, Clayton D: Individual variation between general practitioners in labelling of hypertension. BMJ 300:74–75, 1990.
9. Watson RDS, Lumb R, Young MA, et al: Variation in cuff blood pressure in untreated outpatients with mild hypertension: Implications for initiating antihypertensive treatment. J Hypertens 5:207–211, 1987.
10. Weiland SK, Keil U, Spelsberg A, et al: Diagnosis and management of hypertension by physicians in the Federal Republic of Germany. J Hypertens 9:131–134, 1991.
11. White WB, Lund-Johansen P, Omvik P: Assessment of four ambulatory blood pressure monitors and measurements by clinicians versus intra-arterial blood pressure at rest and during exercise. Am J Cardiol 65:60–66, 1990.
12. Wilkinson LS, Perry IJ, Shinton RA, Beevers DG: An emerging consensus among clinicians on treating mild hypertension but persistent uncertainty as to how blood pressure should be measured. J R Coll Physicians Lond 25:116–119, 1991.

3. THE SKIN

Debra J. Grossman, M.D., M.P.H., and Cynthia Guzzo, M.D.

The power of making a correct diagnosis is the key to all success in the treatment of skin diseases; without this faculty, the physician can never be a thorough dermatologist, and therapeutics at once cease to hold their proper position, and become empirical.

Louis A. Duhring (1845–1913)

Beauty's but skin deep.—John Davies of Hereford (1565–1618)

TOPICS COVERED IN THIS CHAPTER

CONVENTIONAL TEACHING WATCH

Skin lesions are frequently encountered and quite important in general practice. If left unrecognized, some of these disorders may cause serious consequences for the patient; early detection becomes imperative. Simple inspection, palpation, and astute clinical interpretation are often the only tools required to reach a diagnosis. Hence, the importance of physical examination for the evaluation of skin disorders remains clear and incontrovertible. Most lesions reviewed in this chapter, therefore, have received a high pass.

FINDING		CONVENTIONAL TEACHING REVISITED
Lesion classification	⇑	ABCs of dermatology; essential roadmap to diagnosis.
Herpes simplex, zoster, and varicella	⇔	Common and overall benign problems; therapy now available.
Pemphigus and pemphigoid	⇑	Serious and important disorders; need to be recognized.
Acne	⇔	Usually not a diagnostic dilemma, but therapy is available and recognition is necessary.
Warts	⇔	As above.
Basal cell carcinoma	⇑	Very important to recognize.
Squamous cell carcinoma	⇑	As above.
Actinic keratosis	⇑	Important for its possible consequences.
Nevi	⇔	Relatively common and quite important findings because of differential diagnosis.
Atypical and dysplastic nevi	⇑	Important because of possible consequences.
Melanoma	⇑	Mandatory for all physicians: early recognition is key to patient's survival.
Lentigines/freckles	⇔	Common, benign lesions, but beware of lentigo maligna.
Seborrheic keratoses	⇔	Benign and common lesions.
Xanthomas/xanthelasmas	⇔	Usually not a diagnostic dilemma.
Staphylococcal scaled skin syndrome	⇑	Dermatology emergency.
Toxic epidermal necrolysis	⇑	As above.
Stevens-Johnson syndrome	⇑	As above.
Urticaria	⇔	Common but rarely serious.
Psoriasis	⇔	Common, important problem; usually not a diagnostic dilemma.
Dermatophytosis	⇔	As above.
Pityriasis rosea	⇔	Usually benign condition; may present diagnostic dilemma
Lichen planus	⇔	As above.
Atopic dermatitis	⇔	As above.
Stasis dermatitis	⇓	Not a diagnostic dilemma.
Seborrheic dermatitis	⇔	Benign, common lesion; recognition is key to treatment.
Kaposi's sarcoma	⇔	Still not too common but increasingly easier to recognize.
Syphilis	⇑	Still around; treatable and important.
Insect infestations	⇑	Common even in our society; recognition is key.
Skin manifestations of systemic disorders	⇑	Important topic for primary care physicians.

BASIC TERMINOLOGY AND DIAGNOSTIC TECHNIQUES

1. What are the key categories of skin lesions?

Skin lesions are commonly divided into two main groups: primary and secondary. **Primary lesions** result only from disease and have not been changed by any other event (such as trauma, scratching, or medical treatment). **Secondary lesions** have been altered by outside manipulation or medical treatment or, over time, by their own natural course.

2. What are the major primary skin lesions?

- **Macules:** flat, nonpalpable, circumscribed areas of discoloration smaller than 1 cm in diameter. Typical macules are the familiar freckles.

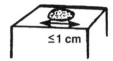

- **Patches:** flat, nonpalpable areas of skin discoloration larger than 1 cm in diameter. The patch associated with vitiligo is typical.

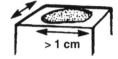

- **Papules:** raised, palpable skin lesions smaller than 1 cm in diameter that may or may not have a different color from the surrounding skin. A raised nevus is a typical papule.

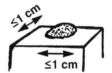

- **Plaques:** raised, palpable lesions larger than 1 cm in diameter. They are usually confined to the superficial dermis and may result from confluence of papules.

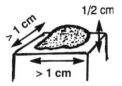

- **Nodules:** raised, palpable lesions larger than 1 cm in diameter. Unlike plaques, nodules either go deeper into the dermis or project outward from the skin surface. Because they are located below the surface of the skin, the overlying cutis is usually mobile.

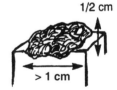

- **Tumors:** nodules that are either larger than 2 cm in diameter or poorly demarcated.

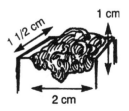

- **Wheals:** raised, circumscribed, edematous plaques that usually are pink or pale and tend to be present only transiently. The classic wheal is the lesion produced by a mosquito bite.

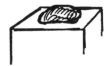

- **Vesicles:** fluid-filled, circumscribed, raised lesions that contain clear serous fluid and are smaller than 1 cm in diameter. Vesicles are the typical lesions of herpes simplex.

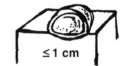

- **Bullae:** vesicles that measure more than 1 cm in diameter. They are commonly seen in patients with second-degree burns.

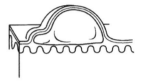

- **Cysts:** raised, encapsulated, fluid-filled lesions.

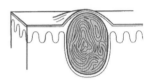

- **Pustules:** papules filled with pus (yellow fluid, viscous to solid in consistency). They represent localized collections of inflammatory cells and serum. Pustules are commonly seen in patients with impetigo or acne.

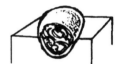

- **Purpura:** general name for the escape of red blood cells into the skin. Based on size, purpura may present as petechiae or ecchymoses. Palpable purpura is never normal and usually implies an antigen-antibody complex.

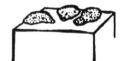

- **Petechiae:** reddish-to-purple discolorations that are small and flat. If it were not for their color, they would resemble macules and papules. They usually occur in groups and are smaller than 0.5 cm in diameter.

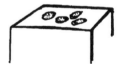

- **Ecchymoses (bruises):** reddish-to-purple lesions that are larger than petechiae. If it were not for their color, they would resemble patches and plaques. They are typically located below an intact epithelial surface.

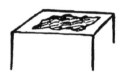

Figures adapted from Willms JL, Schneiderman H, Algranati PS: Physical Diagnosis. Baltimore, Williams & Wilkins, 1994, with permission.

3. What are the major secondary lesions?

- **Excoriations:** scratch marks (i.e., lesions produced by scratching). They are often raised and linear but also may present as a crust on top of a primary lesion that has been in part scratched off.

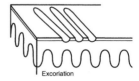

Excoriation

• **Lichenification:** a typical thickening of the skin seen in patients with chronic pruritus and recurrent scratching. It resembles the process of callus formation in the palms and soles of people exposed to chronic and recurrent trauma. The lichenified skin is hardened and leather-like, with accentuation of the skin markings and some scaling.

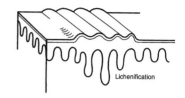

• **Scales:** raised lesions presenting as flaking on the upper surface of the skin. Scales represent thickening of the uppermost layer of the epidermis, the stratum corneum. They may be white, gray, or tan. They also may be quite small or relatively large. Scales provide the squamous component in what are commonly called papulosquamous diseases. They are common in dandruff and psoriasis.

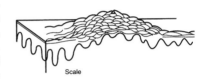

• **Crusts:** raised lesions produced by dried serum and blood cell remnants. The most familiar form of a crust is the scab, commonly seen in impetigo.

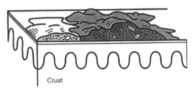

• **Erosions:** depressed lesions produced whenever the epidermis is either removed or sloughed. Erosions are moist, usually red, and well circumscribed. Classic erosions are seen in patients with chickenpox after rupture of a vesicle.

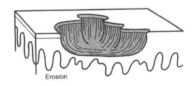

• **Ulcers:** depressed lesions produced whenever not only the epidermis but also part (or all) of the dermis is gone. Ulcers are concave lesions, often moist and at times inflamed or even hemorrhagic. A classic ulcer is the syphilitic chancre.

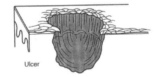

• **Fissures:** depressed lesions that present as narrow and linear skin cracks. They penetrate through the epidermis and reach at least part of the dermis. Classic fissures are the lesions seen in athlete's foot.

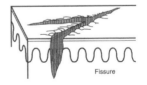

• **Atrophy:** usually the nonspecific end-product of various skin disorders. It is characterized by a pale and shiny area with loss of skin markings and full skin thickness.

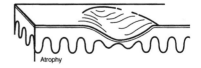

• **Sinuses:** connective channels between the surface of the skin and deeper components.

(Figures from Fitzpatrick JE, Aeling JL: Dermatology Secrets. Philadelphia, Hanley & Belfus, 1996, with permission.)

4. Are there other ways to classify skin lesions?

Skin lesions may be classified in quite a few ways. One particularly useful system divides skin lesions into four groups based on their relationship with the surrounding skin:

1. **Flat, nonpalpable lesions**

Macules	Purpura	Spider angioma
Patches	Ecchymoses (bruises)	Venous spider

2. **Raised, solid, palpable lesions**

Papules	Nodules	Wheals	Crust
Plaques	Tumor	Scale	

3. **Raised, cystic, palpable lesions**

Vesicles	Pustules	Bullae	Cysts

4. **Depressed lesions**

Atrophy	Erosion	Ulcer	Fissure

5. What terms are used most commonly to describe the distribution (body location) of multiple skin lesions?

Multiple skin lesions have a distribution that may be helpful diagnostically; therefore, it should be recognized and documented. In general, the distribution of skin lesions may be described as follows:

1. **Scattered (generalized) lesions** are spread throughout the body.
2. **Localized lesions** involve only selective parts of the body:
   - Palms or soles
   - Intertriginous areas
   - Extensor surfaces
   - Trunk
   - Face and neck or malar area
   - Selective dermatomes (see below)
   - Pressure areas
   - Any combination of the above

6. What do we mean by the configuration and pattern of distribution of a skin lesion? What terms are used most commonly to describe them?

The **configuration** of a skin lesion refers to its outline as seen from above. Lesions may present with the following configurations:

1. *Annular:* ring-shaped lesions. Cutaneous fungal infections often present as red rings with a scaly surface.
2. *Linear:* lesions arranged in a line. Streaks of small vesicles are seen on an erythematous base. The most common example of a linear lesion is rhus dermatitis (poison ivy rash). *Rhus* is the Greek word for sumac, which describes various shrubs or small trees. Some species of sumac (or rhus) include poison ivy and poison oak, which cause an acute itching rash on contact.
3. *Reticular:* net-like cluster of lesions.
4. *Gyrate:* lesions with a serpentine (or polycyclic) configuration, as in gyrate erythema.

The **pattern of distribution** refers to the relationship of the lesions to each other:

1. *Clustered (grouped):* lesions in close proximity to one another, occurring in a group or series of groups.
2. *Confluent (coalescent):* multiple lesions that blend together.
3. *Dermatomal:* lesions typically distributed along neurocutaneous dermatomes. The most classic example is herpes zoster (shingles), in which blisters are grouped along a dermatome.

7. How should an initial cutaneous exam be done?

Ideally, any initial exam should be conducted from head to toe. The patient should disrobe fully. With the patient wearing a hospital gown, one should inspect the entire body, including palms and soles, scalp, and mouth.

8. How should a specific lesion be examined to determine its classification?

Not only by looking at it, but also by touching it. Indeed, beyond the obvious gross visual inspection, palpation of a particular lesion often yields the most valuable information. For example, it may allow determination of whether the lesion is papular, sclerotic, soft, mobile, rough, or smooth.

9. What should the general approach to a dermatology diagnosis include?
It should include the following four key components:
1. **Morphology:** assessment of lesion characteristics
   • Dimensions (both width and height, if necessary)
   • Elevation or depression
   • Palpable features (such as smoothness, induration, tenderness)
   • Color
2. **Distribution (body location)**
   • Generalized   • Localized
3. **Configuration**
   • Annular   • Reticular
   • Linear   • Gyrate
4. **Pattern of distribution**
   • Clustered   • Confluent (coalescent)   • Dermatomal

10. What skin appendages should be part of a thorough dermatologic examination?
Fingernails, toenails, and hair (including eyebrows and eyelashes).

11. How should fingernails and toenails be assessed?
Fingernails and toenails should be examined for color, shape, lunula characteristics, and condition of the cuticle (the thin skin adherent to the nail at its proximal portion) and perionychium (the epidermis forming the ungual wall behind and at the sides of the nail).

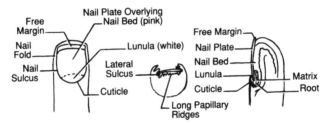

Anatomy of the fingernail. (From DeGowin RL: DeGowin and DeGowin's Diagnostic Examination, 6th ed. New York, McGraw-Hill, 1994, with permission.)

Lesions characteristic of the nails include the following:
1. **Clubbing** (see chapter 23)
2. **Onycholysis:** separation of the nail plate from the nail bed (loosening of the nails in Greek), beginning at the nail's distal tip and usually incomplete. Onycholysis may be seen in thyrotoxicosis, psoriasis, various eczematous disorders, and mycosis of the nails (onychomycosis).
3. **Paronychia:** inflammation of the perionychium, which becomes red, swollen, and often tender.
4. **Leukonychia** (literally, white nails in Greek): characterized by the occurrence of white spots or patches between the nail and its bed. The spots are due to the presence of subungual air bubbles. The white discoloration may involve the entire nail (total leukonychia) or present as lines (striate leukonychia) or dots (punctate leukonychia). Total leukonychia is a congenital dominant disorder. Striate or punctate leukonychias result from trauma.
5. **Spooning** or **koilonychia**: typical malformation of the nails characterized by concavity of the outer surface. It is often seen in patients with severe iron deficiency anemia.
6. **Lindsay's nails** (from the American physician who first described them in 1967) are also called half-and-half nails: the proximal half of the nail is white, whereas the distal half is darker (usually brownish but may be reddish or pink). They are seen in patients with chronic renal failure.

7. **Terry's nails** (from the British physician who first described them in 1954): characterized by whitening of the proximal 80% of the nail, leaving a small rim of peripheral reddening. They are seen in older people or patients with heart failure, cirrhosis, or non–insulin-dependent diabetes.

8. **Red half-moons in nail beds** (variety of Terry's nails, also described by Terry): characterized by a lunula that is not white but red. They also are called the nails of cardiac failure.

9. **Azure half-moons in nail beds:** the nails of Wilson's disease (hepatolenticular degeneration). The lunulae are not white but light blue.

10. **Muehrcke's lines** (from the American nephrologist who first described them in 1956): two arcuate white lines parallel to the lunula and separated by normal nail. Because they are located in the nail bed (not in the nailplate), Muehrcke's lines do not progress with the growth of the nail. They are seen in patients with hypoalbuminemia (< 2 gm/100 ml) and disappear with its resolution.

11. **Beau's lines:** transverse grooves on the fingernails of patients recovering from a serious illness such as myocardial infarction. They were first described by the French physician Joseph H.S. Beau (1806–1865).

12. **Mees' lines** (also called Reynolds or Aldrich lines): transverse white lines distal to the cuticle. They are seen in arsenical or thallium poisoning, cancer chemotherapy, Hodgkin's lymphoma, and other systemic disorders, such as severe cardiac or renal disease. They were first described by the Dutch physician R.A. Mees.

13. **Nail pitting:** an early (but nonspecific) sign of psoriasis.

14. **Yellow nail syndrome:** characterized by a yellowish color of the plates due to abnormal lymphatic circulation.

15. **Brittle nails:** seen in various dysmetabolic states such as hyperthyroidism, malnutrition, and iron or calcium deficiency. They are characterized by irregular, frayed, and torn nail borders.

16. **Splinter hemorrhages:** linear red hemorrhages, extending from the free margin of the nail bed toward the proximal margin. Traditionally considered a typical finding of subacute bacterial endocarditis or trichinosis, they result much more commonly from trauma.

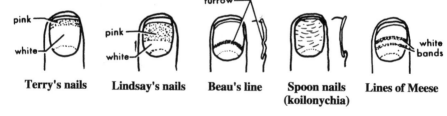

| Terry's nails | Lindsay's nails | Beau's line | Spoon nails (koilonychia) | Lines of Meese |

12. How is the hair assessed?

Hair should be examined region by region, both the scalp and the body, including the pubic region, axillae, and extremities. Attention should be given to the quantity and distribution of hair or its thickness and texture.

13. What is folliculitis?

An infection of the hair follicles. It is most commonly due to staphylococci, but it also may be caused by gram-negative organisms and even fungi. In fact, *Pityrosporon*, the organism responsible for tinea versicolor, can overgrow in the follicles of patients with HIV and cause folliculitis.

14. What is eosinophilic folliculitis?

A folliculitis typical of HIV-infected patients. It is highly pruritic and papular.

15. What tools commonly are used to make a dermatologic diagnosis?

1. **Magnifying glass**

2. **Wood's lamp:** a fluorescent, long-wave, ultraviolet light that has been filtered so that most of the radiation is around 360 nanometers in wavelength. This lamp was developed by

Robert Wood (1868–1955) and is commonly used to identify (1) fungal lesions, (2) areas of hypopigmentation, and (3) porphyrin compounds. Examinations with a Wood's lamp are conducted in a darkened room. Fungal infections (such as tinea capitis) appear as sharply marginated patches of bright blue-green. Areas of hypopigmentation appear much more prominently because of the melanin absorption at 360 nanometers. As a result, a *hypopigmented* patch appears pale white, whereas a *depigmented* patch appears bright white. A Wood's lamp, therefore, can be useful to identify lesions of vitiligo or tinea versicolor. Finally, porphyrin compounds under a Wood's lamp also become more visible by acquiring a coral red fluorescence.

3. **Scalpel:** used to obtain scrapings for the identification of fungi or arthropods, such as scabies.

16. How does one do a potassium hydroxide (KOH) preparation for fungus?

A KOH preparation is carried out by scraping a few scales off the skin and placing them onto a glass slide. Potassium hydroxide (10%) is then poured onto the slide, and a coverslip is applied. After the slide is warmed gently (usually over a match), the preparation is examined under the microscope for fungal elements. Hyphae and spores are easily spotted.

17. What is a Tzanck test?

The Tzanck test commonly is used to diagnose a herpes virus infection. It was pioneered by the Russian dermatologist Arnault Tzanck (1886–1954) and is carried out by unroofing a vesicle with a scalpel and then scraping its base. Scrapings are applied to a microscope slide, fixed with 95% alcohol, and stained with a standard Wright or Giemsa stain. If the test is positive, multinucleated giants cells are visible, confirming that the cause of the lesion is either herpes simplex or varicella zoster virus.

18. What are the different types of skin biopsies? How are they performed?

1. A **shave biopsy** is used primarily for the diagnosis of noninflammatory papular lesions that are not suspicious for melanoma. A shave biopsy usually does not allow examination of the entire lesion, which is essential in melanoma because the depth of the lesion is crucial in determining prognosis. Thus, if melanoma is suspected, the entire lesion must be examined. To perform a shave biopsy, the skin is prepared with alcohol and anesthetized with 1% lidocaine mixed with 1:100,000 epinephrine. A number-15 blade is used to shave off the area in question horizontally. Hemostasis is usually achieved by using aluminum chloride.

2. A **punch biopsy** is used in the diagnosis of suspected inflammatory dermatoses or any other lesion in which a deeper sample of the dermis and epidermis is required. A punch biopsy is performed by preparing the lesion with alcohol, locally anesthetizing it, and using a punch biopsy instrument of 2–6 mm to remove the lesion. Nylon skin sutures are used to close the biopsy site.

3. **Incisional or excisional biopsies** are sometimes used for particular lesions, such as suspected atypical melanocytic lesion.

FLUID-FILLED LESIONS

Clear Fluid (Vesiculobullous Diseases)

Herpes Simplex

19. What are the clinical features of herpes simplex?

The onset of lesions is often preceded by pain or tingling. Lesions begin as small erythematous papules and plaques of uniform size and shape that eventually develop into grouped umbilicated vesicles. They may progress to pustules, ulceration, erosions, and crusting. The most common locations are labial (vermilion border of the lip) and genital areas, although lesions may occur anywhere. Other frequently affected areas include the eye and lumbosacral region.

20. Who develops herpes simplex?

Herpes simplex occurs in all age groups. Certain clinical presentations are age-specific, including herpes stomatitis in children, genital lesions in sexually active young adults, herpes labialis in adults, and lumbosacral herpes in adults over age 40.

21. What is the typical clinical course of herpes simplex?

Primary (initial) outbreaks tend to be more severe with pain, edema, and a prolonged course. **Secondary (recurrent) disease** is less severe and generally shorter in duration. Indeed, the hallmark of herpes simplex infections of mucocutaneous areas is the ability to remain dormant in ganglia and to produce recurrent disease in the area of primary infection. The frequency of recurrences varies, but for genital and labial herpes the average is four episodes per year. Approximately 50% of patients with genital herpes have one or more recurrences, which often result from trauma, menses, and even psychologic stress.

22. What are the other clinical presentations of herpes simplex?

1. **Herpetic gingivostomatitis** affects children and young adults. It is associated with fever, malaise, sore throat, painful vesicles, and erosions on the tongue, palate, gingiva, buccal mucosa, and lips.

2. **Herpetic whitlow** (middle English for *white flaw*; also referred to as a felon) is an occupational hazard of medical and dental professionals as a result of exposure to the virus in a patient's mouth. It is characterized by vesicles and edema of a digit, sometimes associated with erythema, lymphangiitis, and lymphadenopathy of the arm. It may last for several weeks.

3. **Herpes simplex infection in immunosuppressed patients** frequently produces more severe and persistent ulceration as well as disseminated cutaneous and systemic lesions.

23. How is herpes simplex diagnosed?

The clinical appearance of grouped umbilicated vesicles on an erythematous base is classic. A Tzanck preparation (a smear of cells from the base of a lesion stained with Wright or Giemsa stain) demonstrates multinucleated giant cells and is diagnostic. Direct immunofluorescent antibody staining of infected cells is an effective and rapid method of diagnosis. Viral cultures grow herpes simplex virus in several days. Biopsy of lesions demonstrates reticular and ballooning degeneration of the epidermis, multinucleated giant cells, and intranuclear inclusions.

Varicella

24. What are the clinical features of varicella?

The classic lesion of varicella is a 2–3-mm elliptical vesicle surrounded by erythema, commonly described as a "dew drop on a rose petal." The vesicle quickly converts to a pustule, umbilicates, and crusts. The crust falls off in 1–3 weeks, leaving a shallow pink depression that may result in scarring. New vesicles appear in successive crops, resulting in the presence of nonclustered lesions in all stages of development. Initial lesions typically appear on the face and scalp; they spread first to the trunk and then centrifugally. Vesicles on arms and legs tend to appear 2–3 days after the first trunk lesions. Mucous membranes are commonly involved, particularly in the mouth.

25. Who develops varicella?

90% of cases occur in children under the age of 10 years; only 5% of cases present in people over the age of 15.

26. What is the typical clinical course of varicella?

Varicella is highly contagious with a household attack rate of 87%. The average incubation period is 15 days. Patients are contagious 1–2 days before the appearance of the exanthem and until all lesions have crusted. The total time from appearance of lesions to resolution of crusting is 2–4 weeks.

27. What are the other clinical presentations of varicella?

Varicella is more severe in adults than children. Fever and constitutional symptoms are common, and pneumonia occurs in up to 4% of adults. Varicella infection during pregnancy can be transmitted to the fetus and produce developmental abnormalities. The morbidity and mortality of varicella are increased in immunocompromised patients, as demonstrated by a more extensive and persistent rash; hemorrhagic complications may develop.

28. How is varicella diagnosed?

Varicella is usually diagnosed by the classic appearance of the rash. Diagnosis often is supported by a history of recent exposure. Methods of diagnosis are the same as for herpes simplex. A culture of the lesion is necessary to distinguish disseminated herpes simplex from varicella.

Herpes Zoster

29. What are the clinical features of herpes zoster?

The hallmark of herpes zoster (from the Greek *zoster* = girdle) is the clustered pattern of lesions (as opposed to the nonclustered pattern of varicella). The rash is usually preceded by pain and paresthesia in the involved dermatome. Symptoms last for several days and may even continue after resolution of the rash as postherpetic neuralgia. The prodromal pain is followed by the appearance of erythematous plaques, which, in sequence, develop into (1) grouped vesicles, (2) pustules, (3) umbilicated pustules, and (4) crusts. The rash is unilateral, does not cross the midline, and generally appears in one dermatome. The skin areas supplied by the trigeminal nerve and the trunk from T3 to L2 are most commonly affected. However, it is not unusual to have a few vesicles appear outside the affected dermatome.

30. Who develops herpes zoster?

The incidence of zoster increases with age. More than two-thirds of cases occur in people over the age of 50; less than 10% appear in people under the age of 20. When zoster occurs in infants, it usually is associated with a history of maternal varicella infection during gestation. It is more frequent in immunosuppressed patients.

31. What is the typical clinical course of herpes zoster?

The rash generally erupts and progresses to complete crusting over a period of 1 week, then resolves over several weeks. Postherpetic neuralgia (pain persisting after all crusts have fallen off) occurs in 15% of patients and is more common in the older population.

32. What are the other clinical presentations of herpes zoster?

1. **Herpes zoster of the eye** involves the ophthalmic branch; lesions appear on the tip of the nose (representing infection of the nasociliary nerve). An immediate ophthalmologic consultation is required.

2. **Ramsay Hunt syndrome** involves the geniculate ganglion with facial paralysis. Thus, motor paralysis also may occur. Herpetic lesions are found over the external auditory canal or tympanic membrane, with or without tinnitus, vertigo, deafness/hyperacusia, unilateral loss of taste, and decrease in tear formation and salivation. The syndrome was first described by James Ramsay Hunt (1874–1937), a Philadelphia neurologist.

3. **Herpes zoster in immunocompromised patients**, particularly those with AIDS or malignancy (especially Hodgkin's disease or lymphocytic leukemia) and those receiving immunosuppressive therapy, is often more severe and associated with an increased risk of dissemination. Zoster is often the first sign of HIV infection and may develop into a chronic eruption with the usual morphologies.

33. How is herpes zoster diagnosed?

The clinical diagnosis is obvious in the presence of a classic rash with umbilicated vesicles and a dermatomal distribution. Diagnostic techniques are the same as for herpes simplex.

PEMPHIGUS AND PEMPHIGOID

34. What are the diagnostic features of pemphigus and pemphigoid?

Pemphigus and pemphigoid (from Greek *pemphix* = blister) are bullous disorders involving not only the face and body but also the mouth. The major difference is that the bullae in pemphigoid are intact, whereas in pemphigus they often are replaced by large and shallow erosions that heal slowly.

35. What is Nikolsky's sign? What is its significance?

Nikolsky's sign refers to the superficial separation of the skin as a result of shearing stress, such as that applied by the sliding pressure of a finger. It owes its name to Pyotr W. Nikolsky (1858–1940), the Russian dermatologist who taught at Warsaw and Rostov. He first described this phenomenon in 1896. A positive Nikolsky's sign is due to the poor adhesion of the cells of the epidermis (acantholysis). It is seen in bullous diseases such as pemphigus, but not usually in pemphigoid, in which the split in the epidermis is much deeper.

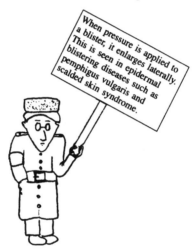

Nikolsky and his sign.

Pustules

Acne

36. What are the clinical features of acne?

The hallmark of acne (from the Greek *akme* = blooming) is the characteristic variety of lesions, both inflammatory and noninflammatory, that literally blossom on the patient's trunk and face. Noninflammatory lesions include closed comedones (whiteheads) and open comedones (blackheads). *Comedo* is the Latin word for glutton. Indeed, a comedo is a big clump of sebum and keratin collected around a hair follicle. Closed comedones are pale and dome-shaped papules, 1–2 mm in diameter. Open comedones are 1–2-mm papules with a central keratinous black plug closing the orifice of a sebaceous follicle. When a comedone opens, its content is exposed to air; an oxidizing reaction makes it black. Inflammatory lesions are papules and pustules of variable size as well as cysts (suppurative nodular lesions). Cystic lesions are more likely to result in scarring if not treated. Scarring may be pitted or hypertrophic and papular. Common sites of involvement include the face and less frequently the chest, shoulders, and back.

37. Who develops acne?

Usually teenagers. The onset of acne in fact is at puberty. Girls may experience their first lesions (usually comedones) 1 year or more before menarche, although women in their third or fourth decade may still suffer from eruptions. Men tend to have more severe involvement.

38. What is the typical clinical course of acne?

After onset in the teens, acne generally persists for several years, then remits spontaneously. However, a significant number of patients have disease well into the third or fourth decade. Women may have persistent flares associated with menses.

39. What are the other clinical presentations of acne?

1. **Acne rosacea** occurs in middle-aged and older people. It is characterized by erythema and telangiectasias over cheeks and nose, with overlying papules and pustules. Rhinophyma also may be present in extreme cases, more commonly in men.

2. **Steroid acne** may begin as early as 2 weeks after administration of systemic corticosteroids. Lesions are monomorphous, generally pustules and dome-shaped papules over the trunk, shoulders, and upper arms.

40. How is acne diagnosed?

The diagnosis is clinical, based on finding a mixture of lesion types in the appropriate location.

SOLID LESIONS

Tan or Pink Papules and Nodules

Warts (Keratotic or Rough-surfaced)

41. What are the major types of warts?

1. **Common wart:** a rough-surfaced, circumscribed papule most commonly located on the trunk and extremities. Often present are the so-called black seeds, which represent thrombosed blood vessels.

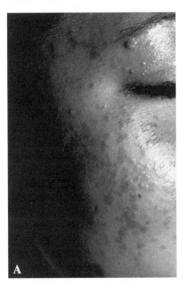

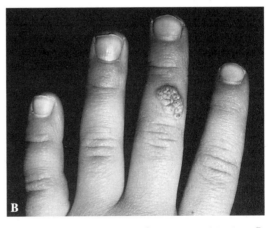

Some common types of warts. *A,* Flat warts of the face. *B,* Wart of the hand. (From Fitzpatrick JE, Aeling JL: Dermatology Secrets. Philadelphia, Hanley & Belfus, 1996, with permission.)

2. **Condyloma:** a genital wart, usually located on the anus, vulva, or glans. It most commonly presents as a flat-topped papule with an irregular surface. Condylomata may be pink at first but turn tan or brown over time.

3. **Plantar wart:** typically found on the sole or dorsum of the foot or even on the toes. It is often callused but may appear as a white, irregularly surfaced area with or without black dots.

42. How are warts treated?

Because no one treatment is universally effective, there is a large variety of treatment modalities.

1. Initial treatment is often either **cryosurgery** with liquid nitrogen or **topical therapy** with various combinations of salicylic or lactic acids, which may be applied as a plaster or liquid.

2. The next level of treatment includes **electrodesiccation and curettage**.

3. When the first and second modalities fail, patients may be referred for **laser therapy** for excision or vaporization with the continuous wave carbon dioxide laser or for yellow pulsed dye laser, which thromboses blood vessels and also acts by heating the wart.

4. Patients may undergo **immunotherapy**, which involves sensitizing them to a particular compound and then painting it on the warts in the hope that the immune system will see the warts as foreign and attack them. Immunotherapy also may consist of injections of alpha interferon, which is approved for use in genital warts as well as common warts.

5. Last but not least, a small amount of **diluted bleomycin** may be injected repeatedly into the wart. This modality must be used with care, especially on the distal extremities, because of the risk of local circulatory compromise.

Other reportedly successful treatments include making an appointment for a painful treatment, applying a raw potato, and various homemade brews. These modalities are not reimbursable under most insurance plans.

Basal Cell Carcinoma (Nonkeratotic or Smooth-surfaced)

43. What are the major clinical features of basal cell carcinoma?

Basal cell carcinoma (BCC) typically presents as a papule that is pink, pearly, and smooth. It is accompanied by telangiectasias (dilated small blood vessels); has a rolled, translucent border; and is located on sun-exposed areas of the face and ears.

44. What are the other major morphologic types of BCC?

1. Morpheiform (scarlike)
2. Cystic
3. Superficial

45. What is the usual clinical course of BCC?

BCC is a benign-behaving skin cancer; it used to be called basal cell epithelium because of its relatively tranquil behavior. If left untouched, it continues to grow locally (with the potential of becoming highly destructive) but rarely metastasizes.

46. What treatments are available for BCC?

1. **Electrodesiccation and curettage** (for primary, small, well-localized lesions)
2. **Excision**
3. **Radiation therapy** initially causes erythema, but it eventually fades. Over many years some telangiectasia or atrophy may develop. Treatment is usually fractionated into 20–30 sessions to avoid unwanted skin changes.
4. **Cryotherapy** is carried out with cryoprobes only on small, well-localized lesions and only in selected areas.
5. **Mohs microscopically controlled surgery** is a staged technique using horizontally cut frozen sections. It has the highest cure rates and conserves normal tissue as much as possible. It is used in cosmetically or functionally important areas and also for lesions that are poorly defined, large, recurrent, or located on mucous membranes.

Squamous Cell Carcinoma (Keratotic or Rough-surfaced)

47. What is an actinic keratosis?

Actinic keratosis (literally "sun-induced"; *aktis* = ray in Greek) is a pink and scaly macule or papule induced by protracted sun exposure. It typically is located over exposed surfaces, such as face, bald scalp, hands, and arms. It represents a partial-thickness atypia of the epidermis and, if left alone, may degenerate into squamous cell carcinoma (SCC). It is treated most frequently by cryotherapy with liquid nitrogen. If a large number of lesions are present, however, topical 5-flu-orouracil or one of the pulsed carbon dioxide lasers also may be used.

48. What is Bowen's disease?

Bowen's disease, or full-thickness atypia of the epidermis, is considered equivalent to SCC in situ. Clinically, Bowen's disease presents as erythematous, scaly, relatively flat plaques ranging in diameter from 2–6 cm. Lesions originate on sun- and non–sun-exposed skin. Bowen's disease was first described by John T. Bowen (1857–1941), professor of dermatology at Harvard, shy lecturer, and reclusive bachelor.

49. What is the typical appearance of SCC?

Although SCC has a myriad of morphologic variants, it is classically described as a scaly plaque, often with ulceration and lacking a defined translucent border. SCC is often found in sun-exposed areas of the face, ears, arms, and hands and in a background of actinic keratosis.

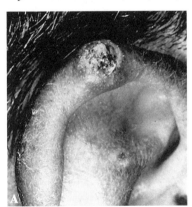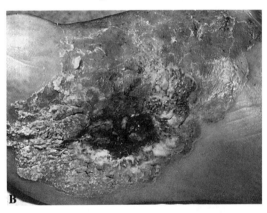

A, Squamous cell carcinoma of the ear, demonstrating a nodule with central scale and crust. *B,* Large verrucous carcinoma of the sole of the foot. Verrucous carcinomas often reach large sizes before diagnosis because they are often treated as warts. (From Fitzpatrick JE, Aeling JL: Dermatology Secrets. Philadelphia, Hanley & Belfus, 1996, with permission.)

50. Where in the skin does SCC arise?

SCC arises in the epidermis of the skin above the basal layer from cells called keratinocytes.

51. Describe the evolution of SCC. Why is it important?

SCC originates in sun-exposed areas when a number of cells become atypical. At this early stage the lesion appears as a flat, scaly, pink macule and is usually called an actinic keratosis (see above). The lesion is precancerous but may not evolve into SCC. As the atypical cells fill the entire epidermis but do not breach the basal layer, the lesions become SCC in situ (Bowen's disease). The next and final step is progression to invasive SCC, in which the atypical cells penetrate below the basement membrane and into the dermis.

52. What is the course of SCC?

When it arises in actinically damaged skin, SCC rarely metastasizes. Risk factors for spread include depth of invasion, degree of cellular differentiation, and origin in a mucous membrane.

53. How is SCC treated?

Treatment modality depends on the severity and location of the SCC. **SCC in situ**, especially when not on the face, is often treated by electrodesiccation and curettage. On the face the same lesion often is treated with Mohs microscopically controlled surgery or excision. **Invasive SCC** is treated with scalpel removal, including excision and Mohs microscopically controlled surgery. If the lesion is at high risk for metastasis, scalpel removal often is followed by local irradiation.

White Lesions

Vitiligo

54. How does vitiligo present?

Vitiligo presents as milky white, nonscaly macules and patches of variable size with sharp borders. They often are symmetrically located, commonly involving the periorificial areas (eyes, nose, ears, mouth, and anus), elbows, knees, dorsal hands and feet, and axillae. Mucosal surfaces also may be involved; the extent of involvement varies greatly. Lesions also may appear at sites of injury, a phenomenon known as koebnerization (see below). Hair growing in areas of vitiligo may be white. Other associated cutaneous findings include prematurely gray hair, piebaldism (from old English = *spotted*, a reference to the congenital appearance of a white patch of hair that remains stable in size over the years), halo nevi, alopecia areata, and ocular abnormalities, including chorioretinitis, retinal pigmentary abnormalities, and iritis.

55. Who develops vitiligo?

Vitiligo can occur at any age but most commonly begins in the first two decades of life. It is considered an autoimmune phenomenon, a mechanism corroborated by its association with other autoimmune diseases (see below). People with darker skin types are affected more prevalently, but they also may be more apt to seek treatment because of the greater cosmetic impact. The male-to-female ratio is equal. A genetic component also is involved; 30% of patients report another family member affected by the disease. Vitiligo affects 1–2% of the population in the United States.

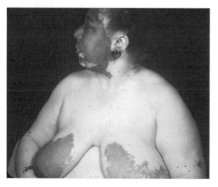

Extensive vitiligo in a black woman. (From Fitzpatrick JE, Aeling JL: Dermatology Secrets. Philadelphia, Hanley & Belfus, 1996, with permission.)

56. What is the typical clinical course of vitiligo?

The natural course is unpredictable but generally is characterized by slow progression, which may be interrupted by periods of stability. Spontaneous repigmentation also may occur but generally is incomplete.

57. What are the other clinical presentations of vitiligo?

1. **Segmental vitiligo** is characterized by unilateral depigmented macules and patches in a dermatomal or quasi-dermatomal distribution. It generally has a stable course.

2. **Focal vitiligo** presents as one or more depigmented macules in an area that is single but not segmental.

3. **Universal vitiligo** results in total or nearly total body involvement.

58. How is vitiligo diagnosed?

The diagnosis generally is clinical. In patients with fair skin the lack of contrast between normal and diseased areas may make the identification of vitiligo lesions more difficult; use of the Wood's lamp may be necessary. A biopsy may be helpful by demonstrating absence of melanocytes, but the presence of melanocytes does not eliminate the diagnosis.

59. Are any systemic diseases associated with vitiligo?

Yes. In fact, at least 10% of all patients with vitiligo may have serologic or clinical evidence of associated autoimmune disorders. The most common are autoimmune thyroid diseases, particularly hypothyroidism of the Hashimoto variety (especially in females). Diabetes mellitus, Addison's disease, pernicious anemia, alopecia areata, and uveitis (Vogt-Koyanagi's syndrome) also may occur with increased frequency. A careful history and appropriate screening tests to rule out associated diseases are therefore recommended, but treatment of concomitant diseases does not influence the course of vitiligo.

Brown Lesions

60. List and describe the different types of common nevi (moles).

Melanocytic nevi are classified according to histology:

1. A **junctional nevus** is usually a macule or slightly raised papule with well-circumscribed borders and homogeneous brown pigment. Cells are located at the dermoepidermal junction.

2. A **compound nevus** is a raised papule, often brown or tan with even pigmentation and border. Cells are located at the dermoepidermal junction and upper dermis.

3. A **dermal nevus** is a dome-shaped, pedunculated, or warty-surfaced papule, brown, pink, or flesh in color; cells are located primarily in the dermis.

61. Describe an atypical nevus.

An atypical nevus is usually larger than 6 mm and has an irregular border with variegated color, usually shades of dark brown to light tan.

62. What is the difference between an atypical nevus and a dysplastic nevus?

This terminology has been the subject of much controversy. Several years ago a National Institutes of Health consensus conference recommended replacement of the term *dysplastic nevus* with the term *atypical nevus*. Familial atypical melanocytic nevus syndrome describes members of families who have multiple dysplastic nevi and an increased chance of developing melanoma. The exact incidence is still to be determined. Atypical nevi have been estimated to occur in at least 2–6% of the population. Their significance is unknown.

63. Describe the morphology and significance of seborrheic keratoses.

Seborrheic keratoses are well-circumscribed, rough-surfaced, flat-topped, brown papules. They are sharply marginated, 5–20 mm in diameter, and most commonly located on the trunk or face, although they may appear anywhere. They are benign lesions that appear at mid-life and increase with aging (senile verruca or senile warts). On the face of African-Americans, lesions may be multiple and are called dermatosis papulosis nigrans.

64. What is the sign of Leser-Trélat?

It is the hallmark of an important paraneoplastic syndrome, usually related to the presence of an internal malignancy (commonly of the gastrointestinal tract). The sign of Leser-Trélat consists of the explosive blooming of hundreds and hundreds of seborrheic keratoses on the chest, back, or face. The sign was first described by two surgeons, the German Edmund Leser (1828–1916) and the French Ulysse Trélat (1828–1890).

65. What is solar lentigo?

Solar lentigo is a sun-induced, well-circumscribed, light brown or tan macule that persists even when a tan or sunburn fades. It usually is located over the sun-exposed areas of the face, hands, and shoulders, where it may range in diameter between 5–20 mm. A solar lentigo usually has no potential for neoplastic degeneration, but a lentigo with black, pinhead-sized speckles (**lentigo maligna**) may degenerate over the years into **lentigo maligna melanoma**. Thus, lentigo maligna is an important precancerous lesion and should be recognized. It often is called Hutchinson's freckle from the English surgeon who first described it (the same surgeon who described Hutchinson's triad of congenital syphilis).

66. What is a freckle?

A freckle is a sun-induced brown lesion that resembles a solar lentigo except that (1) it appears early in life (lentigines do not occur until mid-adulthood); (2) it usually is smaller (only 1–2 mm in diameter); and (3) it may disappear with time. It has no malignant potential. Clustered freckles, however, especially over the lips and fingertips, should raise the possibility of Peutz-Jeghers syndrome.

67. What are the morphologic warning signs of melanoma?

A commonly used mnemonic for the warning signs of melanoma is the ABCD checklist:

A = **A**symmetry (if the lesion is bisected, one-half should not be identical to the other half)
B = **B**order irregularity (a border that is uneven or ragged as opposed to smooth and straight)
C = **C**olor variegation (more than one shade of pigment)
D = **D**iameter increase (defined as a diameter greater than 6 mm)

A suggested addition to this list is a final **E** for **E**levation above the skin surface. But because elevation is also a feature of many benign nevi, E is often excluded.

68. How good is the ABCD(E) checklist?

Two studies have assessed its diagnostic accuracy. In one study the checklist was considered positive if the lesion had one or more of the five features. In this case, the sensitivity was 92%. Another study evaluated the accuracy of using only the BCD features of the checklist. In this retrospective analysis, the checklist had a sensitivity of 100% and a specificity of 98%. In another study, the requirement of a diameter greater than 6 mm lowered the sensitivity of the checklist considerably.

69. What other criteria are used to diagnose melanoma?

The British have proposed a different checklist based on four major and three minor criteria. The three major criteria are historical: (1) change in size; (2) change in shape; and (3) change in color of a lesion. The four minor criteria are primarily physical and tend to be late signs: (1) inflammation, (2) crusting or bleeding, (3) sensory change, and (4) diameter ≥ 7 mm. A scoring system assigns 2 points for each of the major criteria and 1 point for each of the minor criteria. Any patient with at least one major criterion should be referred to a dermatologist. Similarly, any patient with a score of 3 points or more should be referred for evaluation.

70. How good is the 7-point checklist?

Several studies have found a sensitivity of 79–100% and a specificity of 30–37%.

Pearl. *The ABCD checklist (particularly when positivity does not require the presence of all four features) and the 7-point checklist appear to be sensitive tools that lack specificity.*

71. What are the major morphologic types of melanoma?

1. **Lentigo maligna**, which is considered a precursor to melanoma (see above), is a flat and hyperpigmented area with variegated pigment and irregular border. It appears most commonly on sun-exposed areas (especially head and neck) of people in their 50s and 60s. Estimates of the incidence of transformation into melanoma range between 5% and 30%. The growth pattern is radial rather than vertical.

2. **Lentigo maligna melanoma** is the rarest form of melanoma. It appears almost exclusively on the face and neck of people in their 60s and 70s. It is usually quite large, easily over 3 cm in diameter. Pigment and color are more varied than in lentigo maligna.

3. **Superficial spreading melanoma** is the most common form of melanoma, accounting for over 70% of cases. Its usual locations are the back of men, the legs of women, and the trunk of both sexes. It is the type of melanoma that is most frequently found close to existing nevi.

4. **Nodular melanoma** is typically papular with no macular portions. Its color is usually black or bluish-black. The lesion originates at the dermoepidermal junction and grows into the dermis (less commonly into the epidermis as well). It is characterized by vertical growth with little radial extension.

5. **Acrolentiginous melanoma** is the most common form of melanoma on palms, soles, and digits. It resembles somewhat lentigo maligna melanoma, presenting as one or more dark papules against a pigmented and unevenly speckled background.

72. What are the major prognostic characteristics of stage I melanoma?

The best prognosis is in young women with lesions on the extremity rather than the trunk or head. The histologic level of the lesion is also of paramount importance: the thinner and higher in the skin, the better the prognosis. Lesions < 0.75 mm have a 5-year survival rate greater than 98%. Lesions over 4 mm in thickness have survival rate less than 50%. Overall, lesions greater than 1.0 mm in thickness carry a worse prognosis. Other factors associated with a worse prognosis are vertical growth phase, high mitotic rate, ulceration and decreased lymphoid infiltrates, involvement of blood vessels, and presence of microscopic satellites.

73. What are the characteristic signs of sun damage?

1. **Lentigines** (from the Latin *lentigo* = lentil) are brown macules resembling freckles except that the border is usually regular and microscopic proliferation of the rete ridges is present. Scattered solitary nevus cells are seen in the basal cell layer.

2. **Freckles** (from the old English *freken* = ephelis) are yellowish or brownish macules that develop on the exposed parts of the skin, especially in people of light complexion (typically with red or blonde hair). Lesions increase in number on exposure to the sun. The epidermis is microscopically normal except for increased melanin.

3. **Rhytides** (Greek for wrinkles) are the familiar wrinkles of the skin that are so common in sun-exposed people such as farmers, fishermen, and ski instructors who do not believe in sunscreen.

4. **Hyperpigmentation or hypopigmentation** (including localized areas of hyperpigmentation, such as the solar lentigo; see above).

5. Evidence of **sun-induced cellular atypia** such as actinic keratoses, basal cell carcinoma, or squamous cell carcinoma.

Of course, the risk of developing melanoma should be included among the effects of sun damage. Melanomas recently have become almost epidemic. In 1930, for example, the lifetime risk of a person in the United States developing melanoma was 1 in 1500. In 1996 this risk was 1 in 87, and the projected risk for the year 2000 is 1 in 75. Moreover, 6 of 7 deaths due to skin cancer are due to melanoma, and melanomas are the most common malignancy reported in white people between the age of 25 and 29. The median age of onset for a superficial spreading melanoma (the most common type of melanoma) is quite low: 44 years.

Pearl. *Early detection is imperative to curb the potential for metastasis and death. The importance of the physical examination is clear and incontrovertible.*

Yellow Lesions

74. What are the most common yellow lesions of the skin?
1. **Xanthomas:** smooth-surfaced yellow papules and nodules of various sizes, typically found in patients with hyperlipidemia. They usually are located around tendons and over joints but also may be found on the palms.

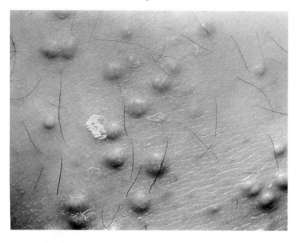

Eruptive xanthomas. Typical yellow-brown papules. White material was applied by the patient to remove these "warts." (From Fitzpatrick JE, Aeling JL: Dermatology Secrets. Philadelphia, Hanley & Belfus, 1996, with permission.)

2. **Xanthelasmas:** soft, sharply marginated papules and plaques, usually flat-topped and of various sizes. Typically they are confined to the eyelids. Around 40% of patients with xanthelasmas have hyperlipidemia.
3. **Necrobiosis lipoidica diabeticorum:** yellow and asymptomatic plaques 2–10 cm in diameter, located over the anterior shins of patients with diabetes. The borders of the plaques may acquire a violaceous hue due to atrophy of the skin that makes the underlying veins visible. The cause of such lesions is unknown, although they are believed to originate from diabetic microangiopathy.

Drug Reactions

75. How does one differentiate between staphylococcal scaled skin syndrome (SSSS) and toxic epidermal necrolysis (TEN)?
TEN is characterized by a deeper split in the epidermis (i.e., at the dermoepidermal junction). The split in SSSS is higher, just inferior to the stratum corneum (the uppermost layer of the epidermis). Frozen section is usually used to differentiate the lesions. Clinically the lesions of SSSS are more superficial and heal more quickly. SSSS, which is induced by a staphylococcal toxin, commonly is treated with antibiotics. TEN, on the other hand, often is treated in burn units because of the extensive sloughing of skin. TEN may be fatal in as many as 50% of cases.

76. What is the difference between Stevens-Johnson syndrome (erythema multiforme major) and TEN?
Although many consider them to be separate entities, controversy still exists as to whether they represent two extremes along a spectrum of the same disease.
Stevens-Johnson syndrome (SJS; described by the American pediatricians Albert Stevens and Frank Johnson) is characterized not only by skin lesions but also by vesicles and bullae typically located on the mucosae of eyes, mouth, and genitalia. The location on the mucous membranes upgrades the disease from simple erythema multiforme (in which the lesions are papules involving usually the skin of the trunk but also palms and soles) to bullous (or major) erythema

multiforme. Involvement of the mucous membranes is diagnostic of SJS. On glabrous skin, SJS also may present with target lesions (characterized by three concentric rings) or purpuric patches.

TEN is characterized by a much more extensive blister formation. The bullous lesions of the trunk become confluent; as a result, sheets of skin may lift off as in a severe thermal burn. TEN also is called toxic epidermal necrolysis of the Lyell type (from the British dermatologist who first described it) to distinguish it from toxic epidermal necrolysis of the Ritter type (from the Austrian dermatologist who described it in 1878), which is another name for SSSS. TEN is lymphocyte-mediated cutaneous destruction, with full-thickness loss of the skin. Thus, it is extremely painful. It also carries a high risk for sepsis, which is usually the cause of death. Other systems also may be involved, such as eyes, lungs, gastrointestinal tract, and kidneys. TEN represents the worst imaginable skin disease. Prompt referral to a burn center is key to survival. In fact, referral in less than 7 days after onset has a mortality rate of 4%, whereas referral beyond 7 days has a mortality rate of 83%.

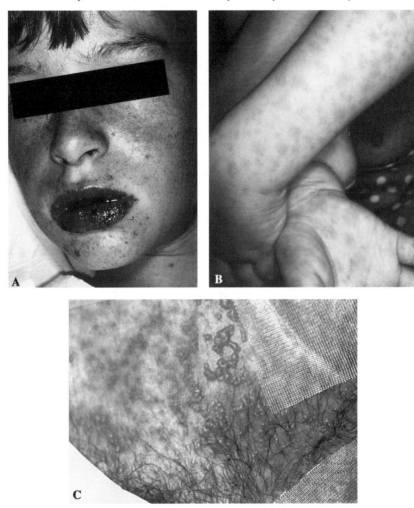

A, Stevens-Johnson syndrome. Typical mucosal inflammation of the mouth, lips, and conjunctiva. *B,* Erythema multiforme or Stevens-Johnson syndrome. The eruption consists of annular and papular erythema over the acral areas. *C,* Toxic epidermal necrolysis. The patient demonstrates the typical "telangiectatic" blanching erythema and blistering that progress to denuding of the epidermis. (From Fitzpatrick JE, Aeling JL: Dermatology Secrets. Philadelphia, Hanley & Belfus, 1996, with permission.)

77. What drugs are most commonly responsible for TEN?

The usual suspects: sulfonamides, phenytoin and other anticonvulsants, penicillins, and non-steroidals.

78. What are the major cutaneous manifestations of drug reactions?
1. Urticaria (hives)
2. Morbilliform rash
3. Phototoxic reaction
4. Erythema nodosum (panniculitis most commonly in the pretibial areas)
5. Pigmentary changes
6. Fixed drug eruptions
7. Vasculitis
8. Bullous drug eruptions
9. Lichenoid drug eruptions
10. Nail changes such as onycholysis

Urticaria (Flat-topped Vascular Reactions)

79. What are the clinical features of urticaria?

The characteristic lesion is the wheal, an elevated, pink, annular or polycyclic plaque usually surrounded by a halo and associated with pruritus. Size varies from several millimeters to 10 cm. The trunk, buttocks, and chest are involved most frequently, but urticaria may occur anywhere. Lesions are transient, lasting from minutes to hours. Swelling in subcutaneous tissue is termed angioedema. It occurs in the distensible tissue of the eyelids, lips, and oral mucosal membranes (including tongue). It may result in respiratory distress.

80. Who develops urticaria?

Urticaria occurs in all ages and in both sexes.

81. What is the clinical course of urticaria?

1. By definition, **acute urticaria** resolves in 4–6 weeks. It usually is associated with a drug (penicillin, sulfonamides, aspirin), food allergens (e.g., chocolate, shellfish, nuts, peanut butter, tomatoes, strawberries), or infections (upper respiratory infection, especially streptococcal in children).

2. **Chronic urticaria** persists for more than 6 weeks and may last for years. One-half of patients are free of lesions in 1 year, but 20% have persistent lesions for more than 20 years. The cause remains undetermined in 80% of patients, but possibilities include the causes of acute urticaria as well as cryoglobulins, food additives, viruses (hepatitis B), parasites, inhalants, and neoplasms.

82. What are the other clinical presentations of urticaria?

1. **Hereditary angioedema** is transmitted in an autosomal dominant pattern, appears in the second to fourth decade of life, and is associated with sudden attacks of angioedema that last for days. It is often life threatening. Hereditary angioedema results from a low or nonfunctional C1 inhibitor. The diagnosis is suggested by a low C4 level.

2. **Physical urticarias** appear in response to a stimulus such as cold, sunlight, or trauma:
- Dermatographism (urticaria at site of skin stroking)
- Pressure urticaria (severe swelling with deep pain several hours after localized pressure is applied, most commonly on the feet and buttocks)
- Aquagenic urticaria (urticaria elicited by water)
- Cold urticaria (urticaria appearing on rewarming of skin exposed to cold, most commonly on the hands and feet)
- Solar urticaria (urticaria on unshielded skin after exposure to sunlight)
- Cholinergic urticaria (highly pruritic, 1–3-mm wheals located on the face and trunk and induced by exercise and emotional stress)

83. How is urticaria diagnosed?

By viewing classic lesions and obtaining a history of their fleeting nature. After obtaining a thorough history with special focus on medicine intake, food exposure, recent illness, and physical stimuli associated with lesion onset, work-up for underlying causes should be delayed until the problem becomes chronic. A work-up then may include a complete physical exam, complete blood count and differential, biochemistry screen, urinalysis, hepatitis B surface antigen, sinus films, oral examination, stool specimens for ova and parasites, and an elimination diet. A biopsy is indicated if the duration of an individual lesion is prolonged (> 24 hr) to rule out urticarial vasculitis.

Red Lesions (Scaling)

Psoriasis (Papulosquamous Disease with Prominent Plaque Formation)

84. What are the clinical features of psoriasis?

Classic psoriasis vulgaris (from the Greek *psoriasis* = itch) presents as sharply demarcated erythematous papules and plaques of widely varying size with a white overlying scale. Removal of the scale results in tiny bleeding droplets (Auspitz sign). Associated pitting and dystrophy of the nails are quite common. Areas of predilection include the elbows, knees, scalp, genitals, and lumbar region, but any area may be involved. The extensor surfaces of the extremities are a typically preferred site. The degree of involvement, however, is variable.

Newly developed lesions tend to be small (1–3 mm) but easily coalesce, resulting in large plaques often with a gyrate pattern. Psoriasis, lichen planus, vitiligo, and warts are the only skin diseases characterized by Koebner's phenomenon, in which lesions are lined up along a site of cutaneous trauma, such as scratching. The phenomenon was first described by the German dermatologist Heinrich Koebner (1838–1904), a fellow with a unique penchant for melodrama. Koebner was famous for self-inoculating with various kinds of skin infections from his patients. He then exposed parts of his anatomy to demonstrate typical skin lesions during his lectures. This approach, of course, preceded invention of the auditorium projector and Kodachrome slides and is no longer required of academicians.

85. Who develops psoriasis?

Psoriasis may appear at any time in life. The peak incidence of onset is in the third decade; a smaller group of patients develop disease in the sixth decade. There is a strong as yet undefined genetic influence, particularly in patients with earlier age of onset. Sex ratios are equal. One to two percent of the United States population is affected.

86. What is the typical clinical course of psoriasis?

Psoriasis is usually a lifelong disease. Spontaneous remissions occur with varying and unpredictable frequency. Patients also may move from one clinical form to another.

87. What are the other clinical presentations of psoriasis?

Psoriasis is a heterogeneous disorder with a spectrum of clinical variants:

1. **Intertriginous psoriasis** involves the axillae, inframammary, inguinal, and perianal regions. It usually lacks scales as a result of maceration.

2. **Guttate psoriasis** is characterized by the sudden explosion of hundreds of small, erythematous, and nonconfluent papules that are widely distributed and not very scaly. Guttate psoriasis often occurs in young adults and children and may be triggered by a streptococcal infection.

3. **Erythrodermic psoriasis** presents as total body erythema with scaling. It also may be associated with hypothermia and congestive heart failure.

4. **Pustular psoriasis** is the most serious form, presenting with severe erythema and overlying pustules, fever, and leukocytosis. It is a generalized and systemic form (Von Zumbusch type) associated with fever, anemia, and leukocytosis. A more localized form of pustular psoriasis, however, involves primarily the palms and soles and has no systemic symptoms (Barber type).

88. How is psoriasis diagnosed?

Clinical appearance is usually sufficient for diagnosis. Distribution (scalp, elbows, knees, and gluteal folds), Koebner phenomenon, and nail pitting are classic clues. A skin biopsy may be performed when the diagnosis is in doubt and classically shows acanthosis, parakeratosis, neutrophils in the stratum corneum, and a lymphohistiocytic infiltrate in the papillary dermis.

89. What other disease is associated with psoriasis?

Five to 8% of patients with psoriasis have psoriatic arthritis. When the arthritis appears before the psoriasis, it is important to do a complete cutaneous exam, looking at nails for characteristic changes and the scalp and genital region for hidden plaques.

Dermatophytes (Papulosquamous Disease with Prominent Plaque Formation)

90. What are dermatophytoses?

Dermatophytoses (from the Greek *dermato* = skin and *phyton* = plant) are fungal infections of the skin, hair, and/or nails. Their hallmark is to attack keratinized tissues.

91. What are the clinical features of dermatophyte infections?

Lesion morphology includes papules, scaly plaques, maceration, vesicles, and bullae. The clinical presentation and the specific name applied to the individual infection depend on the area of the body involved. The most common are listed below.

DISEASE	LOCATION	CLINICAL PRESENTATION
Tinea corporis (ringworm)	Body	Circular lesions with central clearing and elevated, erythematous, and at times vesicular border.
Tinea faciale	Face	Red scaly plaques sometimes lacking central clearing and elevated border.
Tinea cruris (jock itch)	Groin	Plaques with papular scaly border and central clearing involving inguinal fold and adjacent skin but usually sparing scrotum.
Tinea pedis (athlete's feet)	Feet	Interdigital spaces (most commonly 3 and 4) with scaling, erythema, and maceration. Scaling and hyperkeratosis may extend to instep of foot. Variations include bilateral moccasin distribution with scaling over soles or vesicopustules on instep.
Onychomycosis	Nail	Yellow-brown discoloration of nail plate associated with subungual hyperkeratosis.
Tinea manus	Hand	Annular plaque on dorsum of hand; hyperkeratosis of palms.
Tinea capitis	Scalp	Areas of alopecia and scaling with broken hairs. Kerion, an inflammatory variant, produces tender nodules with purulent drainage and may result in scarring.

92. Who develops dermatophyte infections?

Tinea corporis occurs in any age group. Tinea faciale is more common in children, and tinea capitis occurs primarily in children. Tinea cruris is more common in males and first appears in adolescence. Tinea pedis is frequent in adults (10% of the population), particularly those who use communal showers or pools. Onychomycosis (fungal infection of the nail) also affects adults, and the incidence increases with advancing age.

93. What is the typical clinical course of dermatophyte infections?

The clinical course depends on the area involved. Tinea corporis and tinea faciale resolve with antifungal therapy (topical for localized disease and oral for widespread disease). Tinea cruris responds to topical antifungal therapy but may recur, particularly in warm environments. Oral antifungal therapy is necessary to cure tinea capitis. Tinea pedis, particularly the moccasin type, is difficult to eradicate; it frequently recurs and sometimes is chronic. Onychomycosis is a chronic problem, and treatment failure has been the rule. However, with the advent of more effective oral antifungal agents (fluconazole and itraconazole), cure is now possible in many cases.

94. How are dermatophyte infections diagnosed?

The diagnosis may be established rapidly by microscopic examination with potassium hydroxide (KOH) of scrapings from cutaneous lesions or clippings from nails that reveal hyphae or examination of hairs from scalp infection that demonstrate spores involving the hair shaft. If the KOH examination is negative, a culture should be planted on Sabouraud's dextrose agar with an antibiotic. Four weeks' incubation at room temperature is required.

Pityriasis Rosea (Predominantly Papular Papulosquamous Disease)

95. What are the clinical features of pityriasis rosea?

Pityriasis rosea (from the Greek *pityron* = bran, dandruff) is a dermatosis marked by branny desquamation. It begins with a herald patch in at least one-half of all cases. The herald patch is an oval or round lesion, 2–3 cm in size, with a peripheral collarette of scale. It is usually located on the trunk. Because of its annular shape, the lesion may be mistaken for tinea corporis. Thus, a KOH preparation is necessary to separate the two processes. The herald patch is followed in 1–2 weeks (average: 7–10 days) by a diffuse eruption on the trunk, neck, and inner aspects of proximal extremities. During this eruption (which usually lasts for 2 weeks) 50–100 isolated, nonconfluent papules may appear. These lesions are similar in morphology to the herald patch (oval or football-shaped) with much less (if any) scaling. Lesions typically are distributed with the long axis along the lines of cleavage of the skin parallel to rib lines, forming a Christmas-tree pattern. Most patients are asymptomatic, but a few complain of severe itching.

96. Who develops pityriasis rosea?

The incidence of the disease is equal in both sexes and generally affects children and young adults; it is seen almost exclusively between 10 and 35 years of age.

97. What is the typical clinical course of pityriasis rosea?

The rash generally resolves without sequelae. The average duration of the eruption is 6 weeks, but it may vary from 2–10 weeks. Recurrence of the eruption is unlikely (5% of patients). In darker-skinned people, residual postinflammatory hyperpigmentation may remain after resolution of active lesions. The disease is noncontagious and of unknown etiology.

98. What are the other clinical presentations of pityriasis rosea?

Localized forms commonly affect the axillae and groin. The following variations in lesion morphology more frequently occur in children:
- Vesicular pityriasis rosea (may involve palms and soles)
- Urticarial pityriasis rosea
- Purpuric pityriasis rosea
- Facial involvement

99. How is pityriasis rosea diagnosed?

The diagnosis is made by clinical observation of the characteristics of the eruption:
1. Distribution of lesions (trunk and proximal extremities but not lower extremities)
2. Oval shape
3. Lesions parallel to the rib lines (Christmas-tree pattern)
4. Herald patch

The biopsy is nondiagnostic. Serology is recommended to rule out secondary syphilis.

Lichen Planus (Nonscaling)

100. What are the diagnostic features of lichen planus?

The typical lesions of lichen planus are summarized by five Ps: planar, purple, polygonal, pruritic, and papular. Basically, lichen planus lesions are shiny, flat-topped, violaceous, and pruritic papules that are 2–4 mm in diameter and located on the trunk (especially sacral areas), extremities (tibial areas and wrists), and penis. Over the extremities the lesions are found most commonly on flexor surfaces. Lesions generally occur in clusters, often with either an annular configuration or coalescence in small plaques that are 1–2 cm in diameter. They are called lichen planus because they are discrete and flat (*planus* in Latin) papules or aggregates of papules arranged in a configuration resembling lichens growing on rocks. Morphology, however, is highly variable. Bullous, verrucoid, and mucosal lesions are among the many variations. The white streaks on the buccal mucosa are termed Wickham's striae from the French dermatologist, Louis Wickham (1860–1913), who first described them. Remember that lichen planus is one of the few skin diseases characterized by Koebner's phenomenon.

101. Who gets lichen planus?

Usually men and women in their 40s. Approximately 10% of patients have a positive family history, suggesting some genetic predisposition. Lichen planus often is associated with hepatitis B or C and occasionally may occur as a drug reaction.

102. What is the course of lichen planus?

In most cases, it resolves with treatment within 1 year. It may recur, however. Some cases are resistant to treatment and may persist for years.

Atopic Dermatitis (Eczematous Disease)

103. What are the clinical features of atopic dermatitis?

Atopic dermatitis is characterized by uncontrolled scratching in response to itching. This itch-scratch cycle leads to the classic lesions. The primary lesion of atopic dermatitis has been debated, and indeed multiple skin findings may coexist:

1. Erythematous papules and plaques, which at times may be follicular, are common.
2. The appearance of vesicles, pustules, weeping, and crusting may be associated with secondary infection with herpes simplex or *Staphylococcus aureus.*
3. Secondary changes resulting from chronic excoriation include linear erosions and lichenification (thickening and accentuation of skin markings).

104. What is the distribution of atopic dermatitis lesions?

The distribution of lesions is age-related (see figure on facing page). In **infants** the face, particularly the cheeks, and the extensor surfaces are typically involved. In **children** the disease may be more localized to the antecubital and popliteal fossae and the hands and feet. **Adults** show continued involvement of the flexures (including the genitalia) and, in more generalized cases, the face (eyelids and forehead), neck, hands, and feet. Generalized involvement may develop at any age.

105. Who develops atopic dermatitis?

The onset of atopic dermatitis usually occurs in childhood; 60% of patients develop disease in the first year of life and 30% between 1 and 5 years of age. Patients frequently have a personal or family history of allergic rhinitis or asthma. Commonly associated cutaneous findings include dry, lackluster skin, an extra infraorbital eyelid fold, and hyperlinear palms.

106. What is the typical clinical course of atopic dermatitis?

In general, atopic dermatitis is more severe and persistent in childhood; improvement is noted as the patient ages. However, 50% of patients have persistent disease as adults. A family history of atopy, early disease in childhood, and severe cutaneous lesions are associated with persistence into adult life.

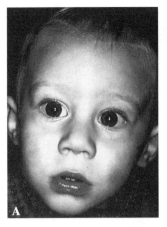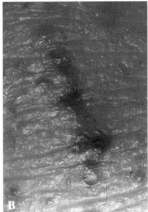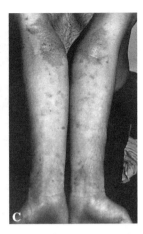

Phases of atopic dermatitis. A, Infantile phase. Typical erythematous, oozing, and crusted plaques seen on the cheek of an infant with atopic dermatitis. B, Childhood phase. Close-up view of a lichenified, excoriated, crusted, and secondarily infected plaque on the right knee of a 5-year-old girl. C, Adolescent or young adult phase. Classic lichenified flexural plaque in a young man. (From Fitzpatrick JE, Aeling JL: Dermatology Secrets. Philadelphia, Hanley & Belfus, 1996, with permission.)

107. What are the other clinical presentations of atopic dermatitis?

The most severe cases of atopic dermatitis may progress to erythroderma, which is characterized by generalized scaling and redness and associated with systemic symptoms of fever, high-output cardiac failure, systemic infection, and heat loss. It is a severe complication and may require hospitalization.

108. How is atopic dermatitis diagnosed?

The diagnosis of atopic dermatitis is primarily clinical. Major criteria include typical morphology and distribution, chronic or chronically relapsing course, and personal or family history of atopy and pruritus. Elevated serum IgE levels and specific IgE-mediated sensitization as measured by skin test or radioallergosorbent tests support the diagnosis. The biopsy is nondiagnostic with varying degrees of acanthosis, at times spongiosis, and a mixed dermal infiltrate.

109. What other diseases are associated with atopic dermatitis?

Cutaneous infections are more common in atopic patients. Infection with *S. aureus* is particularly frequent, often manifested by oozing and crusting. Herpes simplex infections are also common and may progress to Kaposi's varicelliform eruption, a disseminated form of the disease. Other frequent infections include warts, molluscum contagiosum, and dermatophytosis.

Stasis Dermatitis

110. What is the clinical presentation of stasis dermatitis?

Patients with stasis dermatitis commonly have erythematous scaly plaques associated with brown hyperpigmentation and edema of the lower legs and ankles. In severe cases, ulceration (often on the medial lower leg and ankle) may develop. An aching discomfort of the limbs is usually present, but severe pain is infrequent.

111. Who develops stasis dermatitis and ulceration?

The disease is more common in women, occurs in adults over the age of 50, and is associated with a history of phlebitis.

112. What is the typical clinical course of stasis dermatitis and ulceration?

The disease is chronic and, if left untreated, may become quite severe with large recalcitrant ulcerations. The dermatitis responds to mid-potency steroids and compression stockings, and the ulcers heal with elevation and compression bandages.

113. How are stasis dermatitis and ulceration diagnosed?

The diagnosis is based on typical clinical findings and confirmed by vascular evaluation to rule out arterial disease. Pulses should be normal.

Seborrheic Dermatitis

114. What are the clinical features of seborrheic dermatitis?

Lesions frequently occur in people with oily-looking skin. Indeed, the word *seborrhea* is Greek for overflow of sebum. The lesions of seborrheic dermatitis are erythematous papules and plaques, with greasy-appearing yellow scales and crusts (inflammatory dandruff). The yellow color usually is produced by serum that exudes on the surface of the scale. Lesions may occur in both hairy and nonhairy skin. Common locations include the scalp, eyebrows, glabella, beard, nasolabial folds, retroauricular area, and ear canal. More severe disease may involve the central chest (midsternum), back, and intertriginous regions. Blepharitis also may be associated, and pruritus is common.

115. Who develops seborrheic dermatitis?

The disease occurs in both sexes with a slight increase in males. In adults the onset is often between the fourth and seventh decade. The disease also is common in infants under 6 months of age.

116. What is the typical clinical course of seborrheic dermatitis?

In adults the disease is chronic with periods of exacerbation and remission.

117. What are the other clinical presentations of seborrheic dermatitis?

The disease occurs in infants in the first 6 months of life. Lesions consist of erythematous plaques covered with greasy-appearing scales and crusts involving the scalp and intertriginous areas. Spontaneous resolution is the rule. The incidence of seborrheic dermatitis is increased in patients with AIDS, in whom the disease is generally more severe, widespread, and resistant to treatment.

118. How is seborrheic dermatitis diagnosed?

The diagnosis is based on clinical appearance. The biopsy is nondiagnostic.

OTHER DISORDERS

Kaposi's Sarcoma

119. What are the major types of Kaposi's sarcoma? Describe each.

1. The classic form, which is now relatively rare, is usually located on the pretibial areas or feet of older men of Mediterranean origin. It begins as purplish papules and progresses to plaques. It is rarely fatal.

2. The AIDS-associated variant may be present in over one-third of patients with AIDS. Lesions are more varied and widespread than in the classic form, and the spectrum ranges from macular to papular to plaque or ulcerating red-to-purple lesions.

3. Mucous membranes, including genital, oral, and other gastric mucosa, are often involved.

4. In Africa an endemic form of the disease may be cutaneous and/or lymphatic.

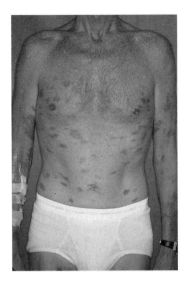

Kaposi's sarcoma. Multiple violaceous plaques following the lines of skin cleavage in a pityriasis rosea-like pattern are seen on the trunk of an HIV-positive patient. (From Fitzpatrick JE, Aeling JL: Dermatology Secrets. Philadelphia, Hanley & Belfus, 1996, with permission.)

120. Who was Kaposi?

Moritz Kaposi (1837–1902) was a Viennese dermatologist. He was born Moritz Kohn in the small town of Kaposvar, Hungary. When he converted to Catholicism, he chose to name himself after his native town. A conceited fellow famous for never saying, "I don't know," Kaposi linked his name not only to sarcoma but also to one of the earliest descriptions of lupus erythematosus and dermatitis herpetiform.

Lupus Erythematosus

121. What are the clinical features of lupus erythematosus?

The word *lupus* is Latin for wolf and was used originally to describe diseases that literally gnaw and devour the skin. The term is now used, with modifying adjectives, to designate chronic discoid lupus erythematosus (CDLE), a mainly cutaneous disease, and systemic lupus erythematosus (SLE), in which cutaneous findings are associated with systemic manifestations.

Discoid lesions begin as sharply demarcated erythematous papules and plaques with adherent scales and progress to areas of atrophy, telangiectasia, and follicular plugging. The end stage results in pink or white depressed scars, which may include hyperpigmentation. Commonly affected regions include sun-exposed parts, such as the malar areas, scalp, nose, and external ears, although any site on the head may be involved. In severe disease, lesions may be present on the upper chest, back, and arms; on rare occasions, the legs are involved.

Cutaneous findings are present in 85% of patients with SLE. The butterfly rash, characterized by an erythematous blush located on the cheeks and bridge of the nose, may be the first sign of the disease. A maculopapular eruption resembling a drug eruption is located more commonly above the waistline. Discoid lesions, urticarial vasculitis, purpuric lesions of vasculitis (palpable purpura, which may result in ulceration), mucosal ulcerations, and livedo reticularis develop. Associated findings in SLE include periungual erythema and telangiectasia and alopecia.

122. Who develops lupus erythematosus?

CDLE generally affects people between 25 and 45 years old and is twice as common in women as in men. The most common age of onset for SLE is between ages 30–40 years, but it may occur in children and elderly people. It is more frequent in African-Americans and eight times more common in females than in males. In about 10% of patients a genetic component is present.

123. What is the typical clinical course of lupus erythematosus?

Most patients with CDLE do well; progression to systemic disease occurs in 5% or less of all patients. SLE may be associated with multisystem involvement, most commonly arthritis, renal disease, nervous system and gastrointestinal manifestations, and hematologic abnormalities. Careful management with corticosteroids, immunosuppressants, and antimalarials may allow patients to lead normal productive lives. The five-year survival rate is 95%.

124. What are the other clinical presentations of lupus erythematosus?

1. Patients with **subacute cutaneous lupus erythematosus** have widespread, nonscarring photosensitive erythematous lesions that are annular or psoriasiform and lack atrophic scarring and follicular involvement. Lesions are more common in light-exposed areas. A low-titer antinuclear antibody (ANA) with antibodies to Ro/SS-A antigen is characteristic. Patients usually meet criteria for diagnosis of SLE.

2. **Lupus profundus** develops when lupus erythematosus involves the adipose tissue. It is characterized by multiple subcutaneous nodules, usually with normal overlying skin but sometimes with overlying discoid lesions distributed on the face, proximal arms and legs, breasts, buttocks, or trunk. They may ulcerate and heal with subcutaneous atrophy. Calcification may occur. Most patients have a positive ANA and antibodies to double-stranded DNA. However, the lesions may occur with CDLE or SLE.

125. How is lupus erythematosus diagnosed?

For **CDLE** the clinical appearance with confirmation by biopsy is diagnostic. The biopsy usually reveals hyperkeratosis, epidermal atrophy, follicular plugging, and liquefaction degeneration of the basal cell layer with a perivascular inflammatory infiltrate. A lupus band test is positive in 90% of active lesions. An evaluation for systemic involvement also should be done.

The diagnosis of **SLE** is made in the presence of multisystem disease together with antinuclear antibodies, particularly a positive ANA, a low serum complement, and increased antidouble-stranded DNA antibodies. Only 50% of patients at the time of diagnosis meet the Revised Criteria for Classification of SLE proposed by the American Rheumatism Association. Cutaneous lesions may display characteristic findings on biopsy (see above) but also may be nonspecific. Direct immunofluorescence may be helpful. The presence of subepidermal immunoglobulin and complement in uninvolved skin is evidence for systemic disease.

126. Are drugs associated with the onset of lupus erythematosus?

Yes. Drugs such as hydralazine, procainamide, isoniazid, methyldopa, sulfonamides, phenytoin, and penicillamine may induce a lupus-like illness.

Purpura

127. What are the two major types of purpura?

- **Noninflammatory**. Noninflammatory purpura, which is due to red cell extravasation, is nonindurated and nonpalpable. The most common example is a bruise.
- **Inflammatory**. Because it is due to extravasation not only of red blood cells but also of white cells, inflammatory purpura is peculiarly indurated and palpable.

Pearl. Inflammatory purpura is palpable purpura, and palpable purpura, by definition, is vasculitis involving the small vessels.

128. What are the causes of palpable purpura?

The most common causes of small vessel vasculitis are drug reactions, infections, collagen vascular diseases, and various vasculitides. Overall, the etiology varies depending on the age of the patient:

- In **children** the most common cause is Henoch-Schönlein purpura, followed at a great distance by leukocytoclastic hypersensitivity (i.e., drug reaction).

• In **adults** leukocytoclastic hypersensitivity (i.e., drug rash) is still by far the most common cause, followed by collagen vascular diseases, periarteritis nodosa, cryoglobulinemia, endocarditis, Wegener's granulomatosis, and malignancy.

A prominent livedo pattern (purplish streak-like net of vessels) and subungual splinter hemorrhages are other features of vasculitis. If a patient has vasculitis of the skin, he or she also may have vasculitis in other systems (e.g., brain, kidneys). Thus a thorough exam and work-up are necessary.

Syphilis

129. What are the clinical features of syphilis?

The lesion varies depending on the stage of the disease:

1. The classic lesion of **primary syphilis** is the chancre, which appears at the site of treponemal penetration. The chancre is a 1–2-cm, round, firm, painless ulcer with raised indurated borders. The induration is key. In fact, the lesion can almost be flipped between the fingers of the examiner as if it were a coin being buried under the skin. Genital lesions are most common, but the chancre may occur anywhere.

2. Lesions of **secondary syphilis** are generally red to ham-colored, circular or ring-shaped papules with sparse scaling. Lesions are distributed diffusely and often involve the palms and soles. Flat, white plaques occur on the oral and genital mucosae. Lymphadenopathy is common.

3. **Benign tertiary syphilis** appears after untreated resolution of secondary lesions. Gummas, which may occur anywhere, are nontender rubbery nodules that may ulcerate and heal with noncontractile scarring.

130. Who develops syphilis?

Early syphilis (primary and secondary disease) may occur in any age group but is more common during the sexually active years. The male-to-female ratio is 2:1. In the past decade the incidence has increased. The increase initially occurred in homosexual males, but with changes in sexual practices to reduce the incidence of HIV infection, people now at greatest risk are inner-city, African-American heterosexual males and females involved in drug use.

131. What is the typical clinical course of syphilis?

The chancre develops an average of 20 days after inoculation. If untreated, it resolves in 1–6 weeks. Secondary syphilis lesions usually erupt 2–4 months after appearance of the chancre and, if untreated, resolve in the same amount of time. Relapses of secondary lesions may occur. Only one-third of patients manifest signs of tertiary syphilis, which are divided among cutaneous gummas (16%), cardiovascular disease (9.6%), and central nervous system disease (6.5%).

132. What are the other clinical presentations of syphilis?

1. **Syphilis in HIV-infected patients** may result in difficulty in diagnosis with negative serology, increased incidence of neurosyphilis, and persistence of disease even with adequate treatment.

2. **Congenital syphilis** appears when syphilis is transmitted by the mother to the fetus in utero. The clinical manifestations are divided into early prenatal syphilis (before age 2) and late prenatal syphilis (after age 2). They are associated with multiple congenital anomalies.

133. How is syphilis diagnosed?

In early primary syphilis a dark-field examination of the chancre should be performed. Subsequently, serologic tests are the primary method of diagnosis. Nontreponemal serologic tests (Venereal Disease Research Laboratory, rapid plasmin reagent) become positive 3–4 weeks after infection. Specific treponemal antigen tests (fluorescent treponemal antibody absorbed test, *Treponema pallidum* hemagglutination, and microhemagglutination *T. pallidum*) are positive at

6 weeks after infection. Nontreponemal tests are screening procedures, whereas specific treponemal tests are used to confirm diagnosis. Biopsy may demonstrate spirochetes with the special Dieterle stain.

Insect Infestations

134. What are the most common insect infestations?

The most common are lice and mites:

1. **Pediculosis capitis**, infestation of the scalp by the head louse, is characterized by pruritus of the back and sides of the scalp, which may result in excoriation, secondary infection, and cervical lymphadenopathy. Nits (1-mm, oval egg capsules) are firmly attached to the hair and may number in the thousands. Live lice are few in number.

2. **Pediculosis pubis** affects the hairy regions, most commonly the pubic area, but may involve the chest, axillae, and upper eyelids; it is associated with pruritus. Physical findings include lice, 1–2-mm, brownish-gray specks in the hair and skin, and nits, tiny white-gray specks attached to the hair.

3. **Scabies** is an infestation by the mite *Sarcoptes scabiei*. It presents with intractable pruritus, particularly nocturnal, and is associated with linear ridges, vesicles, nodules, excoriation, and crusting involving the web spaces, wrist, genitalia, axilla, buttocks, waist, and ankles.

135. Who develops insect infestations?

Infestations occur at any age. Pediculosis capitis is more common in children; pediculosis pubis occurs often in young adults and frequently is spread by sexual contact; and scabies may occur in epidemics in nursing homes and hospitals. Infestation is spread by close physical contact with an infected person or clothing.

136. What is Norwegian scabies?

Norwegian scabies produces diffuse crusting involving large areas of the body, including the palms and soles. It occurs in debilitated and immunosuppressed patients, including those with AIDS. In the AIDS population, infection may be persistent and difficult to treat.

Skin Manifestations of Systemic Disorders

137. What is necrobiosis lipoidica diabeticorum?

A skin disorder associated with diabetes mellitus (although still relatively rare: only 2% of diabetics have it) and characterized by pink-yellow, telangiectatic, scaly, and asymptomatic plaques usually located over the anterior shins. Lesions are 2–10 cm in diameter with borders that often acquire a violaceous hue because the skin atrophy makes the underlying veins visible. Of all patients with this condition, 67% have diabetes, 16% have abnormal glucose tolerance test, and 8% have a family history of diabetes; only 9% have no link to diabetes. The cause is unknown although believed to originate from diabetic microangiopathy.

138. What is porphyria cutanea tarda (PCT)?

PCT is an autosomal dominant, symptomatic porphyria associated with liver dysfunction and photosensitive cutaneous lesions. The lesions are characterized by hyperpigmentation, scleroderma-like changes in the skin, fragility in sun-exposed areas, milia (tiny white cysts), and hypertrichosis. Typical lesions are blisters on the back of the hands. The underlying biochemical mechanism is increased excretion of uroporphyrin caused by a deficiency of uroporphyrinogen decarboxylase. Contributing environmental factors include alcohol, estrogens, hepatitis C, and HIV infection.

139. What are the skin manifestations of sarcoidosis?

The most common skin manifestation is clusters of small, nonscaling, skin-colored, dome-shaped papules, usually located on the face and neck. Lesions may coalesce and form larger nodules and plaques, especially on the trunk and extremities. Biopsy confirms the presence of typical noncaseating granulomas.

140. What is lupus pernio?

Another skin manifestation of sarcoidosis, lupus pernio is characterized by lesions resembling those of frostbite (*pernio* in Latin). They usually involve ears, cheeks, nose, hands, and fingers.

141. What is erythema nodosum?

A skin manifestation of sarcoidosis and many other diseases, erythema nodosum is characterized by large, red, nonscaling, and painful lesions on the pretibial areas (shins and ankles mostly, usually bilaterally but initially even unilaterally). Lesions are nonspecific inflammatory nodules or plaques (*not* the typical noncaseating granulomas of sarcoid). Lesions usually resolve, but other lesions may appear. The course of the disease may last for months. Healing leaves residual hyperpigmentation but no scarring.

142. Is erythema nodosum pathognomonic for sarcoidosis?

No. It may be associated with a myriad of other disorders, including (1) medication reactions (e.g., oral contraceptives, sulfonamides, iodides, bromides); (2) infections (particularly fungal infections but also streptococcal infection and tuberculosis); and (3) autoimmune diseases (especially the inflammatory bowel diseases).

143. What is Behçet's syndrome?

It is a syndrome characterized by the presence of aphthous ulcers of the mouth and genitalia. The ulcers are associated with arthritis, uveitis, and various neurologic disorders. The syndrome was first described by the Turkish dermatologist Hulusi Behçet (1889–1948) based on the observation of 3 patients followed between 1924 and 1936.

144. What are the dermatologic manifestations of dermatomyositis?

The most common is a violaceous edema of the upper eyelids associated with redness and edema of the entire face. The lesions are not as well marginated and circumscribed as those of lupus erythematosus. Patients also may present with reddish/violaceous patches and plaques of the elbows, knees, dorsal surfaces of the knuckles, palmar surfaces of the fingertips, and hypothenar eminence. Skin lesions are encountered in as many as 50% of patients with dermatomyositis and do not correlate with severity of the myositis.

145. What are the skin manifestations of scleroderma?

The most typical is sclerodactyly, which is characterized by thickening and tightening of the skin over fingers and hands. Fingertips may be scarred, pitted, and tapered. Hyperpigmentation of the dorsum of hands and arms at times may be associated with patches of vitiligo. Finally, telangiectasias of the face, upper chest, and arms also may be seen.

146. What are the skin manifestations of hyperthyroidism?

Graves' disease is associated with a typical pretibial myxedema, consisting of thickened, bumpy, and colored plaques located over the lower pretibial areas and usually asymptomatic. In addition, patients with hyperthyroidism tend to have thin hair; they may have onycholysis of the fingernails and clubbing (thyroid acropachy) and even areas of vitiligo (5–10% of patients).

147. What is Sweet's syndrome?

Sweet's syndrome is seen in patients with leukemias or other proliferative disorders. It is characterized by the presence of dark red nodules, often ulcerated and with a purulent base, localized over the hands, face, arms, and legs (see figure). It is similar to erythema multiforme but is caused by a neutrophilic infiltrate. It was first described by the British dermatologist Robert D. Sweet.

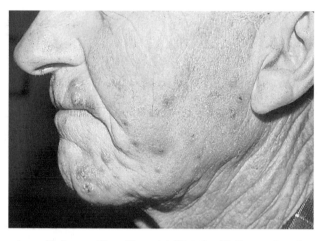

Sweet's syndrome in an elderly man. (From Fitzpatrick JE, Aeling JL: Dermatology Secrets. Philadelphia, Hanley & Belfus, 1996, with permission.)

148. Which cancers metastasize to the skin?

The most common are cancers of breast, gastrointestinal tract, prostate, kidney (especially involving the scalp), and head and neck. Melanomas, of course, also may metastasize to the skin. All of these cancers usually appear as firm and rapidly growing skin nodules, often covered with fine telangiectasias (due to the neoplastic angiogenesis) and even ulcers (due to inability of the vasculature to catch up with the rapid growth of the tumor). Another interesting feature of these tumors is the zosteriform pattern of metastasis (with clusters of papules that merge into a zoster-like plaque). Once metastasis to the skin has occurred, the prognosis is poor.

BIBLIOGRAPHY

1. Arnold HL, Odom RB, James WD: Andrews' Diseases of the Skin: Clinical Dermatology, 8th ed. Philadelphia, W. B. Saunders, 1990.
2. Fitzpatrick TB, Johnson RA, Polano MK, et al: Color Atlas and Synopsis of Clinical Dermatology, 3rd ed. New York, McGraw-Hill, 1997.
3. Freedberg IM, Eisen AZ, Wolff K, et al (eds): Fitzpatrick's Dermatology in General Medicine, 4th ed. New York, McGraw-Hill, 1999.
4. Lynch PJ: Dermatology for the House Officer. Baltimore, Williams & Wilkins, 1982.
5. Whited JD, Grichnik JM: Does this patient have a mole or a melanoma? JAMA 279:696–701, 1998.
6. Willms JL, Schneiderman H, Algranati PS: Physical Diagnosis. Baltimore, Williams & Wilkins, 1994.

4. EYE EXAMINATION

Sylvia R. Beck, M.D., Richard Tipperman, M.D.

The eye is the light of the body.—Matthew 6:22

TOPICS COVERED IN THIS CHAPTER

Fundus *(continued)*
 Posterior eye structures *(continued)*
  Retinal circulation
   Retinal veins vs. retinal arteries
   Light reflex
   Hypertensive retinopathy
   Arteriovenous nicking
   Malignant hypertension
   Central retinal artery occlusion
   Central retinal vein occlusion
   Branch retinal vein occlusion
   Hollenhorst plaques
   Retinal neovascularization
  Retinal background
   Light-colored spots
    Cotton-wool spots
    Hard exudates
    Drusen
    Myelinated nerve fibers
   Red spots
    Microaneurysms
    "Blot" and "dot" hemorrhages
    "Flame and splinter" hemorrhages
    "White-centered" hemorrhages
      (Roth spots)

Fundus *(continued)*
 Posterior eye structures *(continued)*
  Retinal background *(continued)*
   Black spots
    Laser scars
    Healed chorioretinitis
    Retinitis pigmentosa
    Retinal pigment epithelium
      hypertrophy
    Melanomas/benign choroidal
      nevi
  Diabetic retinopathy
   Background diabetic
     retinopathy
   Proliferative diabetic
     retinopathy
  Retinal detachment
  Macula
   Macular degeneration
Red Eye
 Definition
 Structures involved
 Signs and symptoms
 Differential diagnosis

CONVENTIONAL TEACHING WATCH

Conventional teaching has often bypassed the eye. Yet certain physical findings are extremely important and should be recognized by all practicing physicians. Indeed, from measurement of visual acuity to funduscopy, all parts of the eye exam yield valuable "wheat" and may help to unlock important secrets not only of the eye but also of the body.

PART OF EYE EXAM		CONVENTIONAL TEACHING REVISITED
Visual acuity	⇑	Like vital signs, vision should be measured and recorded at the beginning of the eye exam.
Visual fields testing	⇑	This maneuver detects (and separates) important neurologic or ocular disease.
Pupillary exam	⇑	Examining pupils can yield invaluable clinical information.
External eye	⇑	Much of the external exam can be done with a penlight and thoughtful observation of patient's orbits, eyelid position, conjunctiva, anterior portion of globe, and corneal light reflex.
Ophthalmoscopy	⇑	Practice is the key: the more you do it, the better you get at it.
Red eye	⇑	Common problem worth special attention

VISUAL ACUITY

The visual acuity exam assesses the vital signs of the eye. Nothing meaningful can be said about the status of the eye without first measuring vision.

EYE LESIONS		CONVENTIONAL TEACHING REVISITED
Measurement of visual acuity	⇑	Essential tool in every physician's armamentarium.
Ophthalmoscopy in reduced visual acuity	⇑	Armed with only an ophthalmoscope, you can go a long way toward identifying the cause of decreased vision.
Hand movements (HM), counting fingers (CF), light perception (LP), and no light perception (NLP)	⇔	It is important to know the alphabet soup of visual acuity to understand what the consultant is talking about.
Dyschromatopsia	⇔	Important to consider; *acquired* color vision deficiency (as opposed to congenital color blindness)

1. What equipment is needed to measure visual acuity?
Four simple and easily available tools are needed:

1. Snellen chart
2. Pinhole occluder
3. Pocket-size near-vision test card
4. Color vision screening plates

2. What is a Snellen chart?
It is a standard, wall-mounted eye chart imprinted with lines of black characters (letters, numbers, or illiterate Es), ranging in size from smallest (on the bottom) to largest (on top).

3. Who was Snellen?
Hermann Snellen (1834–1908) was a Dutch ophthalmologist who graduated from and later taught at the University of Utrecht. He created his famous chart in 1862 as a first attempt to standardize measurement of visual acuity.

4. How is visual acuity measured?
Covering one eye at a time, the patient is asked to read a well-illuminated Snellen chart at a distance of 20 feet (6 m). By convention, the right eye is tested and recorded first. Testing should be carried out with the patient's distance glasses. The smallest line on which the patient can distinguish more than one-half of the letters is the visual acuity. The number of letters missed on the same line also should be recorded, such as 20/20 − 1 or 20/40 − 2.

5. What does 20/20 mean?
20/20 means that the patient can read at a distance of 20 feet a letter that was designed to be read at 20 feet; 20/40 means that the patient can distinguish at 20 feet a letter that normally can be read at 40 feet, and so on. The numerator of the visual acuity fashion represents the distance at which the Snellen chart is placed, whereas the denominator represents the distance at which the letter can be recognized by a person with standard acuity. The denominator also identifies the smallest line on the chart on which the patient was able to read more than one-half of the letters.

6. Can visual acuity be better than 20/20?
Yes. Although 20/20 is the standard visual acuity, most normal people can actually see better than 20/20. The patient's vision should be recorded accordingly (such as 20/15, 20/12, and so on).

7. How is vision measured in illiterate patients?
For illiterate patients or children, one should use the single E chart. The patient is asked to designate the direction of the strokes of the E.

8. How is vision measured in bedridden patients?
Near visual acuity can be measured (one eye at a time) with a pocket-size near-vision test card, such as the Rosenbaum Pocket Visual Screener, which can be purchased at any medical supply store. The card is held 14 inches (35 cm) from the patient's eye while the other eye is

occluded by the examiner. The smallest legible characters indicate visual acuity. Reading or distance glasses should be worn during testing. If the patient does not have them available or cannot
see the near card, one may substitute counting fingers (CF) (see below).

9. How is vision measured in patients who cannot read any letters on the chart?

When a patient cannot read any letter on the chart, the distance between patient and chart
should be reduced. The shortened distance should be recorded as the numerator of the new visual
acuity measurement (e.g., 5/70). This fraction may be translated into a more conventional visual
acuity recording (e.g., 20/280). If the patient cannot read the largest letters on a Snellen chart
placed at 3 feet, vision may be measured in terms of counting fingers. The examiner records the
distance at which counting is accurate. If even this measurement is not possible, vision may be
measured as ability to see hand motions (HM) or a flashlight (light perception [LP]) or finally as
no light perception (NLP).

10. What is pinhole vision?

It is vision through a pinhole occluder. If a patient cannot read the 20/20 line, an occluder
with a small opening can be placed over the eye. The pinhole occluder admits only axial light
rays; it eliminates peripheral rays that are responsible for blurring of the vision secondary to refractive errors of the eye. Thus, the pinhole occluder improves the vision of patients with problems correctable by glasses but does not modify the vision of patients with other ocular or
neurologic disorders (such as retinal diseases or opacities of the light-transmitting media).
Problems correctable by glasses include hyperopia (in which the axial length of the eye is too
short), myopia (in which the axial length is too long), and astigmatism (in which the refracting
power of cornea and lens are different in one meridian compared with the other).

11. Who should have visual acuity testing? When?

Measuring vision is like taking the vital signs of the eye. Nothing intelligent can be said
about the status of the eye without measuring vision. Because normal vision requires not only
normal eye function but also integrity of the eye's vascular and neurologic supply, testing of
visual acuity is an excellent tool in the armamentarium of any practicing physician. Visual acuity
should be measured in all patients with visual complaints. Because it can detect painless loss of
vision in one or both eyes, visual acuity also should be part of the screening physical examination
of all adult patients. Visual loss is usually painless, with the exception of disorders presenting
with red eye (see below). In children, visual acuity should be measured as early as possible (usually after the third birthday) to allow early detection of amblyopia.

12. What is the significance of reduced visual acuity?

Reduced visual acuity may indicate the presence of any of the following processes:
- Refractive and correctable errors of the eye, such as myopia, astigmatism, and presbyopia
- Treatable and reversible blinding eye disease, such as cataracts or uveitis
- Ocular manifestations of systemic diseases, which are progressive if left untreated, such as
  diabetes or hypertension
- Neurologic disorders that may be both vision-impairing and life-threatening, such as multi-
  ple sclerosis or gliomas
- Congenital disorders such as rubella or toxoplasmosis
- Infectious disorders such as cytomegalovirus retinitis or toxoplasmosis

13. How can one confirm the cause of reduced visual acuity?

- **Uncorrected refractive errors** of the eye are usually suspected whenever vision improves
  with the use of a pinhole occluder.
- **Opacities of the light-transmitting media** are usually diagnosed by examining the red
  reflex or by ophthalmoscopy.
- **Neurologic or retinal disorders** are usually revealed by ophthalmoscopy, the swinging
  flashlight test, or visual field testing.

• **Amblyopia** is usually suggested by a childhood history of reduced visual acuity and is often accompanied by strabismus.

14. When should newly discovered reduced visual acuity be referred to an ophthalmologist?
• Patients with visual symptoms
• Asymptomatic patients with visual acuity of 20/40 or worse in one or both eyes
• Patients with a visual acuity difference between eyes of two lines or more
• Middle-aged or elderly patients with presbyopia, even if distance visual acuity is preserved (for prescription of reading glasses), and for glaucoma screening
• Patients with an afferent pupillary defect

15. What are color vision screening plates?
Color vision screening plates are pseudoisochromatic tables (i.e., pseudo-similarly colored tables) that present numbers or figures against a background of colored dots. This combination of colors is usually confusing and illegible to a person with abnormal color discrimination.

16. How is color vision tested?
Color plates are presented consecutively to the patient, one eye at a time, and results are recorded as a fraction (the numerator indicates the number of correct responses and the denominator the number of total plates presented). In testing for unilateral dyschromatopsia, a simpler and still reliable method is to ask the patient to cover the affected eye and then look at a red object, such as the red cap of a mydriatic solution bottle. The patient is then asked to look at the same object with the other eye (while the unaffected eye is covered) and to report whether the red color appears the same. In patients with dyschromatopsia, the red object appears gray or washed-out when presented to the affected eye.

17. What is dyschromatopsia?
Dyschromatopsia (from the Greek *dys* = abnormal, *chroma* = color, opsis = *vision*) is an abnormality of color vision. Dyschromatopsia is used to describe an acquired deficiency in color vision as opposed to congenital color blindness.

18. What causes dyschromatopsia?
Optic nerve diseases or toxic or degenerative diseases of the macula.

VISUAL FIELDS

CONVENTIONAL TEACHING WATCH

Visual field testing may reveal important neurologic or ocular diseases, but the terminology may be confusing.

EYE LESIONS/FINDINGS		CONVENTIONAL TEACHING REVISITED
Visual fields testing	⇑	With confrontation of fields one can find previously undetected occipital strokes and chiasmal tumors.
Visual field defects due to neurologic or ocular diseases	⇑	This distinction is important and can be easily made at bedside.
Ophthalmoscopy for visual field defects	⇑	Important in interpretation of visual field defects.
Hemianopia(s)	⇑	Important concepts and findings.

19. How do you test visual fields?
The examiner sits 3 feet away from the patient and asks him or her to cover one eye with the palm of one hand while fixating on either the examiner's nose or opposite eye. While the patient is

fixating on the reference point, the examiner outstretches an arm and briefly holds up 1, 2 or 5 fingers. The fingers are held in each quadrant while the patient is asked to report how many fingers he or she can see. The test is repeated for the opposite eye. Checking visual fields thus relies on confrontation (i.e., a rough comparison of the fields of the examiner with the fields of the patient). (See Fig. p. 409.)

20. What is the difference between visual field defects due to a neurologic lesion and visual field defects due to an ocular lesion?

Visual field defects due to **neurologic lesions** respect the vertical midline of the patient's vision and are usually bilateral. Visual field defects due to **ocular lesions** are primarily unilateral (monocular) and often respect the horizontal midline.

21. What is the most important step after finding a monocular visual field defect?

Test the visual field of the other eye. As stated above, monocular visual field defects are usually due to a problem in the affected eye, whereas binocular visual field defects are usually caused by intracranial (neurologic) processes.

22. What is bitemporal hemianopia?

Hemianopia refers to loss of vision for one-half of the visual field of both eyes (from the Greek *hemi* = half, *an* = lack of, and *opsis* = vision). A bitemporal hemianopia is a visual defect in which the temporal fields of both eyes (bitemporal) are cut. It is typically seen in patients with a chiasmal tumor (craniopharyngiomas in children and pituitary tumors in adults).

23. What is homonymous hemianopia?

It is a visual defect in which fields of the same side (homonymous) are cut in both eyes. For example, if the cut in the left eye involves the temporal region (the left portion of the left eye's visual field), the cut in the right eye affects the nasal region (the left portion of the right eye's visual field). Homonymous hemianopia is typically seen in patients with a lesion in the cerebral cortex.

24. What are tunnel fields?

Tunnel fields are severely constricted visual fields and may be seen in advanced glaucoma, retinitis pigmentosa, and other more unusual conditions. They also may be due to malingering.

PUPILS

CONVENTIONAL TEACHING WATCH

Attention to pupillary shape, size, and response to external stimuli provides extremely valuable clinical information.

EYE LESIONS/FINDINGS		CONVENTIONAL TEACHING REVISITED
Response to light and accommodation	⇑	If pupils react to light, they also react to accommodation (thus there is no need to check for it).
Anisocoria	⇑	Before drilling holes in people's skulls, remember that the most common form of anisocoria is physiologic.
Swinging flashlight test	⇑	Sensitive test for pathologic causes of decreased vision in one eye.
Marcus Gunn pupil	⇑	Discovery of an afferent pupillary defect should prompt referral to an ophthalmologist.
Hippus	⇔	Important in the differential diagnosis of a Marcus Gunn pupil.
Argyll Robertson pupil	⇔	Nice to ask medical students about it, but hard to find in practice.
Adie's pupil	⇔	More common than above, but still unusual

25. How does one examine the pupils?

Ideally, in a somewhat darkened room. The patient fixates his or her gaze on something in the distance while the examiner shines a penlight from below to ensure that the pupils are round and equal in size.

26. What are the major features to identify in a pupillary exam?

There are major pupillary features to identify: (1) shape, (2) size, and (3) responses to external stimuli. These responses, in turn, include (1) response to light (both direct and consensual) and (2) response to accommodation.

27. What are the most common abnormalities in pupillary shape?

- The most common abnormality is probably the irregular, pear-shaped contour of pupils that have undergone an intraocular surgical procedure (such as cataract excision).
- Eyes subjected to blunt trauma may suffer tears in the iris sphincter, causing the affected pupil to appear larger and slightly irregular.
- Inflammatory disease of the iris (iritis) may lead to adhesions (synechiae) of the iris to the anterior capsule of the lens and thus to an irregular pupil.
- A coloboma of the iris is a congenital defect caused by incomplete closure of the embryonic fissure of the optic cup. The involved iris usually has a keyhole shape, with the defect located most commonly in an inferonasal position.

28. What is hippus?

Hippus is a physiologic condition characterized by constant change in pupillary size. The expression comes from the Greek word *hippos* (horse), chosen to convey the up-and-down movements of a galloping horse. As is the case for other normal pupils, the initial reaction to light of a pupil with hippus is constriction. This response separates hippus from an afferent pupillary defect (see below).

Pearl. A pupil with an afferent pupillary defect initially dilates in response to the back-and-forth swinging of the penlight. In hippus, on the other hand, the pupil initially constricts.

29. What are the most common causes of unequal pupils?

1. The most common cause is **physiologic anisocoria** (from the Greek *an* = lack of, *iso* = equal, and *core* = pupils), a normal variant (present in 20% of the population) characterized by a physiologic difference in muscular tone between the right and left pupillary sphincters. In physiologic anisocoria, the difference between the pupils does not change with different levels of illumination. Physiologic anisocoria is not associated with ptosis or light-near dissociation.

2. Another common cause of anisocoria is **pharmacologic dilation**. The patient has either knowingly or inadvertently instilled a mydriatic (dilating drop) into the eye, causing the pupil to dilate. Pupils that are pharmacologically dilated do not constrict to light or after instillation of a cholinergic eye drop (e.g., pilocarpine).

3. Anisocoria also may be seen in patients with **Horner's syndrome** (see figure at top of following page) The pupil of the affected eye is smaller (miotic). In addition to miosis, patients also have ipsilateral ptosis and anhidrosis. In anisocoria created by Horner's syndrome, the difference between the pupils varies with illumination. For example, the difference is greater in the dark (revealing defective dilation) and less in bright illumination (demonstrating intact constriction).

4. Anisocoria in patients with **third-nerve palsy** is due to mydriasis (i.e., dilation) of the pupil on the affected side. Other findings associated with third-nerve palsy are (1) ptosis and (2) weakness of all extraocular muscles with the exception of the lateral rectus and the superior oblique. The dilated pupil constricts if a cholinergic drop is instilled. In anisocoria secondary to third-nerve palsy, the difference between the pupils is greater in bright illumination, demonstrating defective constriction.

5. **Other reasons** for developing anisocoria include (1) inflammatory processes (e.g., unilateral iritis), (2) old trauma, (3) acute angle closure glaucoma, (4) previous intraocular surgery, and (5) various neurologic disorders.

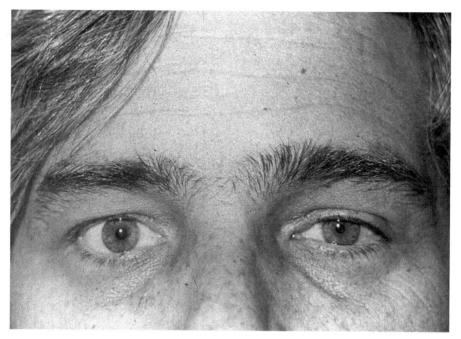

Horner's syndrome with ptosis and miosis on the left. Note that the left lower lid is higher than the right lower lid. This inverse ptosis is due to interruption of sympathetic innervation to the analog of Mueller's muscle in the lower lid. (From Vander JF, Gault JA: Ophthalmology Secrets. Philadelphia, Hanley & Belfus, 1998, with permission.)

30. What is the response to accommodation?

It is the pupillary constriction that follows the shift in focus from a distant to a closer object. The test is conducted by asking the patient to look at a far-away point and then to focus rapidly on a much closer object, such as the examiner's finger. Looking back a far-away point again leads to a brisk pupillary dilation.

31. What is the response to light?

It is the pupillary constriction that follows the shining of a light into the eye. The response to light can be either direct (when it occurs in the same eye in which the light is shined) or consensual (when it occurs in the contralateral eye).

32. What are Argyll Robertson pupils?

Argyll Robertson pupils constrict only in response to accommodation but not in response to light (light-near dissociation). Typically described in tertiary syphilis, they also may be seen in diabetics, alcoholics (Wernicke encephalopathy), and other patients with various neoplastic, infectious, and degenerative processes of the central nervous system. The Argyll Robertson pupil is always pathologic.

33. Who was Argyll Robertson?

Douglas M.C.L. Argyll Robertson (1837–1909) was a Scottish physician and surgeon. An avid and skilled golfer who studied in Berlin with Von Graefe, Argyll Robertson eventually returned to his native Scotland, where he founded and chaired ophthalmology at the University of Edinburgh. He was the teacher and mentor of Marcus Gunn (see question 39).

34. What is Adie's pupil?

It is a tonic pupil that usually fails to constrict in response to both accommodation *and* light. After a prolonged attempt at accommodation, an Adie's pupil eventually constricts but always sluggishly. When the near-effort is relaxed, the pupil redilates slowly. Adie's pupils tend to be unilateral, often mydriatic, frequently oval, and always benign. They demonstrate a supersensitivity to dilute (0.125%) pilocarpine.

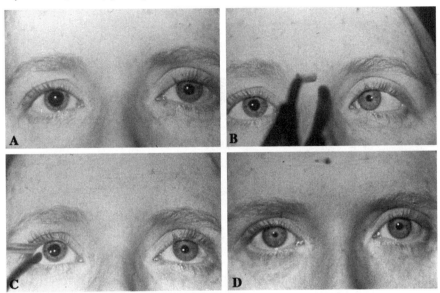

Adie's tonic pupil right eye. *A,* Anisocoria with right pupil larger than left pupil. *B,* Right pupil constricts with near response. *C,* Right pupil reacts poorly to light. *D,* Right pupil constricts markedly in response to ⅛% pilocarpine, whereas the left pupil does not. (From Tasman W, Jaeger EA (eds): The Wills Eye Hospital Atlas of Clinical Ophthalmology. Philadelphia, Lippincott-Raven, 1996, p 298, with permission.)

35. Who was Adie?

William J. Adie (1886–1935) was an Australian who studied medicine in Edinburgh and graduated just in time for World War One. Drafted into the army, he fought with honor in France, where he saved several fellow soldiers from a gas attack by improvising a mask with cloth soaked in urine. Thanks to a well-timed attack of measles, he managed to survive the subsequent slaughter of his entire regiment and returned to England, where he taught and practiced until his death. His name is linked not only to the description of Adie's pupil but also to the first description of narcolepsy. Adie was a charismatic teacher, an avid skier, and an amateur ornithologist. He died prematurely at the age of 49 of a myocardial infarction.

36. What is the swinging flashlight test?

It is a test of pupillary response to light used to screen for a Marcus Gunn pupil or afferent pupillary defect. The patient is asked to gaze at something in the distance. A penlight is shined first in one eye and then in the other. As the light swings from one eye to the other, each pupil should briskly constrict. If one eye has an optic nerve lesion or a massive retinal lesion, it dilates to the light instead of constricting.

A Marcus Gunn pupil has a normal efferent system, but an abnormal afferent pathway. Because the afferent stimulus from the contralateral eye is much stronger than the afferent stimulus from the affected eye, shifting the light from the unaffected eye to the affected eye removes the stimulus to constrict (which comes from the good eye). As a result, when the light is removed from the normal eye and applied to the affected eye, the affected eye dilates. Such patients are usually described as having a Marcus Gunn pupil (MGP) or an afferent pupillary defect (APD).

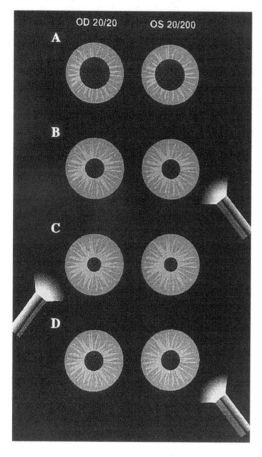

Left APD. *A,* The pupils in dim light are equal. *B,* Light directed into the left eye results in partial and sluggish constriction in each eye. *C,* Light directed into right eye results in a brisk and normal reaction in each eye. *D,* The light quickly directed into the left eye results in a dilatation of both pupils. (From Tasman W, Jaeger EA (eds): The Wills Eye Hospital Atlas of Clinical Ophthalmology. Philadelphia, Lippincott-Raven, 1996, p 297, with permission.)

37. What is the response of a Marcus Gunn pupil when the light is shined on it first?

If the penlight is shined on the affected pupil first (step 1 of the swinging flashlight test), the pupil constricts, although poorly. On the other hand, as the light is swung back and forth, the Marcus Gunn pupil dilates.

38. What is a common cause of Marcus Gunn pupil?

A common cause of Marcus Gunn pupil is optic neuritis. However, any asymmetric optic neuropathy may cause an afferent pupillary defect, as may a massive retinal lesion, such as central retinal artery occlusion.

39. Who was Marcus Gunn?

Robert Marcus Gunn was a Scottish ophthalmologist. He was a contemporary of another famous Scot, Robert Louis Stevenson, whom he personally knew. Marcus Gunn was attracted to the study of ophthalmology by Argyll Robertson (see above). He became highly regarded for his skillful use of the ophthalmoscope.

EXTERNAL EYE

CONVENTIONAL TEACHING WATCH

Much of the external exam can be done with a penlight and thoughtful observation of the orbits, eyelid position, conjunctiva, anterior portion of the globe, and corneal light reflex.

EYE LESIONS/FINDINGS		CONVENTIONAL TEACHING REVISITED
Schirmer's test	⇔	Internists usually do not have Schirmer's strips, but it is still important to know what the consultant is talking about.
Xanthelasmas	⇓	Not as pathognomonic for hyperlipidemia as conventional teaching might lead you to believe.
Exophthalmos	⇑	Important to know its differential diagnosis in both children and adults.
Enophthalmos	⇑	Not as common as exophthalmos but still important to recognize.
Thyroid ophthalmopathy	⇑	A plethora of important findings, often carrying complicated, unpronounceable German names. It is important to recognize stare and lid lag, along with proptosis.
Ptosis	⇑	Important to identify and to differentiate possible etiologies.
Preseptal and orbital cellulitis	⇑	Important to be able to assess and separate these entities.
Subconjunctival hemorrhage	⇑	Common, scary, but often benign eye problem.
Conjunctivitis	⇑	As above; important in differential diagnosis of red eye.
Preauricular node	⇑	Important clue in differential diagnosis of conjunctivitis.
Extraocular movements	⇔	Testing usually has low yield, unless patient complains of double vision.
Nystagmus	⇑	Important clue to oculomotor, cerebellar, or vestibular dysfunction.
Scleral (conjunctival) icterus	⇑	Yellow sclerae are more important than blue sclerae (see below). Sensitivity of scleral icterus depends on amount of natural light illuminating patient's eyes.
Blue sclerae	⇔	Common in newborns; in children and adults suggests osteogenesis imperfecta.
Arcus cornealis (partial or full)	⇓	Much taught, but of dubious clinical significance.
Ciliary flush	⇑	Important sign in diagnosis of uveitis and differential diagnosis of red eye.
Anisocoria in iritis	⇔	Patients with iritis can be so photophobic that it may be difficult to compare pupil size.
Hyphema (blood in anterior chamber)	⇑	Together with hypopyon, a finding that is too important to miss.
Hypopyon (pus in anterior chamber)	⇑	Same as above.
Narrow anterior chamber (penlight test)	⇓	Inaccurate procedure, not worth performing.
Corneal light reflex	⇑	Important bedside test for corneal integrity.
Hirschberg's test	⇑	Important test for ocular misalignment; direct extension of corneal light reflex.

Tear Film

40. What is Schirmer's test?

Schirmer's test is a measurement of tear production. It can be used to assess the dry eyes of patients with keratoconjunctivitis sicca or Sjögren's syndrome, an autoimmune disorder consisting of dry eyes and dry mouth and often accompanied by other autoimmune disorders.

41. How is Schirmer's test performed?

After anesthetizing the eyes with a topical anesthetic, the examiner inserts a small strip of filter paper in the recess of the lower lid (the fornix). The strip should be placed either medially or laterally, not in the center of the eye. The strip is removed after 5 minutes, and the wetting produced by the tears is measured in millimeters. Normal distances are 15 mm (below the age of 40) and 10 mm (above the age of 40). A distance less than 5 mm is usually diagnostic of decreased tear production, whereas a distance between 5 and 10 mm is suspicious.

42. Who was Schirmer?

Otto W.A. Schirmer (1864–1917) was a German ophthalmologist.

Eyebrows

43. What is the significance of thinning or absence of the lateral eyebrows?

Thinning or absence of the lateral eyebrows is a traditional sign of hypothyroidism (often referred to as Queen Anne's sign from the name of a celebrity patient), but it also may be a normal variant of nonhypothyroid patients. In addition, thinning of the eyebrows also may represent personal cosmetic practices (such as plucking). Other etiologies include drugs, skin diseases, and lupus erythematosus.

Eyelids and Orbit

44. What are xanthelasmas?

Xanthelasmas (from the Greek *xanthos* = yellow and *elasma* = beaten metal plate) are yellowish fatty deposits localized over the eyelids. Most patients with xanthelasmas have no lipid abnormalities, but xanthelasmas are encountered in as many as 25% of patients with type III hyperlipoproteinemia and also may be seen in other more common types (such as types II and IV). Xanthelasmas can be removed surgically if they are a cosmetic problem.

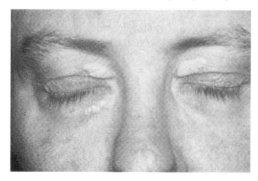

Patient with xanthelasma in all four lids. (From Tasman W, Jaeger EA: The Wills Eye Hospital Atlas of Clinical Ophthalmology. Philadelphia, Lippincott-Raven, 1996, with permission.)

45. What is an ectropion?

It is the eversion (i.e., outward rolling) of the lower eyelid, often encountered in elderly patients. This eversion exposes a rim of tarsal conjunctiva to external stimuli and may lead to eye irritation secondary to corneal exposure and keratinization of the exposed conjunctiva.

46. What is an entropion?

It is the inversion (i.e., inward rolling) of the lower eyelid. It is not uncommon in the elderly. It also may lead to mechanical irritation of the eye by contact with the eyelashes.

47. What is a stye?

It is a focal, acute, inflammatory process localized to one of the eyelid margin glands (e.g., hair follicle gland or meibomian gland). The classic findings are redness, swelling, tenderness, and sometimes a purulent discharge.

48. What is blepharitis?

It is a diffuse inflammatory process involving the margin of the eyelid, which may appear swollen and erythematous. Blepharitis is usually associated with *Staphylococcus aureus* or *Staphylococcus epidermidis* and also may have a hypersensitivity component. Crusting is usually present at the eyelid margin, with cuffing of the cilia; patients may complain of dry eyes.

49. What is ptosis?

Ptosis *(falling* in Greek) is the drooping of the upper eyelid; it may occur unilaterally or bilaterally.

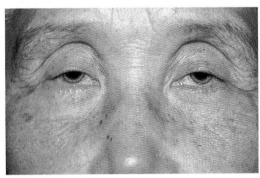

Involutional (aponeurotic) ptosis characteristically is mild to moderate with high lid creases. Levator function is usually normal. (From Tasman W, Jaeger EA: The Wills Eye Hospital Atlas of Clinical Ophthalmology. Philadelphia, Lippincott- Raven, 1996, with permission.)

50. What are the possible causes of ptosis? How can they be differentiated?

Common causes are (1) aging, (2) changes secondary to surgery or trauma, and (3) congenital ptosis. Less common causes include (1) myasthenia gravis, (2) Horner's syndrome, and (3) third-nerve palsy. The less common causes can be separated from the more common causes by identifying the associated clinical findings, such as change in pupillary size or weakness of other cranial nerves.

51. What is proptosis?

Proptosis (or exophthalmos) is the abnormal protrusion of one or both eyeballs (the Greek word *proptosis* indicates a falling forward). The limit for a normal protrusion varies between 19–24 mm, depending on race and sex. Unilateral exophthalmos is an asymmetry in prominence between the eyes of more than 2 mm.

52. What is the most common cause of exophthalmos in adults?

The most common cause of unilateral exophthalmos is thyroid ophthalmopathy (Graves' disease). The next most common cause is a space-occupying lesion (such as metastatic tumor or primary tumor, either benign or malignant). The most common cause of bilateral exophthalmos remains Graves' disease, followed by tumors.

53. What are the other ocular manifestations of thyroid ophthalmopathy?

• Eyelid retraction (thyroid stare)
• Upper lid lag on downgaze (von Graefe's sign)

- Conjunctival edema (chemosis) and hyperemia
- Infrequent blinking and proptosis (Stellwag's sign)
- Fine tremor of the gently closed eyelids (Rosenbach's sign)
- Failure of ocular convergence following close accommodation at a distance of 5 inches (Moebius' sign)
- Impairment of extraocular motility
- Corneal exposure with ulceration
- Optic nerve compression resulting in optic nerve edema and visual loss

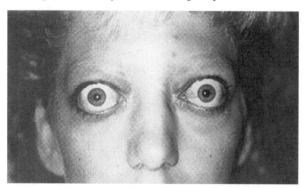

Thyroid-related ophthalmopathy with proptosis and lid retraction. (From Vander JF, Gault JA: Ophthalmology Secrets. Philadelphia, Hanley & Belfus, 1998, with permission.)

54. What is the most common cause of unilateral exophthalmos in children?

The most common cause is orbital cellulitis. The most common space-occupying lesion responsible for unilateral exophthalmos in children is rhabdomyosarcoma.

55. What is the difference between preseptal cellulitis and orbital cellulitis?

Preseptal cellulitis involves only the eyelids, which are erythematous and swollen. Therefore, the process violates neither the orbital septum nor the contents of the orbit. Patients with preseptal cellulitis do not appear systemically ill; vision, pupils, conjunctiva, and ocular motility are entirely normal.

Orbital cellulitis, on the other hand, is a medical emergency. It involves not only the eyelids but also the orbital contents. Patients with orbital cellulitis look systemically ill and have a host of symptoms and signs, including (1) pain on eye movement, (2) erythema and edema of the eyelids, (3) conjunctival injection and chemosis (swelling), (4) limitation of ocular motility on the affected side, (5) proptosis, (6) decreased vision, and, possibly, (7) an afferent pupillary defect.

56. What are the signs of a blow-out fracture?

A blow-out fracture is a fracture of the floor of the orbit (which is also the roof of the maxillary sinus). The inferior rectus muscle may become entrapped. In patients with blunt orbital trauma, therefore, the rim of the orbit should be palpated for step-offs or discontinuities. The surrounding soft tissue also should be palpated gently for subcutaneous crepitus, caused by air from the fractured sinus. Subconjunctival air bubbles sometimes may be seen with a penlight. Patients also should be tested for numbness on the side of the injury in the distribution of the fifth nerve; if numbness is present, it may indicate a fracture. With entrapment of the inferior rectus muscle, the patient will be unable to look up or will have diplopia on upgaze.

57. What is enophthalmos?

Enophthalmos is the opposite of exophthalmos (literally, a falling inward). The eye is sunken into the orbit rather than protruding from it. Enophthalmos may result from a large blow-out fracture.

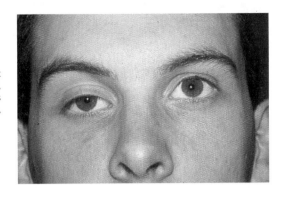

Pseudoptosis in a patient with a blow-out fracture of the right eye. (From Tasman W, Jaeger EA: The Wills Eye Hospital Atlas of Clinical Ophthalmology. Philadelphia, Lippincott- Raven, 1996, with permission.)

Extraocular Movements

58. How valuable is testing of extraocular movements?

Not very. Although no ocular examination is complete without this measurement, the yield is quite low (particularly if the patient has no complaints of double vision). Conversely, if an adult patient has a new ocular misalignment or complains of diplopia, such signs and symptoms may herald a serious illness. Hence, such patients merit prompt referral to the appropriate consultant. For strabismus and pseudostrabismus, see Corneal Light Reflex section on p 86.

Nystagmus

59. What is nystagmus?

It is a neurologic sign characterized by an abnormal, rhythmic movement of the extraocular muscles. The Greek word *nystagmos* literally means nodding. This nodding movement may take place on either the horizontal or vertical plane and includes both a quick and a slow phase.

60. What is the clinical significance of nystagmus?

It usually indicates dysfunction of one or more of three structures: (1) cerebellum, (2) vestibularis, or (3) oculomotor system. This dysfunction may be due to toxic-metabolic causes or an anatomic lesion. It also may be congenital.

61. What are the major types of nystagmus?

Nystagmus is usually classified on the basis of the direction of eye movement; the three varieties are horizontal, vertical, and rotatory. Physiologic nystagmus, on the other hand, represents the quick and slow eye movement that can be seen in travelers (typically train travelers) whose gaze is fixed on rapidly approaching objects (such as telephone poles). This eye response is normal and can be tested by having the patient gaze at a rapidly rotating drum covered with vertical stripes (optokinetic nystagmus).

Sclera

62. What are blue sclerae?

Blue sclerae are often the hallmark of osteogenesis imperfecta. Bluish sclerae, however, also may be seen in many other conditions, including (1) 7% of patients with anemia (87% of those with iron-deficiency anemia), (2) 3% of patients with Marfan's syndrome, and (3) 15% of patients with pseudo-pseudohypoparathyroidism. Finally, blue sclerae also may be encountered in normal people. For example, they are the norm, not the exception, in newborns and small children.

63. What bilirubin level is necessary to produce icteric sclerae?

It depends on the amount of natural light illuminating the patient's eyes. In bright daylight one can probably detect hyperbilirubinemia (icterus) of as little as 1.5–1.7 mg/dl. In artificial light, however, one probably can detect bilirubin levels of only ≥ 4 mg/dl. The same is true for other areas of the body normally checked for icterus, such as the roof of the palate or palm of the hands.

64. Does scleral icterus look any different in dark-skinned patients?

No. It is important, however, not to interpret as icterus the brownish color normally present in the bulbar conjunctiva of black patients. This finding is usually the result of exposure to sunlight and should not be confused with a sign of hyperbilirubinemia. To avoid this mistake, ask the patient to look upward and then inspect the inferior conjunctival recess, which should be entirely white in nonicteric patients.

Conjunctiva

65. What is a pinguecula?

It is a small, rounded, yellowish collection on the conjunctiva (from the Latin *pinguiculus* = fattish). This degenerative lesion of the bulbar conjunctiva is secondary to actinic exposure and is found nasal and sometimes temporal to the limbus in the interpalpebral space.

66. What is a pterygium?

Pterygium (from the Greek *pteros* = wing) is similar to the pingueculum in histology and etiology. A pterygium, however, extends from the conjunctiva onto the cornea. The pterygium may compromise vision if it continues to grow over the cornea and into the visual axis.

67. What is a subconjunctival hemorrhage?

It is a well-demarcated hemorrhage in the subconjunctival layer. Although it may be quite an impressive sight (and a common cause of red eye), a conjunctival hemorrhage remains a relatively trivial problem, destined to yellow over a few days and eventually resolve. The redness from a subconjunctival hemorrhage is confluent and thus can be distinguished from other causes of a red eye.

68. What are the common causes of a subconjunctival hemorrhage?

The most common, of course, is trauma. Hemorrhages also may result from a sudden increase in venous pressure (as after a paroxysm of coughing). In many cases, however, subconjunctival hemorrhages occur without a clear-cut predisposing factor, reflecting fragility of the vessel wall (as may result from aging or diabetes) or a defect in hemostasis.

69. What does the conjunctiva look like in conjunctivitis?

Both scleral and palpebral conjunctivae appear inflamed. The palpebral conjunctiva lines the eyelid. Typical signs include (1) redness, (2) discharge, and (3) conjunctival edema. Patients report discomfort (but never true pain), usually scratchy with a feeling of sand in the eye.

70. What is the significance of a palpable preauricular node?

Viral conjunctivitis often is accompanied by a tender, palpable preauricular node. If enlarged, this lymph node can be palpated just anterior to the tragus of the ear.

71. How can the character of the conjunctival discharge help to differentiate causes of conjunctivitis?

Bacterial conjunctivitis has a purulent or mucopurulent discharge, whereas viral and chemical conjunctivitides have a watery discharge. Allergic conjunctivitis is often accompanied by a stringy, white discharge.

72. How can one differentiate the injected vessels of uveitis from the injected vessels of conjunctivitis?

Uveitis is associated not with discharge from the eye (which is always present in conjunctivitis) but instead with prominence of the vessels around the cornea (at the limbus). Such circumcorneal injected vessels suggest a diagnosis of anterior uveitis (i.e., iritis). In addition, patients with uveitis complain of photophobia and a deep, aching pain.

73. What is chemosis?

Chemosis is edema of the bulbar conjunctiva. The conjunctiva is visibly swollen, at times even protruding anteriorly and encroaching on the cornea. The word comes from the Greek *chemos*, which means not only yawning but also cockle. The opening of affected eyes is reduced to a slit, like the gaping shell of a cockle. Chemosis is typically seen in patients with allergic conjunctivitis.

Iris

74. What is iris heterochromia?

Iris heterochromia is characterized by a difference in pigmentation between the irises of the two eyes (from the Greek *eteros* = different and *chroma* = color). In congenital Horner's syndrome, the affected iris is lighter, whereas in acquired Horner's syndrome heterochromia is rare. Other causes of heterochromia include a ferrous intraocular foreign body, which causes the affected iris to appear darker, and various ophthalmic conditions beyond the scope of this text.

Cornea

75. What is arcus senilis?

Arcus senilis is corneal stromal lipid deposition near the limbus, the interface between cornea and sclera. It appears as a whitish line in the peripheral cornea, which usually starts as an arc (hence the name) and eventually grows into a complete ring, fully encircling the limbus, with a clear zone between the arcus and the limbus.

76. What is the clinical significance of arcus senilis?

Probably not great. Traditional teaching suggests that an arcus senilis should be considered a sign of underlying atherosclerotic cardiovascular disease. This conclusion, however, has not been supported by epidemiologic data. The prevalence of arcus senilis increases with age and probably is not of pathologic significance in people over the age of 40.

Pearl. An arcus should be considered the result of the normal aging process. Therefore, it should be absent in the young and quite common in the elderly.

Anterior Portion of the Globe

77. What is uveitis?

Both uveitis and iritis are commonly used to describe inflammatory processes affecting the eye's middle coat (from the Greek *uvea* = grape). When the outer coat of the eye (i.e., the sclera) is peeled away, the middle or vascular coat appears as a dark and grapelike layer.

78. What is ciliary flush?

It is the result of inflammation of the ciliary body, a part of the uveal coat of the eye. The ciliary body encircles the limbus, and when it is inflamed, the overlying conjunctiva also is inflamed. This circumcorneal erythema is called ciliary flush and helps to distinguish a red eye caused by uveitis from the more diffuse redness associated with conjunctivitis.

79. What are the other distinguishing features of uveitis?

Patients with uveitis are not only much more uncomfortable than patients with conjunctivitis but also so photophobic as to wear dark glasses at all times, even in the examining room. Often the pupil of the affected eye is smaller and the intraocular pressure lower. A helpful sign is that pain from uveitis (often described as a deep ache) is not relieved by a topical anesthetic, whereas discomfort from external eye problems, such as conjunctivitis, is relieved. In addition, conjunctivitis is always associated with a discharge, whereas with uveitis no discharge is present.

80. What is a hypopyon?

It is the accumulation of white cells (in Greek *pyon* = pus) in the dependent portion (in Greek *upo* = lower) of the anterior chamber. When a penlight is shined tangentially over the eye, the accumulation appears as a white layer in the inferior portion of the anterior chamber. Hypopyons may be seen in both infectious (such as endophthalmitis after cataract surgery) and noninfectious inflammatory processes (such as Behçet's disease).

81. What is a hyphema?

A hyphema (from the Greek *hyphaimos* = suffused with blood) is blood in the anterior chamber, typically from trauma. When bleeding is significant, the blood can be seen with a penlight as a dark red layer in the inferior portion of the anterior chamber.

82. What is an eight-ball hyphema?

An eight-ball hyphema is a hyphema that entirely fills the anterior chamber so that the eye appears black like an eight-ball. Often such hyphemas do not clear with conservative management and require surgical evacuation.

83. What are the eye findings in acute or angle closure glaucoma?

Patients with acute (angle closure) glaucoma have a red eye, decreased vision in the affected eye, a cloudy cornea with an irregular corneal light reflex, and a pupil that is mid-dilated and unresponsive. All of these findings are due to an extremely high intraocular pressure, causing the globe to feel rock-hard on palpation. The mid-dilated, unresponsive pupil is an important sign.

Pearl. A briskly reactive pupil usually excludes the diagnosis of acute angle closure glaucoma.

84. What is the value of gauging the anterior chamber with a penlight?

Little. This procedure is extremely inaccurate. The anatomic predisposition for acute angle closure glaucoma in the United States is rare; in general, it is safe to dilate patients who need to be dilated.

Corneal Light Reflex

85. What is the corneal light reflex?

When a penlight is shined on an eye, the light is reflected off the cornea as a bright, crisp, round reflex. If the surface of the cornea is not smooth, whether from scarring, corneal drying, or corneal edema, the light reflex appears irregular or broken up.

86. What is the Hirschberg test?

This bedside test was devised by Leonard K. Hirschberg (a Baltimore neurologist) as a way of assessing ocular misalignment. It is carried out by measuring the degree by which the corneal light reflex is deviated from the center of the pupil in the nonfixating (turned) eye.

87. What is pseudostrabismus?

In pseudostrabismus the eyes appear to be misaligned, whereas in reality they are straight. It differs from strabismus, a condition in which the eyes are not straight but truly misaligned. Pseudostrabismus is usually due to a prominent epicanthal skin fold that obscures part of the nasal sclera and makes the eyes appear to be turned in. In pseudostrabismus the corneal light reflex is centered in both eyes (Hirschberg test).

OPHTHALMOSCOPY

CONVENTIONAL TEACHING WATCH

Ophthalmoscopy is a fundamental skill. Practice, as always, is the key to success.

EYE LESIONS/FINDINGS		CONVENTIONAL TEACHING REVISITED
Abnormal red reflex	⇑	Important bedside maneuver for identification of abnormalities in light-transmitting media of eye.
Cataracts	⇑	Too common not to receive high importance.
Leukocoria	⇑	Important to recognize, particularly in children.
Disruption of corneal epithelium	⇑	Newer ophthalmoscopes have cobalt blue filter. When used on high magnification and with fluorescein, corneal abrasions can be visualized with this light.
Ciliary flush	⇑	Important sign in diagnosis of uveitis and differential diagnosis of red eye.
Anisocoria in iritis	⇑	Patients with iritis may be so photophobic that it is difficult to compare pupil size.
Angle closure glaucoma	⇑	Always consider angle closure glaucoma in patients with headache, nausea, vomiting, and red eye.
Open angle glaucoma	⇑	It is extremely important to know patients with open angle glaucoma are asymptomatic until it is too late. Screening for glaucoma by caregiver competent in evaluating optic discs is essential.
Schiotz tonometry	⇓	Of questionable utility; often inaccurate and provides misleading results. Patients who need intraocular pressure monitoring should be referred to ophthalmologist.
Optic disc	⇑	It is essential to detect pathologic changes in color, cup, and size of disc.
Fundus in papilledema	⇑	Essential that all practicing physicians can recognize.
Retinal microaneurysms	⇑	Important retinal lesions.
Retinal exudates	⇑	As above.
Retinal hemorrhages	⇑	As above.
Retinal black-colored spots	⇔	Nice to know but difficult to see.
Drusen	⇑	Earliest feature of age-related macular degeneration.
Hollenhorst plaques	⇑	Misnomer (more an embolus than a plaque) but important clue to severe generalized atherosclerosis.
Retinal venous pulsations (spontaneous)	⇑	Important when present, less important when absent.
Hypertensive retinopathy (four stages)	⇔	Nice to know; much less important now that hypertension can be treated.
Arteriovenous nicking (crossing defect)	⇔	Nice to recognize, but prevention is much more important (through treatment of underlying hypertension).
Retinitis pigmentosa	⇔	Important but cannot be seen with direct ophthalmoscopy.
Retinal detachment	⇔	One can appreciate loss of red reflex but cannot see retinal detachment with direct ophthalmoscopy.
Choroidal melanomas and benign choroidal nevi	⇓	Nice to know but rare and difficult to see with direct ophthalmoscopy.
Red eye	⇑	Important to be familiar with its bedside evaluation and differential diagnosis.

Technique

88. What is the clinical value of ophthalmoscopy?

Tremendous. When properly used, ophthalmoscopy provides outstanding information about the various structures of the ocular fundus, such as (1) the anterior end of the optic nerve (optic disc) and (2) the retina and its blood supply (retinal vessels and choroid). Ophthalmoscopy also helps to evaluate the red reflex and thus provides information about all clear media of the eye, such as (1) the cornea, (2) anterior chamber, (3) lens, and (4) vitreous.

89. Who should undergo ophthalmoscopy? When?

All comprehensive examinations should include ophthalmoscopy. Particular attention, however, should be given to (1) all patients complaining of altered vision; (2) patients older than 40 (because of the higher incidence of glaucoma with age); (3) patients suffering from neurologic disorders that may lead to increased intracranial pressure; and (4) patients with systemic diseases (such as diabetes and hypertension) which may be associated with vascular degeneration.

90. How does one perform ophthalmoscopy?

Ideally, the room lights should be dimmed and the patient's pupils dilated (see below). Glasses should be removed, whereas contacts may stay in place. Similarly, if the examiner wears glasses, they also should be removed (contacts may stay in place). The examiner asks the patient to fix his or her eyes straight ahead, usually gazing at a light as a reference point (fixation light), and then approaches the patient's eyes from the temporal side (never from the front). This approach is necessary to avoid direct (and painful) stimulation of the macula. The examiner then should look into the patient's right eye, using his or her right eye and holding the ophthalmoscope in the right hand. Afterward the examiner should hold the ophthalmoscope in the left hand and look into the patient's left eye, using his or her left eye.

91. How close should one get to the patient?

One should start 2–3 feet away from the eye so that the red reflex can be visualized and any abnormalities of the clear media of the eye identified. For a proper viewing of the eyeground, however, one should follow the law of Robert Capa, the famous World War II photographer who said that "if a picture is not good enough, it is because you did not get close enough." Thus, to see the fundus adequately, you should get as close to the patient as possible (in other words, if you are not uncomfortably close, you are not close enough).

As a measure of proximity, you should place your hand on the patient's forehead and then place your head on your hand. While you do so, your index finger should be on the focusing dial of your ophthalmoscope, and the knob should be actively turned until any part of the retina is in focus. At that point, you should follow the vessels inward (using the natural "arrows" formed by their bifurcations) until you can see them merge into the optic disc. At this point, refocusing becomes necessary. From the optic disc, you should explore the four quadrants of the eyeground (superior temporal, superior nasal, inferior nasal, and inferior temporal). Finally, you should examine the macula.

Pearl. *Ophthalmoscopy is a dynamic process, requiring the examiner to be continuously refocusing and repositioning the ophthalmoscope to find whatever part of the fundus is sought.*

92. What is the best way to examine the macula?

Traditionally the patient is asked to look into the light. This technique, however, is not only quite painful (it causes intense photophobia) but also quite wrong. In fact, the glare from the cornea is so bright that it is impossible to inspect the macula properly. One should approach the macula from the disc by rotating the ophthalmoscope temporally a few degrees. Because the macula is light-sensitive (and its inspection is always a bit painful), this exam should be done last and quickly.

93. How can one dilate the pupils pharmacologically?

The two most commonly used mydriatics are Mydriacyl ophthalmic (tropicamide), 0.5% or 1%, and Neo-Synephrine ophthalmic (phenylephrine), 2.5% or 10%. The 10% phenylephrine is no longer commonly used because of possible systemic side effects.

94. Do mydriatic drugs have systemic effects?

Both mydriatic drugs are absorbed systemically. Thus, systemic responses may be noted. Hypertension, for example, has been described after use of phenylephrine, an alpha$_1$-adrenergic agonist. If concerned about a cardiovascular reaction, one should use tropicamide (a short-acting antimuscarinic agent).

95. Are there any local contraindications to dilation of the pupils?

Very few. The most important *absolute* contraindication is the need to monitor pupillary signs in patients with suspected neurologic disease or trauma. Another contraindication is the presence of an old intraocular lens implant in patients who have undergone cataract extraction (such implants, no longer used, were supported by the iris and thus tended to dislocate after pharmacologic mydriasis). A *relative* contraindication is narrow angle glaucoma. Paradoxically, the precipitation of an attack of acute angle closure glaucoma may be beneficial to the patient. Indeed, precipitating an attack in a previously undiagnosed patients unmasks an important and treatable condition.

Red Reflex

96. What is the red reflex?

The red reflex represents light that is reflected from the retina (red because of the rich retinal vascular supply). It looks much like the red eye effect commonly seen in flash photography. The red reflex is important clinically because it signifies the transparency of all light-transmitting media of the eye.

97. How is the red reflex viewed?

Through an ophthalmoscope by using a plus lens (high plus, black or green). One should look at the pupil from a distance of at least 1 foot, focusing the ophthalmoscope until a bright red pupil is clearly visualized.

98. What is leukocoria?

Leukocoria literally means white pupil (in Greek *leukos* = white and *core* = pupils) and indicates total loss of the red reflex. Leukocoria in children is a cause of concern, usually indicating a serious underlying condition, such as retinoblastoma. Other causes of leukocoria in children include cataract, severe intraocular inflammation, retinopathy of prematurity, and other congenital lesions. Leukocoria is also seen in patients with retinal detachment. Its detection should prompt immediate referral to an ophthalmologist.

99. What common conditions may cause an abnormal red reflex?

Any condition that causes an opacity in one of the clear light-transmitting media of the eye also produces an irregular or partially darkened red reflex by projecting its shadow as a black silhouette. The most common opacities affect the anterior eye structures (such as opacities of the lens and cornea). Posterior eye opacities are much less common.

Anterior Eye Structures

100. Which are the most common opacities of the anterior eye?

Lenticular opacities, such as cataracts, are much more common than corneal opacities, such as corneal scars or abrasions. Cataracts are particularly common in the elderly.

101. What is a cataract?

Any opacity of the lens.

Posterior Eye Structures

102. What is the posterior cavity of the eye?

Behind the lens and iris is a large posterior cavity. This cavity is filled primarily with vitreous, a clear, gel-like substance consisting of hyaluronic acid, collagen, and water.

103. What are the most common opacities of the vitreous?

Hemorrhages. A vitreous hemorrhage usually results from proliferative retinopathy (e.g., diabetes, sickle cell disease, or retinopathy of prematurity) or tearing of a retinal vessel. It may appear acutely and be either massive (totally obliterating the red reflex) or subtle (consisting of only a few erythrocytes, presenting as "floaters" in the vitreous gel). A vitreous hemorrhage is a reason for immediate referral to an ophthalmologist because it may accompany serious disorders, such as retinal detachment.

104. After visualization of the red reflex, which eye structures should be examined?

The optic disc, retinal blood vessels, retinal background, and macula.

Optic Disc

105. What is the optic disc?

The optic disc (or nerve head) is the point at which the axons of the retinal ganglion cells form the optic nerve.

106. How does one find the optic disc?

By approaching the patient's eye closely and focusing the ophthalmoscope. The examiner should then focus on the retina and follow its blood vessels toward the optic disc. Refocusing is necessary throughout. It also may be necessary to rotate the ophthalmoscope slightly around its vertical axis to find the disc.

107. In following the blood vessels toward the disc, how does one know that the direction is right?

If the caliber of the vessels increases. Another way is to follow the "arrowheads" formed by the bifurcations of the retinal vessels.

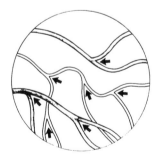

108. What does a normal optic disc look like?

It has an oval contour, sharp margins, and a yellowish-pinkish color.

109. Are there any normal optic disc variants?

There are several normal variants. Some people may have a hypopigmented crescent surrounding the optic disc (particularly in its temporal side, as commonly encountered in myopic patients). This crescent is caused by the failure of the eyeground's pigmented layers (i.e., retina and choroid) to reach the optic disc margins. Other people may have an excess of pigment, which usually appears as a hyperpigmented rim surrounding the optic discs.

110. What is the optic cup?
It is the whitish central excavation of the disc. It is also the site where the retinal vessels enter and exit the eye. Located in the center of the disc, this physiologic cup should constitute about 30% or less of the total disc diameter; it should not exceed more than 50% horizontally.

111. What pathologic changes can be detected in the optic disc?
Pathologic changes may involve (1) the color of the disc (either pallor or hyperemia); (2) the size of the cup (i.e., cupping, as in glaucoma); (3) the elevation of the disc (papilledema or papillitis); and (4) the presence or absence of retinal venous pulsations.

Changes in Color

112. What causes redness of the disc?
Vascular engorgement, such as in retinal vein occlusion, papilledema, or polycythemia. Redness also may result from neovascularization of the disc.

113. What causes pallor of the disc?
It usually results from death of the axons of the retinal ganglion cells. The paleness is caused by the loss of the supplying blood vessels, no longer needed after the axons have died.

114. Should everyone with pallor of the disc be considered as having disc atrophy until proved otherwise?
Not at all. Paleness (or even whitening) of the disc often represents a normal variant, particularly in myopic people.
Pearl. A diagnosis of disc atrophy should be based not only on the presence of pallor but also on loss of function (decreased visual acuity, visual field defect, dyschromatopsia, or afferent pupillary defect).

115. What are the common causes of optic atrophy?
Any condition causing damage to the retina, optic disc, optic nerve, optic chiasm, or optic tracts may lead to optic atrophy. Examples include (1) previous optic neuritis (such as that encountered in patients with multiple sclerosis); (2) previous ischemic optic neuropathy (e.g., from temporal arteritis); (3) compression of the nerve by a mass (tumor, meningioma, or aneurysm); and (4) toxicity from drugs or toxins (e.g., ethambutol, ethylene gycol, methanol).

Changes in Cup Size

116. What is the aqueous humor?
It is the fluid produced by the ciliary body. This fluid normally flows through the pupil, bathes the anterior chamber, and from there drains into the venous system via the trabecular meshwork and Schlemm's canal.

117. Under normal conditions, does the aqueous humor produce intraocular pressure?
Yes. Because drainage of the aqueous is usually a bit slower than its production, intraocular pressure on the order of 21 mmHg or less is normally present.

118. What is glaucoma?
A disease characterized by an excessive increase in intraocular pressure due to poor drainage of the aqueous humor at the level of the trabecular meshwork. The increase in intraocular pressure leads to loss of neuronal tissue at the optic disc and corresponding loss of vision.

119. What does glaucoma mean?

The word *glaucoma* was first introduced in reference to the shining of the eyegrounds of patients blinded by the disease (*glaukos* = sparkling in Greek) as opposed to the opacity of the eyegrounds of patients blinded by cataracts who therefore have lost their red reflex.

120. What are the symptoms of open angle glaucoma?

None. In open angle glaucoma (the more common, nonacute variety and also the vast majority of glaucoma seen in the United States) there are no symptoms. Thus it is so important to screen patients for glaucoma. In open angle glaucoma the increase in intraocular pressure is quite insidious. The first visual changes affect peripheral vision; central vision usually remains preserved until the very end. Thus, although visual fields are affected by glaucoma, visual acuity is not. Because of its insidious nature, open angle glaucoma remains the number one treatable cause of blindness in the United States.

Pearl. A thorough funduscopic exam (coupled with intraocular pressure measurement and possibly visual field testing) is the only way to ensure an early diagnosis.

121. What are the symptoms of acute angle closure glaucoma?

Acute angle closure glaucoma (in which the trabeculum becomes suddenly occluded by the iris) is associated with a rapid build-up in intraocular pressure, which leads to a dramatic clinical presentation: pain, nausea, abnormal visual acuity, and a red, teary eye. The cornea is usually hazy (due to corneal edema), with injection of the surrounding deep conjunctival and episcleral vessels (ciliary flush). The pupil is mid-dilated and unreactive. If the pupil is reactive, it is *not* an attack of angle closure glaucoma.

Pearl. The visual complaint of the appearance of halos (rainbow-colored fringes around points of light), caused by corneal edema, is an important symptom for the diagnosis of acute glaucoma.

122. How does the optic disc look in glaucoma?

Glaucomatous discs have an abnormally increased cup-to-disc ratio, a phenomenon commonly referred to as **cupping**. The cup is usually enlarged in a vertical or oblique direction, and asymmetry between the two eyes is common.

Pearl. An optic cup ≥ 50% of the entire disc diameter should be considered suspicious for glaucoma until proved otherwise. A cup > 70% strongly suggests the diagnosis of glaucoma.

123. Are there any other funduscopic findings in glaucoma?

Splinter hemorrhages on the optic disc margin are highly suggestive of glaucomatous damage. The hemorrhages may be one of the earliest signs of glaucoma before significant cupping. It is estimated that up to one-third of patients with glaucoma have splinter hemorrhages of the optic disc at some point during the course of the disease.

124. How accurate is the funduscopic exam in diagnosing glaucoma?

It depends on the examiner's skills. Studies have shown sensitivities and specificities that vary, respectively, between 48% and 89% and between 73% and 93%. The American Academy of Ophthalmology recommends that patients should be screened by an ophthalmologist for glaucoma according to the following guidelines: age 65 or older, every 1–2 years; age 40–64, every 2–4 years; age 20–39 (African-Americans), every 3–5 years (because glaucoma has a higher incidence and earlier onset in this population). Others should be screened less frequently.

125. What is the utility of Schiotz tonometry?

Questionable. Schiotz tonometry has been advocated as the nonophthalmologist's method to measure intraocular pressure. Yet it is often inaccurate and may provide misleading results.

Pearl. Patients who need intraocular pressure monitoring should be referred to an ophthalmologist.

Changes in Disc Size

126. What is papilledema?

Papilledema is the swelling (edema) of the head of the optic nerve (i.e., disc or papilla) in the setting of increased intracranial pressure. The finding of papilledema often is associated with brain tumors and therefore should set into motion a set of neurodiagnostic procedures.

127. What are the funduscopic findings of papilledema?

The funduscopic findings of papilledema are by definition bilateral. The earliest findings are (1) blurred disc margins, (2) swelling of the disc without loss of physiologic cupping, and (3) loss of spontaneous retinal venous pulsations. Later findings include (4) disc hyperemia, (5) engorgement of retinal veins, and (6) peripapillary hemorrhages (splinter hemorrhages surrounding the papilla) and cotton-wool spots (nerve fiber layer infarcts). As disc edema progresses, the disc appears enlarged, and circumferential retinal folds (Paton's lines) may be seen in the retina around the swollen disc.

Papilledema in a 24-year-old obese woman with pseudotomor cerebri. The patient complained of severe headaches and transient visual obscurations. (From Tasman W, Jaeger EA: The Wills Eye Hospital Atlas of Clinical Ophthalmology. Philadelphia, Lippincott-Raven, 1996, with permission.)

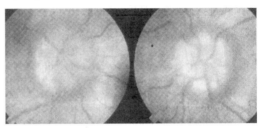

128. What are spontaneous retinal venous pulsations (SRVPs)?

SRVPs are the visible collapse and refilling of the largest branches of the central retinal vein (in the retina veins, *not* arteries, pulsate). SRVPs usually are detected at the point at which the vessels emerge from the cup and cross the disc. They occur in synchrony with the arterial pulse and are never seen beyond the central optic disc.

129. What is the clinical significance of absent SRVPs?

Not much. SRVPs are absent in 20% of normal people. Thus, their absence does not represent a significant negative finding. Presence of SRVPs, on the other hand, is much more helpful: it suggests that the patient's intracranial pressure (ICP) is *not* pathologically elevated. SRVPs cease whenever the ICP goes above 200 ± 25 mmH$_2$O. Thus, in a patient with blurred optic disc margins (in whom papilledema is considered in the differential diagnosis), presence of SRVPs indicates that ICP is probably normal.

Pearl. *As opposed to papilledema (which may take as long as 24–48 hours to develop after a rise in ICP, SRVPs can disappear in a matter of seconds (and return just as quickly after prompt management of increased ICP).*

130. Is there any loss of visual activity in papilledema?

No. Visual acuity is usually well preserved, unless the papilledema is long-standing.

131. What is the clinical significance of papilledema?

Papilledema is one of the most dramatic and important funduscopic findings. It reflects conditions that are both life- and vision-threatening. As such, it should be identified by all practicing physicians.

132. What are the most common causes of papilledema?

Conditions associated with increased ICP, such as tumors, abscesses, meningitis, hematomas, subarachnoid or intracranial hemorrhages, and pseudotumor cerebri (idiopathic intracranial hypertension).

133. What other conditions may make the optic disc appear swollen?

Many entities cause the optic disc to swell without a concomitant increase in ICP. Swollen discs may be congenital (anomalous discs); due to local eye disease (e.g., central retinal vein occlusion); metabolic (e.g., thyroid eye disease); inflammatory; infiltrative (e.g., secondary to lymphoma); due to systemic diseases (e.g., malignant hypertension); or due to local vascular problems (e.g., ischemic optic neuropathy).

134. What is papillitis?

Papillitis is inflammation and swelling of the optic disc unassociated with increased ICP. Unlike papilledema, the chief complaint of papillitis is unilateral acute loss of vision, accompanied by eye pain. The loss of vision is also accompanied by an afferent pupillary defect and an acquired defect in color vision.

135. What is optic neuritis?

Optic neuritis is a form of papillitis.

136. What is retrobulbar optic neuritis?

It is an inflammatory condition of the optic nerve in which the inflammation occurs behind the globe (retrobulbar). Retrobulbar optic neuritis is characterized by a scotoma (i.e., blind spot, from the Greek *skotos* = darkness) and has *no* visible optic disc findings (no disc swelling). As with other forms of optic neuritis, patients with the retrobulbar variant also exhibit impairment of color vision and an afferent pupillary defect.

137. What does optic neuritis look like funduscopically?

The disc usually looks much like the disc in papilledema. However, as stated above, optic neuritis is associated with an acute, unilateral, painful loss of vision and an afferent pupillary defect.

138. What is AION?

AION, or anterior ischemic optic neuropathy, is an infarction of the optic nerve head or disc. Patients with AION present with profound, sudden, and painless monocular loss of vision.

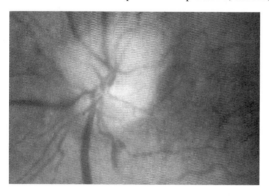

Superior segmental pale swelling of the optic disc in a patient with nonarteritic ischemic optic neuropathy. (From Tasman W, Jaeger EA: The Wills Eye Hospital Atlas of Clinical Ophthalmology. Philadelphia, Lippincott-Raven, 1996, with permission.)

139. Describe the eye exam of patients with AION.

AION is characterized by an afferent pupillary defect (i.e., Marcus Gunn pupil) on the affected side. Ophthalmoscopy reveals a pale, swollen optic nerve head. Dyschromatopsia also may be present.

140. What is an important cause of AION?

Giant cell arteritis, a granulomatous inflammation of medium-sized arteries that can result in blindness by causing AION.

Retinal Circulation

141. What is the normal organization of the retinal circulation?
The retinal circulation includes branches of the central retinal artery and central retinal vein. The arterial branches originate at the optic disc, move centrifugally toward the four retinal quadrants, and distribute themselves in the superficial nerve fiber layer. The venous branches are arranged similarly but follow an opposite direction, converging centripetally toward the optic disc. Because there is a blood-eye barrier, just as there is a blood-brain barrier, retinal vessels autoregulate flow in response to changes in blood pressure, just like vessels in the central nervous system.

142. How can one differentiate retinal veins from retinal arteries?
Retinal veins are larger (the normal vein-to-artery diameter ratio is 3:2) and darker. Retinal arteries, on the other hand, have a unique light reflex.

143. What is the light reflex?
A reflection of light typical of only retinal arteries. Normal retinal vessels have walls that are transparent. In fact, what is normally viewed on ophthalmoscopy is the column of blood contained within the transparent walls. This column is larger and darker in veins and smaller and brighter in arteries. Arteries also reflect the light that they receive. This bright light reflex is normally narrow, occupying about one-fourth of the diameter of the arterial column of blood.
   Pearl.   Changes in the width of the artery and its light reflex may occur as a result of chronic hypertension or as a normal part of arteriosclerosis with aging. As the hypertension becomes more chronic, the anterior walls progressively thicken. As they thicken, the walls reflect more light (increased light reflex), resembling at first copper wires and eventually silver wires.

144. What kind of changes affect the caliber of retinal vessels?
   • **Retinal veins** may become dilated, usually as a result of either obstruction (e.g., papilledema) or increased blood viscosity.
   • **Retinal arteries**, on the other hand, may become narrowed, usually as a result of chronic hypertension.

145. What is hypertensive retinopathy?
Hypertensive retinopathy indicates the visible changes in retinal vasculature and tissue as a result of hypertension. Many grading systems have been proposed, but as pharmacologic ability to alter the course of hypertension improves, the prognostic significance of the classifications has become less important than the efficacy and rapidity of treatment. Hypertensive retinopathy is divided into four phases:
   1. In the **vasoconstrictive phase**, the retinal blood vessels respond to increased blood pressure by autoregulating and increasing tone. This constriction is difficult to appreciate without photographs and usually occurs at the second or third branching point of the arteries (which may be difficult to view with a direct ophthalmoscope).
   2. In the **sclerotic phase**, if the blood pressure is not lowered, sclerotic changes occur in the arteries. These changes lead to narrowing, arteriovenous nicking, and alteration of the light reflex.
   3. In the **exudative phase**, insult to the vessel walls leads to a breakdown of the blood-eye barrier, flame hemorrhages, hard exudates, and cotton-wool spots. This phase may accompany or follow the other two phases.
   4. **Complications of the sclerotic phase** include central retinal artery occlusion (CRAO), branch retinal artery occlusion (BRAO), central retinal vein occlusion (CRVO), and branch retinal vein occlusion (BRVO).

146. What is arteriovenous (AV) nicking?
AV nicking refers to an abnormal AV crossing, characterized by narrowing of a retinal vein at the point where the arteriole crosses it. As the changes progress, the vein may seem to be

deflected and to disappear on either side of the arteriole. When the nicking has reached the occlu-sive stage, the vein is dilated distal to the crossing; flame hemorrhages and hard exudates also are present.

147. What is the mechanism of AV nicking?

Retinal arterioles have walls that are thin and ophthalmoscopically transparent. As a result, a vein crossed by an artery may be seen up to the point of intersection. Chronic and moderate hy-pertension, however, induces thickening of the arteriolar wall, which, in turn, leads to compres-sion of the venule.

148. What is the clinical significance of AV nicking?

AV nicking indicates chronic, moderate hypertension. Statistically significant relationships have been observed between the degree of AV crossing changes and left ventricular hypertrophy. The condition of the blood vessels in the retina probably reflects the condition of the arterioles elsewhere in the body.

149. Does AV nicking revert with control of hypertension?

No. It is permanent. Thus, it provides valuable and indelible information about the patient's medical history. AV nicking also may help to understand the timing of a hypertensive disease. For example, because the changes usually take years to develop, a hypertensive patient presenting with renal failure but no AV nicking is more likely to have primary nephropathy with secondary hypertension than primary hypertension with secondary renal failure.

150. What are the funduscopic findings in central retinal artery occlusion?

CRAO causes profound, painless loss of vision in one eye. The fundus of the affected eye shows pallor and swelling of the retina with the exception of the macula, which appears cherry-red. This features is usually diagnostic and is due to the visualization of the normal choroidal cir-culation through the fovea. The affected eye also demonstrates an afferent pupillary defect.

151. What are the causes of CRAO?

The most common cause is an embolus from the carotid artery, although giant cell arteritis or other sources of embolization also may be responsible.

152. What are the funduscopic findings in central retinal vein occlusion?

CRVO also may cause an acute, painless loss of vision in one eye. Common fundus find-ings include (1) venous engorgement and dilation, (2) multiple intraretinal dot or flame hemor-rhages in all quadrants of the retina, (3) microaneurysms close to the retinal veins, (4) multiple cotton-wool spots, and (5) even optic disc edema.

153. What is malignant hypertension?

It is a condition related to severe and precipitous rise in blood pressure. Fibrinoid necrosis of the retinal blood vessels results and in turn leads to exudates, flame hemorrhages, cotton-wool spots, and swelling of the retina. When the optic disc also becomes swollen, the clinical picture is called malignant hypertension.

154. What is a Hollenhorst plaque?

A Hollenhorst plaque (or cholesterol embolus) is a bright, refractile arteriolar deposit. It is bright yellow, usually wedged at the bifurcation of a peripheral arteriole, often appearing larger than the vessel in which it sits. At times it may even be seen migrating down the vessel; report-edly, this migration may be facilitated by gently massaging the eyeball. All of these characteris-tics suggest that a Hollenhorst plaque does *not* represent a true retinal artery plaque but rather an arterial embolus originating from ulceration of an atheromatous plaque in a more proximal vessel (usually the internal carotid).

155. What is the clinical significance of a Hollenhorst plaque?

A Hollenhorst plaque is a sign of severe generalized atherosclerosis. Indeed, patients with a Hollenhorst plaque are much more likely to die of either stroke or myocardial infarction; their 10-year survival rate is one-half that of age-matched controls. In addition, Hollenhorst plaques may complicate as many as 14% of all carotid endarterectomies.

156. What causes CRVO?

Almost all CRVOs are caused by thrombosis of the central retinal vein at the level of the lamina cribrosa. Usually there is associated atherosclerotic and hypertensive disease, but hyperviscosity syndromes (e.g., blood dyscrasias and dysproteinemias) also may contribute to the formation of CRVO.

157. What are the findings in branch retinal vein occlusion (BRVO)?

Only the quadrant of the retina corresponding to the occluded vein demonstrates the findings of flame hemorrhages and cotton-wool spots; the vein distal to the occlusion is dilated and tortuous.

158. What causes BRVO?

BRVO is almost always caused by hypertension, as described in the section on hypertensive retinopathy.

159. What is retinal neovascularization?

It is the formation of new retinal vessels and is always abnormal. New vessels tend to occur around the disc but also may begin in the peripheral retina. They tend to be friable and may bleed into the vitreous.

160. What conditions cause neovascularization?

The most common cause is diabetes mellitus. In addition, other conditions that lead to retinal ischemia (such as hemoglobinopathies) also may cause neovascularization.

Retinal Background

161. What type of lesions can be seen in the retina?

Retinal lesions come in various types, sizes, and shapes. Color, however, is commonly used for classification. Thus, retinal lesions are divided into three groups: (1) light-colored spots, (2) red spots, and (3) dark-colored spots.

162. What is the significance of light-colored and red retinal lesions?

Exudates (light-colored lesions) and hemorrhages (red lesions) are always pathologic.

Light-colored Spots

163. What types of light-colored spots may be seen in the retina?

The four most common types are (1) cotton-wool spots, (2) hard exudates, (3) drusen, and (4) myelinated nerve fiber layer.

164. What are cotton-wool spots?

Cotton-wool spots (often misnamed soft exudates) appear as white, indistinct, opaque areas of the superficial (inner) retina. Because they are superficial, cotton-wool spots can obscure nearby vessels. They represent small retinal infarcts, all secondary to microvascular disease. These infarctions involve the nerve fiber layer of the retina and are caused by occlusion of the end-arteriole.

165. What conditions cause cotton-wool spots?

Usually, conditions that damage the retinal microvasculature, such as (1) diabetes, (2) hypertension, (3) leukemias/lymphomas, (4) collagen vascular diseases (e.g., systemic lupus erythematosus), (5) infections (including bacterial endocarditis and, rarely, cytomegalovirus retinitis in patients with AIDS), (6) increased intracranial pressure with papilledema, (7) microembolic disease, and (8) severe anemia. Cotton-wool spots are encountered in as many as one-third of all patients with hemoglobin concentrations lower than 7 gm/dl.

166. What are hard exudates?

Hard exudates are yellowish/whitish, well-demarcated retinal lesions. They are located deeper in the retina than cotton-wool spots. Hard exudates are the result of microvascular retinal disease. As opposed to cotton-wool spots, however, they are due not to microinfarcts but rather to leaky and damaged vessel walls. Leakage of serum residues and various lipid aggregates eventually leads to accumulation of lipoproteins in the middle retinal layers.

Pearl. *Soft and hard exudates always indicate an underlying pathologic process.*

167. What conditions cause hard exudates?

The same conditions that cause cotton-wool spots (i.e., processes affecting the retinal microvasculature). The most common are (1) diabetes and (2) hypertension.

168. What are drusen?

Drusen are discrete, round, yellowish deposits of subretinal pigment epithelium (RPE). They can be located in the macula or peripheral retina. The number of drusen increases with age, and drusen alone rarely cause a visual disturbance. They are the earliest feature of age-related macular degeneration.

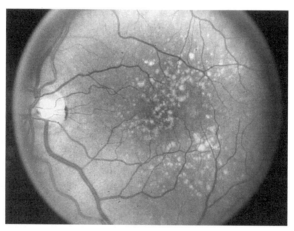

Drusen are the byproduct of retinal metabolism and manifest as focal yellow-white deposits deep to the retinal pigment epithelium. They serve as a marker of nonexudative age-related macular degeneration. (From Vander JF, Gault JA: Ophthalmology Secrets. Philadelphia, Hanley & Belfus, 1998, with permission.)

169. What are myelinated nerve fibers?

They are congenitally myelinated (i.e., medullated) nerve fibers. Normally, the optic nerve becomes myelinated as it leaves the lamina cribrosa, but occasionally patches of nerve fiber layer within the eye become myelinated. These myelinated fibers are a bright white color and variable in size; they have feathery borders and, because they are superficial, obscure blood vessels. They have no pathologic significance.

Red Spots

170. What are the most common red lesions of the retina?
1. Microaneurysms
2. Blot and dot hemorrhages
3. Flame and splinter hemorrhages
4. Preretinal hemorrhages, including subhyaloid hemorrhages

171. What causes retinal hemorrhages?
All are due to leaky and damaged retinal capillaries, such as may be encountered in chronic microvascular diseases such as diabetes.

172. What other lesions may be associated with red spots?
Light-colored spots are also common. They are usually hard exudates, particularly common in the perimacular area. Indeed, the damaged retinal vessels leak not only blood (responsible for red spots) but also serum (responsible for hard exudates).

173. Why do red lesions have different shapes and sizes?
Shape and size depend on the location of the hemorrhage:
- When the hemorrhage occurs in the **superficial nerve fiber layer** of the retina, it is parallel to the radial orientation of nerve fibers from the optic disc and assumes a linear shape (flame or splinter hemorrhage). Red lesions of this type are seen most commonly in hypertension.
- When the hemorrhage occurs in the **middle retinal layer**, it assumes a circular shape (dot and blot hemorrhage). Red lesions of this type are seen most commonly in diabetes mellitus.

174. What are microaneurysms?
Microaneurysms are small, round, well-demarcated, red dots representing saccular outpouchings of the retinal capillaries (from the Greek *aneurysma* = dilatation). They may be seen in association with other manifestations of microvascular disease (such as hard exudates; see question 172) and almost always are associated with diabetes mellitus.

175. Which processes are associated with dot and blot hemorrhages?
The most common cause is diabetes mellitus, but dot and blot hemorrhages also may be encountered in (1) severe hypertension, (2) collagen vascular diseases, (3) infections, and (4) various hematologic disorders (leukemias or severe anemia).

176. Which processes are associated with flame and splinter hemorrhages?
It depends on the location of the lesions. When localized around the disc, splinters and flames usually suggest a major ophthalmologic or neurologic emergency, such as (1) increased intracranial pressure and papilledema, (2) intracranial hemorrhage, or (3) poorly controlled glaucoma. When localized outside the disc, they usually carry the same differential diagnosis as dot and blot hemorrhages (although they are not as commonly linked to diabetes).

177. What are white-centered hemorrhages?
Red spots with white centers are often called Roth spots (even though Roth did not exactly describe them). They represent hemorrhages with a fibrinous (e.g., whitish and pale) center. White-centered hemorrhages are typical of endocarditis but also common in diabetes; they also may be seen in (1) intracranial hemorrhage, (2) leukemias, and (3) various infectious processes.

178. Who was Roth?
Moritz Roth was a Swiss pathologist, born in Basel in 1839, and a graduate of the University of Basel. He became professor of pathology in Basel, where, in addition to his retinal spots, he also became famous for a biography of the Renaissance pathologist Andreas Vesalius.

Dark-colored Spots

179. What are the most common pigmented retinal lesions?

The most common pigmented retinal lesions are (1) laser scars from treatment of proliferative diabetic retinopathy, (2) healed chorioretinitis, (3) retinitis pigmentosa, (4) retinal pigment epithelium hypertrophy, and (5) melanomas/benign choroidal nevi.

180. What is retinitis pigmentosa?

It is a degenerative disease of the retina. In the United States, 19% of all cases are autosomal dominant, 19% are autosomal recessive, 8% are X-linked, 46% are isolated, and 8% are undetermined. Only in a few cases is it secondary to a known disease process and thus treatable. An example is retinitis pigmentosa secondary to vitamin A deficiency.

181. What does retinitis pigmentosa look like ophthalmoscopically?

The retina is covered with aggregations of pigment, usually arranged in a bony spicule formation. The pigment, however, may not always be present. Indeed, in 10% of cases of retinitis pigmentosa there is no pigment at all. The bone spicules are usually in the midperipheral retina and are difficult to see with direct ophthalmoscopy.

182. What is retinal pigment epithelium hypertrophy?

This congenital "grouped" pigmentation results from hypertrophy of pigment cells in the retinal pigment epithelium (the same cells responsible for the red-orange color of the retinal background). The color of the normal retinal background is also the result of the blood and pigment of the choroid. Indeed, the darker fundus color of the pigmented races is produced by the increased choroidal pigment content of their fundi. Retinal pigment epithelium hypertrophy often is seen in patients with Gardner's syndrome, in which multiple bilateral pigmented lesions have a sensitivity of 78% and a specificity of 95%.

183. What does retinal pigment epithelium hypertrophy look like ophthalmoscopically?

The retina is covered with many (> 4) bilateral pigmented lesions of different sizes and shapes. These lesions are never larger than an optic disc and do not compromise vision. Their typical grouping resembles animal tracks (bear track lesions). The number of lesions is key to the diagnosis of retinal pigment epithelium hypertrophy; although normal people may have a few pigmented lesions, they never have more than four. Such lesions are usually in the peripheral retina and therefore may be difficult to see with direct ophthalmoscopy.

184. What are melanomas of the choroid and benign choroidal nevi?

Melanomas of the choroid are the most common malignancies of the eye. They appear as raised and highly pigmented lesions, which are often asymptomatic. **Benign choroidal nevi** consist of clumps of choroidal melanocytes, presenting ophthalmoscopically as flat, grayish/greenish pigmented lesions with indistinct borders. They do not compromise vision.

Diabetic Retinopathy

185. Is there any correlation between diabetic retinopathy and diabetic nephropathy?

The correlation is strong. Diabetic nephropathy (i.e., the glomerular disease of Kimmelstiel-Wilson) is almost always associated with diabetic retinopathy. Thus, absence of retinal disease in a patient with renal changes suggestive of diabetes should call into question the diagnosis of diabetic nephropathy. Conversely, a patient with diabetic retinopathy may not have glomerulopathy because diabetic retinopathy usually *precedes* diabetic nephropathy.

186. What are the findings in background diabetic nephropathy?

Background diabetic retinopathy consists of dot and blot hemorrhages, hard exudates, and cotton-wool spots. The hallmark of diabetic retinopathy, however, is the presence of microaneurysms.

Pearl. *Microaneurysms are so typical of diabetic retinopathy that the diagnosis should be considered until proved otherwise. Conversely, absence of microaneurysms calls into question a diagnosis of diabetic retinopathy, even in the presence of retinal hemorrhages and exudates.*

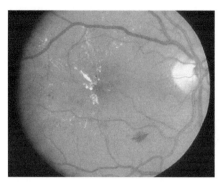

Background diabetic retinopathy with exudate, hemorrhages, and edema. (From Vander JF, Gault JA: Ophthalmology Secrets. Philadelphia, Hanley & Belfus, 1998, with permission.)

187. What is proliferative diabetic retinopathy (PDR)?

PDR is the most advanced stage of diabetic retinopathy. It is characterized by proliferation of new vessels over the optic disc and/or retina. These new vessels (neovascularization) appear tiny and irregular, often with a fibrous component. They may develop rapidly, even within 1 year after the initial appearance of an isolated cotton-wool spot. New vessels not only lead to preretinal or vitreous hemorrhages but also cause traction retinal detachments. Patients with PDR are candidates for photocoagulation. Patients with diabetes should be referred at least yearly for ophthalmologic evaluation.

Retinal Detachment

188. What is retinal detachment?

It is the shearing of the retina into two layers: (1) an outer layer (composed of the retinal pigment epithelium) and (2) an inner layer (i.e., the sensory retina). Embryologically, there is a potential space between the two layers, which may become separated under certain circumstances, resulting in retinal detachment.

189. What are the causes of retinal detachment?

- The most common cause is a degenerative tear in the retina, which, in turn, allows the entry of fluid from the vitreous cavity and subsequent dissection of the retina into two layers.
- The second most common cause is mechanical traction on the retina, as in the eyes of diabetics with PDR. The contracting neovascular membranes pull the retina away from the retinal pigment epithelium.

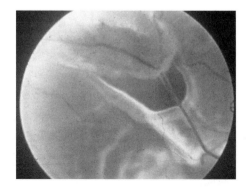

Horseshoe retinal tear with a bridging vessel. (From Vander JF, Gault JA: Ophthalmology Secrets. Philadelphia, Hanley & Belfus, 1998, with permission.)

190. Who is at risk for retinal detachment?

Usually middle-aged patients (peak incidence: 55–65 years), particularly if they are severely myopic. Retinal detachment, however, may occur at any age.

191. What are the most common complaints in patients with retinal detachment?

The initial complaint is usually the sudden appearance of floaters, or opacities that float in the vitreous of the affected eye. Each floater may represent a red cell released at the time of retinal tear or a condensation in the vitreous. Subsequently the patient reports flashes of light (i.e., phospheni, from the Greek *phos* = light and *phaino* = to show). These "shows of light" represent mechanical activation of the retinal sensory layer, stretched by traction from the vitreous. Finally, if the detachment progresses, the patient gradually experiences a curtain that obscures vision. The curtain may occur as early as a few hours or as late as a few weeks after the initial event.

192. What are the ophthalmoscopic findings in retinal detachment?

Loss of red reflex if the entire retina is detached. If only part of the retina is detached, the affected area appears whiter, with fine folds on its surface.

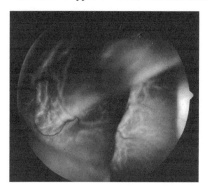

Bullous rhegmatogenous retinal detachment with mobile, corrugated appearance. (From Vander JF, Gault JA: Ophthalmology Secrets. Philadelphia, Hanley & Belfus, 1998, with permission.)

Macula

193. How does a normal macula look?

Like a little spot (indeed in Latin *macula* = little spot). The macula is temporal to the optic disc and approximately one-fourth of its size, darker than the surrounding retina (macular cells are taller and more heavily pigmented), with small vessels converging toward it (but not entering it), and with a little dipping in the center. This dipping is the fovea centralis. The central depression of the fovea may function as a concave mirror and thus reflect the light of the ophthalmoscope (foveal reflex). In some people the macula may even appear yellowish (macula lutea) because of the presence of a yellow retinal pigment.

194. What are the most common macular abnormalities?

In addition to specific lesions, such as macular degeneration, the macula should be examined carefully for the presence of microaneurysms and hard exudates.

195. What is macular degeneration?

Macular degeneration is the leading cause of severe visual loss in people over 50 years of age. The classic symptom of age-related macular degeneration is loss of central vision (which is concentrated in the macula) with preservation of peripheral vision. Thus, patients with macular degeneration cannot read but have normal ambulatory vision. Alternatively, patients may complain of metamorphopsia, a distortion in perceived shape of objects (from the Greek words *meta* = after, *morphe* = shape, and *opsis* = vision), or of micropsia, a reduction in perceived size of images (from the Greek words *micros* = small and *opsis* = vision).

196. How many types of macular degeneration are there?

There are two major types: (1) a dry form, characterized by drusen (see above) and degeneration of the retinal pigment epithelium but without choroidal neovascularization, and (2) a wet form, characterized by choroidal neovascularization.

197. How does macular degeneration look ophthalmoscopically?

Appearance may vary greatly. The **dry type** is associated with drusen, as precursors, and then pigmentary changes in the retinal pigment epithelium. Loss of pigment may be total, with prominent choroidal vessels showing through. The **wet type** is associated with thickening of the retinal pigment epithelium and a choroidal neovascular membrane, which appears as a gray-green area deep to the retina. Hemorrhage and exudates may emanate from the choroidal membrane, leading to a disciform scar in the macula.

RED EYE

198. What is a red eye?

It is a hyperemic and congested eye. Vascular congestion may be due to involvement of any of the major eye layers. Although a red eye is usually the result of trivial disorders, in a few cases it may herald serious and possibly vision-threatening conditions. Thus, a red eye should always be evaluated thoroughly.

199. What eye structures may be involved in a red eye?

All of the major eye layers, if involved, may produce a red eye. The most important are as follows:

1. **Conjunctiva.** Conjunctivitis, allergic, viral, or bacterial, is a common and usually benign cause of a red eye. The same is true for subconjunctival hemorrhage.

2. **Cornea.** Inflammation of the cornea or keratitis (from the Greek *keras* = horn or cornea) is also common but potentially a much more serious disorder.

3. **Episclera.** Episcleritis is inflammation of the connective tissue between the sclera and conjunctiva. It is a less common and usually benign condition.

4. **Sclera.** Inflammation of the sclera (scleritis) is also less common but more serious. It usually indicates an underlying systemic disease, such as connective tissue disease.

5. **Iris and ciliary body.** Acute iridocyclitis (from the Greek *irid* = iris and *kyklos* = circle or ciliary body) is inflammation of both the iris and ciliary body.

6. **Adnexal structures**, such as tear or sebaceous glands. Both dacryocystitis and styes are common disorders.

Pearl. In addition to the above conditions, a red eye should prompt consideration of acute glaucoma.

200. What other ocular signs may accompany a red eye?

The most important signs in patients with a red eye include the following:

1. **Ciliary flush** is the injection of the deep conjunctival and episcleral vessels that surround the cornea. When injected, these vessels remain indistinct enough to appear as a deep red ring encircling the cornea. Ciliary flush is a serious sign, probably indicating one of three disorders: (1) iridocyclitis, (2) acute glaucoma, or (3) keratitis. It is typically absent in more benign conditions, such as conjunctivitis.

2. **Corneal opacities** are always serious findings in patients with a red eye. Corneal opacities may be either localized (as in keratitis or corneal ulcers) or diffuse (as in acute glaucoma, in which the edema of the cornea creates a haze that obscures the iris). They also may result from cellular deposits on the cornea (as in iridocyclitis).

3. **Disruption of the corneal epithelium** usually results from trauma. Corneal abrasions are easily visualized under cobalt blue light and after application of fluorescein. Sometimes they can even be detected by noticing a distortion of the corneal light reflex.

4. **Anisocoria** is usually a sign of iridocyclitis. The pupil of the involved eye is smaller (because of a reflex constriction of the iris sphincter muscle) and may be distorted (because of inflammatory adhesions between the lens and iris).

5. **Proptosis** is usually a serious sign, indicating involvement of either the cavernous sinus or orbit.

6. **Eye discharge** is usually a benign finding, most commonly associated with a process such as conjunctivitis. A watery, clear discharge usually indicates viral conjunctivitis, whereas a purulent discharge suggests a bacterial etiology.

7. **Preauricular lymph node enlargement** is much more common in viral than in bacterial conjunctivitis (see under conjunctiva). Hence, it may provide a clue to the etiology of the conjunctivitis.

201. What other ocular symptoms may accompany a red eye?

Several symptoms may be present in patients with a red eye. Five important symptoms almost always indicate serious ocular emergencies:

1. **Blurred or reduced vision** is always absent in conjunctivitis but frequently present in disorders such as keratitis, iridocyclitis, or acute glaucoma. The key maneuver is to ask the patient to blink. An improvement in vision indicates the cleaning of inflammatory debris from the cornea (as in the case of conjunctivitis), whereas persistent blurring indicates a much more serious disorder.

2. **Pain** is always absent in conjunctivitis (in which patients usually complain of a scratchy, itchy feeling but never of pain) and common in three serious conditions associated with ciliary flush: keratitis, iridocyclitis, or acute glaucoma.

3. **Halos** are indicative of corneal edema, usually resulting from a sudden increase in intraocular pressure (as seen in acute glaucoma). Patients with this complaint describe a rainbow-like ring surrounding a point of light (i.e., the halo).

4. **Photophobia** is also absent in conjunctivitis but common in serious conditions such as iritis.

5. **Mid-dilated and unreactive pupil** is associated with acute angle closure glaucoma; the eye is red.

BIBLIOGRAPHY

1. Federman J, Gouras P, Schubert H, et al: Retina and vitreous. In Podos S, Yanoff M (eds): Textbook of Ophthalmology, vol. 9. St. Louis, Mosby, 1991.
2. Hitchings RA, Spaeth GL: The optic disc in glaucoma. II: Correlation of the appearance of the disc with the visual field. Br J Ophthalmol 61:107–113, 1977.
3. Hollenhorst RW: Significance of bright plaques in the retinal arterioles. Trans Am Ophthalmol Soc 59:252–273, 1961.
4. Pfaffenback DD, Hollenhorst RW: Morbidity and survivorship of patients with embolic cholesterol crystals in the ocular fundus. Am J Ophthalmol 75:372–375, 1973.
5. Traboulsi EI, Krush AJ, Gardner EJ, et al: Prevalence and importance of pigmented ocular fundus lesions in Gardner's syndrome. N Engl J Med 316:661–667, 1987.
6. Tso M, Abrams G, Jampol L: Hypertensive retinopathy, choroidopathy, and optic neuropathy: A clinical approach to classification. In Singerman L, Jampol L (eds): Retinal and Choroidal Manifestations of Systemic Disease. Baltimore, Williams & Wilkins, 1991.
7. Vander JF, Gault JA: Ophthalmology Secrets. Philadelphia, Hanley & Belfus, 1998.
8. Wood CM, Bosanquet RC: Limitations of direct ophthalmoscopy in screening for glaucoma. BMJ 294:1587–1588, 1987.

5. THE EAR

Katherine Worzala, M.D., M.P.H., and Dale Berg, M.D.

The ears should be kept perfectly clean; but it must never be done in company. It should never be done with a pin, and still less with the fingers, but always with an ear-picker.
St. John Baptiste de la Salle (1651–1719),
The Rules of Christian Manners and Civility, I

TOPICS COVERED IN THIS CHAPTER

Normal anatomy
Cerumen and its removal
Otoscopy
  Landmarks of the normal tympanic membrane
  Otoscopic features in pathology
    Purulent otitis media
    Serous otitis media
    Bulging of the tympanic membrane
    Perforation of the tympanic membrane
    Angel's sign
    Bullous myringitis
    Ramsay Hunt syndrome
    Cholesteatoma
    Otitis externa
    Pneumatic otoscopy

Otoscopy *(continued)*
  Auricle
    Normal anatomy
    Ecchymosis of the auricle
    Vesicles of the auricle
    Sturge-Weber syndrome
    Pre- and postauricular lymph
      nodes
    Battle's sign
    Auscultation of the auricle
Assessment of hearing loss
  Weber test
  Rinne test

CONVENTIONAL TEACHING WATCH

The ear is an important site for physical examination; abnormalities may reflect either local or systemic disease. It is also an extremely important sensory organ, the function of which can be assessed (albeit in a rudimentary manner) with basic bedside tools.

FINDING		CONVENTIONAL TEACHING REVISITED
Otoscopy	⇑	Still a valuable part of physical examination.
Hemotympanum	⇑	Important finding in assessment of head trauma.
Bullous myringitis	⇔	Not as specific for *Mycoplasma pneumoniae* as often reported.
Pneumatic otoscopy	⇔	More advanced; not necessarily part of the routine exam.
Auricular lesions	⇑	Wide array, some with systemic significance.
Pre- and postauricular lymph nodes	⇔	Useful to identify site of infection.
Earlobe creases	⇔	Probably not as valuable as initially reported.
Rinne and Weber tests	⇔ ⇔	Rudimentary, albeit still valuable tools for bedside interpretation of hearing loss.
Auscultation of the ear	⇔	Valuable, at times, in work-up of tinnitus.

OTOSCOPIC EXAMINATION

1. What is the best way to visualize the tympanic membrane effectively?

The examiner should grasp the superior aspect of the auricle and gently pull it posteriorly and superiorly. This maneuver reduces the curvature of the external canal, making it easier to introduce the speculum. It also may elicit pain, thereby alerting the clinician to the presence of inflammatory processes in the canal. Once this maneuver has been completed, the examiner should gently insert the speculum. If cerumen obstructs the view, it should be removed.

2. What is the best way to remove cerumen?

There are various schools of thought. The first relies on a number of proprietary substances, all purportedly able to soften the cerumen when administered as a solution into the external canal. An alternative method consists of using a metal loop to remove the wax mechanically, bit by bit. The effectiveness depends in great part on the skills of the examiner. Of course, the patient should be instructed not to insert various probes (especially cotton-tipped swabs) to remove wax by him- or herself. The authors' favorite method is to flush the canal with warm tap water using a syringe armed with a 16- to 14-gauge plastic IV catheter.

3. Other than cerumen, what else may prevent visualization of the tympanic membrane?
- **Otitis externa**, also known as swimmer's ear, is characterized by swelling and erythema of the ear canal.
- **Exostosis** consists of one or more bony protuberances, covered by normal skin, that project into the lumen of the canal and make visualization difficult. They tend to be bilateral.
- A **furuncle** is an exquisitely tender and erythematous inflammatory nodule arising from the canal's wall.

4. What is the normal surface anatomy of the tympanic membrane?

The normal tympanic membrane is pale, gray, translucent, and surrounded by a ring (*anulus* in Latin). The ring should be inspected carefully because it may be the site of tiny perforations.

The normal surface structures of the membrane include the visible projections of the **malleus** (hammer in Latin), which is the largest of the three auditory ossicles. The malleus actually resembles a club more than a hammer. It is composed of a **head (caput)**, below which is the **neck (collum)**. From the neck diverge the **handle (manubrium)** and slender anterior process. From the base of the manubrium arises the short lateral process. The manubrium and lateral process are attached firmly to the tympanic membrane (with the lateral process projecting anteriorly and superiorly), whereas the head articulates with a saddle-shaped surface on the body of the incus.

Otoscopically one can visualize not only the short lateral process and manubrium but also the **umbo** of the malleus (from the Latin *umbo* = boss of a shield, knob). The umbo coincides with the head of the hammer and presents as an inferior and posterior projection through the tympanic membrane. One also sees a reflective triangular cone of light, located inferiorly and anteriorly to the umbo. Finally, anteriorly and superiorly to the manubrium is the flaccid portion of the tympanic membrane (**pars flaccida**); posteriorly to the manubrium is the **pars tensa**. These terms reflect the greater or lesser mobility of the corresponding areas of the tympanic membrane. (See figure on facing page.)

5. What are the otoscopic features of the tympanic membrane in patients with purulent and serous otitis media?

Purulent otitis media (usually bacterial) presents with a rim of redness, prominent vessel dilation, and outward bulging of the eardrum. Resultant findings include loss of markings for the umbo, loss of the cone of light reflex, and decreased mobility on pneumatic otoscopy (see opposite page). At times, spontaneous perforation of the eardrum may occur, leading to discharge of purulent material into the canal. The patient presents with earache, a fever that may be quite high, and hearing loss of the conductive type. Purulent otitis media is much more common in children than in adults.

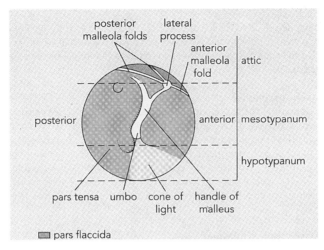

Anatomy of normal tympanic membrane. (From Epstein O, Perkin GD, de Bono DP, Cookson J: Clinical Examination, 2nd ed. St. Louis, Mosby, 1997, with permission.)

Serous otitis media (usually viral) often presents with an air/fluid level and at times even bubbles behind the eardrum due to the presence of retromembrane fluid, usually amber in color. The bulging from the fluid may lead to loss of the cone of light and retraction of the tympanic membrane. As a result the malleus becomes prominent and white. The tympanic membrane, in turn, acquires a yellowish hue. The patient presents with some earache, low-grade fever, and hearing loss of the conductive type.

6. How do you tell an earache due to otitis media from an earache due to otitis externa?

In otitis media movement of the auricle or tragus is painless. Conversely, the same movement is exquisitely painful in otitis externa.

7. What does bulging indicate?

Bulging is the result of fluid (either purulent or serous) behind the tympanic membrane that pushes the membrane outward, causing a loss of markings for the umbo and disappearance of the cone of light reflex. It is a nonspecific sign of fluid accumulation, independent of the nature of the fluid.

8. What is a hemotympanum? What are the other manifestations of basilar skull fracture?

Hemotympanum is the presence of blood behind the tympanic membrane and usually results from a basilar skull fracture. It was first described by the English surgeon William H. Battle (1855–1936), along with a plethora of other signs of similar significance, including (1) Battle's sign (hematoma over the mastoid process; see question 19), (2) periorbital ecchymoses, and (3) rhinorrhea and otorrhea, which represent leakage of cerebrospinal fluid through the fractured planes.

9. What does a perforation of the tympanic membrane look like?

It looks like a hole in the center of the tympanic membrane (i.e., pars tensa) with a nonerythematous diffuse loss of tympanic membrane markings. The edges of the perforation are usually smooth if trauma-related (in which case bloody material also may be present). Conversely, they are ragged if related to an infectious cause (in which case purulent material also may be present). Traumatic or infectious perforations can be easily differentiated from iatrogenic perforations (such as tympanoplasty tubes). Indeed, patients with tympanoplasty have a plastic or metallic orifice in the inferior aspect of the eardrum, usually immediately inferior to the tip of the umbo.

10. What is Angel's sign?

This procedure, described by Rick Angel in 1994, consists of performing an otoscopic examination while the patient is blowing against a pinched nose. The maneuver increases the sensitivity of otoscopy for the detection of a perforated tympanic membrane by demonstrating fluid or pus in the external canal.

11. What is bullous myringitis?

It is an inflammation of the tympanic membrane (from the Greek *myrinx* = tympanum) characterized by the presence of one or more vesicles on the tympanic membrane. These vesicles are filled with fluid that may be clear, blood-tinged, or even purulent. Each vesicle usually has one or more petechiae adjacent to the base. Patients usually complain of earache, hearing loss, and bloody discharge. By conventional teaching this finding is considered pathognomonic for *Mycoplasma pneumoniae* infection. In reality, bullous myringitis also may result from various other infections (either viral or bacterial) and may occur even in Ramsay Hunt syndrome.

12. What is Ramsay Hunt syndrome?

Ramsay Hunt syndrome is herpes zoster involvement of the geniculate ganglion. The patient presents with facial paresis, hyperacusia, and unilateral loss of taste. In addition, salivation and tear formation are reduced, and pain in the ear is accompanied by vesicles on the ear canal and eardrum (see below).

13. Who was Ramsay Hunt?

Ramsay Hunt (1874–1937) was a Philadelphia neurologist. A graduate of the University of Pennsylvania, he studied in Paris, Vienna, and Berlin and eventually settled in New York, where in 1907 he described the syndrome bearing his name while working at Cornell University.

14. What is a cholesteatoma? What does it look like?

It is a benign, tumor-like mass of keratinizing squamous epithelium and cholesterol in the middle ear (from the Greek *cholesterol* = biliary-like mass, *steat* = tallow, and *toma* = tumor). It is usually the sequela of chronic otitis media. It presents as an exophytic papular lesion of yellow-white color and keratin-like composition. Histologically it is characterized by squamous metaplasia or inward extension of squamous epithelium to line an expanding cystic cavity. Cholesteatomas are usually adjacent to a posterosuperior perforation of the tympanic membrane and may grow into the external canal. They also may involve the mastoid and erode surrounding bone.

PNEUMATIC OTOSCOPY

15. How is pneumatic otoscopy performed?

This procedure, which is not a mandatory part of the routine exam, is performed by first visualizing the tympanic membrane. The clinician then attaches a pneumatic bulb to the head of the otoscope and squeezes it to observe any movement of the tympanic membrane. The principle behind this maneuver is that the normal eardrum is mobile, albeit slightly. Therefore, when air is introduced into the external canal, the normal membrane and its light reflex move inward. When air is removed, the membrane moves outward. Any decrease in mobility is abnormal.

Pearl. *Lack of mobility usually results from perforation, middle-ear adhesions, blocked eustachian tube, or acute otitis media.*

16. What if I do not have a pneumatic bulb?

A poor man's way to test the mobility of the eardrum is to ask the patient to pinch his or her nose and then swallow. This maneuver may create enough of a pressure change to elicit visible movement of the membrane.

17. Is there any utility to performing pneumatic otoscopy?

The procedure assists the clinician in differentiating the pathologic from the normal eardrum. It is particularly important in children, in whom the tympanic membrane invariably becomes red as the result of crying. Thus, the clinician attempting to differentiate reddening due to crying from reddening due to otitis media will find pneumatic otoscopy quite helpful: a mobile eardrum, even if red, is much more likely to be normal and vice versa. Moreover, identification of decreased eardrum mobility may be crucial in children because it may be linked to hearing and language impairments.

18. Should one routinely inspect and palpate the postauricular space?

Palpation of the postauricular space is indicated in every patient with an ear complaint to rule out mastoiditis. Patients with mastoiditis have exquisite tenderness in the 1-cm crescent-shaped depression immediately posterior to the external auditory canal. They also may have (1) a palpable posterior auricular node (presenting as a nodule in the area of the mastoid process) and (2) a positive Battle's sign (ecchymosis over the mastoid, most often due to trauma and indicative of basilar skull fracture).

19. When does Battle's sign occur?

It usually occurs approximately 48 hours after the traumatic event.

AURICLE

20. What is the auricle?

The auricle (pinna) is the part of the ear external to the canal. It is a cartilaginous structure, quite soft, flexible, and malleable.

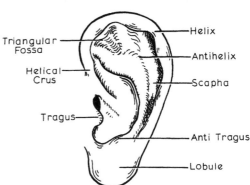

Anatomy of the auricle. (From Lee KJ: Essential Otolaryngology—Head and Neck Surgery. Norwalk, CT, Appleton & Lange, 1995, p 2, with permission.)

21. What may result in the presence of bumps on the auricle?

Papules or nodules on the surface of the auricle are quite common. Although the vast majority are benign and of no clinical significance, some may be early malignant neoplastic lesions. They also may assist in the diagnosis of systemic diseases. Specific etiologies include the following:

1. **Darwin's tubercle** is a completely benign and congenital nodule, located near the superior aspect of the auricle (approximately two-thirds of the way from the bottom of the helix). It was described by Charles R. Darwin of evolutionary fame. The tubercle is nontender and usually unilateral, although at times it may even be bilateral.

2. **Tophi** are one or more nontender (or mildly hard) nodules located on the edges of the auricles. The name derives from the Latin tufa, a calcareous and volcanic deposit from springs. Tophi may be present on both the helix and antihelix and are usually indicative of hyperuricemia and gout.

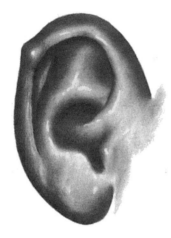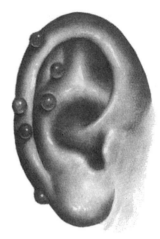

Darwin's tubercle (left) and tophi (right). (From Seidel HM, Ball JW, Dains JE, Benedict GW: Mosby's Guide to Physical Examination, 3rd ed. St. Louis, Mosby, 1995, with permission.)

   3. **Earlobe keloids** are one or more smooth, flesh-colored papular growths on one or both sides of the earlobe. They may be either unilateral or bilateral.

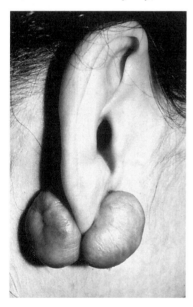

Keloids of the earlobe. (From Fitzpatrick JE, Aeling JL: Dermatology Secrets. Philadelphia, Hanley & Belfus, 1996, with permission.)

22. Can I really diagnose gout by looking at an ear?
   Yes. The presence of one or more hard, painless-to-mildly tender nodules on the edges of the auricles (either the helix or antihelix) should lead the clinician to query the patient about episodes of monoarticular arthritis, particularly podagra, chiragra, or gonagra. These medieval monikers for arthritis, involving, respectively, the great toe, hand, or knee, were not uncommon among the well-fed (and drunk) aristocracy of the times. The presence of similar nodules over the elbows or extensor surfaces of hands or feet is also quite consistent with tophaceous gout. Because gouty crystals precipitate more easily in the colder areas of the skin, the auricles and nasal cartilages are often the first sites of tophi formation (at least in Wisconsin).

23. What is so malignant about otitis externa maligna?

Because it occurs only in patients who either are neutropenic or have a severe deficit in neutrophil function (such as poorly controlled diabetics or patients taking high-dose corticosteroids), the prognosis is often guarded. *Pseudomonas aeruginosa* infection usually spreads directly into adjacent structures and eventually spills into the bloodstream, causing gram-negative sepsis, shock, and death if not promptly treated. It is, therefore, a diagnosis that the primary care physician should not miss.

24. Distinguish among vesicles, bullae, and pustules.

Vesicles are blisters that contain clear fluid; bullae are blisters larger than 0.5 cm in diameter; and pustules are blist. rs that contain purulent fluid.

25. What may cause vesicles in the auricle?

Vesicles of the auricle are not too common and carry a relatively narrow differential diagnosis. They may result from (1) severe contact dermatitis, such as poison ivy; (2) varicella, as part of the pruritic rash over the face, trunk, and extremities; and (3) Ramsay Hunt syndrome, which is characterized by a unilateral painful, vesicular rash of the inferior portion of one auricle and due to herpes virus infection of the geniculate ganglion (see above). Ramsay Hunt syndrome requires treatment with acyclovir.

26. What may cause ecchymoses of the auricle?

Ecchymoses of the auricle are uncommon but quite concerning to the patient (or the patient's parents, considering that this condition is often found in children). The causes of ecchymoses include the following:

1. **Port wine stain**, which usually is congenital and of cosmetic importance only. One of the most famous port wine stains in history, not to mention in political cartoons, was on the forehead of Soviet President Michal Gorbachev.

2. **Sturge-Weber disease**, which is characterized by a port wine nevus on the upper part of the scalp and other vascular abnormalities, both intracranially and in other parts of the body (such as cerebellar calcifications and recurrent seizures).

3. **Pugilistic activity** also may result in auricular ecchymoses and even in hematoma formation (see above).

27. Who were Sturge and Weber?

William A. Sturge (1850–1919) was a native of Bristol, England. A devout Quaker, a passionate liberal, and a strong supporter of women's rights (including free access to medical education), he married a physician, Emily Bovell, with whom he eventually shared practice in London. An excellent speaker and teacher and a compassionate physician, Sturge contracted rheumatic fever at the age of 44. Because of his declining health, he eventually moved to the French Riviera, considerably reducing his practice (although he still found time to look after Queen Victoria during her four visits to France). After his second marriage to a young archeologist, he studied early Greek art and became the founder and first president of the East Anglia Society of Prehistoric Archaeology. He collected more than 100,000 archeologic pieces, which he donated to museums upon his death. Throughout his life he wrote only four medical papers.

Frederick Parkes Weber (1863–1962) is the English physician associated with Rendu-Osler-Weber disease. In addition to these two conditions, he also described Weber-Christian disease and Weber-Klippel syndrome. He was an avid climber (like his father) and an enthusiast of physical exercise. He lived well into his nineties, spending the last parts of his life collecting ancient coins and vases, which, upon his death, he donated to the British Museum.

28. Why palpate the pulse anterior to the tragus?

The pulse anterior to the tragus, so often overlooked in the routine examination, corresponds to the temporalis artery, a branch of the external carotid artery. The temporalis artery runs immediately in front of the tragus and supplies the temporalis area of the scalp. It is an important artery to palpate in patients with profound proximal muscle weakness and jaw claudication because the temporalis is affected by polymyalgia rheumatica or temporal arteritis (which is an external carotiditis, involving all branches of the external carotid). The presence of tenderness and/or nodularity in this artery may be an important clue to the presence of external carotiditis.

29. Where are the preauricular and postauricular lymph nodes? What may result in their enlargement?

The preauricular lymph node is located immediately anterior to the tragus. The postauricular lymph node is located over the mastoid process. A tender enlargement of the preauricular node is seen most often in patients with conjunctivitis or periorbital inflammation, whereas tender enlargement of the postauricular node is seen most often in patients with otitis externa or mastoiditis.

30. What is a tender and swollen auricle?

It is an uncommon but dramatic event. A diffusely swollen auricle is usually due to one of the following three causes:

1. A **traumatic etiology** can be easily identified in patients with a history of a recent altercation (especially in the presence of other signs of trauma, such as a broken nose or black eye). Indeed, a swollen auricle has been an occupational hazard of boxers for many centuries. A beautiful statue from the Hellenistic period depicts a resting boxer with a typical "cauliflower" ear. Unless evacuated, the traumatic hematoma to the auricle usually leads to fibrotic evolution; hence the cauliflower deformity. A cauliflower ear may even result in mild hearing loss. It has been stated that the hearing loss of Thomas Alva Edison was the result of his being picked up by the ears as a child. There is, however, no evidence that he had a cauliflower ear. President Johnson, on the other hand, contributed to our advance in veterinary medicine by demonstrating that cauliflower ears do not occur in dogs, especially beagles. In fact, he used to pick up his beagle by the ears and toss him around, often to the amusement (or chagrin) of the press corps. LBJ had no ear problems of which we know, with the possible exception of selective deafness to war protesters in nearby Lafayette Park.

2. **Relapsing polychondritis** usually affects all facial cartilages, including the alar cartilage of the nose and the auricular cartilage of either or both ears.

3. **Otitis externa maligna** is usually seen in patients with impaired neutrophil function because of either quantitative or qualitative disorders. It results in *Pseudomonas aeruginosa* infection of the auricle, which causes diffuse swelling and an exquisitely tender auricle.

31. Can I diagnose coronary artery disease by looking at the auricle?

Probably not. Earlobe creases (oblique fissures of the earlobe) were first described by the American physician Sanders T. Frank as a sign of coronary artery disease, hypertension, and diabetes. Among adults they are an acquired finding and therefore different from the congenital creases of newborns with Beckwith syndrome or from the ear crease occasionally present in normal children.

The crease has been the target of several investigations and has high positive predictive value for coronary artery disease in patients undergoing cardiac catheterization (i.e., in patients with a high prevalence of coronary artery disease). Other studies, however, have indicated a similar frequency of coronary atherosclerosis in men with and without creases. This suggests that selection bias and the effect of age may lead to misinterpretation of this finding. In other words, because both coronary artery disease and earlobe creases (or wrinkles in general) are common in elderly patients, the two appear to be unrelated events. A related but even more interesting sign is hair in the canal, which is associated with coronary artery disease in retrospect but has no relation to pathogenesis.

AUSCULTATION OF THE AURICLE

32. When should a clinician auscultate over an auricle? (Laennec, are you listening?)

In patients presenting with tinnitus in one ear, often paroxysmal and without associated vertigo, nausea, or nystagmus. In patients with a negative work-up (including magnetic resonance imaging of the posterior fossa and audiogram), auscultation of the ear during tinnitus may reveal a bruit consistent with an arteriovenous malformation of the carotid artery. Further work-up with a magnetic resonance arteriogram or angiogram may be indicated. Of interest, whenever the symptom disappears, so does the bruit.

33. How is auscultation of the auricle performed?

By placing the diaphragm of the stethoscope over the auricle. One should listen for bruits or crepitus. Bruits are clues to the presence of arteriovenous fistulas, whereas crepitus suggests temporomandibular disease.

34. How do you test hearing at the bedside?

The most common way is by using a tuning fork to perform the Weber and Rinne tests. In combination these tests distinguish between conductive and sensorineural hearing loss. Conductive loss involves the transmission of sound, whereas sensorineural loss involves the perception of sound.

35. What is the Weber test?

The Weber test consists of placing the base of a vibrating tuning fork (1024- or 512-Hz tool) over the midline of the skull at an equal distance between the two ears. The patient is asked to state where the buzzing of the tuning fork is best perceived. Normal patients perceive it best in the midline. Patients with disease, on the other hand, perceive it best in only one ear (lateralized Weber sign). In conductive hearing loss (from impacted cerumen, for example), the Weber sign is lateralized to the bad ear (which is not distracted by ambient noise). Conversely, in sensorineural loss, the Weber sign is lateralized to the good ear.

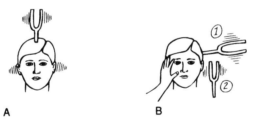

Tests of hearing perception and conduction. *A,* Weber test. *B,* Rinne test. (From DeGowin RL: DeGowin and DeGowin's Diagnostic Examination, 6th ed. New York, McGraw-Hill, 1994, with permission.)

36. What is the Rinne test?

The Rinne test consists of placing the base of the vibrating tuning fork directly over the patient's mastoid process and keeping it in place until the patient can no longer hear any sound. At that point the tuning fork is placed as close as possible to the patient's ear. A normal patient is still able to hear sound (because air conduction lasts longer than bone conduction). A patient with a conduction defect (such as an external canal impacted with cerumen) has normal bone conduction but impaired air conduction and therefore cannot hear any sound when the tuning fork is placed close to the ear. Conversely, in a patient with a sensorineural loss (due to involvement of the inner ear receptors) both air and bone conduction are equally affected. Thus the normal pattern prevails: air conduction still lasts longer than bone conduction.

37. Who were Weber and Rinne?

E.F.W. Weber (1806–1871) was the proponent of the physiology behind the test, even though the test is usually credited to a later German otologist, F.E. Weber-Liel (1832–1891). The Rinne test was the brainchild of Heinrich A. Rinne (1819–1868), a German ear, nose, and throat surgeon.

BIBLIOGRAPHY

1. Brady PM, Zive MA, Goldberg R, et al: A new wrinkle to the earlobe crease. Arch Intern Med 147:65–66, 1987.
2. Elliot WJ: Ear lobe crease and coronary artery disease. Am J Med 75:1024–1032, 1983.
3. Frank STM: Aural sign of coronary artery disease. N Engl J Med 289:327–328, 1973.
4. Jafek BW, Stark AK: ENT Secrets. Philadelphia, Hanley & Belfus, 1996.

6. NOSE AND MOUTH

Dale Berg, M.D., and Katherine Worzala, M.D., M.P.H.

TOPICS COVERED IN THIS CHAPTER

NOSE

"How do you know that I've told a lie?" Pinocchio asked the Fairy.
*"Lies, my dear boy, are quickly discovered; because they are of two kinds. There are lies
with short legs, and lies with long noses. Yours is clearly of the long-nosed variety."*
Carlo Collodi, *The Adventures of Pinocchio*

CONVENTIONAL TEACHING WATCH

If you can excuse the pun, it is wise to be nosy about the nose. Examination of this important facial appendix in fact may reveal unsuspected abnormalities that lead to diagnosis of either systemic diseases or capital sins (such as cocaine abuse).

FINDING		CONVENTIONAL TEACHING REVISITED
Rhinophyma	⇔	Interesting and obvious finding; hard to miss.
Saddle nose	⇓	Rare finding thanks to the very low incidence of congenital syphilis.
Lupus pernio	⇔	Uncommon but important clue to diagnosis of sarcoidosis.
Septal hematoma/abscess	⇔	Important complications of nasal fracture.
Septal perforation	⇑	Think of cocaine, vasculitis, and trauma (including nasal rings).
Nasal polyps	⇑	Common complications of chronic atopic rhinitis.
Anosmia	⇔	Important problem but rarely pursued during routine history and physical examination.

1. What are the normal structures of the external nose?
1. **Bridge:** located superomedially and representing the bony upper third of the nose.
2. **Alae** (= *wings* in Latin): cartilages that make up the inferior, medial, and lateral two-thirds of the nose.
3. **Nares:** paired orifices.
4. **Tip and columella**

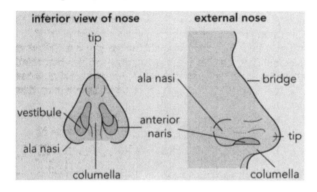

From Epstein O, Perkin GD, de Bono DP, Cookson J: Clinical Examination, 2nd ed. St. Louis, Mosby, 1998, with permission.

2. What is rhinophyma?
Rhinophyma (from the Greek *rhino* = nose and *phyma* = tumor) is thickening of the nasal skin, which becomes indurated, nontender, modestly erythematous, and often covered with multiple telangiectasias. As a result, the nose may appear bulbous and quite prominent. Rhinophyma is also called **hypertrophic rosacea** (rhinophyma is, in fact, a variety of acne rosacea). More colorful lay terms for the same condition include brandy nose, rum nose, and toper's nose (all in reference to the reported association between rhinophyma and generous alcohol intake); copper nose; hammer nose; and potato nose.
Pathologically, rhinophyma is characterized by nasal hypertrophy with follicular dilation. It is caused by hyperplasia of the sebaceous glands with fibrosis and hypervascularity and associated with the development of basal cell carcinoma.

3. What is the cause of rhinophyma?
Possible culprits include exposure to climate and chronic excessive ethanol ingestion. Although the association with ethanol is loose at best, the telangiectasias are often called rum blossoms or gin blossoms. Perhaps the best example of rhinophyma with gin blossoms is the great comedian W.C. Fields, a man whose nose size was directly proportional to his affinity for liquor in general and gin in particular. Rhinophyma is not uncommon among politicians, retired baseball players, and department chairs (go figure). If this observation prompts you to wonder whether even Pinocchio had rhinophyma, the answer is no. Pinocchio had variable rhinomegaly, a peculiarly reversible condition related to telling lies.

4. What is a saddle nose? Does it really exist outside of board questions?
Saddle nose is the congenital or acquired development of an erosive indentation in the area corresponding to the nasal bone. As a result, the distal tip of the nose appears to be turned upward and outward. A true saddle nose (due to destruction of the bony portion of the nose) is traditionally described in congenital lues but is seen more commonly as either a subacute or old manifestation of Wegener's granulomatosis. With increasing availability of good therapy for both lues and Wegener's disease, the saddle nose is encountered less and less frequently. As a result, it is becoming more of a finding for the birds (and the boards) than for real life. A **pseudo-saddle nose** also may be seen in relapsing polychondritis as a result of the destruction of the cartilaginous (not bony) part of the nose.

5. What are the manifestations of a nasal fracture?

Nasal fractures are the most common trauma-related disorders involving the nose. They are characterized by severe pain and significant anterior epistaxis, often originating from both nares. Over the ensuing 24 hours periorbital ecchymoses invariably develop, along with one or more significant sequelae, such as septal hematoma and septal deviation. Because the fractures are open, antibiotics are necessary to prevent osteomyelitis.

6. What is a septal hematoma?

A septal hematoma is a purple and painful nodule in the nasal septum. It is usually quite easy to spot. Conversely, displacement of the nasal bone or septum as a result of trauma (i.e., septal deviation) may be difficult to see until later. The edema of the early stages makes physical exam more difficult. Both of these traumatic complications require referral to an ear, nose, and throat specialist for drainage or reduction.

7. What is lupus pernio?

Lupus pernio is the chronic, nonblanching, diffuse purple discoloration of the skin of the external nose. Although the nose is not actually enlarged (as in rhinophyma), other sarcoid lesions often are present and may involve the ears, cheeks, hands, and fingers. The term *lupus* in old medical nomenclature referred to any disfiguring skin condition that, like a wolf (= *lupus* in Latin) literally devoured the facial features. It is therefore used with various modifying terms to designate disfiguring skin diseases, such as lupus erythematosus, lupus verrucosus, lupus tuberculosus, lupus vulgaris, and, of course, lupus pernio. The word *pernio* is Latin for frostbite. It refers to the peculiar violet-bluish hue of the condition. Lupus pernio is a sign of active sarcoidosis and thus may present in association with erythema nodosum, Achilles' enthesitis, uveitis, and pulmonary infiltration.

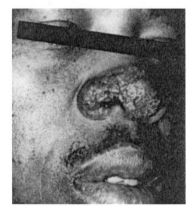

Lupus pernio. (From Fitzpatrick JE, Aeling JL: Dermatology Secrets. Philadelphia, Hanley & Belfus, 1996, with permission.)

8. What did Rudolph the Red-nosed Reindeer really have?

Probably rhinophyma, but that begs the question: did Santa spill some of the grog while feeding the reindeer?

Inspection of the Nares and Internal Nose

9. What are the normal structures of the internal nose?

1. **Vestibules:** paired internal widenings located immediately beyond each naris. They are delimited as follows:
   - Medially by the **septum.** Like the external nose, the septum is partly bone and partly cartilage. The word *septum* is an anglicized adaptation of the Latin verb *saepire*, which means

to erect a hedgerow. Indeed, the function of the septum is to provide the medial boundary for each vestibule.
• Laterally by a wall of **cartilage**.

2. Deeply beyond the vestibules are the **turbinates**, which are curving bony structures that project into the internal nose. There are three turbinates on each side: inferior, middle, and superior. Their main function is to increase the nasal surface dedicated to the humidification, temperature control, and filtering of inhaled air. To carry out this function, the turbinates are covered by a well-vascularized mucosa.

Pearl.   On routine examination conducted by either otoscope or Vienna speculum, one can inspect only the vestibule, anterior portion of the septum, and inferior and middle turbinates.

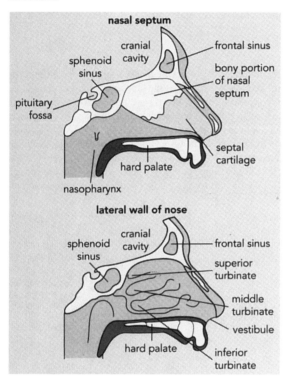

From Epstein O, Perkin GD, de Bono DP, Cookson J: Clinical Examination, 2nd ed. St. Louis, Mosby, 1997, with permission.

10. What is the significance of flaring of the nostrils?

Flaring of the nostrils (that is, flaring of the alae of the nose) is a sign of increased work of breathing. It is usually seen in patients with impending respiratory failure. Thus, it is often associated with other bedside findings of respiratory distress and respiratory muscle fatigue, such as respiratory alternans and abdominal paradox. It also may be seen, however, in patients with acute abdomen and peritonitis, usually as a result of impaired excursion of the diaphragm caused by pain.

11. What are the best tools for inspecting the nares and internal structures of the nose?

1. The **otoscope** can be mounted with a nasal speculum (instead of an ear speculum) and used to shine light directly into each vestibule.

2. A **handheld Vienna nasal speculum** opens on closure of the handles. It is usually used with a head mirror.

In the absence of these tools, the physician may use simply a penlight and his or her fingers. In all situations the patient first should be instructed to blow the nose gently but forcibly to remove any mucus.

12. What results in swelling or bumps in the nasal septum?
The most common causes include (1) septal hematoma (see above); (2) septal abscess, an erythematous, tender, fluctuant nodule in the septal mucosa; and (3) nasal polyp, a fleshy, pink, pedunculated lesion derived from the mucosa of the septum. Any of these three conditions may present with nasal airway obstruction. An untreated hematoma or abscess may even result in septal perforation. Polyps, on the other hand, tend to be typically associated with chronic atopic rhinitis or asthma. All three conditions require referral to an ear, nose, and throat specialist.

13. Is inspection of nasal secretions useful?
Yes indeed. Actually there is quite a bit of value in snot, the colloquial term to indicate excessive flow from the nasal mucosa. Although quite common and even vulgar, snot is actually noble in origin, descending directly from the old English term *gnotte*. Snot has high diagnostic value because different disease processes produce different types of nasal discharge. A clear discharge, for example, is nonspecific but consistent with viral or atopic rhinitis. A yellow discharge is also nonspecific but may indicate an early suppurative process. A green discharge is quite consistent with purulent sinusitis. Obviously a bloody discharge is consistent with anterior epistaxis. A dark and almost black discharge (particularly in a comatose patient) may indicate mucormycosis.

14. What does a nasal septal perforation look like?
It looks like a hole in the septum and is demonstrable (1) on visual inspection; (2) by shining a light source into one naris and transilluminating both sides; or (3) by demonstrating airflow in the nares even when the contralateral side is pinched closed.

15. What is the usual cause of nasal septal perforation?
Traditionally it results from an untreated septal hematoma or abscess, but now it more frequently results from chronic snorting of cocaine, which is a profound alpha agonist that leads to severe mucosal and septal ischemia and necrosis of the septum. Another unique and increasingly frequent cause of nasal perforation is nasal piercing. Depending on the area of placement of the ring, this procedure may lead to abscess formation and perforation of either the cartilaginous septum or alae.

16. What are less common causes of nasal perforation?
Infections, such as tuberculosis, syphilis, and (more rarely) leprosy. In addition, many collagen vascular diseases also may lead to nasal perforation, including Wegener's granulomatosis, midline granuloma, systemic lupus erythematosus, rheumatoid arthritis, progressive systemic sclerosis, and mixed connective tissue disease. Finally, trauma also may cause septal perforation, although usually trauma causes septal deviation.

17. What are the nasal manifestations of a basilar skull fracture?
In addition to direct trauma to the face, patients with a basilar skull fracture often present with evidence of nasal fracture, such as periorbital ecchymoses, swelling and tenderness of the nasal bridge, and anterior epistaxis. Patients may even have cerebrospinal fluid (CSF) rhinorrhea, which represents leakage of CSF through the fracture site. CSF rhinorrhea is a tremendous risk factor for the development of meningitis and requires prompt surgical attention.

18. How do you recognize CSF rhinorrhea?
By placing a drop of nasal secretions over a paper towel. In cases of CSF rhinorrhea a clear halo surrounds the nasal secretions. This bedside test is a poor man's paper chromatography and confirms the presence of spinal fluid. Alternatively, the glucose content of the secretions may be

measured at bedside by using, for example, the Chemstrip method. In cases of CSF rhinorrhea, the test reveals glucose in levels close to those of of the spinal fluid (40–80 mg/dl).

19. What are the nasal manifestations of the common cold?

The cold, one of the most common human afflictions, is a viral infection of the upper respiratory tract. It is usually characterized by a preponderance of manifestations in the nose. The nasal mucosa is swollen, often to the point of obstruction, and the patient has a stuffy feeling with either serous or yellow discharge from both nares. Concurrent manifestations often include serous otitis, nonexudative pharyngitis, and shotty nodes. Treatment has been, is, and for the foreseeable future will be supportive.

20. What results in swelling of the nasal mucosa?

Swelling of the nasal mucosa is due to one of three causes:

1. **Viral causes** include infection of the nasal and oropharyngeal mucosa by either rhinoviruses or adenoviruses.

2. **Atopic causes** include pollen or dander exposure that results in congestion, serous conjunctivitis, and sneezing.

3. **Vasomotor causes** are a response to a specific inhalant. The response consists of a boggy edema of the mucosa with marked tearing. The inhalant may be either noxious to all people (such as tear gas) or idiosyncratic, in which case only certain people are affected. For example, an idiosyncratic response is elicited by some perfumes, which result in swelling in a few predisposed people.

21. What are the most common causes of obstruction to airflow in one or both nares?

The most common causes are (1) nasal mucosa edema, (2) nasal polyps, (3) septal deviation, and (4) foreign bodies. All of these causes are demonstrable and diagnosable by simple physical examination. Foreign bodies are particularly common in children, who have a unique penchant for inserting rocks, twigs, and crayons into the nares. Obviously visual inspection provides the diagnosis, and a fine forceps may allow the clinician to clinch and extricate the incarcerated foreign body.

22. What is a nasal polyp?

It is a fleshy, red, pedunculated, and friable structure that hangs from the lateral or medial mucosa of the nose. Polyps can be distinguished from other internal structures of the nose by the fact that they are not tender when touched by the speculum. Polyps may be quite large and often are multiple; they may even protrude from the vestibule of the nares. The patient usually has a sensation of nasal fullness, frequently accompanied by obstruction to nasal airflow and associated with a definable and visible lesion on examination.

23. What causes polyps?

Polyps usually are due to chronic or recurrent edema of the mucosa, most commonly caused by either severe chronic atopic rhinitis or aspirin hypersensitivity (often in association with asthma).

24. Can a clinician diagnose the cause of a gastrointestinal bleed by looking into the nose?

Although the exciting response is yes, this situation tends to be quite rare and uncertain. Two nasal entities may be linked to gastrointestinal bleeding. The most common is simple epistaxis, in which the patient swallows nasal blood with resulting guaiac-positive stools and even melena. More intriguingly, however, some patients may present with multiple telangiectasias in the nasal or oral mucus and on the face, neck, and chest. They should be considered part of multiple hereditary hemorrhagic telangiectasia, such as the autosomal dominant Osler-Weber-Rendu syndrome.

25. Who was Rendu?

Henry J.L. Rendu (1844–1902) was the grandson of a distinguished Parisian painter and the son of an agricultural inspector. A lover of art, Rendu was so fascinated by his father's profession that he pursued a medical career only after a stint in agriculture, geology, and botany. He never lost his passion for plants, however, and eagerly maintained it as a hobby throughout his life. At the age of 43 he finally joined the staff of the Necker Hospital in Paris (the same hospital where Laennec had been chief of chest medicine), where he rapidly gained fame as a charismatic lecturer and gifted clinician.

26. Who was Weber?

Frederick P. Weber (1863–1962) was a British physician. Educated in Cambridge, Vienna, and Paris, he cultivated throughout his life a keen interest in medical philosophy and the arts, which he expressed in many books and articles. He was the son of Herman D. Weber (1823–1918), also a famous and long-lived physician (he is the same Weber who described the midbrain syndrome that still carries his name). Weber senior was a charming man with many interests who taught himself English so that he could read Shakespeare. He befriended, among others, Thomas Addison, Thomas Carlyle, and several British Waterloo veterans, including the famous Sir Peregrine Maitland ("Now it's your time, Maitland, now it's your time!"). Increasingly fascinated by England, Weber moved there in 1854, married an Englishwoman, and eventually became a member of the Royal College of Physicians. Both Weber senior and his son were avid alpinists and great advocates of physical exercise as the essential key to a long and productive life (which, incidentally, seems to have served them quite well). Weber senior climbed several mountains in the Italian Alps (including one for his 80th birthday) and walked 40–50 miles per week. In his later years, he developed a keen interest in numismatics and became an authority on ancient Greek coins.

27. Who was Osler?

Sir William Osler (1849–1919) is such a legend that a few lines in this chapter do him a disservice. The son of a missionary, born in the woods of Canada, Osler was so spiritual that early in life he even considered joining the clergy. A charming and compassionate man, he was a charismatic teacher, a superb bedside diagnostician, and a good person who never lost his respect for patients as fellow humans in need of help. After teaching in Canada and the United States, he moved to England, where he became Regius Professor of Medicine at Oxford. The last part of his life was unfortunately quite sad and tormented by the memory of his only son, who died in Flanders toward the end of World War I.

28. What is anosmia?

Anosmia is the absence of the sense of smell (from the Greek *an* = lack of and *osme* = sense of smell). It may be acquired or congenital.

Acquired anosmia may result from a long list of disease processes, affecting either the central nervous system or nose. Among them are multiple sclerosis, Parkinson's disease, diabetes mellitus, pernicious anemia, liver cirrhosis, chronic renal insufficiency, Cushing's syndrome, cystic fibrosis, sarcoidosis, allergic rhinitis, nasal polyposis, and zinc deficiency. Sequelae of a viral infection, however, seem to be the most common reasons for acquired reversible anosmia.

Congenital anosmia almost always results from Kallmann's syndrome. Described by the German psychiatrist Franz J. Kallmann (1897–1965), this syndrome consists of familial hypogonadotropic hypogonadism with or without anosmia (usually characterized by congenital absence of olfactory lobes). Kallmann's syndrome is inherited through sex-linked recessive or autosomal transmission with expression only in males. It is currently treatable through the administration of exogenous gonadotropins.

29. Is perception of alcohol odor an indication that the sense of smell is intact?

No. Alcohol is an irritant. Thus, it stimulates the trigeminal nerve rather than the olfactory endings of the nasal mucosa. Even patients without olfactory lobes (e.g., patients with Kallmann's syndrome) can "feel" an alcohol sponge. The same is true for other irritants, such as ammonia and pepper. Thus, for testing the sense of smell one should use nonirritating substances with strong odors. Coffee or spices (such as cinnamon, cloves, nutmeg) are excellent choices.

OROPHARYNX

Americans may have no identity, but they do have wonderful teeth.
Jean Baudrillard, *Astral America*

CONVENTIONAL TEACHING WATCH

If it is true that you should not look a gift horse in the mouth, it is also true that patients are not horses. Always take a good look at their mouth. In fact, a close examination of the oropharynx may provide a wealth of information. Among the abnormalities that you may detect are important mouth and tongue lesions that may be clues to the diagnosis of systemic disorders. Even the lowly teeth may become important diagnostically. Indeed, they not only represent risk factors for serious anaerobic infections of the respiratory system but also may assist in the diagnosis of otherwise unsuspected systemic and psychiatric disorders. Lead poisoning, congenital syphilis, and bulimia can be recognized by an astute dental examination. It is a sad reality that far too many patients have gone undiagnosed because of a poor or incomplete examination of the mouth.

FINDING		CONVENTIONAL TEACHING REVISITED
Pharyngitis	⇑	Common finding. Physical exam helps to sort viral from bacterial etiologies.
Crimson crescents	⇑	Recently described finding in patients with chronic fatigue syndrome.
Leukoplakia	⇓	Poor and nonspecific term; should be abandoned.
White spots of the mouth	⇑	Common and important.
Red spots of the mouth	⇓	Uncommon and, overall, unimportant.
Dark spots of the mouth	⇓	Very uncommon but important in right setting.
Yellow spots of the mouth	⇔	Fordyce spots are not that important clinically, but occasional hypochondriac patient may need reassurance.
Ulcers and erosions of the mouth	⇑	Common and important; wide differential diagnosis.
Ranula	⇓	Little clinical value other than need to recognize it.
Torus	⇓	As above.
Macroglossia	⇔	Important clue to a few important systemic disorders.
Scrotal tongue	⇓	Common in the elderly; no clinical value.
Hairy tongue	⇓	As above; variety of black tongue.
White hairy tongue (hairy leuko-plakia)	⇑	Much more important, given its association with AIDS.
Geographic tongue	⇔	Common but benign form of white tongue.
Red tongue	⇑	Always rule out atrophic glossitis.
White tongue	⇑	Common and usually important; occasionally serious.
Black tongue	⇓	Of all tongue colors, probably the least clinically useful.
Sublingual varicosities	⇓	Varicose veins of the tongue; little clinical significance.
Tongue biting	⇑	Poorly sensitive but highly specific sign of seizure.
Cheilosis and cheilitis	⇔	Common findings; occasionally clues to systemic disorders.
Ulcers and erosions of the lips	⇑	Look at vermilion border to diagnose herpes.
Pigmented lesions of the lips	⇓	Freckles are more common than Peutz-Jeghers lesions. Know how to tell them apart.
Gum hypertrophy	⇔	Common finding with finite differential diagnosis.
Hutchinson's teeth	⇓	Rare finding, thanks to very low incidence of congenital syphilis.
Burton's lines (lead lines)	⇔	Important clue to diagnosis of lead poisoning.
Halitosis	⇑	Common and important sign.

Pharynx

30. Name the structures of the posterior pharynx.
The posterior pharynx is divided into a hard and a soft palate, which are supported by the anterior and posterior pillars.

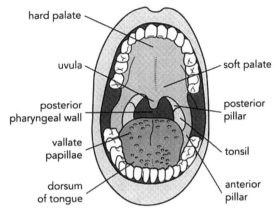

Anatomy of the oropharynx. (From Epstein O, Perkin GD, de Bono DP, Cookson J: Clinical Examination, 2nd ed. St. Louis, Mosby, 1998, with permission.)

hard palate

uvula

soft palate

posterior pharyngeal wall

posterior pillar

vallate papillae

tonsil

dorsum of tongue

anterior pillar

31. What is the uvula? What disease processes may manifest in the uvula?
The uvula (in Latin = little grape) is the midline structure projecting from the roof of the posterior pharynx. Its main function is probably to prevent fluids from entering the nasopharynx with swallowing. Interesting features of which one should be aware during the physical examination of the uvula include the following:

1. **Absence of the uvula.** The most common reason is surgical removal as part of a uvulopalatinopharyngoplasty (UPPP) to treat obstructive sleep apnea.

2. A **bifid uvula** is a fascinating but benign normal variant in which the uvula is congenitally forked. Because a bifid uvula may be associated with an occult cleft palate, it is an important finding to look for.

3. The uvula of patients with severe and chronic aortic insufficiency may have a **rhythmic pulsatile movement**, which is the equivalent of the de Musset sign (bobbing motion of the head; see below) and is called Mueller's sign. It has become a rare finding, thanks to timely treatment of valvular disease.

32. What is the differential diagnosis for uvulomegaly?
At least two important entities may result in a swollen and elongated uvula. One is common (pharyngitis), whereas the other is exceptionally rare (gamma-heavy chain disease). In both conditions the uvula may become sufficiently enlarged to cause cough, snoring, and even gagging. If caused by pharyngitis, uvulomegaly often is associated with other manifestations. If caused by heavy chain disease, on the other hand, uvulomegaly is often associated with B symptoms of lymphoproliferative disorders and pancytopenia.

33. What are the causes of a diffuse reddening of the oropharynx?
The most common causes are viral and bacterial infections. Viral etiologies include rhinovirus, adenovirus, human immunodeficiency virus (HIV), Epstein-Barr virus (EBV), cytomegalovirus (CMV), and coxsackie virus. Bacterial causes include group A streptococcus, *Neisseria gonorrhoeae*, and, in the olden days, diphtheria.

34. What are the causes of a localized reddening of both anterior pharyngeal pillars?
This condition (which is different from diffuse inflammation of the oropharynx) recently has been described in association with chronic fatigue syndrome (CFS) and dubbed the *crimson*

crescents. As many as 80% of patients with CFS present with a peculiar purplish discoloration of the two anterior pharyngeal pillars. These crescents have a vivid crimson color and demarcate quite briskly. The patient has no pain, no sore throat, and no other evidence of pharyngitis. The crimson crescents eventually fade over a period of 3–6 months.

35. What are the causes of an exudate on the posterior pharynx?

Exudative pharyngitis may be due to a large number of different etiologies, including the following:

1. **Group A beta-hemolytic streptococcal infection** is marked by pharyngeal exudate, minimal cough and rhinorrhea, high fever, mild nausea, enlarged jugulodigastric nodes, and increased risk of rheumatic fever.

2. **EBV or CMV infection** (also called infectious mononucleosis) is associated with severe exudative pharyngitis, significant swelling, diffuse lymphadenopathy, splenomegaly, hepatomegaly, hemolytic anemia, and profound fatigue.

3. **Acute HIV infection** also may manifest with an infectious mononucleosis syndrome. Because the stage is early, the patient is viremic (and therefore highly infectious) but HIV-antibody negative.

4. **Gonorrhea** may result in exudative and ulcerative pharyngitis. Risk factors are fellatio and cunnilingus. Therefore, pharyngitis refractory to standard therapy should lead to queries about the patient's sexual activities plus a Thayer-Martin culture of the throat.

36. Can strep throat be diagnosed by history and physical examination?

History and physical exam are the best method of diagnosis. History provides a significant amount of data to diagnose strep throat; invariably the patient reports no rhinorrhea, cough, or earache. Symptoms include modest nausea and vomiting with headaches, fever, and moderate-to-severe sore throat. Physical exam reveals a moderate-to-severe amount of exudate in the posterior pharynx and presence of jugulodigastric node tenderness. Although culture may be confirmatory, the diagnosis is usually established on the basis of history and physical findings (presence of exudate with fever and adenopathy). Pharyngitis caused by EBV may resemble closely the findings of strep throat.

37. What are the causes of a nodule in the posterior pharynx?

1. A warty lesion on the tonsils or tonsillar pillars is usually the result of an infection with human papilloma virus (HPV), which has an increased risk of degenerating into squamous cell carcinoma.

2. A papule or nodule in the posterior pharynx may represent squamous cell carcinoma, particularly in people with risk factors for cancer, such as smoking, chewing tobacco, heavy ethanol ingestion, and HPV infection.

3. A tender nodule that is associated with erythema and uvular displacement and follows exudative pharyngitis is highly consistent with quinsy (peritonsillar abscess). Although the term *quinsy* goes back a long time (Middle English from the original Greek word *kunankhê* = dog collar), we like to think of it as a more modern reference to the fictional television character, Dr. Quincy (Jack Klugman). Quincy is the medical examiner that you inevitably end up visiting if you do not receive prompt surgical drainage of quinsy.

Inspection of Oral Mucosa

38. What is the magic of "Ahhhh"?

Asking the patient to say "Ahhhh" has aided more clinicians in the examination of the oral mucosa and posterior pharynx than anything else in medicine, with the possible exception of the penlight and tongue blade. The technique is so common that even toddlers, who have an inborn aversion to physicians and throat examinations, often spontaneously agree to say "Ahhhh." Saying "Ahhhh" is effective for two reasons:

1. It permits the clinician to visualize the greatest amount of the oropharynx because of the active elevation of the soft palate, which allows assessment of the base of the tongue, uvula, tonsillar pillars, and even hypopharynx.

2. It permits adequate assessment of the motor division of cranial nerves IX (glossopharyngeal) and X (vagus). In cases of bilateral damage to these nerves, the uvula is not elevated by saying "Ahhhh." In cases of unilateral damage, on the other hand, "Ahhhh" makes the uvula deviate toward the intact side (it also prevents the soft palate of the paralyzed side from rising).

Some controversy surrounds the best sound and tongue position to use. Options include (1) the traditional falsetto "Ahhhh" with tongue protruded, (2) "Ae" rather than "Ah," and (3) "Ha" with the tongue maximally pulled in. Although no studies have assessed the predictive values for these maneuvers, the controversy is best settled by the universal rule: use whatever works best for you, and make sure that you can visualize the patient's tonsils and oral mucosa.

39. What is the descriptive nomenclature of lesions in the oral mucosa?
The nomenclature is not too dissimilar to that of skin lesions. It relies on size and characteristics of lesions:
  • Macules (if flat and < 1 cm)
  • Patches (if flat and > 1 cm)
  • Papules (if palpable and < 1 cm)
  • Plaques (if palpable and > 1 cm)
Other terms, such as *vesicles* and *bullae* (for fluid-filled lesions), are used in a similar fashion.

40. What color are lesions of the oral mucosa?
It depends on the lesion. Colors range from white to red to black.

41. What causes white spots in the oral mucosa?
1. The most common white spots result from **thickening of the oral mucosa**, usually due to chronic minor trauma, such as biting of the sides of the mouth. The linea alba, for example, is the horizontal white line in the buccal mucosa originating from the juxtaposition of upper and lower teeth (*linea alba* = Latin for white line). The linea alba stretches between Stensen's duct and the angle of the mouth. White thickenings of the buccal mucosa also may be seen adjacent to a broken tooth or ill-fitting denture.

2. The second most common cause is **squamous cell carcinoma** of the oral mucosa. In the past such lesions were termed leukoplakia (from the Greek *leukos* = white and *plax* = patch). Because it is impossible to differentiate benign from malignant lesions solely on the basis of inspection and palpation, leukoplakia has been recently abandoned as a diagnostic term (see below).

3. White lesions made by multiple papules and plaques, often surrounded by a rim of erythema, may represent **oral thrush** (candidal infection of the oral and oropharyngeal mucosa). Candidal lesions are easily scraped off with a tongue blade or cotton-tipped swab, leaving an underlying mucosa that is highly inflamed and often bleeding. Diagnosis is usually confirmed by performing a KOH preparation on the material.

4. A less common cause for white lesions of the mouth is **Koplik's spots**, a cluster of tiny white macules on the buccal mucosa adjacent to the first and second molars. They are consistent with early rubeola and precede the skin rash by a day.

5. A white lesion on the lateral aspects of the tongue (and occasionally on the buccal mucosa of the cheeks) should raise the suspicion of **HIV seropositivity**. This distinctive lesion is called hairy leukoplakia (see figure on following page). The term refers to the raised appearance of the lesion and its corrugated or hairy surface caused by keratin projections.

42. Are Koplik's spots specific for rubeola?
No. Koplik's spots also may be seen in echovirus and adenovirus infections. Thus, the finding is an interesting, albeit minor, feature of systemic viral infection.

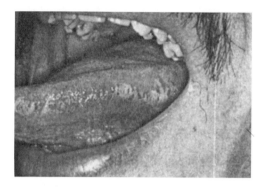

Oral hairy leukoplakia. (From Fitzpatrick JE, Aeling JL: Dermatology Secrets. Philadelphia, Hanley & Belfus, 1996, with permission.)

43. Who was Koplik?

Henry Koplik (1858–1927) was an American pediatrician. Born in New York and trained in Berlin, Vienna, and Prague, Koplik practiced at the Mt. Sinai Hospital of New York. In addition to being one of the founding fathers of the American Pediatric Society, Koplik was also instrumental in developing the first sterilized milk deposit for American infants.

44. How do you distinguish monilial spots from leukoplakia?

The best way is to grab a cottontip swab or tongue blade and attempt to scrape the lesion. Unlike monilial spots, leukoplakia cannot be scraped from the buccal mucosa. It is, in fact, part of the mucosa and not an overlay. The patient's history is also of some assistance. Patients with oral thrush are either immunocompromised (as a result of chemotherapy, AIDS, or high-dose steroids) or taking inhaled corticosteroids. Hairy leukoplakia is also a feature of AIDS (although not exclusively, as once thought).

45. What is Wickham's sign?

Wickham's sign (or Wickham's striae) is a lacy, white, reticulated pattern on the surface of lesions in patients with lichen planus. Lesions are flat-topped, shiny, pruritic, and violaceous. They are located not only on the buccal mucosa but also on flexor surfaces and male genitalia. At times they may form linear groups and thus give a patterned configuration that resembles lichens growing on rocks.

46. Who was Wickham?

Louis F. Wickham (1860–1913) was a French dermatologist and one of the early promoters of radium as treatment of skin cancer. His name is linked to a special knife that he designed for scarification of lesions in patients afflicted by lupus vulgaris.

47. Why is leukoplakia a "garbage can diagnosis" that should be abolished from medical parlance?

In the past all white lesions were termed leukoplakia (which, quite conveniently, means *white lesions* in Greek). Subsequently the term was unjustly elevated to the rank of diagnosis. Because it is absolutely impossible to differentiate benign from malignant white lesions solely on the basis of inspection and palpation, leukoplakia should not be used as a diagnostic term but as a descriptor. Hence, any white lesion not otherwise diagnosed should be suspected of being neoplastic and thus biopsied.

48. What features of a white lesion increase its chance of being malignant?

1. Presence of risk factors for malignancy, such as past or present history of smoking, chewing tobacco, or ethanol abuse.

2. Lesions that are palpable, indurated, bleeding, and associated with a concurrent ulcer have a much greater likelihood of malignancy. The risk is even higher in the presence of lymphadenopathy.

Of interest, in a large review of oral and oropharyngeal carcinomas, neoplastic lesions were much more frequently red than white (64% vs. 11%). Thus, erythroplakia more than leukoplakia is a clue to the diagnosis of malignancy.

Pearl. *In the final analysis, the only way to differentiate a malignant from a benign oral lesion is to perform an excisional biopsy.*

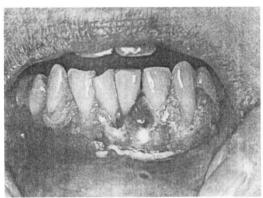

Squamous cell carcinoma presenting as leukoplakia with erythematous and verrucous areas. (From Sonis ST: Dental Secrets, 2nd ed. Philadelphia, Hanley & Belfus, 1999, with permission.)

49. What causes pigmented spots in the oral mucosa?

Pigmented spots in the oral mucosa are relatively common and may result from several causes. A far from exhaustive list includes the following:

- Amalgam tattoo (see below)
- Peutz-Jeghers syndrome (see below)
- Smokers' melanosis (see below)
- Hemochromatosis (15–25% of patients have a bluish-gray pigmentation of the hard palate with a lesser degree of pigmentation in the gingiva)
- Malignant melanoma (pigmented lesion with irregular borders, which may be palpable; often ulcerates)
- Addison's disease. Primary adrenal insufficiency is characterized by increased pigmentation of both skin (think of JFK and his chronically tanned look) and mucosae. Thus, the buccal mucosa (as well as the lips, tongue, and gingiva) may have a few scattered melanotic spots. The buccal mucosa of normal African-Americans also may have one or more pigmented patches. This condition, termed *melanoplakia* (black spots in Greek), is of little clinical significance.

50. Who was Addison?

Thomas Addison (1793–1860) was a contemporary of Bright and Hodgkin. Born in Newcastle and educated in Edinburgh, Addison taught and practiced at Guy's Hospital in London, where he gained a reputation as a brilliant teacher and astute bedside clinician. His shy and introverted personality, however, and his emphasis on diagnosis more than treatment adversely affected his popularity. Even his work on primary adrenal insufficiency (published in London in 1855) was almost discounted as fiction by many of his contemporaries. Plagued by recurrent bouts of depression, Addison eventually jumped to his death at the age of 67.

51. What is an amalgam tattoo?

It is the presence of a blackish-grayish stain in the buccal mucosa adjacent to an area of tooth restoration. It is due to accidental exposure of the mucosa to dental amalgam.

52. Do smokers have specific types of pigmented lesions in the oral mucosa?

Yes. In addition to an increased risk of carcinoma of the oral cavity, smokers also may develop pigmentary changes in the oral mucosa. Smoker's melanosis is a diffuse increase in mucosal pigmentation, particularly localized over the anterior mandibular areas and gingiva. The mucosa may even have a few pigmented nevi. Yellow staining of teeth and fingernails is often associated.

53. What is Peutz-Jeghers syndrome? Will I ever see it?

Peutz-Jeghers syndrome (named after the Dutch John Peutz and the American Harold Jeghers) is an autosomal dominant disease characterized by intestinal, pigmented, hamartomatous polyps. It is associated with multiple melanin deposits on the mucocutaneous junctions of the mouth and, occasionally, of the anus. Pigmented spots (1–5 mm in diameter) also may be seen on the lips, oral mucosa, and dorsa of fingers and toes. With age the perioral lesions tend to fade, whereas lesions on fingers, toes, and oral mucosa become more prominent. Peutz-Jeghers syndrome is associated with a slightly higher risk of gastrointestinal malignancies, although not as high as the risk for patients with Gardner's syndrome. The chance of seeing a case of Peutz-Jeghers syndrome depends, as in other areas of physical diagnosis, on the clinician. Although the syndrome is rare, you are never going to see it unless you look for it.

54. How do you distinguish Peutz-Jeghers syndrome from plain freckling?

In Peutz-Jeghers syndrome the pigmented spots are not only more prominent on the lips than on the surrounding skin but also present in the buccal mucosa. This is not the case with simple freckling.

55. What causes red spots in the oral mucosa?

In addition to inflammation adjacent to other oral lesions, various specific entities may manifest with red spots on the oral mucosa:

1. **Pyogenic granuloma** is usually a red, small, well-defined, and rounded nodule in an area of recurrent trauma. It is made of highly vascular granulation tissue, frequently with an ulcerated surface, and projects from the buccal mucosa. Histologically it resembles a capillary hemangioma.

2. **Erythema migrans** is associated with multiple, flat, irregularly shaped, red patches with raised white rims. They are usually located on the buccal mucosa, ventral tongue, and gingiva. They often are correlated with a geographic tongue (also called erythema migrans lingualis, i.e., erythema migrans of the tongue).

3. **Palatal petechiae** are also typical lesions, usually scattered near the border of the hard and soft palates. Although not entirely pathognomonic of infectious mononucleosis, palatal petechiae are highly suggestive of the diagnosis. They can be seen in almost two-thirds of patients with mononucleosis toward the end of the first week of illness.

4. **Kaposi's sarcoma** is associated with deeply purplish lesions that may be either raised or flat. They typically involve the palate in patients with AIDS but not in the form affecting elderly, nonimmunocompromised patients of Mediterranean origin. Incidentally, Moritz Kaposi was a Viennese dermatologist. Of interest, his family name was Kohn, but he changed it to Kaposi upon his conversion to Catholicism. He chose the name as a reference to the Hungarian town of Kaposvar, where he was born in 1837.

56. What causes yellow spots in the oral mucosa?

Yellow (or sometimes white) spots on the mucosa of lips, cheeks, or tongue were first described in 1896 by the American dermatologist John Fordyce. They still carry his name. Fordyce spots are tiny (1 mm in diameter) spots that represent normal mucosal sebaceous cysts.

57. What causes flesh-covered palpable lesions in the oral mucosa?

The most common examples are normal anatomic structures, such as Wharton's or Stensen's ducts, which drain, respectively, the submaxillary glands and parotid salivary glands.

1. **Wharton's ducts** (described by Thomas Wharton, one of the personal physicians to Oliver Cromwell and an active presence during the 1665 great plague of London) appear as two tiny papules located on the floor of the mouth, just under the tongue and approximately 5 mm lateral to the frenulum. They represent the opening of the submaxillary glands.

2. **Stensen's ducts** (often called Steno's ducts from the italianized version of Stensen's name) are located on both sides of the buccal mucosa, directly opposite to the second upper molar. They represent the opening of the parotid glands.

3. A **ranula** (Latin for small frog) is a unilateral, painful, dome-shaped, fluctuant nodule in the floor of the mouth. It represents the sequela of a salivary duct obstruction, usually involving one of the sublingual or submandibular glands. The resulting mucus retention leads to a tumor-like swelling that often requires referral to an ear, nose, and throat specialist for resection.

4. **Torus mandibularis or torus palatinus** (see below).

58. Who was Stensen?

Neils Stensen was a Danish anatomist who moved to Italy in 1666 as court physician to Ferdinand II. There he was converted to the Catholic faith by a nun and eventually became a priest. In addition to his description of the parotid gland's duct, he is also famous for describing the tetralogy of Fallot more than two centuries before Fallot himself.

59. What is a torus?

A torus is a benign, cartilage-capped, and mucosa-lined exostosis. Based on its origin, a torus may be called (1) torus mandibularis or (2) torus palatinus. Torus mandibularis is usually smaller and located over the mandible. Torus palatinus is a bit larger, originating from the midline of the hard palate and also nontender. The term *torus* is Latin for protuberance. It is used most commonly to indicate the bony structures of the skull. Tori are uniformly benign and require only clinical recognition.

60. What are the causes of ulcers and erosions in the oral mucosa?

The most common causes are (1) thermal injuries (such as hot coffee burns) and (2) aphthous ulcers (canker sore). Aphthous ulcers (from the Greek *aphthae* = ulcerations) are among the most painful mucosal erosions. They are small, round or oval, with a whitish-yellowish color and a reddened rim. They are extremely common and painful. Although benign and spontaneously healing in a few days, they tend to recur. Less common and ominous causes include the following:

1. Viral gingivostomatitis due to either herpes or coxsackie virus (see below).

2. Autoimmune gingivostomatitis, such as pemphigus, phemphigoid, and Stevens-Johnson syndrome, causes a tender, painful inflammatory sloughing of mucosa, which is usually preceded by vesicles or bullae.

3. Painless solitary ulcers may result from either carcinoma or primary syphilis.

61. How do you differentiate between a canker and a chancre?

Although both may result in oral mucosal ulcers, there is a significant difference between them. *Canker* (a Middle English term for a malignant, spreading, invading, and ominous lesion) has become a modern colloquialism for canker sore, a quite painful but entirely benign aphthous ulcer. Conversely, a *chancre* (an Old French term subsequently adopted in modern French) still refers to a much more serious lesion: the painless ulcer of primary syphilis.

Of interest, both terms derive from the Latin *cancer* (crab) or the Sanskrit *karkata* (crab) and *karkara* (hard). Their gloomy connotation reflects the ominous significance of an ulcer in the mouth in medieval times. Syphilis was dubbed *morbus gallicus* (French disease) by the Italian physician Girolamo Fracastoro in his 1530 poem "Syphilis." It kept its historical association with France for quite some time. Ironically, the French had acquired the disease in Italy during their 1494–1515 invasion (and indeed had tried to dub it *the Italian disease*, a term that never took hold). The Italians, in turn, had acquired the epidemic from the Spanish sailors who had visited their ports after returning from America. Considering where syphilis probably originated, a more appropriate term is *the American disease*.

62. Can the vermilion border of the lip help to differentiate specific causes of oral mucosal ulcers and vesicles?

Yes. If the lesions cross over the vermilion border of the lip and involve the skin, the causative agent is invariably herpes simplex. Conversely, if the lesions are limited to the lip and do not cross the vermilion border, the cause is more likely to be either coxsackie virus infection or an autoimmune process.

63. Where is Coxsackie? Who there has the disease?

Coxsackie is a city in New York state, the proud hometown of patients in whom the virus causing herpangina (infection of the oropharynx) was first isolated. The virus is also responsible for aseptic meningitis, pericarditis, myocarditis, and pleurodynia. Of course, the coxsackie virus is not uniquely limited to Coxsackie, New York; it crosses both interstate and international borders (see below).

64. Why is Bornholm in indirect geographic competition with Coxsackie?

Bornholm is a Danish island in the Baltic Sea and the site where the syndrome of epidemic pleurodynia (appropriately called Bornholm disease) was first described. The intriguing aspect of this syndrome (characterized by sore throat, cough, and attacks of severe pain, usually pleuritic but often abdominal) is that it is caused by a virus named after another geographic location, coxsackie virus.

65. Why should a clinician examine the palms and soles of a patient with oropharyngeal vesicles and erosions?

Often patients, particularly children with severe herpangina due to coxsackie virus, may present with vesicles on the palms and soles. This finding may assist the clinician in diagnosing a particularly vexing case of sore throat.

Tongue

66. Describe the anatomy of the tongue.

The tongue consists of skeletal muscle covered with mucosa. On the dorsum of the tongue are many exophytic structures of three different types: filiform, fungiform, and circumvallate papillae. Filiform and fungiform papillae are relatively small and cover the entire dorsal tongue surface; circumvallate papillae are larger, located on the posterior dorsum of the tongue, and arranged in a semicircle. All of these papillae increase the surface area of the tongue and, more importantly, contain the taste buds for gustatory sensation.

67. What is dysgeusia?

It is the altered perception of taste (from the Greek *dys* = abnormal and *geusis* = taste). It may reflect abnormalities that are either local (such as those involving the tongue) or central (i.e., involving the central nervous system).

68. What is the best way to inspect the tongue visually?

Visual inspection requires effective protrusion of the tongue, which is best accomplished by asking the patient to say "Ahhhh" or "Aeee" (but definitely not "Ha"; see question 38) while protruding and curling upward the tongue. This maneuver allows the examiner access to the sublingual surface of the tongue. Examination of the far interior and lateral aspect can be accomplished by placing gauze on the tip of the tongue, gently grasping it, and pulling it out. Unilateral paralysis of cranial nerve XII (hypoglossal nerve) is associated with asymmetric protrusion of the tongue.

69. What are the causes of a diffusely enlarged tongue?

Although politicians are at greater risk for development of an occupational variety of this condition, macroglossia (large tongue in Greek) is a relatively rare physical finding. Patients often present with a typical indentation on the sides of the tongue, caused by pressure from the lateral teeth. They also may have a history of thickened speech, snoring, or full-blown sleep apnea. Macroglossia is often associated with various systemic manifestations of underlying disorders, such as hypothyroidism, acromegaly, Down syndrome, amyloidosis, and various thesaurismoses. In all of these conditions, enlargement of the tongue is caused by either proteinaceous infiltration or hypertrophy of the muscle. The exceptions, of course, are politicians, whose macroglossia is due to idiopathic tongue in cheek, and some normal people who present with a simple lateral indentation of the tongue without clear-cut macroglossia or concurrent systemic illness.

70. What is a scrotal tongue?

A relatively common finding in the elderly, the scrotal tongue has many ugly-looking fissures (hence the colorful term scrotal tongue, which otherwise has little or no clinical significance).

71. What is a hairy tongue?

It is a tongue characterized by brownish-to-blackish discoloration of the papillae, usually as the result of antibiotic therapy. It also may occur for no specific reason. Like the scrotal tongue, a hairy tongue is usually of little clinical significance. It should not be confused with hairy leukoplakia.

72. What is a geographic tongue?

See question 75.

73. What causes a smooth red tongue?

The most common cause is atrophic glossitis, which is the final stage of glossitis, an entity characterized initially by papillary hypertrophy, then by papillary flattening, and finally by loss of all but the circumvallate papillae. As a result of this process, the initially shiny red color (beefy tongue) changes to a paler hue accompanied by a smooth, shiny, and often sore tongue (indicative of atrophy).

74. What are the causes of atrophic glossitis?

The most common cause is a profound deficiency of B-complex vitamins, such as niacin, pyridoxine, thiamine, riboflavin, folate, and B_{12}. Of interest, physical examination helps to differentiate folate from B_{12} deficiency by testing proprioceptive sensation. In folate deficiency the patient has glossitis but normal proprioception; in B_{12} deficiency (and, therefore, in pernicious anemia) the glossitis is accompanied by abnormal proprioception. Other causes of glossitis include regional enteritis, iron-deficiency anemia, alcoholism, severe malnutrition (particularly protein-calorie), and malabsorption.

75. What is the differential diagnosis of a white tongue?

Although the surface of the tongue may appear whitish as the result of ingested foodstuffs, several entities may result in a truly white color:

1. **Geographic tongue** is a migratory atrophic glossitis characterized by multiple, smooth, and red glossy patches, each with a rim of surrounding white. These patches resemble the islands of an archipelago; hence the nickname geographic. It is a relatively common condition (1–3% of the general population). Unlike atrophic glossitis, a geographic tongue is not associated with nutritional deficiency but is idiopathic. A psychosomatic relation has been suggested. Indeed, histologically these lesions are similar to the lesions of psoriasis or the mucocutaneous lesions of Reiter's syndrome. A geographic tongue is almost entirely asymptomatic, quite benign, and usually self-limited. The patches of glossitis change over time (hence the adjective "migratory") and eventually return to normal. Reassurance of the patient is usually the best management.

2. **White hairy tongue** (hairy leukoplakia) manifests with multiple white, warty, and painless plaques, usually located on the lateral aspects of the tongue and inner mucosa of the cheeks. Each of these plaques has hair-like projections, which give the condition its name. Unlike candidal infection,

hairy leukoplakia cannot be scraped off. Hairy leukoplakia occurs in severely immunocompromised patients, usually as a result of HIV infection. However, it has been described recently in patients without AIDS.

  3. **Oral thrush** is a common cause of white tongue. As with thrush elsewhere, it manifests with white plaques that may be easily scraped off and stained with KOH.

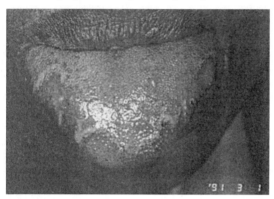

Geographic tongue. (From Sonis ST: Dental Secrets, 2nd ed. Philadelphia, Hanley & Belfus, 1999, with permission.)

76. What is the differential diagnosis of a black tongue?

  The most common cause, of course, is temporary discoloration due to the ingestion of dark-colored candy or black licorice. A more permanent condition suggests (1) use of substances containing bismuth, such as Pepto-Bismol; (2) colonization of the tongue by *Aspergillus niger* (usually associated with a few black and hairy patches on the tongue surface); (3) a hairy tongue (see above); or (4) use of charcoal for gastrointestinal decontamination of overdose patients (a not uncommon event in the emergency ward).

77. Can I diagnose the cause of gastrointestinal bleeding by inspecting the tongue?

  If the patient has multiple red-purple macules and telangiectasias on the tongue surface, the diagnosis of Osler-Weber-Rendu syndrome should be considered (see above).

78. What may cause palpable papules and nodules in the tongue?

  Several entities may cause papules or nodules in the tongue. Most are benign variants of normalcy, but some can be harbingers of malignancy.

  1. **Benign entities** include the circumvallate papillae, which are normal structures arranged in a semicircle on the posterior dorsum of the tongue. They can be easily visualized by having the patient protrude the tongue. Other benign but slightly more abnormal entities include a lingual thyroid, which is a smooth, round, and red nodule located in the midline of the base of the tongue. It consists of vestigial remnants of the embryologic site of the thyroid gland before it migrated inferiorly. A radionuclide scan may confirm uptake of iodine. Nodular and soft structures located at the posterolateral base of the tongue may represent normal, albeit hypertrophied, lingual tonsils.

  2. A **papilloma** of the tongue is a soft, well-circumscribed, and pedunculated nodule that originates in the mucosa of the tongue and may achieve a relatively large size. It is usually caused by the human papilloma virus.

  3. Any nontender and firm plaque, papule, or nodule (or even ulcer) should be considered a **carcinoma** until proved otherwise. Carcinomas, especially squamous cell carcinomas, have a proclivity to involve the lateral aspects of the tongue. Therefore, they may be missed on a less-than-thorough examination.

  4. Conversely, a midline, indurated ulcer of the tongue is unlikely to represent cancer but suggests a **granulomatous disorder** (such as tuberculosis or histoplasmosis).

  5. An ulcer located on the inferior surface of the tongue suggests the diagnosis of **Behçet syndrome**, which was first described by the Turkish dermatologist Hulusi Behçet in 1937 and

consists of oral and genital ulcers associated with ocular and joint manifestations. Oral ulcerations may be of three types: (1) herpetiform-like, (2) minor aphthae, and (3) major aphthae. The larger lesions may be deeply punched out, 1 cm or more in diameter, and may involve the palate, pharynx, and even esophagus.

79. What are sublingual varicosities? What do they indicate?

They are enlarged and purplish varicose veins located on the undersurface of the tongue. Because they resemble little drops of purple-black caviar, they are often called caviar lesions. Varicosities of this type tend to be an entirely normal byproduct of age, although in some patients they may indicate chronic increase in right-sided pressures. In this case a diagnosis of either superior vena cava syndrome or congestive heart failure should be entertained.

80. What is the significance of tongue biting?

In patients presenting with a history of syncope, tongue biting is an insensitive but highly specific sign for the diagnosis of generalized tonic-clonic seizures, particularly when the biting involves the side of the tongue. In a study of 106 consecutive patients admitted to an epilepsy monitoring unit, tongue biting had a sensitivity of 24% and a specificity of 99% for the diagnosis of generalized tonic-clonic seizures. Lateral tongue biting had a specificity of 100%.

Lips

81. What is the difference between cheilosis and cheilitis?

Cheilosis is a reddening and cracking of one or both angles of the mouth (angular cheilosis or angular stomatitis). It is usually encountered in edentulous patients with ill-fitting dentures. The condition in fact is caused by recurrent leakage of saliva from the mouth, leading to maceration of the surrounding tissues (hence the French term *perleche* = excessive licking) and superimposed infection with endogenous organisms. In patients with dentures, a candidal infection is usually the culprit. Conversely, in dentate patients the responsible agent tends to be *Staphylococcus aureus*. Cultures and antibiotics, respectively, lead to diagnosis and therapy. Concomitant nutritional deficiencies (such as B_{12}, pyridoxine, riboflavin, or folate) as well as iron-deficiency anemia and Plummer-Vinson syndrome also may contribute to the development of cheilosis.

Cheilitis results from accelerated tissue degeneration, usually due to excessive exposure to wind and especially sunlight (actinic cheilitis). Cheilitis is characterized by painful vertical fissures that are perpendicular to the vermilion border and tend to affect predominantly the lower lip. It represents a risk factor for the development of squamous cell carcinoma of the lip. Cheilitis also may be an early sign of Crohn's disease and may be caused by the nutritional deficiencies listed above. Prevention includes use of ultraviolet blockers in lip balm and lipstick.

Unfortunately, the terms cheilosis and cheilitis are often used interchangeably (as in the hybrid angular cheilitis), thus generating a bit of confusion.

82. What are the causes of lip ulcers or erosions?

The most common causes are squamous cell carcinoma and herpes labialis. Squamous cell carcinoma presents as a solitary, nontender, firm ulcer involving the lip. Herpes labialis, on the other hand, results in a cluster (*herpes* = cluster in Greek) of tender vesicles and erosions.

83. What causes a diffusely enlarged lip?

Other than trauma (fat lip), the most common cause of an enlarged lip is angioedema. Angioedema results in marked, nonpitting swelling of one or both lips, which may develop rapidly and disappear rapidly over a period of only a few hours. Angioedema is usually allergic in origin; it may have concurrent pharyngeal swelling and even stridor.

84. What are the causes of pigmented areas on the lips?

The most esoteric cause, of course, is Peutz-Jeghers syndrome (characterized by multiple pigmented macules on the lips and oral mucosa plus gastrointestinal polyps). A much more common cause in the simple presence of ephelides (i.e., freckles). These pigmented macules, 2–3 mm in diameter, may be solitary or multiple and involve the lips. Ephelides are usually benign, but if any changes occur, they should be excised.

85. What lip lesion may result in an ophthalmologic emergency?
A red, painful eye in a patient with an antecedent or concurrent lesion of herpes labialis suggests a diagnosis of herpes keratitis. The diagnosis is confirmed by a positive corneal uptake of fluorescein with a characteristic dendritic pattern.

Gums and Teeth

86. What causes diffuse thickening of the gums?
1. The most common cause is **gingivitis vulgaris** in association with periodontal disease.
2. Another important cause of gum hypertrophy and bleeding is **scurvy**; vitamin C deficiency, although rare, is still an important cause of morbidity and even mortality. The gums are diffusely swollen, friable, thickened, and bleeding with concurrent petechiae in the perifollicular areas and dysmorphic, corkscrew-type hair. All of these manifestations are easily preventable and reversible by vitamin C. When the association between lack of vitamin C and scurvy became known, British sailors earned the nickname "limeys" because of their fondness for citrus fruits.
3. **Certain medications** also may result in marked gingival hypertrophy. The two most common are phenytoin and cyclosporin A.
4. The most ominous cause of gum hypertrophy and bleeding is **leukemic infiltration** in patients with acute monomyelocytic leukemia. This tumor has a proclivity to involve and diffusely invade the gingiva so that bleeding and hypertrophic gums may be the presenting manifestation.

87. What are the complications of gingivitis vulgaris?
The most common complication is tooth loss. In addition, the patient may develop severe gingival infections that present with pain, fever, gum erosions (trench mouth), and severe halitosis (halitosis paramaligna). Finally, severe gingivitis may lead to anaerobic pneumonias and abscesses as a result of recurrent aspiration.

88. What is "long of tooth"?
The expression is based on a common observation: with age teeth tend to look longer. This finding used to be considered a normal feature of aging. It is now interpreted as due not to lengthening of teeth (as in sharks) but to regression of gums caused by gingivitis. In other words, a person who is long of tooth will rapidly become short of teeth without prompt treatment.

89. What are the causes of tooth loss?
Most clinicians think of tooth loss as due to either extraction or fracture. In reality there are three other important causes:
1. **Tooth abrasion** is due to localized grinding, as on a toothpick or pipe. It may result in notches on the occlusal surfaces of the affected tooth.
2. **Tooth attrition** is usually due to decades of mastication and results in the diffuse wearing down of teeth as if a file had been used (like Nurse Diesel in Mel Brooks' *High Anxiety*). As a result of attrition, the yellow-brown dentin becomes surrounded by only a rim of worn-down enamel; thus, the entire tooth assumes a yellowish hue.
3. **Tooth erosion** is the diffuse wearing down of teeth caused by exposure to corroding chemicals. It often is seen in people who consume large quantities of freshly squeezed citrus fruits or even sugar-sweetened carbonated beverages. It is, however, more typically described in bulimic patients as a result of exposure to regurgitated gastric acid. For example, Jones et al. found dental erosion in 69% of bulimics. Erosion usually affects the posterior (lingual) aspect of the teeth, particularly of the incisors. Similar erosions also may occur in nonbulimic patients as a result of

simple acid reflux disease. Thinning of the enamel, as a result of erosion, results in exposure of the yellow-brown dentin and yellow discoloration of the teeth. Patients may have concurrent caries.

90. If you plumb a sulcus and it is normal, can the patient still have plumbism?

Yes indeed. A clinician plumbs a gingival sulcus to detect the severity of gingivitis. If the sulcus is inappropriately deep, the physician can diagnose moderate-to-severe gingivitis but certainly not plumbism. Plumbism is chronic lead intoxication. Although plumbism is much rarer than gingivitis, it can be diagnosed by examining the tooth gingival margin: if serum lead levels are chronically and markedly elevated, the patient has lead lines (also called Burton's lines from Henry Burton, a physician at St. Thomas Hospital in London and a victim of the great cholera epidemic of 1849). Lead lines are dark blue and are made by a series of tiny dots that circle the tooth at its point of insertion in the gum. Lead lines are produced by synthesis of lead sulfide (which is bluish-black) by tartar bacteria. Hence, lead lines are absent in patients who have no concomitant gingival infection (such as edentulous patients). Similar dark lines also may be seen with chronic exposure to bismuth.

Other manifestations of plumbism include renal insufficiency, peripheral neuropathy, saturnine gout (monoarticular arthritis), and, in young patients, a cognitive delay that may be quite profound.

91. What are Hutchinson's teeth?

They are part of Hutchinson's triad of congenital syphilis (interstitial keratitis, labyrinthine deafness, and Hutchinson's teeth). The upper incisors are smaller than normal and notched.

92. Who was Hutchinson?

Sir Jonathan Hutchinson (1828–1913) was an English surgeon and a Quaker. He was so interested in syphilis that he was rumored to have seen as many as one million patients with the disease. He also was famous for his ten-volume classic, *Archives of Surgery*, a textbook that he wrote entirely by himself. In 1908 he was knighted for his distinguished service to medicine.

93. What is halitosis?

Halitus is Latin for breath and *osis* is a Greek suffix indicating an abnormal condition. Thus, halitosis literally means bad breath. In the olden days, physicians used to draw a distinction between fetor oris (a smell originating from the rhino- or oropharynx, including the paranasal sinuses) and true halitosis, interpreted as a systemic odor exhaled from the lungs. This difference is almost entirely disregarded today.

94. What is the importance of halitosis?

Aside from its social and psychological implications, halitosis is an important sign of underlying disease awaiting recognition and treatment. Although usually not picked up by the patient, halitosis is rarely missed by the poor innocent bystander. Thus, unless you are blessed with Kallmann's syndrome (see question 28), you cannot escape halitosis medically or socially.

95. What are the causes of halitosis?

1. **Nonpathologic causes** include changes with age, so-called morning breath (due to reduced nocturnal wash-out by the saliva), hunger breath, menstrual breath (mostly quoted by German texts from the late 1800s), tobacco breath, and various foods and drugs (such as garlic, onions, fish, metronidazole, and paraldehyde).

2. **Pathologic causes** may be local or systemic. The most common **local causes** are (1) disorders of the oral cavity, such as retained food, stomatitis, glossitis, periodontal disease, poorly cleaned dentures, and even decreased saliva with development of dry mouth (xerostomia); (2) disorders of the nose and sinuses, such as atrophic rhinitis, chronic sinusitis, nasal septal perforation, ozena (an atrophic disease involving the nose and turbinates), and retained foreign bodies (especially in children); (3) disorders of tonsils and pharynx, such as recurrent infections of tonsils and

adenoids, pharyngitis, and especially Zenker's diverticulum; (4) disorders of the digestive organs (esophagus, stomach, and small intestines), such as achalasia and gastroesophageal reflux; and (5) disorders of the lungs, such as anaerobic lung abscesses, bronchiectasis, pneumonia, and empyema. **Systemic conditions** presenting with a particular odor of the breath include (1) the fruitish, sweet smell of acetone in diabetic ketoacidosis and (2) the ammoniacal odor of fetor hepaticus and uremia.

3. In **psychiatric conditions** the "bad smell" is perceived by the patient but not substantiated by an observer. Patients with a psychiatric condition also may perceive odors emanating from an external source. Causes of extrinsic olfactory hallucinations include schizophrenia and temporal lobe epilepsy. Conversely, psychiatric patients who perceive odors emanating from themselves (such as bad breath) have intrinsic olfactory hallucinations. A common cause is the olfactory reference syndrome (ORS), which is a hypochondriacal psychosis characterized by excessive preoccupation with body image. Patients with ORS are sensitive, insecure, mildly paranoid, compulsive, and depressive; they are so obsessed with the thought that other people may detect their smells that they prefer to isolate themselves. Providing reassurance is usually not enough. Patients are so convinced of their bad smells that frequently they seek confirmation by a different doctor.

BIBLIOGRAPHY

1. Cunha BA: Crimson crescents—A possible association with the chronic fatigue syndrome. Ann Intern Med 116:347, 1992.
2. Drinka PJ, Langer E, Scott L, Morroe F: Laboratory measurements of nutritional status as correlates of atrophic glossitis. J Gen Intern Med 6:137–140, 1991.
3. Eisenberg E, Krutchkoff D, Yamase H: Incidental oral hairy leukoplakia in immunocompetent persons: A report of two cases. Oral Surg Oral Med Oral Pathol 74:332–333, 1992.
4. Friedman IH: Say "ah" [letter]. JAMA 251:2086, 1984.
5. Johnson BE: Halitosis, or the meaning of bad breath. J Gen Intern Med 7:649–656, 1992.
6. Jones RR, Cleaton-Jones P: Depth and area of dental erosions and dental caries in bulimic women. J Dent Res 68:1275–1278, 1989.
7. Kidd DA: Collins Gem Dictionary: Latin-English, English-Latin. London, Williams Collins Sons, 1979, as quoted in Sapira JD: The Art and Science of Bedside Diagnosis. Baltimore, Urban & Schwarzenberg, 1990.
8. Mashberg A, Feldman LJ: Cinical criteria for identifying early oral and oropharyngeal carcinoma: Erythroplasia revisited. Am J Surg 156:273–275, 1988.
9. Moore MJ: Say "ah" [letter]. JAMA 251:2086, 1984.
10. Nenbadis SR, Wolgamuth BR, Goren H, et al: Value of tongue-biting in the diagnosis of seizures. Arch Intern Med 155:2346–2349, 1995.
11. Redman RS, et al: Psychological component in the etiology of geographic tongue. J Dent Res 45:1403–1408, 1966.
12. Roenigk RK: CO_2 laser vaporization for treatment of rhinophyma. Mayo Clin Proc 62:676–680, 1987.
13. Savitt JN: Say "ae." N Engl J Med 294:1068–1069, 1976.
14. Schroeder PL, Filler SJ, Ramirez B, et al: Dental erosion and acid reflux disease. Ann Intern Med 122:809–815, 1995.
15. Talbot T, Jewell L, Schloss E, et al: Cheilitis antedating Crohn's disease: Case report and literature update of oral lesions. J Clin Gastroenterol 6:349–354, 1984.
16. Vilter RW: Sore tongue and sore mouth: Systemic diseases that may cause sore tongue and sore mouth. In MacBryde CM, Nlacklow RS (eds): Signs and Symptoms: Applied Pathologic Physiology and Clinical Interpretation. Philadelphia, J.B. Lippincott, 1970, pp 142–146.

7. NECK EXAMINATION

Janice Wood, M.D.

Better bend the neck than bruise the forehead.—American proverb

TOPICS COVERED IN THIS CHAPTER

Anatomic Landmarks
  Anterior triangle
  Posterior triangle
Abnormal Anatomy
  Pterygium colli
    Turner's syndrome
    Noonan's syndrome
    Bonnevie-Ullrich syndrome
  Short neck
    Klippel-Feil syndrome
    Sleep apnea syndrome
  Buffalo hump
Swellings of the Neck
  Midline neck swellings
    Thyroid
    Benign congenital cyst
      Thyroglossal cysts and fistulas
      Dermoids
  Lateral neck swellings
    Laryngocele
    Branchial cysts and fistula
    Branchial hygroma
  Inflammatory neck swellings
    Lymphonodal in origin
    Neck abscesses
    Ludwig's angina
    Submental sinus
    Neoplastic masses
  Masseter muscle hypertrophy (congenital)
  Torticollis

Salivary Glands
  Anatomic landmarks
  Methods of examination
  Swelling of salivary glands
    and differential diagnosis
  Parotitis
  Parotid cancer
  Frey's syndrome
Trachea
  Palpation of the trachea
  Deviation of the trachea
    and its interpretation
  Oliver's sign
  Cardarelli's sign
  Campbell's sign
  Auscultation of the trachea

CONVENTIONAL TEACHING WATCH

The neck is an important crossroad of various anatomic structures and different organ systems. The most important of these structures is the thyroid (discussed in a separate section).

MANEUVERS/SIGNS		CONVENTIONAL TEACHING REVISITED
Midline neck swellings	⇑	Usually thyroid-related; important.
Lateral neck swellings	⇔	Less common than midline swellings.
Inflammatory neck swellings	⇑	Very important; usually due to swollen and inflamed lymph nodes
Salivary glands	⇑	Important and palpable structures.
Trachea	⇑	Important but often forgotten part of neck exam.

NECK FEATURES AND SWELLINGS

1. What neck features should be identified during inspection?

The most important is the contour of the neck. Several abnormalities can be identified:

1. **Pterygium colli** (from the Greek *pterygion* = wing), also called webbed neck, is usually encountered in patients with one of the following syndromes:
   - *Turner's syndrome.* Henry H. Turner (1892–1970), U.S. endocrinologist at the University of Oklahoma and one of the founders of the Endocrine Society, described a syndrome of ovarian dysgenesis in phenotypic females of short stature, low-set ears, shield chest, congenital heart defect (especially coarctation of the aorta), café-au-lait spots, freckles, and, of course, a webbed neck.
   - *Noonan's syndrome.* This syndrome was described by the American pediatric cardiologist Jacqueline Noonan (b. 1928). Patients are phenotypic males or females with a congenital heart defect (usually pulmonic stenosis), pectus carinatum, short stature, mild mental retardation, hypertelorism, and, of course, a webbed neck. Males tend to be cryptorchic and to have high gonadotropin levels. Females are fertile. Bleeding and dermatologic abnormalities are also common.
   - *Bonnevie-Ullrich syndrome.* Described by U.S. geneticist Kristine Bonnevie (1872–1950) and German pediatrician Otto Ullrich (1894–1957), this syndrome includes both skeletal and soft tissue abnormalities, such as lymphedema of hands and feet, nail dystrophy, laxity of the skin, short stature, and, of course, a webbed neck. When associated with Klippel-Feil syndrome (see below), the same constellation of findings is named Nielsen disease.

2. A **short neck** may be seen in patients with one of the following syndromes:
   - *Klippel-Feil syndrome.* Described by Maurice Klippel and André Feil, French neurologists of the turn of the century, Klippel-Feil syndrome is the congenital fusion of two or more cervical vertebrae, producing a low posterior hairline and a short neck that displaces the head anteriorly and inferiorly. At times it may lead to neurologic compromise, such as platybasia (a developmental anomaly of the skull that causes the floor of the posterior cranial fossa to bulge upward in the region of the foramen magnum).
   - *Sleep apnea syndrome*

3. A **buffalo hump** at the base of the neck may be seen with Cushing's syndrome.

2. What are the anterior and posterior triangles of the neck?

The anterior and posterior triangles are important regions of the lateral neck, separated from each other by the sternocleidomastoid muscles. These muscles are easily located by inspection and palpation, especially if they are tensed against resistance. The anterior border of the trapezius muscle and clavicle define the remaining borders of the posterior triangle, whereas the mandible and midline define the borders of the anterior triangle (see figure at top of facing page).

3. What are the normally palpable contents of the anterior and posterior triangles of the neck?

The **posterior triangles** contain many lymph nodes in chains that are normally not palpable beneath the superficial fat pad. They become palpable in the presence of a viral upper respiratory illness and pharyngitis. In the **anterior triangles**, the jugulodigastric lymph node is often easily palpable, but smaller nodes are usually not palpable unless enlarged in patients with infection, inflammation, or malignancy.

The subclavian artery often may be felt pulsating in the root of the neck immediately above the clavicle. High in the neck, between the mastoid process and the angle of the mandible, the transverse process of the atlas may be palpated. This hard swelling may be misinterpreted as abnormal. Laterally, along the sternocleidomastoid muscle, the pulsatile common carotid artery and its prominent bifurcation can be appreciated.

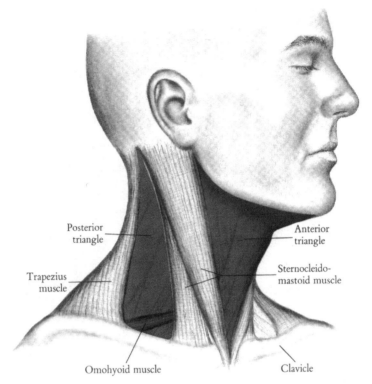

Anterior and posterior triangles of the neck. (From Seidel HM, Ball JB, Dains JE, Benedict GW: Mosby's Guide to Physical Examination, 3rd ed. St. Louis, Mosby, 1995, with permission.)

4. What neck swellings may be encountered during inspection?

Many swellings may be encountered in the neck. Their classification and origin depend on location: midline or lateral.

MIDLINE NECK SWELLINGS

5. What neck swellings occur in the midline of the anterior triangle?

Midline neck swellings are usually of thyroid origin (goiters or nodules). Less commonly they are due to benign congenital cysts that represent remnants of embryonic structures, such as branchial cleft cysts, thyroglossal duct cysts, and dermoids. Nonthyroid swellings are easily differentiated from the thyroid gland on exam (see below and figure at top of following page).

6. What is a thyroglossal cyst? How is it diagnosed?

A thyroglossal cyst may occur in the remnant of the thyroglossal duct, which in the embryo connects the forming thyroid with the tongue. It usually disappears, leaving only a pit in its point of origin: the foramen cecum. However, it may persist as an anomalous tract connecting the isthmus of the thyroid with the foramen cecum. In this case, the tract may harbor a cyst or fistula.

The thyroglossal duct cyst presents as a midline mass, with its bulk at about the level of the thyroid or cricoid cartilages. Because the convexity of the hyoid bone and thyroid cartilage may push the cyst laterally, in some people the thyroglossal cyst may not be exactly in the midline. The thyroglossal cyst moves with deglutination, like any thyroid prominence. Thus it can be differentiated from the thyroid only by its unique ability to rise with protrusion of the

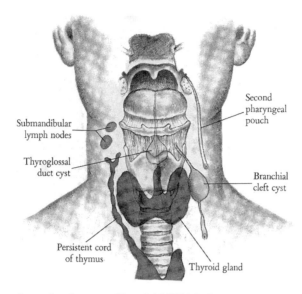

Surface projections of several neck masses. (From Seidel HM, Ball JB, Dains JE, Benedict GW: Mosby's Guide to Physical Examination, 3rd ed. St. Louis, Mosby, 1995, with permission.)

tongue because of its firm attachment to the base of the tongue. To carry out this maneuver, the patient is asked to stick out the tongue as forcefully as possible while the examiner holds the suspected cyst between the thumb and index finger. A good way to force protrusion of the tongue is to ask the patient to try to touch his or her chin with the tongue.

7. What is a thyroglossal fistula? How does it present?

This fistulous opening of the thyroglossal duct is less common than a thyroglossal cyst. It presents as a midline pit at the level of the cricoid that drains mucus intermittently and is subject to recurrent infections.

8. What are dermoids?

Dermoids may occur in any line of embryologic fusion. In the neck they present as midline swellings, usually above the hyoid bone and in the submandibular region. They also may occur lower in the suprasternal regions. In addition to external neck swelling, a dermoid may cause swelling in the floor of the mouth and push the tongue upward. Dermoid cysts usually contain hair and cheesy epithelial debris. They are soft and may be fluctuant. They cannot be transilluminated and are not attached to the skin.

LATERAL NECK SWELLINGS

9. What is a laryngocele?

A laryngocele (from the Greek *kele* = hernia) is a hernia of the larynx that presents as an air-containing diverticular outpouching of the neck. It originates in the larynx and is usually chronic and asymptomatic. Sometimes, however, it may present acutely with hoarseness and stridor or superimposed infection (see below).

10. How does a laryngocele form?

A laryngocele, like a colonic diverticulum, forms as a result of increased intraluminal pressure. Thus, it is often encountered in people who recurrently apply pressure to the laryngeal walls because of disease (e.g., patients with chronic obstructive lung disease who resort to pursed-lip respiration) or job requirements (e.g., glass blowers, trumpet players). The most famous example is the frog-mouthed Dizzy Gillespie. The laryngocele originates as a diverticulum from the ventricle of the larynx because of the intense pressure applied to the walls. As the exterior of the larynx expands through the constrictor muscles, the diverticulum of air becomes evident in the region of the hyoid and thyroid cartilages. Over time there also may be a change in the quality of the voice due to the swelling in the lateral wall of the larynx. The laryngocele may be bilateral and become encysted and complicated by infection, often leading to abscess formation.

11. What bedside maneuver may be used to diagnose a laryngocele?

The Valsalva maneuver, which consists of forced expiration against a closed glottis and nose, results in an increase in both intrathoracic and central venous pressure. It is easily elicited by asking patients to "bear down," as if they were having a bowel movement. The Valsalva maneuver typically inflates a laryngocele as a result of the increased intraairway pressure.

12. What are branchial cysts and fistulas?

Branchial cysts and fistulas are remnants of the branchial arches and clefts. The arches are paired structures that form the lateral and ventral walls of the pharynx of the embryo. They are separated by the branchial clefts externally and the pharyngeal pouches internally. Branchial clefts are reabsorbed in humans, although at times the second branchial cleft may evolve into a branchial cyst or, less commonly, into a fistula. In fish, on the other hand, the branchial clefts become gills (= branchia).

13. Where is a branchial cyst located?

It is usually located between the upper one-third and lower two-thirds of the anterior border of the sternocleidomastoid muscle. It also may continue deep into the muscle.

14. What does a branchial cyst look like?

The most typical presentation is a tense globular swelling, located posteroinferiorly to the angle of a jaw of a young adult. As the swelling enlarges, the cyst bulges characteristically and exclusively around the anterior border of the sternocleidomastoid muscle. A branchial cyst is never located superficial to or posterior to the sternocleidomastoid muscle. It cannot be transilluminated, nor does it move with deglutination. Enlarged lymph nodes are not associated with branchial cysts, which develop slowly from embryonic remnants of the second branchial cleft. If lymph nodes are enlarged, consider the diagnosis of tubercular lymphadenitis (scrofula) or a complicating abscess.

15. How does a branchial fistula present?

A branchial fistula presents as a pit located at the anterior border of the sternocleidomastoid muscle. It usually exits at the level of the hyoid bone but also may open either superiorly (anteroinferior to the earlobe) or inferiorly (near the lower part of the sternocleidomastoid).

16. What is a branchial hygroma?

It is a fluid-filled bursa or sac, originating from the branchial formations. It is usually located in the neck but at times may occur even in the thorax.

INFLAMMATORY NECK SWELLINGS

17. How can a lymph node inflammation be differentiated from other inflammatory neck swellings?

Acute lymph node inflammation is common and easily identified by the presence of swelling and tenderness combined with the identification of the primary infection site. It may be accompanied by systemic symptoms of fever and malaise. In patients with lymph node swelling, knowledge of the drainage patterns of the various lymph nodes is quite helpful in identifying the primary infection site (such as scalp, nose, sinuses, oral cavity, throat, or larynx). An acutely inflamed lymph node over the mastoid process may arise from a scalp infection, simulating acute mastoiditis.

Occasionally the inflammation progresses to a localized abscess and becomes fluctuant. If the suppuration is not well contained, as in the deeper fascial spaces of the neck, there is no fluctuance. This pattern commonly occurs in lateral pharyngeal abscesses and Ludwig's angina (see below).

Chronic enlargement of a lymph node may occur in patients with chronic infection; a persistent hard node requires further analysis for malignancy. Chronic painless enlargement may occur with tuberculous adenitis, although it is rare. Lymphomas, HIV infection, and sarcoidosis also may cause multiple neck lymph node swellings. As noted above, thyroid masses usually can be differentiated from lymph nodes clinically by palpation and observation of ascent with deglutination.

18. Where do neck abscesses typically occur?

Neck abscesses may arise from intensive inflammation and suppuration of a lymph node, as noted above. They may be considerably large and tender, especially in children. Abscesses that occur in branchial cysts or thyroglossal cysts present as a superficially located fluctuant mass. Their specific location on examination facilitates identification (see above).

19. Do neck abscesses always present as a localized fluctuant mass?

No. When an acute abscess forms in one of the deeper fascial planes, such as the lateral pharyngeal space, the patient may present with neither fluctuance nor any obvious portal of entry. The source of the infection may be evident from the presentation of an acute infectious illness and a brawny, diffusely tender swelling in the neck region.

20. What is Ludwig's angina?

Ludwig's angina is an acute cellulitis in the submandibular salivary gland region, deep to the mylohyoid muscle. Most cases represent complications of a mouth or throat infection that has penetrated the neck tissues through the submandibular lymph nodes. Ludwig's angina also may result from suppuration in the submandibular salivary gland itself. The infection is limited by the attachment of the fascial planes deep to the mylohyoid; thus the presence of a severe inflammatory process in this region results in a rapid increase in tension. At times it may be associated with laryngeal edema.

21. How does Ludwig's angina present on physical examination?

It presents as a tender, indurated, nonfluctuant, midline inflammation below the angle of the jaw. Common signs include evidence of edema in the floor of the mouth and dorsal deviation of the tongue (the tongue is pushed upward from the floor of the mouth). Bimanual palpation of this region reveals a characteristic "woody" firmness of the normally soft tissues of the floor of the mouth. A toxic-appearing, drooling patient with a brawny neck swelling is highly suggestive of Ludwig's angina.

22. Who was Ludwig?

Wilhelm F. von Ludwig was a German physician. After his graduation in 1811 from the University of Tubingen, he served as a surgeon in the German allied army that assisted Napoleon in the invasion of Russia. Captured at the battle of Vilna, he spent two years in a Russian prison. Released after Waterloo, he returned to Tubingen, where he became physician to the royal family. He described in Queen Catherine of Wurtemberg the angina that was his ticket to fame but also his only important clinical observation. Upon his death he left most of his fortune to a hospital for the poor, which opened in 1874, nine years after his death.

23. What is a submental sinus?

Chronic granulation tissue forms a sinus around the apical infection of a lower incisor tooth. On exam it presents as a midline pit under the chin.

24. How does a tuberculous cervical abscess typically present?

As a chronic nontender abscess with a draining sinus tract in the posterior triangle of the neck. A tuberculous abscess also may present as firm, nontender cervical lymph nodes without sinus formation. Although relatively common in third-world countries in Asia, cervical tuberculous lymphadenitis is a relatively uncommon cause of chronic cervical lymph node enlargement in the United States.

25. What other generalized inflammatory conditions may occur in the neck?

1. A **sebaceous or intradermal cyst** may occur anywhere as a smooth subcutaneous mass. It may have a central visible punctum. Its superficial location should easily differentiate it from other causes of neck masses and swellings.

2. **Cervical cellulit** is a superficial soft tissue infection. When located in the neck, it frequently results from a dental abscess in the lower molars. No localized swelling or mass is appreciated.

OTHER NECK SWELLINGS

26. What are the most common varieties of neoplastic lateral neck swelling?

1. **Lymphomas** frequently present with enlarged cervical lymph nodes.

2. **Metastatic lymph nodes** from the thyroid, nasopharynx, or postcricoid regions are also important in the differential diagnosis of lateral neck swellings. Lateral neck metastatic masses may cause Horner's syndrome (drooping upper eyelid and constricted pupil of the affected side) due to pressure or direct invasion of the sympathetic chain.

3. **Swellings of neurogenic origin** also should be considered (neurofibromas, neuroblastomas), along with lipomas and cystic hygromas in children.

4. **Paragangliomas or glomus tumors** occasionally occur in the neck at the bifurcation of the carotid or higher in the parapharyngeal region. They may be pulsatile and associated with a bruit.

5. **Other tumors** of the parapharyngeal space include ectopic salivary tumors. In addition to swelling in the neck, such tumors are associated with medial displacement of the pharyngeal wall and tonsil, as are neurogenic tumors and lymphomas.

27. What are the exam features of masseter muscle hypertrophy and torticollis?

Congenital hypertrophy of the masseter muscle may be confused with a parotid mass on inspection but is easily differentiated by careful palpation. **Torticollis**, an acute spasm of the sternocleidomastoid muscle, may present as prominence and deviation of the neck.

Salivary Glands

28. Which salivary glands are palpable?

The parotid glands, submaxillary glands, and sublingual glands.

29. Where are the parotid glands located?

The parotid glands are located below and in front of the ears. On palpation they can be felt just behind the angles of the mandible.

30. Where are the submaxillary glands located?

The submaxillary glands are located medially and anteriorly to the angles of the mandible. They resemble a walnut in shape and size and are best appreciated by asking the patient to swallow, when they can be palpated medially and anteriorly to the angle of the mandible. In young persons with firm tissues, they may be difficult to palpate.

31. Where are the sublingual glands located?

The sublingual glands are located in the floor of the mouth, just beneath the tongue. Although they tend not to be part of the routine assessment of salivary glands, they are in fact palpable.

32. What conditions may produce swelling in the submandibular triangle of the neck?

Conditions affecting the submandibular gland and duct. The submandibular triangle is located inferiorly between the angles of the mandible. Swelling in the submandibular triangle usually arises from swelling of the submaxillary glands or involvement of other structures that extend into the submandibular triangle, such as an upper cervical lymph node chain or the tail of the parotid. Infections and malignant etiologies should be included in the differential diagnosis (see below).

33. What is the differential diagnosis of salivary gland swelling?

The mechanisms are essentially the same for both the parotid and submaxillary glands. It is important to differentiate between unilateral and bilateral swelling. The cause of **unilateral swelling** is usually a ductal calculus and its infectious complications (such as *Staphylococcus* sp. or *Streptococcus viridans*; see below). Inspection of Wharton's duct (located under the tongue, just laterally to the frenulum) for the submaxillary glands and Stensen's duct for the parotids may reveal the stone or simply pus. More rarely, painless swelling of one salivary gland may indicate tumor (see below).

Bilateral swelling, on the other hand, carries a much wider differential diagnosis:

1. Malnutrition, such as starvation, kwashiorkor, and anorexia nervosa. Painless salivary gland swelling may be encountered even in patients who are malnourished but do not look cachectic, such as bulimics.

2. Sjögren's syndrome is a keratoconjunctivitis sicca, characterized by dry eyes (xerophthalmia) and dry mouth (xerostomia). It is caused by a lymphocytic infiltration of the salivary and lacrimal glands and associated with various autoimmune diseases causing arthritis. It was described in 1933 by Henrik Sjögren, the same surgeon who in 1935 developed the technique for corneal transplantation.

3. Mikulicz's syndrome is identical to Sjögren's syndrome in signs and symptoms. Its etiology, however, is not autoimmune but asssociated with a constellation of various processes, such as tuberculosis, Waldenström's macroglobulinemia, systemic lupus erythematosus, or sarcoidosis. It was described by Johann von Mikulicz, a pioneering German surgeon and one of the first to use gloves during surgery.

4. Alcoholism (with or without cirrhosis) also may cause painless enlargement of the salivary glands, usually due to fatty infiltration.

5. Diabetes mellitus

6. HIV infection

7. Thyrotoxicosis

8. Leukemic infiltrates and lymphomas

9. Drugs may cause swelling with or without pain. Examples include sulfonamides, propylthiouracil, lead, mercury, and iodide.

10. Acute parotitis is usually an infectious process, most commonly due to mumps. Bacterial parotitis also may cause the parotids or other salivary glands to become acutely swollen and tender. It tends to be a unilateral process, occurring most commonly in debilitated patients with uncontrolled diabetes, renal failure, dehydration, or severe electrolyte imbalances. It is usually due to staphylococcal infection and may progress to abscess formation, causing the overlying skin to become deep red.

All of the above processes may affect not only the parotids but also the other salivary glands.

34. What are the physical findings in acute parotitis?

The parotids become easily palpable and swollen, to the point of pushing the earlobes forward and laterally. In severe cases swelling may limit jaw mobility.

35. Is parotitis a condition limited exclusively to the parotids?

Not necessarily. Indeed, most conditions causing swelling of the parotid also tend to cause swelling of the other salivary glands.

36. What does parotid cancer look like?

Like a rapidly developing, uncomfortable swelling in the parotid region associated with facial palsy. Pleomorphic adenoma is the most common parotid tumor. Mucoepidermoid carcinoma tends to cause skin ulceration, whereas lymphomas most commonly present with facial palsy.

37. What is Frey's syndrome?

Frey's syndrome, also called auriculotemporal syndrome, is encountered in patients who have suffered either injury or surgery to the parotid gland. It is characterized by sweating, flushing, and feeling of warmth in the ipsilateral area of distribution of the auriculotemporal nerve (i.e., the ipsilateral forehead). It is usually triggered by eating. The syndrome was described by Lucie Frey, a Polish physician who lived and practiced in Warsaw and was killed in 1944 by the Nazis.

Trachea

38. What is the value of palpation of the trachea?

Palpation of the trachea is a fundamental maneuver for the interpretation and recognition of a mediastinal shift. When combined with other methods of chest examination (such as palpation, percussion, and auscultation), tracheal deviation allows the proper interpretation of both ipsilateral and contralateral mediastinal shifts.

39. What is the best method for detecting tracheal deviation?

The tip of the examiner's small finger should be placed in the fossa between the medial aspect of the sternocleidomastoid muscle and the lateral aspect of the trachea, while the patient is in a sitting position, leaning forward with the head straight. By comparing the depth of this fossa with the contralateral fossa, one should be able to appreciate any differences and therefore any deviation of the trachea.

40. How can one distinguish tracheal deviation due to lung collapse from tracheal deviation due to massive pleural effusion?

1. Tracheal deviation due to **lung collapse** is ipsilateral to the atelectasis and associated with decreased tactile fremitus, dullness, and auscultatory silence in the affected lung.

2. Tracheal deviation due to **massive pleural effusion** also is associated with decreased tactile fremitus, dullness, and auscultatory silence in the affected lung, but the deviation is contralateral to this process.

41. What is a tracheal tug?

A tracheal tug (Oliver's sign) can be identified by palpation of the trachea. This sign (described in the 1800s by the British physician William S. Oliver) is a downward displacement of the cricoid cartilage with each ventricular contraction. It can be detected by asking the patient to sit with the head extended, while the examiner grasps the cricoid cartilage and applies a gentle upward pressure with the thumb and index finger. A downward tug of the trachea, synchronous with each systole, reveals the presence of an aortic arch aneurysm. This tug is caused by the anatomic position of the aortic arch, which overrides the left main bronchus. As a result, the force of each systolic ejection is transmitted through the dilated aorta to the left bronchus and from the bronchus directly to the trachea, pulling it downward.

42. What is Cardarelli's sign?

It is another sign of aortic aneurysm, described by the Italian cardiologist Antonio Cardarelli (1831–1926). Cardarelli's sign is elicited by pressing on the thyroid cartilage and gently displacing it toward the patient's left. This displacement increases contact between the left bronchus and aorta, making it possible for the examiner to feel a transverse pulsation of the trachea in patients with aortic arch aneurysm.

43. What is Campbell's sign?

The downward displacement of the thyroid cartilage during inspiration. Although it is a tracheal tug, Campbell's sign is not due to an aortic aneurysm but to chronic obstructive pulmonary disease (COPD). The sign is felt by applying the tip of the index finger over the cartilage, looking for downward displacement of more than 2.5 inches on inspiration. This sign is an accurate indicator of COPD, and tracheal displacement correlates well with the severity of compromise of the forced expiratory volume in one second (FEV_1). The mechanism is an excessive pulling on the trachea during inspiration due to the strong diaphragmatic contraction of patients with COPD.

44. What is the value of auscultation of the trachea?

Auscultation of the trachea allows recognition of stridor, a wheeze found only in inspiration. A true wheeze is usually expiratory or both inspiratory and expiratory. Even an expiratory wheeze should be considered as originating from the upper airways when it is louder over the trachea than over the chest. This finding usually reflects expiratory adduction of the vocal cords (vocal cord dysfunction), and in patients misdiagnosed with refractory asthma may prompt laryngoscopy to confirm the diagnosis of extrathoracic obstruction.

BIBLIOGRAPHY

1. Barnett JL, Wilson JAP: Alcoholic pancreatitis and parotitis: Utility of pilase and urinary amylase clearance determinations. South Med J 79:832–835, 1986.
2. Harris RT: Bulimarexia and related serious eating disorders with medical complications. Ann Intern Med 99:820–827, 1983.

THE NECK AND THYROID IN ART

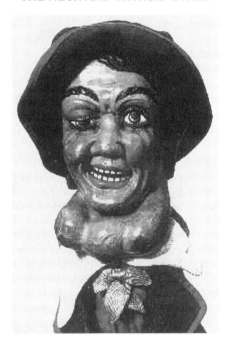

Gioppino, one of the typical masks of the Italian *Commedia dell'Arte*. The character is a hard-headed but good-hearted mountaineer from the northeastern Alpine region. He sports a giant, trilobulated goiter (presumably euthyroid in function) and a Horner's syndrome (presumably due to compression of the right recurrent laryngeal by the goiter). (See chapter 8, question 20.)

8. THYROID GLAND

Janice Wood, M.D.

TOPICS COVERED IN THIS CHAPTER

Inspection
Anatomic landmarks
Techniques of inspection
Marañón's sign
Palpation
Anatomic landmarks
Techniques of palpation
Assessment of goiters
Accuracy of physical examination in detecting a goiter
Auscultation
Indications
Thyroid bruits and their differential diagnosis
Pemberton's sign
Berry's sign
Goiters and their Differential Diagnosis
Graves' disease
Ocular signs of Graves' disease
Plummer's nails

CONVENTIONAL TEACHING WATCH

The thyroid gland may not be the most important organ or system in an internist's practice, but it is second only to the heart in the number of errors in examination technique as well as lack of confidence reported by primary care practitioners. Improvements in examination technique and increased confidence help clinicians to decide whether to order a costly thyroid scan for an HMO patient and how best to determine the likelihood that an anxious young patient has hyperthyroidism.

MANEUVERS/SIGNS		CONVENTIONAL TEACHING REVISITED
Inspection of thyroid	⇑	Essential in two-step approach to thyroid exam.
Palpation of thyroid	⇑	As above.
Swallowing during exam	⇑	Not much studied, but helpful in both inspection and palpation.
Marañón's sign	⇔	Not very popular, but useful little pearl in Graves' disease.
Auscultation of thyroid	⇑	Helpful in all patients with goiter.
Pemberton's sign	⇔	Helpful to unmask retrosternal goiter.
Berry's sign	⇔	Indicative of malignancy; useful to remember.
Ocular manifestations of Graves' disease (and related eponyms)	⇔	Helpful to remember a few (do not worry about eponyms)

THYROID GLAND INSPECTION

1. What normal midline structures in the anterior neck can be used to help locate the isthmus of the thyroid gland?

The midline bony and cartilaginous structures of the neck help the examiner to locate the central isthmus of the normal thyroid gland. Located just below the mandible is the mobile **hyoid bone**. Immediately inferior to the hyoid bone, the **thyroid cartilage** can be readily identified by the notch on the superior edge. This is the most prominent structure in the anterior neck and can be easily observed and palpated. Inferior to the thyroid cartilage is the **cricoid cartilage**. The **isthmus** of the thyroid gland is immediately below the cricoid cartilage. Sometimes it is found as low as the level of the fourth tracheal ring.

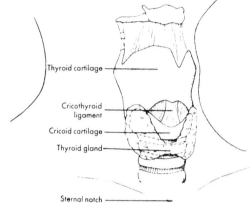

Surface anatomy of the anterior neck.

To feel the isthmus, place your second and third finger in the midline of your own neck and palpate downward from the chin until you feel the most prominent bony structure, the thyroid cartilage with its prominent midline thyroid notch. Two digit spans below the notch of the thyroid cartilage (3 cm) is the cricoid cartilage. Immediately below the cricoid is the thyroid isthmus, which traverses the trachea and connects both lateral lobes of the thyroid.

2. Where are the thyroid lobes in relation to other normal neck structures?

The two lateral lobes of the thyroid gland fan out from the midline isthmus, just below the cricoid cartilage, before curving posteriorly around the sides of the trachea and esophagus. The inferior margins are usually 2 cm above the clavicles. The upper margins (and pyramidal lobe) extend upward to the thyroid cartilage. Except in the midline, the thyroid gland is covered by thin, strap-like muscles, among which only the sternocleidomastoids are visible. The fascial envelope of the thyroid gland is continuous with the pretracheal fascia of the cricoid cartilage and hyoid bone. The thyroid isthmus ascends and descends with the laryngeal structures during deglutition because of this attachment of the fascial envelope. This important feature of the thyroid helps to distinguish it from other neck structures on physical examination.

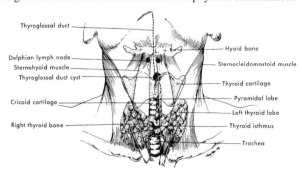

Midline structures of the anterior neck.

3. What is the best way to inspect the thyroid gland?

The patient should be either standing or sitting, looking forward with relaxed neck muscles and a slightly extended neck. Recalling where the normal gland lies, one should then inspect the neck 2 cm above the clavicles, looking for the inferior margins of the thyroid lobes (just within the sternocleidomastoid muscles). One should then look for the isthmus of the gland (below the cricoid cartilage). Finally, one should inspect the superior margins of the lobes (just touching the prominent thyroid cartilage) and, possibly, the pyramidal lobe.

Cross-lighting with a pen light is quite helpful in accentuating shadows and detecting nodules. Occasionally, having the patient tip the head slightly backward (10° of extension) can move a low-lying gland upward and tighten the skin over the gland to enhance visualization. Similarly, slight contralateral flexing may accentuate a mass, nodule, or gland asymmetry. Observing the gland from the side also may help to identify possible abnormalities and protrusions. If protrusions are detected, a ruler can help to quantify the degree. A goiter is effectively ruled out if the gland is not visible on lateral view and with the neck extended. Finally, the examiner should assess the associated venous structures of the neck and record any possible abnormality.

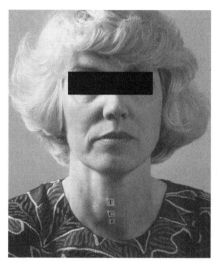 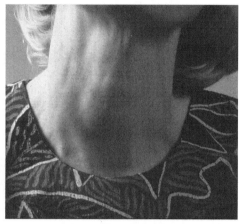

Left, Nodule in the left lobe of the thyroid. *Above,* Accentuation of thyroid nodule with lateral flexion.

4. How helpful is swallowing during inspection or palpation?

The role of swallowing has not been studied, yet conventional teaching considers it a useful adjunct to the thyroid exam. Most skilled examiners ask patients to swallow during inspection (and even palpation). In the opinion of some authors, swallowing may even raise the sensitivity of inspection to values similar to those of inspection and palpation combined. Overall, asking the patient to swallow allows the examiner (1) to modify the shadows of thyroid irregularities or masses, thus enhancing their visual detection; (2) to raise the gland, thus making it more accessible to both inspection and palpation; (3) to slide the gland (or its irregularities) against the hands, thus improving tactile discrimination and recognition; and (4) to locate the abnormality (only a few structures move with swallowing: thyroid, lower trachea, and larynx).

5. Should the patient be given a glass of water?

Probably yes. The degree to which the laryngeal and thyroid structures move upward is proportional to the size of the bolus swallowed. Thus, one should amplify the yield of the maneuver by making fluids available (such as providing patients with a glass of water and asking them to hold a sip in their mouth until given the command to swallow). One should repeat the maneuver if necessary.

6. How much information can be gained by inspection of the thyroid gland?

Quite a bit. Indeed, inspection of the thyroid is valuable because of the gland's superficial location in the anterior neck. Through inspection we can learn about the gland's location, size, shape, symmetry, and surface. In addition, we can learn about the gland's mobility during swallowing. This point is important in distinguishing a thyroid mass from other neck masses.

7. What is Marañón's sign?
Marañón's sign refers to the red (and at times itchy) skin of the neck region overlying the thyroid. It is usually seen in Graves' disease and is named after the Spanish endocrinologist, Gregorio Marañón (1887–1960).

THYROID GLAND PALPATION

8. What are the important aspects of thyroid palpation?
Palpation should confirm the size, location, shape, symmetry, and mobility of the gland, all previously assessed through inspection. Palpation is also important to appreciate the texture and consistency of the gland and whether any focal or diffuse tenderness or fluctuance is present. A hard thyroid, for example, is usually indicative of cancer. Conversely, a rubbery gland is usually typical of Hashimoto's thyroiditis.

It is important to determine whether a solitary nodule or the multiple nodules of a multinodular goiter are present and to assess for diffuse, fine, rounded protuberances like those of a raspberry. Such bosselation is associated with Graves' disease. A diffusely enlarged, soft goiter is highly suggestive of a vascular Graves' gland, whereas a firm goiter suggests a Graves' gland that has become infiltrated, as in a later phase of the disease process. Diffuse tenderness in a firm, diffusely nodular gland suggests subacute thyroiditis.

9. What does the normal thyroid feel like?
The normal thyroid feels like the meat of an almond. Its lobe is the size of a whole almond, no larger than the distal phalanx of the thumb.

10. Should a normal thyroid be palpable?
Not always. Thyroids of 15–20 gm (upper limits of normal) are barely palpable, whereas smaller glands of 10–15 gm are usually *not* palpable. The thyroid size in a specific population is determined largely by the supply of the iodine in the diet, with a tendency toward large glands in iodine-deficient areas. Thus, the previously accepted upper limit of normal (35 gm) has decreased to 20–25 gm with iodine supplementation. More recent studies reveal the upper limit of normal to be 20 gm in the United States, whereas 35 gm may still be appropriate in iodine-deficient regions. Thus, even a "normal" thyroid may be palpable in some areas of the world.

11. What is the average size of the thyroid gland?
The thyroid lobes are 2 cm wide, 5 cm high, and 2.5 cm thick. The isthmus is 1.25–2 cm in width and height and less than 0.6 cm thick. As previously mentioned, the normal thyroid gland weighs 10–20 gm. Overall it is more convenient (for both physician and patient) to categorize thyroid size as normal and palpable or normal and nonpalpable (see above). An experienced examiner can easily palpate a small goiter of up to 1½ times normal size (25–30 gm). In some iodine-deficient regions, a gland of this size may be considered nongoitrous (see above). By the time the gland enlarges to twice normal size, it can weigh up to 40 gm. Even a first-year medical student is able to appreciate a goiter of this size.

12. What is the best technique for palpation of the thyroid gland?
Unlike inspection, palpation of the thyroid gland comes in many forms and techniques, including bimanual or single-hand palpation and anterior or posterior approach.

The **posterior bimanual approach** is the most commonly used. While standing behind the patient, place the second and third fingers of both hands together in the midline. They should be one finger-breadth (2 cm) above the suprasternal notch and one-half cm inside the medial margin of the sternocleidomastoid muscles. Using this position, first attempt to locate the thyroid isthmus (below the cricoid cartilage and above the suprasternal notch), and then palpate the thyroid lobes. In case of a gland asymmetry or nodule, you should then palpate the ipsilateral lobe in detail. This can be done by using one hand to fix the trachea and the other to palpate one lobe of the thyroid at a time.

As for inspection, slight ipsilateral flexing and rotating of the neck may accentuate a mass, nodule, or gland asymmetry. For example, to allow better palpation of the thyroid right lobe, the patient should flex and rotate the neck toward the right. The opposite should be done for the left lobe. Finally, one should ask the patient to swallow repeatedly as you palpate the moving thyroid gland. A slight neck extension (10°) also may be valuable by lifting the top of a substernal thyroid goiter into a palpable position.

Some experts prefer an **anterior approach**. While facing the patient, use thumb and forefinger of one hand to palpate each lobe. This maneuver also should be carried out just inside the sternocleidomastoid muscles, as previously described.

Pearl. *Practice by placing the second and third fingers of both hands at your own sternal notch/manubrium sterni. Move upward 2 cm above the clavicles to the lower poles of the thyroid lobes.*

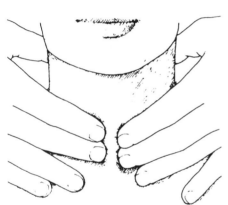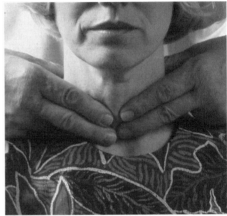

Thyroid palpation, posterior bimanual approach.

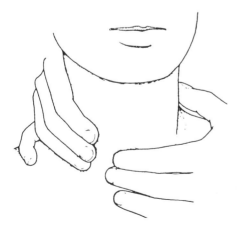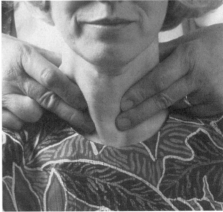

Thyroid palpation of contralateral lobe, posterior approach.

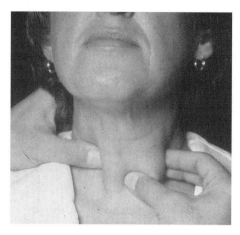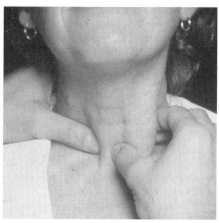

Thyroid palpation, anterior approach.

13. What are the normal variants of size and location?

- Women have larger and more easily palpable glands than men. The right lobe is often larger than the left. In up to 1%, the lower half or entire left lobe is absent.
- A pyramidal lobe may be present in 15% of thyroid glands. A triangular base arises from the isthmus and extends upward as high as the hyoid. It has the consistency of thyroid tissue. Like the thyroid gland, it also moves with deglutition.
- Posterior, extracapsular thyroid tissue may be present in 5% of normal glands. Ectopic tissue may extend superiorly from the posterior aspect of the tongue toward the pyramidal lobe. This lingual thyroid may extend inferiorly to the mediastinum.

14. What are the risks of false-positive and false-negative results in detecting a goiter?

Despite good examination technique, be aware of the following limitations of physical examination in detecting a goiter:

False-positive thyroid enlargement/goiter

1. Accentuated prominence of a palpable but normal gland may occur in the following cases:
   - Thin patients, in whom the thyroid is uniquely and misleadingly accessible.
   - Patients with a long and curving neckline. Despite its normal location and size, the thyroid is misleadingly prominent and palpable. Such pseudogoiters have been dubbed the Modigliani syndrome, after the Italian artist's peculiar style of drawing necks.
   - Whenever the gland is located higher than usual in the neck.

2. The presence of a fat pad in the anterolateral neck is common in obese patients and young women. It is usually differentiated from thyromegaly because, unlike the thyroid, the fat pad does not rise with swallowing.

3. Anterior neck masses must be distinguished from thyroid masses. Other anterior neck masses or swellings are less likely to adhere to the laryngeal structures and usually can be differentiated by their failure to rise with deglutition.

False-negative thyroid enlargement/goiter

1. Inadequate examination skills are the most common reason for a false-negative goiter detection.

2. Short and thick-necked patients, especially if they are obese or elderly or have chronic obstructive pulmonary disease, may yield false-negative results.

3. Atypical or ectopic placement of the thyroid: retrosternal or laterally placed lobes, obscured by the sternocleidomastoid muscles, may yield false-negative results.

15. In summary, what should one do on physical examination to determine whether a goiter is present?

Siminowski recommends the following strategy:

1. Examine the thyroid by carrying out both inspection and palpation.

2. Categorize the thyroid as either normal or goitrous. If a goiter is felt to be present, subcategorize it as either small (1–2 times normal) or large (> 2 times normal).

3. If a small goiter is felt to be present, consider the possibility of overestimation. Determine whether there is any prominence in the neck profile (report it as ≤ 2 mm or ≥ 2 mm) and whether the gland is visible on frontal view with the neck extended.

4. Finally, place the patient into one of the following three categories: (1) goiter ruled out (normal thyroid size or thyroids not visible with the neck extended); (2) goiter ruled in (either a large goiter or a lateral prominence > 2 mm); or (3) inconclusive (all other findings).

PRECISION AND ACCURACY OF THYROID EXAMINATION IN DETECTING GOITER

16. What is a goiter?

A goiter (from the Latin *guttur* = throat) is a chronic enlargement of the thyroid gland. Goiters occur endemically in certain areas (especially mountainous regions) and sporadically elsewhere. As Sapira reminds us, the Latin word for goiter is *struma*, a term that is still occasionally used in medicine. Originally struma did not indicate an enlarged thyroid; it meant scrofula (the widening of the neck that makes the patient look like a female pig (*scrofula* in Latin). Struma became linked to thyroid enlargement (i.e., goiter) only later—in reference to the Struma River in Bulgaria, an area of endemic goiter.

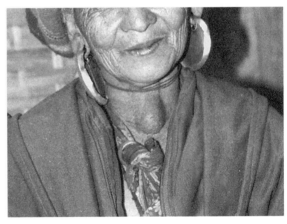

Euthyroid goiter in a Nepalese woman.

17. Is a goiter a neoplastic process?

No. Usually the term goiter refers to a process that is neither neoplastic nor inflammatory but the result of hypertrophy or degeneration of the thyroid gland. From a functional standpoint, a goiter therefore may occur in the presence of either a euthyroid or dysthyroid gland (hypo- or hyperthyroid). Thus, the presence of the goiter does not necessarily reflect the functional status of the gland.

18. Is a goiter common in pregnancy?

A true goiter is uncommon. However, mild hypertrophy of the thyroid gland is quite common as a result of the changed hormonal milieu of pregnancy. In the past this sign was used to detect whether a woman was indeed pregnant. For example, the overbearing and protective fathers of ancient Rome used to keep a keen eye on their daughters' neck. In fact, they used to measure periodically their neck circumferences to detect, as early as they could, any possible "loss of purity."

19. Why is estimating the size of the thyroid gland clinically important?

Not to detect pregnancy, of course, but because in patients with either suspected or known thyroid disorders, thyroid size provides information fundamental to (1) confirming thyroid disease, (2) conducting a differential diagnosis, (3) guiding and interpreting laboratory testing, (4) selecting therapy, and (5) monitoring a patient's response. For example, in patients presenting with symptoms consistent with hyperthyroidism, an enlarged thyroid gland increases the likelihood of thyrotoxicosis, whereas in the absence of a goiter symptoms are more probably due to anxiety.

Determination of thyroid size is important even when a diagnosis of thyroid disease is already established. For example, in patients with Graves' disease, a large goiter favors specific treatment options because larger glands are less likely to undergo immunologic remission during antithyroid therapy. The size of the gland also is taken into consideration in calculating the dose of radioactive iodine.

Finally, clinical evaluation of thyroid size is also important in monitoring adequacy of response to treatment. For example, in patients with a large goiter who are receiving hormonal replacement, shrinking of the gland indicates effective suppression.

20. What is the normal thyroid size?

Normal size depends very much on the supply of iodine in the local diet. In the not-too-distant past (and even today in countries that use noniodinated salt), thyroid glands became progressively larger as one moved away from the sea. As a result, large euthyroid goiters were so common in the mountains of Switzerland and northern Italy that they became part of the local folklore. For example, among the masks of the Italian *Commedia dell'Arte* was a mountaineer named Gioppino, whose trademark sign was a beautiful gigantic and trilobulated goiter.

Of interest, the word *cretin* (in reference to endemic and congenital hypothyroidism) also has something to do with the endemic goiters of mountaineers. Sapira reminds us that long ago a group of Christians was allowed to settle in the French Pyrenees to escape religious persecution. Although they survived unscathed, they all developed hypothyroidism and the mental slowing associated with it. When traveling to different villages they were easily recognized and immediately referred to as *cretins* (*Chretien* = French for Christian).

Extremely large goiters can still be seen but only in remote and mountainous areas of the world (such as the Himalayas), where iodine supplementation is not routinely instituted.

21. What is the prevalence of goiter in iodine-replete countries?

Very low. If we define as normal a thyroid that weighs 10 gm or less (with an upper value of 20 gm), the prevalence of goiter in iodine-replete countries is about 2–5%.

22. Can goiters be easily differentiated from normal thyroid glands?

Yes. Normal thyroid glands are barely visible and only slightly palpable at best because the various surrounding structures (primarily the sternocleidomastoids) normally block access to the gland. Thus, the first sign of a goiter is usually an increase in the size of the lateral lobes of the gland, which become clearly palpable. This is usually followed by visible enlargement of the entire gland, first detected on lateral neck inspection and then on frontal inspection with the neck extended. By the time the goiter is large enough to be palpable, it is easily visible both from the front and the side.

23. Which techniques can be used to assess thyroid size on physical examination?

Various methods have been reported in the literature:

1. Detection of surface abnormalities by either inspection or palpation
2. Estimated volume or weight of the gland
3. Visible prominence of the gland on lateral neck exam
4. Neck circumference, as recorded by tape measure
5. Maximal width of the thyroid lower poles, as measured by calipers or rulers

Little validation supports the use of one method over another. Moreover, most of these techniques share similar features.

24. What is the precision of physical examination in estimating thyroid size based on inspection and/or palpation?

Quite good. Precision data refer to both interobserver and intraobserver variability. For **interobserver variability**, agreement among physicians in either estimating the presence or absence of a goiter and in categorizing gland size into one of three or four groups is usually very good. In fact, the k for combined data from four studies assessing precision in the determination of goiter was a respectable 0.77 (k ranges from +1.0 [two clinicians are in perfect agreement] through 0.0 [chance agreement] to –1.0 [two clinicians are in perfect disagreement]). Agreement tended to be better among examiners with greater experience than among those with varying degrees or duration of training. It was also slightly better for palpation (k = 0.74) than inspection (k = 0.65).

Data are good even for **intraobserver variability**. Inspection (k = 0.73) seems to be slightly better than palpation (k = 0.65).

25. What is the accuracy of physical examination in detecting a goiter?

Good. Combining data from nine separate studies, the **sensitivity** of physical examination in detecting a goiter is 70% (95% confidence interval = 68–73%), whereas its **specificity** is 82% (95% confidence interval = 79–85%). If a goiter is considered present on physical examination, the **positive likelihood ratio** that a goiter is in fact present is 3.8. Conversely, if a goiter is felt to be absent on exam, its **negative likelihood ratio** is 0.37. These likelihood figures are similar (or even better) to those in other areas of physical examination, such as detection of splenomegaly.

26. What is the accuracy of physical examination in assessing thyroid size?

Quite good. The accuracy of physical examination in assigning thyroid sizes to the three categories of normal (0–20 gm), small goiter (1–2 times normal, i.e., 20–40 gm), and large goiter (> 2 times normal, i.e., > 40 gm) has positive likelihood ratios of 0.15, 1.9, and 25, respectively. Overall, glands that are 1–2 times normal tend to be overestimated in size, whereas glands that are 2½ times normal tend to be underestimated.

27. What is the likelihood ratio?

It is another method of describing the accuracy of a diagnostic test (such as a laboratory result, physical finding, or symptom). Although a bit more complex than sensitivity and specificity, the likelihood ratio is a more powerful indicator. Sensitivity means positive in disease (PID), a measure of how often a symptom, sign, or other diagnostic test is present when the target disease is also present, whereas specificity means negative in health (NIH), a measure of how often a symptom, sign, or other diagnostic test is absent when the target disease is not present.

The likelihood ratio, on the other hand, expresses the odds that a given symptom or sign occurs in a patient with, as opposed to a patient without, the target disorder. When the likelihood ratio of a finding is above 1.0, the probability of disease increases (i.e., the finding is more likely among patients with than among patients without the target disorder). Conversely, when the likelihood ratio is below 1.0, the probability of disease decreases (i.e., the finding is less likely among patients with than among patients without the target disorder). Finally, when the likelihood ratio is close to 1.0, the probability of disease is unchanged (i.e., the finding is as likely in patients with as in patients without the target disorder).

28. How do you calculate the likelihood ratio?

The likelihood ratio of a present finding **(positive likelihood ratio)** is equal to sensitivity/(1 – specificity). The likelihood ratio of an absent finding **(negative likelihood ratio)** is equal to (1 – sensitivity/specificity. For a more detailed discussion of likelihood ratios and their advantages in the interpretation of a finding, see Sackett's article on the precision and accuracy of clinical examination.

29. Is the accuracy of detecting a goiter on exam modified by the presence of thyroid nodules?

No, but it is increased by the examiner's experience. As a result, senior examiners tend to have better accuracy than their junior colleagues.

ADDITIONAL COMPONENTS OF THE FOCUSED THYROID EXAMINATION

30. When should I auscultate the thyroid gland?

Definitely in patients with a goiter and findings suggestive of hyperthyroidism. In such patients, a bruit heard over the thyroid indicates the gland's increased vascularity. As such, it is a highly specific finding for Graves' thyrotoxemia. In fact, a bruit is rarely found in other hyperthyroid conditions. Thus, searching for a bruit should be part of the thyroid exam in all patients with a goiter, other signs of Graves' disease, or other manifestations of hyperthyroidism.

31. How do you distinguish a thyroid bruit from other vascular sounds of the neck?

By location:

1. A **venous hum** is heard lower in the neck than a thyroid bruit and is suppressed by compression of the ipsilateral neck veins. The continuous character of a venous hum is not a reliable method of differentiating it from a thyroid bruit. In fact, 20–36% of all hyperthyroid patients have a continuous bruit that is due to the formation of arteriovenous communications within the hyperplastic gland and may be confused with a venous hum. Compression of the neck veins helps to differentiate the two processes.

2. A **carotid bruit** is usually heard lateral to the thyroid. Stridor or hoarseness of the voice may be apparent during auscultation. Carotid bruits also must be differentiated from the thyroid bruit.

3. Finally, a thyroid bruit must be differentiated from the transmitted murmur of **aortic stenosis or aortic sclerosis** by conducting a complete cardiac exam after examining the thyroid.

32. What additional aspects of the neck exam are important in evaluating the thyroid?

The advanced physical examination of the thyroid should include observation of local scars indicative of previous thyroid surgery, erythema, and the venous structures of the neck (such as Pemberton's sign; see facing page). Tracheal position should be noted as well as the presence of lymphadenopathy. Nodules and cysts should be transilluminated.

33. What are the potential complications from a large goiter?

Potential complications consist of obstructive symptoms, such as dysphagia and dyspnea. Although Graves' glands may be up to two times normal size (i.e., 40 gm), multinodular goiters are usually the largest. When a large mediastinal or substernal multinodular goiter obstructs the superior vena cava, engorged veins can be seen over the anterior chest wall and neck. In addition to impairing venous return from upper extremities and chest wall, large goiters also may impair venous return from the head. This obstruction can be detected by Pemberton's sign (see below).

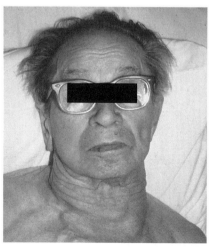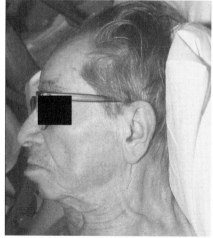

Superior vena cava syndrome.

34. What is Pemberton's sign?

Pemberton's sign is a reversible superior vena cava obstruction produced by a retroclavicular goitrous thyroid rising into the thoracic inlet. In other words, the goiter behaves like a cork, obstructing the thoracic inlet and preventing venous return. The maneuver is carried out by having the patient elevate the arms above the level of the head. If nothing happens after 3 minutes, the test is considered negative. It is considered positive whenever the patient experiences either facial plethora (blue or pink suffusion of the neck and/or face due to venous stasis) or a sensation of head congestion, dizziness, or stuffiness. If severe, the increase in jugular venous pressure may even lead to acute shortness of breath and diminished blood return to the heart.

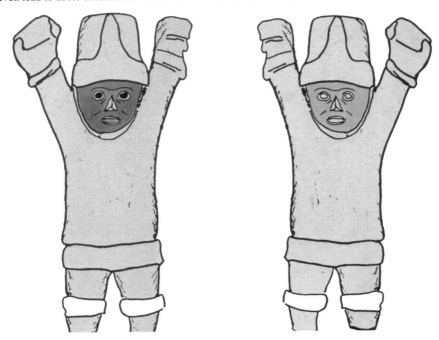

Ancient Toltec statuettes demonstrating Pemberton's sign. (From Sapira JD: The Art and Science of Physical Diagnosis. Baltimore, Urban & Schwarzenberg, 1990, with permission.)

35. Is Pemberton's sign specific for a retrosternal goiter?

No. It may be encountered in other patients with reversible superior vena cava syndrome due to lymphomas or other tumors. It also may be encountered in patients with thoracic outlet obstruction.

36. Who was Pemberton?

John de J. Pemberton, a 1911 graduate of the University of Pennsylvania, became chief of surgery at the Mayo Clinic in 1936. Pemberton had a distinguished career, characterized by several important contributions to both thyroid and general surgery, such as the use of blood transfusions.

37. In the presence of thyroid disease, what additional aspects should be included in the focused examination?

When an autoimmune thyroid disorder such as Graves' disease is suspected, special attention should be directed to the eyes and integument (nails of all digits and skin). It is important to detect extrathyroid involvement (see Graves' disease, below). In addition, a focused search for evidence of noneuthyroid states should be pursued (see hyper/hypothyroidism, below).

38. What is Berry's sign?

Berry's sign is the absence of the carotid pulse in patients with a thyroid malignancy grow-ing into the vascular bundle. It is always a sign of malignant thyromegaly.

39. Who was Berry?

Sir James Berry, an English surgeon born in Canada in 1840, contributed extensively to thyroid surgery. A philanthropist, he assembled a medical team with his first wife and during World War I traveled to Serbia. Captured by the Hungarians, he was forced to repatriate but eventually returned to eastern Europe, where he started his philanthropic work. He died in 1946 at the age of 106.

40. How can one categorize abnormalities of the thyroid gland? With what are they classi-cally associated?

Thyroid finding	Disease process
Diffuse, smooth goiter	Simple goiter, endemic goiter
Diffuse, bosselated goiter	Graves' disease
Multiple nodules	Multinodular goiter
Firm, diffuse tenderness	Subacute thyroiditis
Firm, small, nontender goiter	Chronic thyroiditis
Firm, hard, fixed, nonmoveable gland	Malignancy
Firm, hard, associated with lymphadenopathy	Malignancy
Focal tenderness	Abscess
Transilluminated nodule	Thyroid cyst

Do not forget to assess for non-euthyroid states:

Thyroid finding	Disease process
Toxic with thyroid nodule	Functional adenoma
Focal tenderness, hyperthyroid	Hemorrhage in functional adenoma

41. What are the three major manifestations of Graves' disease?

1. Hyperthyroidism with a diffuse goiter and two other infiltrative processes:
2. Dermopathy
3. Ophthalmopathy

When all three conditions are present, the diagnosis of Graves' disease on physical examina-tion is simple. However, because the three manifestations may have independent courses, the di-agnosis is often more challenging. The dermopathy of Graves' disease is an infiltrative process and is not dependent on or related to the functional state of the thyroid. In other words, it is not associated with or caused by hyperthyroidism. Thus, a patient in fact may be euthyroid with an asymptomatic, diffusely bosselated goiter yet still have other infiltrative manifestations (skin and eyes). Ocular manifestations of Graves' disease should not be confused with the nonfocal myxedema of hypothyroidism. Graves' disease is usually more common in women and tends to occur more frequently in the third and fourth decades of life.

42. Who was Graves?

Robert Graves was born in Dublin in 1797. He studied and practiced in both England and Ireland and became a superb clinician and charismatic teacher with a sarcastic sense of humor. Besides medicine and painting (his main hobby), Graves had many other talents, including a knack for languages (he was once jailed in Austria as a possible German spy because the border guards did not believe that a foreigner could speak German so fluently). He was also a strong leader. During a trip in the Mediterranean, he saved a ship and its mutinous crew by as-suming command in the middle of a storm. Besides describing the association of goiters and exophthalmos that still bears his name, Graves also described many other diseases and their manifestations, including the pin-sized pupils of pontine hemorrhage, scleroderma, and an-gioneurotic edema.

In German-speaking countries Graves' disease is usually referred to as von Basedow's disease in memory of Karl A. von Basedow (1799–1854), a German physician who in 1840 described the triad of goiter, exophthalmos, and palpitations. This syndrome eventually became known as the Merseburg triad after the German town where von Basedow was a general practitioner.

43. What is the dermopathy of Graves' disease?

The dermopathy of Graves' disease is the result of a local infiltrative process of the integument: pretibial myxedema. It is a dermal thickening due not only to lymphocytic infiltration but also to infiltration by other inflammatory cells and mucopolysaccharides. It most commonly affects the anterior aspects of the lower extremities. Although hyperthyroid features also may be present, pretibial myxedema (like the ocular manifestations of Graves' disease) is *not* due to hyperthyroidism.

44. What does pretibial myxedema look like?

The most common presentation of pretibial myxedema is localized, nonpitting edema of the shins. The more classic examples are well-demarcated, raised lesions in the form of a nodule. Lesions may progress to a plaque on the dorsal (anterior) aspects of the shins or elsewhere on the legs; the plaque is less common on the feet.

Pretibial myxedema may be pruritic or hyperpigmented. In about 50% of cases, it occurs in the active states of Graves' disease and is commonly associated with thyroxemia. It is *not* caused by hyperthyroidism. Pretibial myxedema should be easily differentiated from the more general myxedema of hypothyroidism.

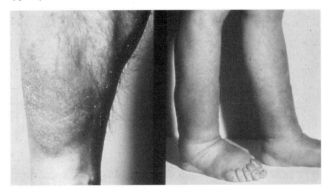

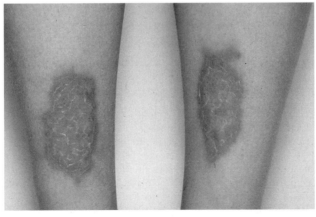

Pretibial myxedema.

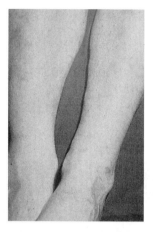
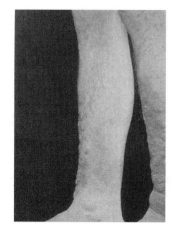

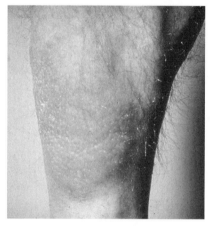

All three photographs show examples of pretibial myxedema.

45. What is thyroid acropachy?

Autoimmune thyroid disease may cause clubbing and bony enlargement of the digits. The periostitis is usually asymptomatic and nonpainful. Unlike the bony enlargement of pulmonary hypertrophic osteoarthropathy, thyroid periostitis occurs in the hands and feet, not the long bones. It is thought to be due to long-acting thyroid-stimulating hormone (LATS).

46. What other autoimmune disorders may be present in patients with Graves' disease?

The advanced exam of the patient with Graves' disease should include a search for other associated autoimmune disorders, such as premature graying, vitiligo, and hyperpigmentation.

47. How are the eyes affected in Graves' disease?

Graves' disease is also associated with an infiltrative condition of the extraocular muscles that causes exophthalmos. The extraocular muscles become enlarged mainly by infiltration of lymphocytes and cause proptosis (abnormal forward protrusion of the eyeball) of the involved eye. When the degree of proptosis is significant, it may cause congestive oculopathy and ophthalmoplegia (see below). Graves' disease of the thyroid is the most common cause of proptosis in adults. It is unilateral in only 5% of patients; therefore, an alternative diagnosis of malignancy should be entertained in cases of unilateral proptosis.

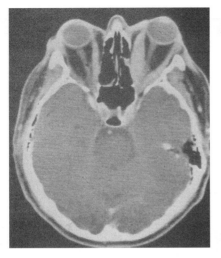
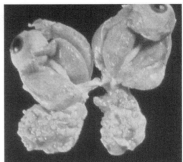
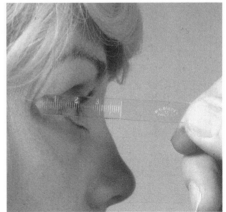

Above left, Exophthalmos, CT image. *Above right and bottom right,* gross pathology.

48. How do you detect and assess the degree of proptosis?

Proptosis is the abnormal forward protrusion of the eyeball (over 18 mm) from the orbit. The poor man's test for proptosis is to have the patient bend the head forward while the examiner looks down on the orbits and estimates the distance to the corneal surface. Usually one can detect whether the distance is greater than normal (> 2 mm). A more accurate measure is made with a Hertel exophthalmometer, a hand-held device designed to quantitate the distance between the lateral orbital rim relative to the anterior corneal surface. For a more detailed description of proptosis, refer to chapter 4.

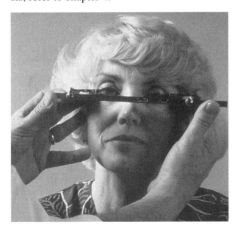
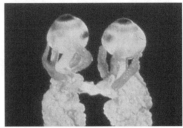

Hertel exophthalmometer.

49. What are the features of congestive oculopathy of Graves' disease?

When exophthalmos is severe, it may cause congestion of multiple layers of the eyeball:

- Conjunctivitis (conjunctival injection and redness)
- Chemosis (conjunctival edema)
- Periorbital edema
- Papilledema and optic atrophy

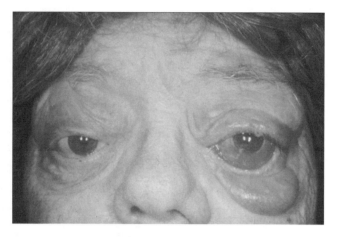

Congestive oculopathy.

50. What extraocular motion defects and impairment occur in exophthalmic ophthalmoplegia?
Inflammation and engorgement of the extraocular muscles preferentially affect the medial rectus and inferior rectus muscles. Overall, the infiltrative ophthalmoplegia of Graves' disease results in a series of extraocular motion defects and impairments, including muscle weakness and amblyopia, impaired upward gaze, impaired convergence, strabismus, restriction of gaze and visual acuity, and visual field competence defects.

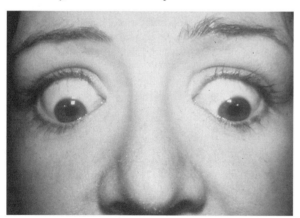

Extraocular muscle impairment

Described mostly in the past century by various German and Austrian physicians (plus a couple of Frenchmen, a Briton, and a Swiss), these signs carry a plethora of eponyms:

Stellwag's sign: infrequent and incomplete blinking.

Möbius' sign: impairment of ocular convergence.

Joffroy's sign: immobility of the facial muscles when the eyeballs are rolled upward (Alexis Joffroy is the first Frenchman on the list).

Graefe's sign: lag of the upper eyelid as it follows the rotation of the eyeball downward.

Sainton's sign: contraction of the musculus frontalis after cessation of action of the musculus levator palpebrae superioris on upward gaze (Paul Sainton is the second Frenchman on the list).

Kocher's sign: on upward gaze, the globe lags behind the movement of the upper eyelid (Theodor Kocher was Swiss; he is also the only Nobel laureate on the list).

Rosenbach's sign: fine tremor of the upper eyelids when the eyes are gently closed.

Topolansky's sign: congestion of the pericorneal region of the eye in patients with Graves' disease.

Jellinek's sign: brownish pigmentation of the eyelids, especially the upper lids.

Dalrymple's sign: retraction of the upper eyelid in Graves' disease, causing abnormal wideness of the palpebral fissure (John Dalrymple is the lonely Briton on the list).

51. What are Plummer's nails?

Onycholysis (separation of the nail from the nailbed) frequently occurs in hyperthyroid states. The eponym Plummer's nails has been applied to this phenomenon, which seems to affect the fourth digits preferentially. Onycholysis is not a specific manifestation of Graves' disease but a result of hyperthyroidism due to many causes.

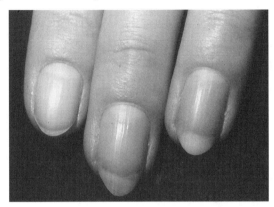

Plummer's nails.

52. Who was Plummer?

Henry Plummer was born in Hamilton, Minnesota in 1874. He practiced at the Mayo Clinic from 1901 until his death in 1936. His creativity and innovation led him to redesign the medical record system of the Mayo Clinic and to create the examination beds that are still commonly used throughout North American offices. Outside medicine, his interests included literature, music, and especially gardening. Plummer's name is linked to a thyroid nodule associated with hyperthyroidism but *not* with ocular manifestations. The condition is sometimes called Plummer-Vinson adenoma in memory of Porter Vinson, a fellow in medicine at the Mayo Clinic and a junior associate of Plummer. Plummer-Vinson adenoma should not be confused with Plummer-Vinson syndrome (sideropenic dysphagia, iron deficiency anemia, dysphagia, esophageal web, and atrophic glossitis). The syndrome is often associated with koilonychia (from the Greek words *koilos* [hollow] and *onyx* [nail]), which is different from the onycholysis of hyperthyroidism and refers to a malformation of the nails in which the outer surface is concave. It is often associated with various hypochromic anemias.

53. What are the manifestations of hyperthyroidism?

- Anxious-appearing, restless, fidgety (nervous, edgy, energetic)
- Tachycardia, wide pulse pressure, weight loss (palpitations)
- Warm, moist, velvety skin; fine silky hair
- Thin, breakable nails; Plummer's nails (onycholysis)
- Palmar erythema (nonspecific); hyperpigmentation at pressure points
- Hyperreflexia
- Fine tremor; palpate hands on outstretched arms (not with paper, which is oversensitive)
- Diarrhea

- Amenorrhea, scant flow
- Frightened facies of hyperthyroidism (sympathetic overstimulation)
- Stare
- Lid retraction, widened palpebral fissures
- Infrequent blinking
- Lid lag
- Failure to wrinkle brow on upward gaze

Hyperthyroidism and thyrotoxicosis in the elderly may present quite differently. Because the following features may predominate in the elderly, older patients who present with new-onset heart failure, atrial fibrillation, or depression should have an evaluation for hyperthyroidism:

- Apathy, depressed mood state
- Myopathy
- Proximal muscle weakness
- Cardiomyopathy or cardiomegaly with high-output congestive heart failure
- Atrial dysrhythmias
- Means-Lerman scratch (high-pitched pulmonic sound similar to pericardial friction rub)
- Flow murmur (increased intensity)

54. What are the manifestations of hypothyroidism?
- Bradycardia, weight gain
- Disinterested, complacent, lethargic
- Hair: coarse, breaks easily
- Skin: coarse, scaling, dry
- Nails: thick
- Periorbital puffiness: edema of facial features
- Doughy, nonedematous swelling (from mucinous deposition of glycosaminoglycan)
- Decreased metabolic rate
- No goiter (usually)
- Menorrhagia
- Constipation
- Good muscle strength (but lethargic)

BIBLIOGRAPHY

1. Graf W, Moller T, Mannheimer E: The continuous murmur: Incidence and characteristics in different parts of the human body. Acta Med Scand 196(Suppl):167–191, 1947.
2. Jarlov AE, Hegedus L, Gjorup T, Hansen JM: Observer variation in the clinical assessment of the thyroid gland. J Intern Med 20:37–42, 1991.
3. Jarlov AE, Hegedus L, Gjorup T, Hansen JEM: Accuracy of the clinical assessment of thyroid size. Dan Med Bull 38:87–89, 1991.
4. Kearns JE: Clinical diagnosis. In Treatment of Hyperthyroidism with Radioactive Iodine: A Twenty-year Review. Springfield, IL, Charles C Thomas, 1967, pp 16–17.
5. Sackett DL: A primer on the precision and accuracy of the clinical examination. JAMA 267:2638–2644, 1992.
6. Sapira JD: The Art and Science of Bedside Diagnosis. Baltimore, Urban & Schwarzenberg, 1990.
7. Siminoski K: Does this patient have a goiter? JAMA 273:813–817, 1995.

9. BREAST EXAMINATION

Carol Fleischman, M.D.

Thy two breasts are like two young roes that are twins, which feed among the lilies.

Song of Solomon 4:5

TOPICS COVERED IN THIS CHAPTER

Inspection
  Anatomic landmarks
  Techniques of inspection
  Haagensen's maneuvers
  Skin dimpling
  Peau d'orange
  Paget's disease of the breast
  Polythelia
  Polymastia
  Athelia

Palpation
  Anatomic landmarks
  Techniques of palpation
  Assessment and description of "lumps"
  Accuracy of physical examination in
    detecting a breast mass
  Nipple discharge
  Breast self-examination
  Gynecomastia
Lymphatic Drainage of the Breasts

CONVENTIONAL TEACHING WATCH

MANEUVER/FINDING		CONVENTIONAL TEACHING REVISITED
Breast self-examination	⇔	Sensitivity and specificity are low, stress created for patient is high. Should still be taught but not elevated to categorical imperative.
Palpation of breast masses	⇑	Yearly breast examination by clinician is important screening test and essential complement to screening mammography.
Dimpling of breast skin	⇑	This sign is usually significant—and ominous.
Peau d'orange of breast skin	⇑	Time-honored and still valuable sign.
Maneuvers to elicit breast discharge	⇓	Discharge that does not occur spontaneously is generally not pathologic.
Nipple inversion, retraction, deviation	⇑	Ominous findings that should prompt work-up.
Erythema of nipple and areola	⇑	Beware of Paget's disease.

1. What is the technique for inspection of the breasts?

The patient should be examined in both supine and seated positions. Breasts should be inspected for asymmetry, swelling, erythema, increase in venous pattern, and skin dimpling. Nipples should be examined for deviation, retraction, and inversion. Palpation of the axillae should follow.

2. Which bedside maneuver can help to detect breast abnormalities by inspection alone?

The most commonly taught and used maneuver is a change in the position of the patient's arms and hands, first described by Haagensen. In sequence the hands should be (1) on the patient's lap (to relax the pectoralis muscles); (2) pressing over the thighs (to tense the pectoralis muscles); (3) raised above the patient's head and clasped behind it (to detect skin dimpling, an important harbinger of breast cancer); and (4) standing up and leaning forward (to allow the breasts to become pendulous). Although these positions are commonly taught and practiced, it is not entirely clear whether they can indeed unmask lesions that are not otherwise detectable by simple palpation.

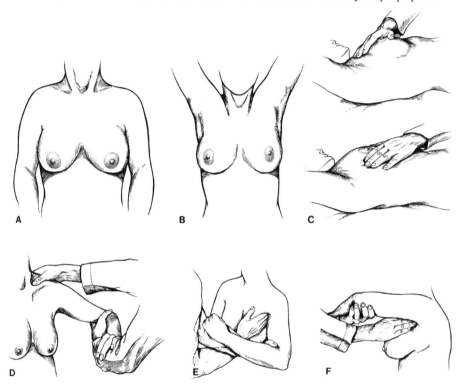

Physical examination of the breast. *A,* Observation with patient sitting and arms resting at side. *B,* Observation with arms raised above head. *C,* Systematic palpation with palm side of hand and fingers while patient is supine. *D,* Palpation of supraclavicular region of sitting patient with examiner supporting and elevating arm. *E* and *F,* Examination of axillae with volar surface of fingers by examiner standing on opposite side and totally supporting patient's arm. (From James EC, Corry RJ, Perry JF: Principles of Basic Surgical Practice. Philadelphia, Hanley & Belfus, 1987, with permission.)

3. What are the most significant abnormalities that can be detected by inspection of the breast?

Noncongenital nipple asymmetry or deviation and nipple retraction and nipple inversion (clues to an underlying cancer). Nipple inversion may actually be normal, but only if long-standing and correctable by gentle manual pulling. Inspection of the skin is also important. One should look for skin dimpling, peau d'orange appearance of the skin, and a scaly red dermatitis of the areola and nipple, which may represent Paget's disease of the breast. The examiner should look for all of these abnormalities in all of Haagensen's positions (see figure at top of facing page).

4. What is skin dimpling?

It is a slight depression or indentation in the breast's surface. It is an important clue to an underlying infiltrating carcinoma.

5. What are the suspensory ligaments of the breast?

Suspensory or Cooper's ligaments are thin fibrous bands that run through the breast and attach stroma to skin. Tension on these ligaments produces the dimpling, which sometimes presents over malignant breast masses.

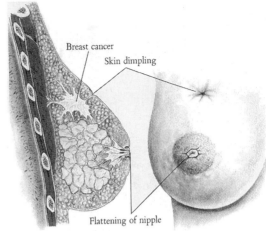

Breast cancer

Skin dimpling

Flattening of nipple

Nipple retraction and skin dimpling. (From Seidel HM, Ball JW, Dains JE, Benedict GW: Mosby's Guide to Physical Examination, 3rd ed. St. Louis, Mosby, 1995, with permission.)

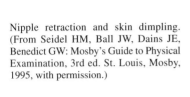

6. What is peau d'orange?

It is French for *orange peel*—an apt description of the breast skin overlying an infiltrating malignancy. This peculiar appearance is caused by the lymphatic blockage produced by the tumor, with resulting localized lymphedema of the skin.

7. What is Paget's disease of the breast?

Paget's disease is a malignant lesion of the areola and/or nipple due to an extension of neoplastic cells from the lactiferous ducts into the epidermis, which eventually becomes irritated. Histologically the tumor is characterized by large cells with a clear cytoplasm. It presents clinically as a scaly dermatitis of the nipple, with itching, crusting, and eventually erosion of the nipple, that eventually may progress to involve the skin extensively. It may occur without a palpable underlying mass. The differential diagnosis includes the other major causes of scaly and excoriative disease of the nipple, such as trauma from nursing and eczema.

Pearl. Redness and thickness of the nipple should be considered suspicious until proved otherwise; biopsy should be done to rule out Paget's disease.

8. Who was Paget?

Sir James Paget (1814–1899) was a British surgeon who stayed for his entire career at the St. Bartholomew's Hospital in London. A tall, brilliant, and charming man, he was so much enamored with clarity and brevity of language that he often quipped, "To be brief is to be wise." He became so famous that Prime Minister Gladstone used to remark that people are divided into two classes: "those who had and those who had not heard of James Paget." His name is linked to the first demonstration of trichinosis in humans (which he reported while still a medical student), osteitis deformans (described the same year in which he was made a baronet), the aforementioned breast disease, and a skin cancer of the apocrine glands presenting with the same cells as Paget's disease of the breast.

9. What is the technique for palpation of the breasts?

The patient should be examined in the supine position, with the arm on the side to be examined raised above and behind the head. Palpation should be systematic and comprehensive, evaluating the full breadth and depth of the breast tissue. The pads of the first two or three fingers of the examiner's hand are used in a circular motion with care to note the tactile quality of skin, subcutaneous fat, and breast tissue. A particular area should be examined carefully and all the way down to the thoracic wall. The examiner can then move to the next area, using a consistent pattern so that no area is missed. The examined areas must include the axillary tail, inframammary area, and anterior chest up to the clavicles. Commonly used patterns for palpation include (1) palpation by quadrants; (2) palpation in concentric circles (or a spiral) centered on the nipple; and (3) palpation in lines radiating from the nipple like the spokes of a wheel.

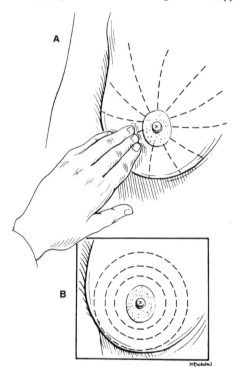

Methods of breast palpation. *A*, "Spokes of a wheel" approach. *B*, "Concentric circles" approach. (From Swartz MH: Pocket Companion to Textbook of Physical Diagnosis, 3rd ed. Philadelphia, W.B. Saunders, 1997, with permission.)

10. What important principles should one follow when palpating the breasts?

Do not skip any areas. Perform the exam in a systematic fashion (see above). Do not neglect to examine the axillary tail of the breast, and remember that breast tissue may extend as high as the clavicles. In each area, be conscious of palpating skin, subcutaneous fat, and breast tissue all the way down to the chest wall. Examine for adenopathy all of the lymphatic stations responsible for the drainage of the breast: axillary, supraclavicular, and infraclavicular nodes. Finally, the nipple should be examined for discharge.

11. What are the characteristics of normal breast tissue?

Variable, depending on the phase of the menstrual cycle. In the pre- and perimenstrual period, breasts are swollen and tender with prominent glands. Benign lesions, such as mastitis or fibrocystic disease, are also tender (which is usually, but not always, a feature of benignity; see question 14).

12. How should a breast lump (or nodule) be described?

1. **Size** is best assessed by using a ruler, tape measure, or, even better, plastic calipers.

2. **Location** is described in relation to the four quadrants of the breast and in relation to the distance from the areolar rim. One may use the clock analogy to report the finding in the patient's record.

3. **Tenderness** is usually a sign of benignity.

4. **Consistency or firmness.** Cancers tend to be rock-hard and firm, whereas benign lesions are compressible, softer, and at times even cystic.

5. **Shape**, including regularity/irregularity and contour. Lesions with indistinct and irregular margins are more likely to be malignant.

6. **Relation to surrounding tissue.** Mobility over superficial and deep planes is often assessed by using Haagensen's maneuver (see question 2). A fixed lesion is much more likely to be carcinomatous.

7. **Character of the overlying skin,** such as increased temperature, redness, swelling, or retraction.

Remember, however, that cancers do not read the books. Indeed, in one study of breast lesions approximately one-half of the cancers were well circumscribed, soft, and movable.

13. What are the characteristics of malignant breast tissue?

A carcinomatous lesion typically is painless, irregular in contour and shape, hard in consistency, not mobile, and not well demarcated from the surrounding tissues. Retraction signs are usually a late event. A serous or serosanguinous nipple discharge can be an important sign of intraductal carcinomas.

14. What are the most common benign breast neoplasms?

1. **Fibroadenomas** are the most common benign neoplasms of the breast. They present as solitary, well-demarcated, rubbery, mobile, nontender breast masses. They are often round but also may be ovoid or oblong. They may occur at any time after puberty but much less frequently after menopause.

2. **Benign cysts**, on the other hand, are the most common breast lump. They are usually part of a fibrocystic pattern and thus tend to occur in association with other cysts. They are round, mobile, and soft with cystic consistency. They vary with the menstrual cycle, becoming smaller immediately after menses (hence the desirability of conducting breast exam only in this phase of the cycle to avoid misdiagnosis). They regress after menopause. Benign cysts may become tender premenstrually.

15. How good is the physical examination in detecting a breast lump?

Variable, depending not only on the examiner's skills but also on the size and location of the lesion. For example, tumors less than 1 cm are palpable only with difficulty (unless very superficial), whereas lesions of 2–3 cm usually are easily detectable. In silicone models the sensitivity of the exam ranges between 17% and 83%, increasing not because of the examiner's experience but because of the exam's duration. In real patients the sensitivity of breast exam to detect a neoplastic lesion has been reported to be as low as 24% and as high as 62%. Because of its much greater sensitivity, mammography should always supplement (but *not* substitute for) physical examination. The false-negative rates of mammography vary from as low as 3% to as high as 63% (usually in the range of 20%). In Hicks' study, for example, 7% of all cancers detected by physical exam were misdiagnosed as benign by mammography, whereas as many as one-fourth of all cancers detected were picked up during self-examinations conducted between mammograms.

16. How high is the interobserver variability in describing a breast lump?

Quite high. For example, in a study of 232 women presenting with a breast lump two observers disagreed on the consistency and margins of the lesions in as many as one-third of the cases. They also disagreed on the presence of axillary nodes in almost one-half of the cases. In another study, four breast surgeons detected a lump in 32 of 42 patients and agreed on biopsy in 11 of the 15 patients eventually diagnosed with cancer.

17. What is the appearance of florid nipple adenoma?

Florid nipple adenoma is a benign lesion that presents as a nodule on the areola. The nodule often becomes ulcerated and may be confused with Paget's disease.

18. What is the differential diagnosis of an inflammatory mass of the breast?

Masses associated with inflammation may be diffuse or localized. Diffuse inflammatory breast masses include acute mastitis and inflammatory breast carcinoma. Localized inflammatory masses are usually due to an acute breast abscess, which is a well-localized, tender, swollen, erythematous, and often fluctuant breast mass. The patient presents with systemic signs and symptoms of infection (such as fever, malaise, and leukocytosis). Inflammatory masses tend to represent the progression of acute mastitis (see below) and therefore tend to occur primarily during lactation.

19. What features may be used to distinguish acute mastitis from inflammatory breast carcinoma?

Both conditions present with diffuse and tender breast masses. **Acute mastitis** is a diffuse infection of the glandular tissue, usually involving only a single breast quadrant and most commonly occurring during lactation. The involved area of the breast is red, swollen, and tender, and the patient presents with systemic signs of infection (such as fever, malaise, elevated white count). **Inflammatory breast carcinoma** generally involves the entire breast and is typically associated with axillary adenopathy (which is usually absent in acute mastitis). Lack of association with lactation and lack of response to a course of antibiotics, therefore, should prompt biopsy.

20. How do you assess for nipple discharge?

To assess for nipple discharge, gentle pressure may be applied at the base of the nipple using the thumb and the first or second finger. A nipple discharge that appears only with nipple compression or squeezing is usually physiologic (see below).

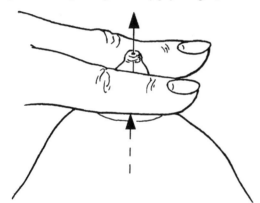

Assessing for nipple secretion. Place fingers beside the areola and begin upward compression of lactiferous ducts, then continuous upward compression of nipple to bring any secretion into view at duct orifices. (From Willms JL, Schneiderman H, Algranati PS: Physical Diagnosis: Bedside Evaluation of Diagnosis and Function. Baltimore, Williams & Wilkins, 1994, with permission.)

21. What is the differential diagnosis of a serous or bloody nipple discharge?

The differential diagnosis should include both benign and malignant etiologies. Benign etiologies include intraductal papilloma, sclerosing adenosis, chronic cystic mastitis, duct ectasia, fibrocystic disease, and tuberculosis. Malignant etiologies include breast carcinoma, adenofibrosarcoma, fibrosarcoma, malignant melanoma, neurosarcoma, and Paget's disease. A nipple discharge, however, is usually not a presenting feature of carcinoma (< 3% of cases); conversely, 6–13% of patients with a nipple discharge eventually are diagnosed with carcinoma. A discharge may be seen in as many as 13% of nulligravida and 22% of parous women between the ages of 16 and 50, with no definite cause in half of the cases. Thus, a nipple discharge is a common problem in premenopausal women. A nipple discharge positive for occult blood has high sensitivity and high negative predictive value but low specificity for a malignant lesion. In a study by Chaudary et al., 16 of 16 patients with carcinoma tested positive for occult blood, but so did 199 of 268 patients with benign lesions. In another study, 27 of 27 cases that tested negative for blood had benign lesions.

22. What is the differential diagnosis of a watery nipple discharge?

This event is not common, occurring only in 2.2% of patients with nipple discharge. In one study, one-half of such patients had cancer.

23. What is the differential diagnosis of a milky nipple discharge?

A milky discharge is usually referred to as galactorrhea (from the Greek *galacto*, milk, and *rhoia*, flow) and indicates discharge of milk in a nonpregnant person. It may occur as a result of disorders that are either local (in which case galactorrhea is usually unilateral) or systemic (in which case galactorrhea is usually bilateral). Mechanical stimulation is also a common cause. Local causes include trauma, surgery, or zoster infection. Systemic causes include hyperprolactinemia, Cushing's syndrome, thyroid diseases, and certain drugs, such as oral contraceptives, phenothiazines, tricyclic antidepressants, and alpha-methyldopa.

24. What is the milk line?

The milk line is the ridge of embryonic tissue from which breasts form. It extends from the axillae to the vulva. Normally, this tissue involutes, leaving only two breasts on the thorax. Persistence of breast tissue along the milk line results in supernumerary (extra) nipples or breasts.

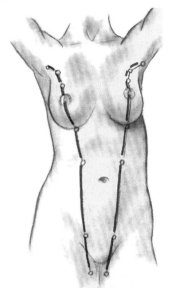

The milk line. (From Bates B: A Guide to Physical Examination and History Taking, 6th ed. Philadelphia, Lippincott-Raven, 1995, with permission.)

25. What is polythelia?

Polythelia (from the Greek *poly*, many, and *thele*, nipple) is the presence of supernumerary nipples along the milk line. They often appear as tiny, raised, and pigmented nevi. They are a rare finding (ranging between 0.22% and 2.5% of the general population). Although in the past extra nipples were considered clues to various underlying congenital abnormalities (such as cardiac diseases), statistically they are associated only with certain renal abnormalities (such as duplicate renal arteries and adenocarcinomas). This association is seen only in Caucasians and not in African-Americans.

26. What is polymastia?

Polymastia (from the Greek *poly*, many, and *mastos*, breast) is the presence of supernumerary breasts. This condition is rarer than polythelia and yet not entirely unheard of. For example, it is rumored that Anne Boleyn (Henry the VIII's unfortunate second wife, famous for being 5′ 4″ tall at the beginning of her reign and only 4′ 6″ tall at the end of it) had four breasts. Considering that she also gave birth to Queen Elizabeth I and, albeit involuntarily, launched the separation of the Anglican Church from Rome, we are left to wonder what the history of England and America would have been if her anatomy had been a touch more correct. Along the lines of historical correctness, Anne Boleyn's breasts should be ranked as high as Cleopatra's nose (which, despite its length, played a major role in launching the civil war between Marc Anthony and Octavius, which eventually gave birth to the Roman Empire).

27. What is athelia?

Athelia (from the Greek *a*, lack of, and *thele*, nipple) is the congenital absence of nipples. This condition is different from the congenital absence of one nipple, which can be seen in adults in association with mitral valve prolapse and in children in association with leukemia. Absence of one nipple also may be part of Poland's syndrome (microsyndactyly or lack of one hand, atrophy of the ipsilateral pectoralis major, and genitourinary abnormalities).

28. Who was Poland?

Alfred Poland (1820–1872) was an English surgeon and quite an interesting character. Utterly disinterested in his own personal appearance, he was once sternly warned by the treasurer of his hospital to dress more "professionally" (advice that was totally ignored). He won, however, the respect and love of colleagues and students alike for being an excellent surgeon, charismatic teacher, and man of encyclopedic knowledge. These qualities, however, did not translate into economic gains (probably because of his habit of scheduling surgery at unusual hours, a custom that kept his practice conveniently small). Afflicted by several bouts of hemoptysis (which did not interfere with his eagerness to teach), he eventually died of consumption.

29. What information can one derive from the chest wall exam of the postmastectomy patient?

The chest wall exam is done to check for recurrent tumor, particularly at the suture line. Generalized induration and tanned appearance of the skin may be present if the patient has undergone local radiation therapy.

30. Describe the lymphatic drainage of the breasts.

The superficial and central areas of the breast are drained by lymphatics that converge on the areola and drain to low and central axillary nodes and subclavian nodes. The deep tissue is drained via pectoral nodes, subclavian nodes, and internal mammary nodes to the mediastinal nodes. Other lymphatics of this system drain into the liver and subdiaphragmatic nodes (see figure at top of facing page).

31. What are level I, II, and III lymph nodes?

This surgical classification of the axillary nodes is based on depth. Level I and II lymph nodes are resected in a modified radical mastectomy for staging of breast cancers.

32. What is the role of the clinician in teaching breast self-examination (BSE)?

BSE is a useful adjunct to breast cancer screening. Physical examination of the breasts has not always been a part of the medical examination of the female patient. Only during the 1950s did the American Cancer Society start to encourage periodic breast examination, prompting women to request to be examined. In the 1960s breast exam became part of the standard periodic physical exam. In the 1970s and 1980s independent self-exam of the breast evolved from the need to achieve early detection. BSE is a complex skill that requires continued reinforcing over time. Women are often ambivalent about doing self-exam but should receive excellent instruction, feedback, and reinforcement.

33. What is the value of BSE?

Often contradictory. Between 1978 and 1987 six studies showed that BSE was associated with smaller cancers at diagnosis, whereas five others failed to demonstrate this effect. Possible reasons for the discrepancy include retrospective design, inconsistent competency and compliance among women, and various tumor sizes. One of the major arguments against BSE is false reassurance with delay in seeking professional examination (supported, in part, by a study from the United Kingdom that showed delays of more than 1 month in establishing a diagnosis among

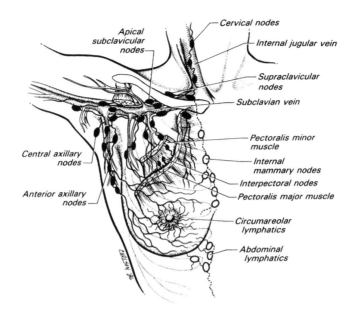

Lymphatic drainage of the breast. The major direction of lymphatic flow is lateral and upward toward the central axillary nodal region. Drainage is then medially to the apical subclavicular nodes, the latter also receiving lymph directly from the interpectoral lymphatics. Lymphatics from the central and medial breast communicate with internal mammary nodes, which drain cephalad and communicate with the deep cervical lymphatic system behind the clavicle. (From James EC, Corry RJ, Perry JF: Principles of Basic Surgical Practice. Philadelphia, Hanley & Belfus, 1987, with permission.)

women who conducted BSE). Even on this point data are conflicting. A study from the World Health Organization (WHO) showed less delay in women doing BSE. Evidence for reduced mortality as a result of BSE is even more scanty. In a study of 18,242 women conducting BSE (classified into good, medium, and poor performers, depending on their skill), BSE had, at best, a sensitivity of 17% and a positive predictive value of 44.5%. Such results are still far from defining BSE as a good screening test. Yet there is still value in teaching patients how to conduct BSE and in increasing their awareness of disease.

34. What are the criteria for BSE?
Published criteria include the following points:
- Visual examination
- Use of three fingers
- Use of finger pad
- Rotary palpation at each site

- Systematic search pattern
- Most of breast examined
- Frequency of 12 times per year

Calendars appear to have little beneficial value as an incentive to do BSE.

35. What is gynecomastia?
Gynecomastia (from the Greek *gyneco*, female, and *mastos*, breast) is a condition of excessive development of male mammary glands. It is characterized by ductal proliferation with periductal edema and is frequently the result of increased estrogen levels or, at least, of an imbalance in the estrogen/testosterone ratio. Thus, mild gynecomastia is often encountered in male neonates (due to the persistence of maternal estrogens) and in normal adolescents at puberty (reported in as many as 65% of healthy boy scouts between the age of 14 and 14.5). Similarly, its prevalence increases with age, becoming as high as 72% in men between 50 and 69 years old. Gynecomastia associated with cirrhosis of the liver may be related to the mechanism of hormonal

imbalance. An increased load of circulating estrogens also may be responsible for the gyneco-mastia reported in 10–40% of hyperthyroid patients, which resolves with restoration of euthyroidism. Finally, abnormal production of estrogens in males (such as that due to adrenal gland tumors or germ cell tumors) may cause gynecomastia. In addition to the above causes, gynecomastia also may be due to the ingestion of certain drugs, including beta blockers, spironolactone, and cimetidine. Gynecomastia also has been reported in association with diabetes, adrenocortical hyperplasia, and a variety of prostatic and testicular disorders.

BIBLIOGRAPHY

1. Atkins H, Wolff B: Discharges from the nipple. Br J Surg 51:602–606, 1964.
2. Baines CJ, Krasowski TP: Breast abnormality detection: Breast self-examination versus nurse-examiners. Prev Med 17:241, 1988.
3. Baines CJ, Wall C, Risch HA, et al: Changes in breast self-examination behaviour in a cohort of 8214 women in the Canadian National Breast Screening study. Cancer 57:1209–1216, 1986.
4. Beller F: Development and anatomy of the breast. In Mitchell GW, Basset L (eds): The Female Breast and Its Disorders. Baltimore, Williams & Wilkins, 1990, pp 1–12.
5. Boyd NF, Sutherland HJ, Fish ED, et al: Prospective evaluation of physical examination of the breast. Am J Surg 142:307–426, 1981.
6. Chaudary MA, Millis RR, Davies GC, Hayward JL: Nipple discharge: The diagnostic value of testing for occult blood. Ann Surg 196:651–655, 1982.
7. De Gowin RL: DeGowin and DeGowin's Diagnostic Examination, 6th ed. New York, McGraw-Hill, 1994.
8. Egan RL, Goldstein GT, McSweeney MM: Conventional mammography, physical examination, thermography, and xeroradiography in the detection of breast cancer. Cancer 39:1984–1992, 1997.
9. Fletcher SW, O'Malley MS, Bumce LA: Physicians' abilities to detect lumps in silicone breast models. JAMA 253:2224–2228, 1985.
10. Hicks MJ, Davis JR, Layton JM, Present AJ: Sensitivity of mammography and physical examination of the breast for detecting breast cancer. JAMA 242:2080–2083, 1979.
11. Leis HP, Greene FL, Cammarata A, Hilfer SE: Nipple discharge: Surgical significance. South Med J 81:20–26, 1988.
12. Mitchell GW: History and physical examination. In Mitchell GW, Bassett L (eds): The Female Breast and Its Disorders. Baltimore, Williams & Wilkins, 1990, pp 13–21.
13. Mushlin AI: Diagnostic tests in breast cancer. Clinical strategies based on diagnostic probabilities. Ann Intern Med 103:79–85, 1985.
14. Newman HF, Klein M, Northrup JD, et al: Nipple discharge: Frequency and pathogenesis in an ambulatory population. N Y State J Med 83:928–933, 1983.
15. Nydick M, Bustos J, Dale JH, Rawson RW: Gynecomastia in adolescent boys. JAMA 178:449–454, 1961.
16. Philip J, Harris WG, Flaherty C, et al: Breast self-examination: Clinical results from a population-based prospective study. Br J Cancer 50:7–12, 1984.
17. Ramzy I: Pathology of benign breast disease. In Mitchell GW, Bassett L (eds): The Female Breast and Its Disorders. Baltimore, Williams & Wilkins, 1990, pp 82–99.
18. Semiglazov VF, Moiseenko VM: Breast self-examination for the early detection of breast cancer: A USSR/WHO controlled trial in Leningrad. Bull WHO 65:391–396, 1987.
19. Yorkshire Breast Cancer Group: Observer variation in recording clinical data from women presenting with breast lesions. BMJ 2:1196–1199, 1977.

10. CARDIOVASCULAR PHYSICAL EXAM

Salvatore Mangione, M.D.

Just when the lamps were lit, a messenger came and brought me to the Emperor as he had bidden. Three doctors had watched over him since dawn, and two of them felt his pulse, and all three thought a fever attack was coming. I stood alongside but said nothing. The Emperor looked first at me and asked why I did not feel his pulse as the other two had. I answered, "These two colleagues of mine have already done so, and as they have followed you ⁓n the journey, they presumably know what your abnormal pulse is, so they can judge its present state better."

When I said this, he bade me, too, to feel his pulse. My impression was that—considering his age and body constitution—the pulse was far from indicating a fever attack, but that his stomach was stuffed with food he had eaten, and that the food had become a slimy excrement. The Emperor praised my diagnosis and said, three times in a row, "That is it. It is just as you say. I have eaten too much cold food."

He then asked what measures should be taken. I replied what I knew of a similar case, saying: "If you were any plain citizen of this country, I would, as usual, prescribe wine with a little pepper. But to a royal patient as in this case, doctors usually recommend milder treatment. It is enough for a woolen cover to be put on your stomach, impregnated with warm spiced salve."

Galen, 129–201 A.D., describing his care of Emperor Marcus Aurelius

TOPICS COVERED IN THIS CHAPTER

CVP and Jugular Venous Pulse *(Continued)*
  Abdominojugular reflux test
    Physiology
    Technique
    Clinical significance
  Kussmaul's sign
    Physiology
    Technique
    Clinical significance
  Venous hum

Precordial Movement and Impulse
  Inspection
  Palpation
Percussion of the Cardiac Area

CONVENTIONAL TEACHING WATCH

The cardiovascular physical examination is centered on five major components. Like the fingers of a hand, all of these components are essential to reach a diagnosis. This chapter discusses general appearance, arterial pulse, central venous pressure and jugular venous pulse, and precordial impulse. Auscultation (the queen of cardiovascular examination) is addressed in chapters 11 and 12.

FINDING/MANEUVER		CONVENTIONAL TEACHING REVISITED
General physical appearance (inspection)	⇑	Often the least used of the five fingers of cardiovascular physical examination, but still important. It can yield a diagnosis at first sight.
Arterial pulse (palpation)*	⇑	Time-honored method, going back 2300 years; still valuable
Central venous pressure and jugular venous pulse (inspection)	⇑	Requires skill and practice but provides wealth of information.
Precordial exam (inspection, palpation, and percussion)	⇑	Also important. Percussion (in olden days included in precordial exam) is fading more and more into the folklore of medicine, although, when accurately performed, it can still be valuable.
Auscultation	⇑	Centerpiece of physical examination; difficult-to-master but highly rewarding skill.

* Evaluation of the arterial pulse also should include assessment of arterial blood pressure (see chapter 2).

1. What are the main components of the general cardiovascular examination?
Physical examination is only one of five general components of the cardiovascular examination; the others are (1) history, (2) office-based studies (e.g., electrocardiography [EKG] and chest radiograph), (3) noninvasive laboratory evaluations (e.g., echocardiography and nuclear medicine), and (4) invasive evaluations (primarily cardiac catheterization).

GENERAL PHYSICAL APPEARANCE

2. What aspects of general appearance should receive particular attention in the evaluation of a cardiac patient?
As suggested by Perloff, one should evaluate in sequence:

1. General appearance and body conformation	5. Extremities
2. Gestures and gait	6. Skin
3. Face and ears	7. Thorax
4. Eyes	8. Abdomen

3. What information can be derived from assessment of body appearance?
1. Struggling, anguished, and frightened look of the patient in pulmonary edema, sitting upright in bed, tachypneic and diaphoretic.

2. Anasarca of congestive heart failure.

3. Tall stature, long extremities, and sparse subcutaneous fat of Marfan syndrome. Patients are prone to mitral valve prolapse and aortic dilatation and dissection.

4. Tall stature and long extremities of Klinefelter syndrome. Patients may have atrial or ventricular septal defects, patent ductus arteriosus, and even tetralogy of Fallot.

5. Long extremities, kyphoscoliosis, and pectus carinatum of homocystinuria. Patients often present with thrombosis of medium-sized arteries.

6. Tall stature and thick extremities of acromegaly (associated with hypertension, cardiomyopathy, and conduction defects).

7. Short stature, webbed neck, low hairline, small chin, wide-set nipples, and sexual infantilism of Turner syndrome (associated with coarctation of the aorta and valvular pulmonic stenosis).

8. Dwarfism and polydactyly of Ellis-van Creveld syndrome (associated with atrial septal defects and common atrium).

9. Morbid obesity and somnolence of obstructive sleep apnea (associated with hypoventilation, pulmonary hypertension, and cor pulmonale).

10. Truncal obesity, thin extremities, moon face, and buffalo hump of hypertensive patients with Cushing syndrome.

11. Mesomorphic, overweight, balding, hairy, and tense middle-aged patient prone to coronary artery disease.

12. Hammer toes and pes cavus of Friedreich ataxia (associated with hypertrophic cardiomyopathy, angina, and sick sinus syndrome).

13. Waddling gait, lumbar lordosis, and calf pseudohypertrophy of Duchenne muscular dystrophy (associated with hypertrophic cardiomyopathy and pseudoinfarction pattern on EKG).

14. Straight back of ankylosing spondylitis (associated with aortic regurgitation and complete heart block).

15. Ataxic gait of tertiary syphilis (associated with aortic aneurysm and regurgitation).

16. Preferential squatting of patients with tetralogy of Fallot.

17. Levine's sign (clenched fist over the chest of patients with acute myocardial infarction).

4. What information can be derived from assessment of the face?

1. Hypertelorism, pigmented moles, and webbed neck of Turner syndrome.

2. Premature aging of Werner syndrome and progeria (associated with premature coronary artery and systemic atherosclerotic disease).

3. Gargoylism of Hurler syndrome (associated with mitral and/or aortic disease).

4. Round and chubby face of congenital valvular pulmonic stenosis.

5. Elfin face (small chin, malformed teeth, wide-set eyes, patulous lips, baggy cheeks, blunt and upturned nose) of congenital stenosis of the pulmonary arteries and supravalvular aortic stenosis (often associated with hypercalcemia and mental retardation).

6. Epicanthic fold, protruding tongue, small ears, short nose, and flat bridge of Down syndrome (associated with endocardial cushion defects).

7. Saddle-shaped nose of polychondritis (associated with aortic aneurysm).

8. Drooping eyelids, expressionless face, receding hairline, and cataracts of Steniert disease (myotonia dystrophica, associated with conduction disorders and mitral valve prolapse).

9. Dry and brittle hair, loss of lateral eyebrows, puffy eyelids, apathetic face, protruding tongue, and thick, sallow skin of patients with myxedema (with pericardial and coronary artery disease).

10. Tightening of skin and mouth, scattered telangiectasias, and hyper/hypopigmentation of scleroderma (with pulmonary hypertension, pericarditis, and myocarditis).

11. Flushed cheeks and cyanotic lips of mitral stenosis (acrocyanosis).

12. Paroxysmal facial and neck flushing of patients with carcinoid syndrome (with pulmonic stenosis and tricuspid stenosis/regurgitation).

13. Deafness and cataracts of rubella syndrome (associated with patent ductus arteriosus or stenosis of the pulmonary artery.

14. Short palpebral fissures, small upper lip, and hypoplastic mandible of fetal alcohol syndrome (associated with atrial or ventricular septal defects).

15. Unilateral lower facial weakness of infants with cardiofacial syndrome, which is encountered in 5–10% of infants with congenital heart disease (usually ventricular septal defect) and often is noticeable only during crying.

16. Pulsatility of the earlobes in patients with tricuspid regurgitation.

17. Macroglossia of Down syndrome, myxedema, and amyloidosis (which is associated with restrictive cardiomyopathy and congestive heart failure).

5. What information can be derived from assessment of the eyes?

1. Lid lag, stare, and exophthalmos of hyperthyroidism (associated with supraventricular tachyarrhythias, angina, and high-output failure).

2. Stare and proptosis of increased central venous pressure.

3. Xanthelasmas of hyperproteinemia and coronary artery disease.

4. Blue sclerae of osteogenesis imperfecta (associated with aortic regurgitation).

5. Icteric sclerae of cardiac cirrhosis.

6. Enlarged lacrimal glands of sarcoidosis (associated with restrictive cardiomyopathy, conduction defects, and, possibly, cor pulmonale).

7. Dislocated lens of Marfan syndrome.

8. Conjunctival petechiae of endocarditis.

9. Conjunctivitis of Reiter disease (associated with pericarditis, aortic regurgitation, and prolongation of the P-R interval).

10. Fissuring of the iris (coloboma) of total anomalous pulmonary venous return.

11. Retinal changes of hypertension and diabetes (associated with coronary artery disease and congestive heart failure).

12. Roth spots of bacterial endocarditis.

6. What information can be derived from assessment of the skin?

1. Jaundice of hepatic congestion.

2. Cyanosis of right-to-left shunt.

3. Pallor of anemia and high-output failure.

4. Bronzing of hemochromatosis (associated with restrictive cardiomyopathy).

5. Telangiectasias of Rendu-Osler-Weber syndrome (at times associated with pulmonary arteriovenous fistulas).

6. Neurofibromas, café-au-lait spots, and axillary freckles (Crowe's sign) of Von Recklinghausen's disease (associated with pheochromocytomas).

7. Symmetric vitiligo (especially of distal extremities) of hyperthyroidism.

8. Butterfly rash of lupus erythematosus (associated with endo-, myo-, and pericarditis).

9. Eyelid with purplish discoloration of dermatomyositis (associated with cardiomyopathy, heart block, and pericarditis).

10. Skin nodules and macules of sarcoidosis (associated with cardiomyopathy and heart block).

11. Xanthomas of dyslipidemia.

12. Hyperextensible skin and joints of Ehlers-Danlos syndrome (associated with mitral valve prolapse).

13. Coarse and sallow skin of hypothyroidism.

14. Skin nodules (sebaceous adenomas), shagreen patches, and periungual fibromas of tuberous sclerosis (associated with rhabdomyomas of the heart and arrhythmias).

7. What information can be derived from assessment of the extremities?

1. Cyanosis and clubbing of central mixing (as in right-to-left shunts, pulmonary arteriovenous fistulas, and drainage of the inferior vena cava into the left atrium).

2. Differential cyanosis and clubbing of patent ductus arteriosus with pulmonary hypertension (the reversed shunt limits cyanosis and clubbing to the feet and spares the hands).

3. Reversed differential cyanosis and clubbing of transposition (aorta originating from the right ventricle): hands are cyanotic and clubbed, but feet are normal.

4. Sudden pallor, pain, and coldness of peripheral embolization.

5. Osler's nodes (swollen, tender, raised, pea-sized lesions of fingerpads, palms, and soles) and Janeway lesions (small, nontender, erythematous or hemorrhagic lesions of palms or soles) seen in bacterial endocarditis.

6. Clubbing and subungual splinter hemorrhages of bacterial endocarditis.

7. Tightly tapered and contracted fingers of scleroderma, with ischemic ulcers and hypoplastic nails (often associated with pulmonary hypertension, myocardial disease, pericarditis, and valvulopathy).

8. Raynaud's phenomenon of scleroderma.

9. Arachnodactyly and hyperextensible joints of Marfan syndrome (associated with aortic disease and regurgitation).

10. Hyperextensible joints of osteogenesis imperfecta (associated with aortic regurgitation).

11. Simian line of Down syndrome (associated with ostium primum defects).

12. Ulnar deviation of rheumatoid arthritis (associated with pericardial, valvular, or myocardial disease).

13. Nicotine stains of chain smokers (clue to underlying coronary artery disease).

14. Leg edema of congestive heart failure.

15. Mainline track lines of intravenous drug abusers (presenting with tricuspid regurgitation, septic emboli, and endocarditis).

16. Liver palms (erythema of thenar and hypothenar eminence) of chronic hepatic congestion.

8. What information can be derived from assessment of the thorax and abdomen?

1. Thoracic bulges of ventricular or atrial septal defects.

2. Systolic and rarely diastolic murmurs of pectus carinatum, pectus excavatum, and straight back syndrome.

3. Pectus carinatum, pectus excavatum, and kyphoscoliosis of Marfan syndrome.

4. Barrel chest of emphysema (often associated with cor pulmonale).

5. Loss of thoracic kyphosis or straight back syndrome (associated with mitral valve prolapse)

6. Cor pulmonale of severe kyphoscoliosis.

7. Right upper quadrant pulsation of tricuspid regurgitation.

8. Ascites of right-sided or biventricular heart failure.

ARTERIAL PULSE

With careful practice the trained finger can become a most sensitive instrument in the examination of the pulse . . . . [F]rom [its] examination we obtain information on three different points: first, concerning the rate and rhythm of the heart's action; second, concerning certain events occurring in a cardiac revolution; third, concerning the character of the blood pressure in the artery . . . . The trained finger can recognize a great variety in the apparent volume of the wave itself. Although the pulse wave occupies such a short space of time, yet the sensitive finger readily recognizes these different features.

James MacKenzie, *The Study of the Pulse*, 1902

CONVENTIONAL TEACHING WATCH

Evaluation of the arterial pulse is a time-honored method of bedside examination. It still provides valuable information about the cardiovascular system. In selective disease processes (such as tamponade, aortic valve disease, and hypertrophic cardiomyopathy), it may even prove essential to securing a diagnosis. Yet assessment of the characteristics of the arterial pulse requires skill and practice and at times can be frustrating. It is still worth the effort, however, and deserves attention even in the era of intraarterial monitoring of the waveform.

FINDING/MANEUVER		CONVENTIONAL TEACHING REVISITED
Pulse deficit	⇑	Another reminder that it is important to measure heart rate both at the precordium and at the arm.
Double-peaked pulse	⇑	Consists of the bisferiens, bifid, and dicrotic pulse; important differential diagnosis.
Hypokinetic pulse	⇑	Important for evaluation of aortic stenosis; may be absent in elderly people.
Hyperkinetic pulse	⇑	Important for evaluation of aortic regurgitation; also known as Corrigan's pulse or water-hammer pulse; wide differential diagnosis.
Pulsus durus	⇑	Compressibility is important aspect of arterial pulse; a hardened pulse may lead to Osler's sign.
Carotid bruit	⇔	Important, but do not rely on it too heavily.

9. What is the history behind examination of the arterial pulse?

Examination of the arterial pulse goes back to Ptolemaic Alexandria, the center of medical knowledge in the Hellenistic world (third and second centuries B.C.). The two leading medical figures of the time were Herophilus of Chalcedon and his rival Erasistratus. Both were Hippocratic Greeks who had moved to Alexandria to practice medicine, perform dissections, and conduct research. Erasistratus gave heart valves the names that they carry today. Herophilus, on the other hand, described the duodenum (which he named after the Greek word for 12 fingers, the measurement of its length), liver, spleen, circulatory system, eye, brain, and genitalia. Herophilus also was the first physician to suggest that the arterial pulse might serve as a diagnostic guide. He counted it by using a portable water clock. Influenced by musical theories, he even developed a classification of pulse characteristics, based on rate, rhythm, strength, and amplitude.

One thousand years later the Chinese expanded this knowledge by developing an even more complex method of classification. Their method required analysis of the pulse at various sites and timing with the physician's own respiration. Four pulsations for each respiratory cycle constituted the normal rate for adults. To avoid possible distractions, physicians were required to banish all extraneous thoughts before examining patients. They also were required to conduct their examination in the morning on an empty stomach.

Things got a little easier in the eighteenth century, when the British physician John Floyer (1649–1734) asked a watchmaker to build a portable clock with a special second hand that ran exactly for 1 minute. This clock allowed him to determine accurately the speed of the pulse and to publish in 1707 *The Physician's Pulse Watch*, in which he suggested that the use of the watch may contribute to a more objective determination of the arterial pulse. Despite Floyer's recommendation, however, practitioners continued to rely more on their "feel" than on objective assessment of rate and rhythm. Only during the middle of the nineteenth century did the practice of measuring the pulse with a watch finally become the standard of care.

10. Which arteries should be examined during the evaluation of the arterial pulse?

It depends on what you are trying to evaluate. If you are simply assessing the presence of peripheral pulses as part of a complete cardiovascular exam, *all* accessible arteries should be examined. The following points are especially important:

1. Arteries on both sides should be compared to detect asymmetries suggestive of embolic, thrombotic, atherosclerotic, dissecting, or extrinsic occlusion.

2. Arteries of upper and lower extremities should be examined simultaneously in patients with hypertension to identify either reductions in volume or pulse delays suggestive of coarctation of the aorta.

If you are trying to evaluate the characteristics of the arterial waveform, you should examine only central vessels—either the carotid or brachial arteries. This section focuses on the bedside examination of the arterial waveform as part of the cardiovascular examination. Evaluation of the peripheral arteries is covered in chapter 23.

11. Is the radial artery the most commonly used vessel to evaluate the characteristics of the pulse?

No—and if so, it should not be. In fact, the radial artery is suited to examine only the rate and rhythm of the pulse. It is particularly well suited to do so in fully clothed patients, a feature that made it quite popular in Victorian times. Conversely, the radial artery is *not* suited to evaluate the contour of the arterial waveform. To do so, one needs a vessel that is as large and central as possible to retain most of the characteristics of the original aortic wave. The optimal choice is the carotid or brachial artery.

12. What alterations occur in peripheral arteries?

The major alterations are an increase in amplitude and upstroke velocity. In fact, as the distance from the aortic valve increases, the primary percussion wave transmitted downward along the aorta begins to merge with secondary waves reverberating backward from more peripheral arteries. This fusion leads to greater amplitude and greater upstroke velocity in peripheral arteries than in central arteries. It also leads to a lowering of the dicrotic notch. The phenomenon of fusion is similar to what occurs in the ocean: waves tend to be higher as they approach the shore. It is also the mechanism behind Hill's sign, the higher indirect systolic pressure in lower extremities than in upper extremities (see chapter 2).

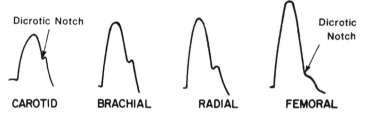

Arterial pulse contour alteration in the peripheral circulation. As the distance increases from the peripheral artery to the central aorta, the amplitude and upstroke velocity of the pulse contour also increase and the dicrotic notch becomes lower. The higher systolic pressure in peripheral arteries is one reason why the arterial pulse is best evaluated at the carotid artery rather than distally. (Adapted from Abrams J: Essentials of Cardiac Physical Diagnosis. Baltimore, Williams & Wilkins, 1987.)

> ***Pearl.*** *The contour of the arterial pulse should* not *be examined in peripheral vessels such as the radial artery. Normal alterations in amplitude and upstroke of these arteries in fact provide misleading information. Conversely, the greater amplitude of distal arteries makes them better suited for the evaluation of subtle findings, such as pulsus paradoxus and pulsus alternans.*

13. What alterations result from decreased arterial compliance?

The same alterations encountered in peripheral arteries. Stiffer arteries conduct the waveform with greater velocity, giving the pulse a greater amplitude and a more rapid upstroke, even in the presence of weak and diminished stroke volume (as in aortic stenosis).

> ***Pearl.*** *The analysis of the arterial pulse for the evaluation of left ventricular outflow obstruction is less reliable in older patients with hypertension or atherosclerosis.*

14. What alterations occur in vasoconstricted patients?

Arteries that are highly constricted may have a diminished pulse even with a normal or increased stroke volume.

15. What is the best technique for evaluating the arterial pulse in carotid arteries?

The arterial pulse should be assessed first by inspecting the carotids in the triangular spaces medial to the sternocleidomastoid muscles. The examiner should look for visible and abnormal pulsations, which often are seen in patients with aortic regurgitation. The examiner then should assess the waveform by applying either the thumb or index finger over the carotids, one at a time. Pressure should be varied for optimal evaluation of pulse characteristics, particularly amplitude and contour. Light pressure is often more valuable than strong pressure. Practice and experience are the keys to success.

16. What is the best technique for evaluating the arterial pulse in brachial arteries?

The best way is first to use the fingers of your left hand to palpate the radial artery of the patient's right arm. Then use the thumb of your right hand to compress the patient's brachial artery until the radial pulse is completely obliterated. At this point, release gently the pressure over the brachial artery until you feel the radial pulse again. This technique allows you to use your thumb as a poor man's transducer, feeling the amplitude and contour of the brachial pulse.

17. What should you evaluate when examining the arterial pulse?

You should evaluate the upstroke, peak, and downstroke of the waveform. More specifically, you should focus on the following characteristics:

1. Rate and rhythm
2. Volume and amplitude
3. Contour
4. Speed (or rate of rise) of the upstroke
5. Speed (or rate of collapse) of the downstroke
6. Stiffness (or distensibility) of the arterial wall
7. Presence of a palpable shudder or thrill
8. Presence of audible bruits or transmitted murmurs

18. What are the characteristics of a normal arterial pulse?

A normal arterial pulse consists of a primary (systolic) and secondary (diastolic) wave, which are separated by a dicrotic notch (*dikrotos* = double-beating in Greek) that corresponds to closure of the semilunar valves (S2). Only the primary wave is palpable. Neither the dicrotic notch nor the secondary wave is normally felt. In certain pathologic conditions, however, a double-peaked pulse may occur (see below). The two spikes are usually located in systole. More rarely the second spike coincides with diastole.

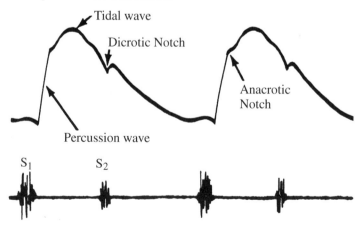

Normal arterial pulse. Note the rapid upstroke, the rounded summit or peak, and the falloff in late systole. (Adapted from Abrams J: Essentials of Cardiac Physical Diagnosis. Baltimore, Williams & Wilkins, 1987.)

19. What mechanisms generate the primary and secondary waves?

The **primary wave** is generated by the ejection of blood into the aorta. Its early portion (percussion wave) reflects ejection into the central aorta, whereas its mid-to-late portion (tidal wave) reflects movement of blood from the central aorta toward the periphery. The two portions are separated by an anacrotic notch that is visible only on tracing and usually is not palpable.

The **secondary wave** is generated by the elastic back-reflection of the waveform from the peripheral arteries of the lower half of the body.

20. What is the meaning of a normal rate of rise of the arterial pulse?

It usually indicates the absence of significant aortic stenosis. This finding is useful, for example, in patients with a benign systolic ejection murmur of aortic sclerosis.

21. What is the meaning of a slow rate of rise of the arterial pulse?

It is usually an indication of aortic stenosis. The stenosis may be either valvular or located above or below the valve. A slow upstroke often is referred to as pulsus tardus (see below).

22. Is there any clinical correlation between the slow rise of the arterial pulse and the degree of severity of aortic stenosis?

Yes. In the presence of good ventricular function, a slow upstroke correlates with a greater and more significant aortic gradient. In patients with left ventricular failure, however, even mild aortic stenosis may have a slow-rising pulse.

23. How can you differentiate supravalvular aortic stenosis from valvular aortic stenosis?

Supravalvular aortic stenosis is associated with right-to-left asymmetry of the arterial pulse. The right brachial pulse is essentially normal, whereas the left brachial pulse resembles the pulse of valvular aortic stenosis. This finding is similar to what occurs in coarctation of the aorta and underscores the importance of routinely examining both pulses.

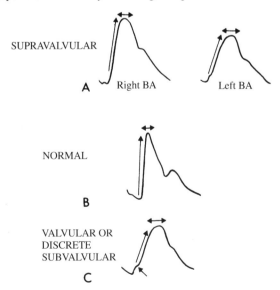

The brachial pulse in supravalvular aortic stenosis *(A)*. In the right brachial artery, the rate of rise is brisker and the pulse pressure greater because of an increase in systolic pressure. The *left* brachial arterial pulse resembles valvular or discrete subvalvular aortic stenosis *(C)*. Normal *(B)* is shown for comparison. (Adapted from Perloff JK: Physical Examination of the Heart and Circulation. Philadelphia, W.B. Saunders, 1990.)

24. What is the clinical significance of a rapid arterial upstroke?

A quick upstroke has useful clinical value. Its significance, however, depends on whether it is associated with a normal or widened pulse pressure.

Normal pulse pressure. If the pulse pressure is normal, a rapid arterial upstroke usually indicates two major conditions:

1. The capacity of the left ventricle to empty either into a high-pressure bed (the aorta) or a lower-pressure bed. The lower-pressure bed can be either the right ventricle (in patients with ventricular septal defect) or the left atrium (in patients with mitral regurgitation). Both diseases allow rapid emptying of the left ventricle, which, in turn, generates a brisk upstroke of the arterial pulse. The pulse pressure, however, remains normal.

2. Hypertrophic obstructive cardiomyopathy (HOCM). Despite its association with left ventricular obstruction, this disease also is characterized by a brisk and rapid upstroke of the arterial pulse, which is due to the delayed ventricular obstruction and hypertrophic ventricle. Even in this case, the pulse pressure is normal.

Widened pulse pressure. A brisk pulse with widened pulse pressure is usually a feature of aortic regurgitation (see below). In contrast to the pulse of mitral regurgitation, ventricular septal defect, or HOCM, the pulse of aortic regurgitation has not only a rapid upstroke but also a quick collapse.

25. What is the differential diagnosis of an arterial pulse with rapid upstroke and widened pulse pressure?

The most common cause is one of the hyperkinetic heart syndromes (high-output states). These include anemia, exercise, thyrotoxicosis, pregnancy, beriberi, Paget's disease, and arteriovenous fistulas. All of these disorders are associated with rapid ventricular contraction and relatively low peripheral vascular resistance.

26. What is pulse deficit?

It is the absence of a palpable arterial pulse despite an audible heartbeat over the precordium. Pulse deficit is a common finding in atrial fibrillation, in which some ventricular contractions may be inadequate to empty into the aorta and originate a waveform. The number of such missing pulses (usually expressed as heart rate minus pulse rate per minute) is the pulse deficit. This finding reminds us of the need to measure the heart rate both over the precoridum and at the arm.

27. What is pulsus paradoxus?

It is the exaggerated fall in systolic blood pressure during quiet inspiration (make sure that the patient is neither hyperventilating nor performing a Valsalva maneuver). Pulsus paradoxus often is due to pericardial tamponade but also may be seen in asthma, emphysema, marked obesity (because of large fluctuations in intrathoracic pressure), and severe congestive heart failure. Rarely (if at all) it may be seen in constrictive pericarditis. Pulsus paradoxus is best assessed in a peripheral artery, such as the radial artery (see above), whereas the contour and amplitude of the arterial pulse are best assessed centrally (over either the carotid or brachial arteries). Optimal assessment of pulsus paradoxus requires a sphygmomanometer (see chapter 2).

28. What is pulsus alternans?

It is the alternation of strong and weak arterial pulses, which at times is encountered in severe left-ventricular dysfunction. Like pulsus paradoxus, pulsus alternans is best assessed in peripheral arteries. Beat-to-beat fluctuations in pulse are paralleled by fluctuation in arterial pressure (see chapter 2).

29. What is bigeminal pulse?

It also is a pulse in which the beats occur in pairs, but the pairs are the result of a bigeminal rhythm.

30. What is double-peaked pulse?

It is a pulse characterized by two palpable spikes. The first peak always occurs in systole. The second peak may occur either during systole as part of the primary wave (pulsus bisferiens and bifid pulse) or during diastole as part of the secondary wave (dicrotic pulse).

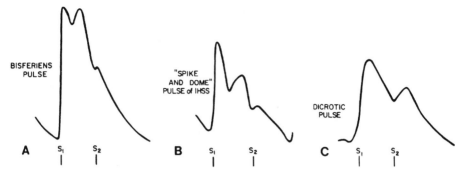

Double-peaked arterial pulses. *A,* Bisferiens pulse, commonly found in severe aortic regurgitation or mild aortic stenosis with moderate aortic regurgitation. *B,* "Spike and dome" arterial pulse of hypertrophic cardiomyopathy or idiopathic hypertrophic subaortic stenosis. This unusual contour is recordable but not readily palpable. *C,* Dicrotic pulse. In this waveform the second palpable component is a diastolic reflection wave. (Adapted from Abrams J: Essentials of Cardiac Physical Diagnosis. Baltimore, Williams & Wilkins, 1987.)

31. Define pulsus bisferiens.

Pulsus bisferiens (from the Latin *bis* = twice and *ferire* = to strike) is an arterial pulse with two palpable peaks, both located in systole. The second usually is equal in strength to the first. Pulsus bisferiens has large amplitude, a quick upstroke, and a rapid downstroke. It typically is encountered in severe aortic regurgitation (with or without aortic stenosis), but it also may be felt in high-output states. In aortic regurgitation this double pulse is not only palpable but often even audible. It may be detected as one of the following:

- **Double Korotkoff sound,** heard at systolic peak while the cuff is being deflated.
- **Traube's femoral double sounds,** detected by light application of the diaphragm of the stethoscope over the femoral artery, coupled with mild arterial compression distal to the stethoscope's head. These sounds are present in approximately one-fourth of patients with aortic regurgitation, resemble normal heart tones (as described by Traube), and may even occur as triple sounds. Lack of arterial compression distal to the head of the stethoscope sharply decreases the sensitivity of the test, confining it to cases of severe left ventricular dilatation.
- **"Pistol shot" femoral sound,** a shotlike systolic sound heard over the femoral artery, can be found in approximately one-half of patients with severe aortic regurgitation but also occurs in other high-output states.
- **Duroziez' double murmur** is a to-and-fro murmur heard over the femoral artery during both systole and diastole. It is elicited by applying gradual arterial compression with the diaphragm of the stethoscope. This compression produces not only a systolic murmur (which is the normal result of arterial compression) but also a diastolic murmur (which is pathologic and typical of aortic regurgitation. Duroziez' maneuver has a sensitivity of 58–100% for aortic regurgitation. False negatives may occur in mild disease, concomitant aortic stenosis, inadequate ventricular filling (due to associated mitral stenosis), inadequate ventricular emptying (due to concomitant mitral regurgitation), or obstruction to waveform transmission (caused by coarctation of the aorta). False positives may occur in all high-output states. In such disorders, however, the double murmurs are due to forward flow. In aortic regurgitation, on the other hand, one murmur is due to forward flow and the other to reverse flow. The two can be differentiated by applying pressure first on the more cephalad

edge of the diaphragm and then on its more caudad end. The murmur of forward flow is enhanced by compressing the cephalad edge. Conversely, the reverse flow murmur is enhanced by applying pressure on the caudad edge. This technique allows identification not only of aortic regurgitation but also of patent ductus arteriosus, the only other high-output state characterized by both forward and reverse flow.

Remember that the typical arterial pulse of aortic regurgitation may disappear when the patient develops left ventricular dysfunction.

32. Define bifid pulse.

It is the classic pulse of HOCM. On tracing it typically presents as a spike and dome, but at the bedside is usually difficult to detect. In fact, most patients with HOCM have a normal carotid pulse. If present at the bedside, a bifid pulse usually reflects severe obstructive cardiomyopathy. The mechanism is rapid early-systolic emptying of the ventricle (causing the first brisk peak), followed by an obstruction and then by another emptying (causing the second peak).

33. Define dicrotic pulse.

It also is a pulse with a double peak (from the Greek *di* = two and *krotos* = beat) except that the second impulse originates in diastole as an accentuation of the dicrotic wave. The dicrotic pulse is the least common of the double-peaked pulses. It can be differentiated from a bifid or bisferiens pulse by the longer interval between the peaks. It has been described in low cardiac output, such as pericardial tamponade during inspiration or severe congestive cardiomyopathy. It also has been reported in young healthy people as a result of fever. It usually requires elastic arteries and therefore is not encountered after the age of 45.

34. What is a hypokinetic pulse?

A hypokinetic pulse (from the Greek *hypo* = diminished and *kinesis* = movement) is a pulse of diminished amplitude. It may be due to (1) obstruction to left ventricular outflow (aortic stenosis), (2) diminished left ventricular contraction (cardiomyopathy), or (3) diminished left ventricular filling (mitral stenosis). A pulse of small amplitude is also referred to as pulsus parvus (small pulse in Latin) and often presents with a slow upstroke (pulsus tardus, delayed pulse in Latin). The combination of slow upstroke and diminished amplitude narrows significantly the differential diagnosis of a hypokinetic pulse.

Pearl.   Diminished amplitude and slow upstroke (pulsus parvus and tardus) are usually features of aortic stenosis. Conversely, a pulse of small amplitude (pulsus parvus) but normal upstroke is a feature of diminished left ventricular contraction or diminished left ventricular filling.

35. What is the carotid shudder?

It is a palpable thrill felt at the peak of the carotid pulse of patients with aortic stenosis, aortic regurgitation, or both. This shudder represents the transmission of the murmur to the artery and is a relatively specific but insensitive sign of aortic valvular disease.

Aortic Stenosis

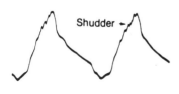

Shudder

Carotid pulse tracing from a patient with significant valvular aortic stenosis. Note the delayed upstroke and shudder that represents the transmitted murmur. (Adapted from Abrams J: Essentials of Cardiac Physical Diagnosis. Baltimore, Williams & Wilkins, 1987.)

S₁   S₂

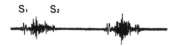

36. What is an anacrotic pulse?

It is another sign of aortic stenosis. The pulse not only is small (parvus) and slow (tardus) but also has a lowering of the anacrotic notch on its ascending limb. This notch is visible on arterial tracings but not palpable at the bedside. Hence it has little clinical relevance. The name derives from the Greek *ana* = upward and *krotos* = impulse and refers to the upstroke (or ascending) limb of the arterial tracing. It is an abbreviation for anadicrotic (twice beating on the upstroke).

37. What is a hyperkinetic pulse?

It is a pulse with large amplitude and rapid upstroke (from the Greek *hyper* = large and *kinesis* = motion). It often is referred to as pulsus celer (*celer* = fast in Latin) to distinguish it from the slow and small pulse (tardus and parvus) of aortic stenosis. The large amplitude of a hyperkinetic pulse reflects increased stroke volume, whereas its quick upstroke reflects increased velocity of contraction. In high-output states (including aortic regurgitation), hyperkinetic pulse usually is associated with a widening of the pulse pressure. Hyperkinetic pulse also may be encountered in mitral regurgitation, but the pulse pressure is typically normal. Finally, hyperkinetic pulse also may be felt in patients with decreased arterial compliance, such as elderly people, especially if they are hypertensive.

38. What is Corrigan's pulse?

It is one of the various names for the bounding pulse of aortic regurgitation. Another common term is water-hammer pulse. Corrigan's pulse may be so brisk that it causes other typical findings, such as De Musset's or Lincoln's signs (see chapter 1).

39. Who was Corrigan?

Sir Dominic J. Corrigan (1802–1880) was an Irish physician, the longest-serving president of the Irish College of Physicians, and a member of Parliament for the city of Dublin. He was also a personal physician to Queen Victoria. In 1832 Corrigan published his observations about aortic regurgitation in a treatise titled "On Permanent Patency of the Mouth of the Aorta, or Inadequacy of the Aortic Valve." He also reported the visible (not palpable) characteristics of his famous pulse. A brisk arterial pulse had been described by De Vieussens 100 years before, but Corrigan first made the correlation between this pulse and aortic regurgitation.

40. What is a water-hammer?

A popular Victorian toy that consisted of a sealed test tube containing water in a vacuum. Because solids and liquids in a vacuum fall at the same rate, the inversion of the tube caused the column of water to fall precipitously, hitting the glass wall with a brisk jolt. This thrust gave great joy to Victorian children, making the gadget almost as popular as today's electronic gizmos. The comparison between the jolt of a water-hammer and the brisk bounding pulse of aortic regurgitation was first made in 1844 by the English physician Thomas Watson. It remains part of medical lore 150 years later.

41. What is pulsus durus?

A pulse so hardened that it is difficult to compress (*durus* = hard in Latin). Usually it is a sign of arteriosclerosis and may be associated with Osler's sign.

42. Can the compressibility of the arterial pulse help to predict the systolic blood pressure?

Yes. It is possible to assess the degree of systolic blood pressure without the aid of a sphygmomanometer by palpating the radial artery with the fingers of your left hand while compressing the brachial artery with the thumb of your right hand. The brachial artery should be compressed until the radial pulse is obliterated. If such compression requires mild force, the blood pressure is probably around 120 mmHg or less. If it requires intermediate force, the blood pressure is probably between 120 and 160 mmHg. Finally, if it requires high force, the blood pressure is probably above 160 mmHg.

43. What are the prevalence and significance of a bruit over the carotid artery?

Bruits of the carotid artery occur in 20% of children less than 15 years old. They are much less common in adults (only 1% of healthy adults). Carotid bruits are commonly heard in high-output states. A relatively typical situation is the creation of a forearm arteriovenous fistula for he-modialysis. In this case the bruits are louder on the side of the fistula and often associated with a subclavian bruit. The major clinical problem posed by a carotid bruit, of course, is to rule out the presence of carotid artery stenosis.

44. How do you auscultate for carotid bruits?

By using the bell of the stethoscope in a quiet room with a relaxed patient. Listen from imme-diately behind the upper end of the thyroid cartilage to immediately below the angle of the jaw.

45. What is the differential diagnosis of a carotid bruit?

1. **Systolic heart murmurs** are only *transmitted* to the neck. Thus, they are easily differen-tiated from carotid bruits because they are louder over the precordium than over the neck.

2. **Venous hums** are innocent murmurs caused by flow in the internal jugular vein. They occur in as many as 25% of young adults. In contrast to carotid bruits, venous hums are loudest in diastole. They also are typically heard in a sitting position with the patient's head turned away from the side of auscultation. Venous hums tend to disappear when the patient is lying down and are always abolished by either compressing the ipsilateral jugular vein (above the stethoscope) or asking the patient to perform a Valsalva maneuver.

Most carotid bruits are heard in systole. Only a few are heard in both systole and diastole. The significance of this phenomenon is unclear.

46. What is the interobserver agreement on carotid bruits?

Quite good for the detection of the bruit but only fair for evaluation of its intensity, pitch, or duration.

47. How common is an asymptomatic carotid bruit?

Both prevalence and incidence of carotid bruits increase with age. The prevalence rises from 2.3% in people aged 45–54 years to 8.2% in people aged 75 years or older. Similarly, the inci-dence of new bruits in adults aged 65 years or older is about 1% per year, twice the rate in people aged 45–54 years.

48. What is the significance of a carotid bruit in an asymptomatic ambulatory patient?

It depends on age. In a 50-year-old man an asymptomatic carotid bruit is associated with increased incidence of both cerebrovascular and cardiovascular events. For example, average annual stroke rates are three times higher in patients with bruits than in patients without. The same is true for transient ischemic attacks (TIAs). There is also a threefold higher risk of death from ischemic heart disease for patients with an asymptomatic bruit. This increased risk decreases sharply with age, becoming essentially nonexistent among people older than 75 years.

49. What is the correlation between presence of a carotid bruit and high-grade stenosis of the artery in a symptomatic patient?

Patients with TIAs or minor strokes in the anterior circulation should be evaluated aggres-sively for the presence of high-grade (70–99%) carotid stenosis. In fact, carotid endarterectomies markedly decrease mortality and stroke rates. The value of the physical exam cannot be underes-timated in such patients. The likelihood of high-grade carotid stenosis is much higher when bruits are present than when they are absent. Yet the relation between bruits and high-grade stenosis is not strong enough to confirm or eliminate disease simply by the presence or absence of a bruit. Moreover, a bruit may be heard even over the bifurcation of the carotid artery when the an-giogram shows either a normal or completely occluded internal carotid artery (in such patients the bruit usually arises from a narrowed *external* carotid artery).

Pearl. The decision concerning surgery in patients with cerebrovascular symptoms in the carotid territory should not be based on physical examination alone; angiography is mandatory.

50. What is the significance of a carotid bruit in an asymptomatic preoperative patient?

Asymptomatic preoperative bruits are relatively common in the surgical population (10% of patients), a prevalence much higher than in the general population (4.4%). Yet such bruits are not predictive of increased risk of perioperative stroke, although they may predict transient postoperative dysfunction and behavioral abnormalities.

CENTRAL VENOUS PRESSURE AND JUGULAR VENOUS PULSE

The visible oscillations in this region consist of a series of filling and collapses, sometimes prominent and easy to recognize . . . . There is found then, aside from the slow oscillations caused by the respiratory movements and simultaneous with them, the following sequence of movements which is repeated with constant and perfect regularity: at first a slow elevation, then two quick elevations, finally two deep depressions, after which the series begins again. Now each series of this kind corresponds to a cardiac cycle. These impulses sometimes have such force and amplitude that at first it might be believed that they represent pulsation of the carotid artery or the subclavian. But after a little attention one is soon convinced that they actually take place in the internal jugular.

Pierre Carl Potain: On the movements and sounds that take place in the jugular veins.
Bull Mem Soc Med Hop Paris 4:3, 1867

We come now to the study of a subject which gives us far more information of what is actually going on within the chambers of the heart. In the study of the venous pulse we have often the direct means of observing the effects of the systole and diastole of the right auricle, and of the systole and diastole of the right ventricle. The venous pulse represents therefore a greater variety of features, and is subject to influence so subtle that it may manifest variations due to the changing conditions of the patient, during which the arterial pulse reveals no appreciable alteration.

James MacKenzie, *The Study of the Pulse, Arterial, Venous and Hepatic, and the Movements of the Heart.* Edinburgh, Young J. Pentland, 1902

The jugular venous pulse should be analyzed clinically in terms of pressure and wave form; it is hard to conceive of any physical sign that is more informative.

Paul Wood, *Diseases of the Heart and Circulation.* Philadelphia, J.B. Lippincott, 1956

CONVENTIONAL TEACHING WATCH

Observation of jugular venous pulse and measurement of central venous pressure are more recent techniques of physical examination than evaluation of the arterial pulse. They provide a wealth of clinical information, particularly about intravascular volume, right ventricular function, integrity of the pulmonic and tricuspid valves, and status of the pericardium. The skills are difficult and at times intimidating, but worth the effort, even in an age of invasive hemodynamic monitoring.

FINDING/MANEUVER		CONVENTIONAL TEACHING REVISITED
Jugular venous pulse	⇑	Analysis of contour of venous pulse is difficult, but its various ascents and descents may be quite valuable in identifying selected cardiac disorders.
Jugular venous pressure	⇑	Poor man's manometry for right-sided pressure. Valuable tool despite its limitations. Technique requires familiarity and proficiency.
Abdominojugular reflux test	⇑	Important for unmasking subclinical right ventricular failure. Proper technique is key.
Kussmaul's sign	⇑	Still valuable finding; important to be aware of its differences from pulsus paradoxus.
Venous hum	⇑	Innocent murmur of children and young adults; important for its differential diagnosis.

Waveform

51. What is the history behind the examination of the cervical venous pulse?

The first report of the venous pulse goes back to the seventeenth century, when the Italian Giovanni Maria Lancisi (1654–1720) described a "systolic fluctuation of the external jugular vein" in a patient with tricuspid regurgitation (i.e., the giant V wave still known as Lancisi's sign). In 1867 Pierre Carl Potain carefully described the jugular waveform in a paper titled "Movements and Sounds that Take Place in the Jugular Veins." Forty years later, the Scottish physician Sir James MacKenzie published *The Study of the Pulse*, which summarized 20 years of clinical assessment of both venous and arterial pulsations and established the jugular venous pulse as an essential element of cardiovascular examination. It also contributed the standard terminology of the waveform (A, C, and V waves and X-Y descent) still in use. But it was only in the 1950s that examination of the jugular venous pulse and pressure became a standard of bedside examination, primarily as a result of the efforts and influence of the British physician Paul Wood.

52. Which veins should be evaluated for the assessment of central venous pressure and venous pulse?

Central veins, as much in direct communication with the right atrium as possible. The ideal vein, therefore, is the internal jugular. As part of a thorough and comprehensive examination, all visible veins also should be evaluated. Because this chapter focuses primarily on the cardiovascular examination, discussion is limited to the jugular waveform and central venous pressure. Evaluation of peripheral veins is covered in chapter 23.

53. What is the clinical value of the jugular venous pulse and pressure?

Evaluation of the jugular venous pressure (JVP) and jugular waveform represents a poor man's monitor of right-heart hemodynamics. It provides an inexpensive and noninvasive assessment of central venous pressure (CVP) and intravascular volume. It also provides information about right ventricular function, status of the tricuspid and pulmonic valves, and presence (or absence) of pericardial constriction.

54. How difficult is evaluation of the jugular veins?

Quite difficult, especially in patients with low CVP or short, fat necks; patients on mechanical ventilation; and patients with wide respiratory swings in CVP (e.g., acute asthmatics). In critically ill patients it is also difficult to assess jugular venous pulse and pressure. In one study of intensive care patients, jugular venous pulsations were adequate for examination in only 20% of cases; moreover, CVP could be measured by physical examination in only one-half of patients. In another study, CVP could be determined accurately in two-thirds of critically ill patients.

Pearl.   *The more severe and acute the condition, the more difficult and inaccurate the bedside determination of jugular venous pulse and pressure.*

55. Should you inspect the right or left internal jugular vein?

The right internal jugular vein. It is in more direct line with the right atrium and thus allows unimpeded transmission of atrial pulsations and pressure. CVP may be slightly higher in the left internal jugular than in the right (although the correlation between the two remains quite high). This discrepancy is caused by compression of the left innominate vein between the aortic arch and the sternum.

56. Can the external jugular veins be used for the evaluation of venous pulse and pressure?

Not really. Only the internal jugular veins (especially the right) provide an ideal site for the evaluation of both venous pulse and venous pressure. The external jugulars are less suited for this task for the following reasons:

1. They often become compressed while going through the various fascial planes of the neck.

2. They have valves that may prevent adequate transmission of right atrial pulsations.

3. In patients with increased sympathetic vascular tone, they may become so constricted that they are barely visible.

4. They are farther away from and form less of a straight line with the right atrium.

57. Is the internal jugular vein too deep for accurate inspection?

It is quite deep and therefore not as visible as the external jugular. But its pulsations are well transmitted to the overlying skin, making its waveform usually recognizable.

58. Describe the anatomy of the internal and external jugular veins.

The **external jugular veins** lie above the sternocleidomastoid muscles, coursing vertically over the muscles posteriorly and laterally to the internal jugular veins.

The **internal jugular veins** lie below the sternocleidomastoid muscles, crossing them in a vertical straight line. At the junction with the subclavian veins, the internal jugulars create a dilatation known as the bulb, which is often visible between the two heads of the sternocleidomastoid muscles.

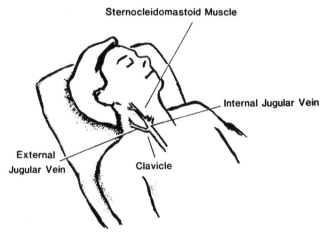

Important landmarks of the venous pulse. The external jugular veins are easily seen lateral to the sternocleidomastoid muscles, extending vertically toward the back of the ear. (Adapted from Abrams JA: Essentials of Cardiac Physical Diagnosis. Baltimore, William & Wilkins, 1987.)

59. How do you examine the internal jugular veins?

By carefully positioning the patient (see below) and by tangentially shining a penlight across the vein. The venous pulse is visible but *not* palpable.

60. How important is the patient's position during examination of the neck veins?

The following guidelines are enormously important:

1. The **head** should be supported so that the neck muscles are fully relaxed and do not impinge over the jugular vein.

2. The **trunk** should be inclined. The angle of inclination must allow the top of column of blood in the internal jugular to reach above the clavicle, yet remain below the jaw. This inclination varies, depending on the CVP:

- In patients with **normal CVP**, the required angle is usually 30–45° above the horizontal.
- In patients with **elevated CVP**, the required angle is above 45°. Patients with severe venous congestion may have to sit upright and take deep inspirations to lower the meniscus into full view. In some patients the level of venous pulsation may still remain behind the angle of the jaw, where it appears to move the earlobes.

- In patients with **very high CVP**, the internal jugular is so full that pulsations may not be visible even when the patient is fully upright. The risk in this case is to overlook the high venous pressure and call it normal.
- In patients with **low CVP**, the required angle is usually between 0° and 30°.
- In patients with **very low CVP**, the neck veins are so empty that pulsations may not be visible at all, even when the patient is horizontal.

61. How do you distinguish the carotid pulse from the jugular venous pulse?

1. **Waveform.** The venous pulsation is diffuse, at least bifid, and has a slow upward deflection. Conversely, the carotid pulse is well localized and single with a fast outward deflection.

2. **Response to position.** The carotid pulsations do not vary with respiration. The venous pulsations classically do so. In fact, as the patient sits up or stands, venous pulsations move downward toward the clavicle and may even disappear below it. Conversely, as the patient reclines, venous pulsations gradually climb toward the angle of the jaw and may even disappear behind the auricle.

3. **Response to respiration.** In the absence of intrathoracic disease, the top of the venous waveform descends toward the heart during inspiration (because of lower intrathoracic pressure and greater venous return). Conversely, the visible carotid pulse does not vary with respiration. The only exception is pulsus paradoxus, and even in this case the variation is rarely visible, at most palpable.

4. **Response to palpation.** The jugular venous pulse is not palpable. In fact, even gentle pressure may compress the vein, engorge its more distal segment, and obliterate the venous pulse. Conversely, the carotid pulse is not only palpable but usually quite forceful.

5. **Response to abdominal pressure.** Sustained pressure on the abdomen (the abdomino-jugular reflux test; see below) does not change the carotid pulse but increases (at least momentarily) even the normal venous pulse.

CHARACTERISTIC	INTERNAL JUGULAR VEIN AND JUGULAR VENOUS PULSE	CAROTID ARTERY AND CAROTID PULSE
Location	Low in neck and lateral	Deep in neck and medial
Contour	Double-peaked and diffuse	Single-peaked and sharp
Character	Undulant, not palpable	Forceful, brisk, easily felt
Response to position	Varies with position	No variation
Response to respiration	Mean pressure decreases on inspiration (height of column falls, but A and V waves become more visible)	No variation
Response to abdominal pressure	Displaces pulse upward and induces transient increase in mean pressure	Pulse unchanged
Effect of palpation	Wave visible but nonpalpable. Gentle pressure 3–4 cm above clavicle obliterates pulse and fills vein	Pulse unchanged; vessel difficult to compress

Modified from Cook and Simel: Does this patient have abnormal central venous pressure? JAMA 275:630–634, 1996, and Abrams J: Essentials of Cardiac Physical Diagnosis. Philadelphia, Lea & Febiger, 1987.

62. How do you evaluate the jugular venous pulse?

With great difficulty and lots of practice:

1. Start by examining the right jugular vein (which is in a more direct line with the right atrium).

2. Position the patient so that the jugular meniscus is well seen (shine a light tangentially).

3. Carefully inspect the level of the venous column and the timing and amplitude of the waveform and its components. Respiratory variations (see below) also should be noted.

4. If you still have difficulty in relating the various venous ascents and descents to the cardiac cycle, you may either auscultate the heart or simultaneously palpate the left carotid artery.

63. What are the components of the jugular waveform?

It depends on whether you are looking at the patient or analyzing the venous tracing. Jugular vein undulations reflect phasic pressure changes in the right atrium. Because the fluctuations in pressure are mild (3–7 mmHg or 4–11 cmH_2O), peaks and troughs of the jugular pulse can be easily recorded, but they are quite difficult to appreciate at the bedside for the following reasons:

1. **On venous tracing** the jugular venous pulse consists of three positive waves (A, C, and V) and three negative descents (X, X_1, and Y).

2. **At the bedside** the jugular venous pulse consists of only two positive waves (A and V) and two negative descents (X_1 and Y). The A wave is followed by the X_1 descent, and the V wave is followed by the Y descent. Neither the C wave nor the X descent is visible (C is usually lost in the A wave, and X is merged with X_1). Remember that descents are easier to spot than ascents.

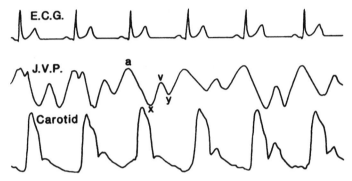

Simultaneous recording of an electrocardiogram *(top tracing)*, jugular venous pressure waves *(middle tracing)*, and carotid pressure waves *(bottom tracing)*. (From Adair OV, Havranek EP: Cardiology Secrets. Philadelphia, Hanley & Belfus, 1995, with permission.)

64. What is the physiology of the jugular venous pulse?

The jugular venous pulse reflects the relationship among volume of blood in the venous system, venous vascular tone, and right-heart hemodynamics. As a result, during diastole it reflects right ventricular filling pressure, whereas during systole it reflects right atrial pressure.

65. What is the physiology of the various ascents and descents of the jugular venous pulse?

It is the physiology of right-sided chambers. Thus, in assessing the jugular venous pulse it is important not only to visualize peaks and troughs but also to relate these undulations to various physiologic and clinical events, such as the EKG, carotid pulse, and heart sounds:

1. The **A wave**, the first and dominant positive wave, is produced by right **A**trial contraction. The A wave follows the P wave on EKG, coincides with the fourth heart sound (if present), slightly precedes the first heart sound, and slightly precedes the carotid upstroke.

2. The **C wave**, the second positive wave, is produced by the bulging of the tricuspid **C**usps into the right atrium. A smaller component of this wave is produced by the transmitted **C**arotid pulsation. This component, of course, is visible only in the neck. The C wave coincides with the ventricular isovolumetric contraction. The interval between A and C waves corresponds to the P-R interval on EKG. (This was one of the methods used by Wenckebach to describe the second-degree heart block that still carries his name.) Because the C wave is poorly visible at the bedside, it is omitted from the remainder of our discussion.

3. The **early X descent** (located between A and C) is produced by right atrial relaxation. The most dominant later trough (X_1) is produced by the pulling of the valvular cusps into the right ventricle. This downward and forward movement of the valve (descent of the base) coincides with right ventricular isotonic contraction and acts as a plunger; it creates a sucking effect that aspirates blood from the great veins into the right atrium. The X_1 descent occurs during systole, coincides with ventricular ejection and the carotid pulse, takes place between S1 and S2,

and ends just before S2. This discussion disregards the X descent and considers only the combined X and X_1 troughs.

4. The **V wave**, the third positive wave, occurs toward the end of ventricular systole and during the early phase of **V**entricular diastole. It coincides with the apex of the carotid pulse and peaks immediately after S2. Because the ventricle relaxes while the tricuspid valve is closed, blood flowing into the right atrium starts to build up. This build-up generates a positive wave.

5. The **Y descent**, the final negative trough, occurs during early ventricular diastole and is produced by the opening of the tricuspid valve and the emptying of the right atrium. The Y trough corresponds to S3.

Pearl. *For practical purposes, the only peaks visible at the bedside are A and V; the only troughs visible at the bedside are X_1 and Y. The A wave usually is more prominent than the V wave, whereas the X descent usually is more prominent than the Y descent. In general, it is easier to time the pulse by using the X and Y descents instead of the A and V waves.*

66. Who was Wenckebach?

Karel F. Wenckebach (1864–1940) was a Dutch physician. Building on an 1873 observation by the Italian physiologist Luigi Luciani, Wenckebach described the phenomenon that still carries his name in 1899, exactly 100 years ago. He reported his findings in a 40-year-old woman who had presented for evaluation of an irregular pulse. Wenckebach based his conclusions on tracings of the patient's arterial pulse, observations of her venous pulse, and intraatrial and intraventricular recordings in a frog. Wenckebach's insight preceded the invention of electrocardiography by two years, the discovery of the atrioventricular node by seven years, and the description of the sinoatrial node by eight years. Despite his genius he remained a simple and unassuming man, full of charm and self-deprecating humor. He was famous for quipping that he was not a great man, just a "happy man." His colleagues loved him and many referred to him affectionately as "Venky." His many friends included Sir William Osler and James MacKenzie (with whom he maintained a long correspondence, praising his 1902 book, *The Study of the Pulse*). A master of physical diagnosis and a pioneer in cardiac arrhythmias, Wenckebach taught at Utrecht, Groningen, Strasbourg, and, finally, Vienna, where he died of urosepsis at age 76.

67. What is the effect of respiration on the jugular venous pulse?

Inspiration tends to make the jugular venous pulse more visible (and the mean jugular venous pressure lower) because respiration increases venous return. This, in turn, distends the right-sided chambers and, because of the Starling effect, makes right atrial and right ventricular contraction stronger. As a result, the X and Y descents become brisker and more visible; even the waveform becomes more accentuated. Conversely, in exhalation the A wave diminishes to a point that the V wave may become the dominant positive deflection. Yet the mean jugular venous pressure remains higher.

68. Which disease processes can be identified by analysis of the jugular venous pulse?

Abnormalities of the Venous Waveforms

WAVEFORM	CARDIAC CONDITION
Absent A wave	Atrial fibrillation, sinus tachycardia
Flutter waves	Atrial flutter
Prominent A waves	First-degree atrioventricular block
Large A waves	Tricuspid stenosis, right atrial myxoma, pulmonary hypertension, pulmonic stenosis
Cannon A waves	Atrioventricular dissociation, ventricular tachycardia
Absent X descent	Tricuspid regurgitation
Prominent X descent	Conditions causing enlarged A waves

Table continued on facing page

Abnormalities of the Venous Waveforms (Continued)

WAVEFORM	CARDIAC CONDITION
Large CV waves	Tricuspid regurgitation, constrictive pericarditis
Slow Y descent	Tricuspid stenosis, right atrial myxoma
Rapid Y descent	Constrictive pericarditis, severe right-heart failure, tricuspid regurgitation, atrial septal defect
Absent Y descent	Cardiac tamponade

Adapted from Cook and Simel: Does this patient have abnormal central venous pressure? JAMA 275:630–634, 1996.

1. In addition to tricuspid stenosis, a **giant A wave** also may be seen in patients with increased right ventricular end-diastolic pressure (because of pulmonic stenosis, primary pulmonary hypertension, pulmonary emboli, or chronic pulmonary disease). In this case the giant A wave reflects a strong atrial contraction against an increased ventricular resistance. Such A waves have a concomitant blunted and small Y descent. A giant A wave also may be seen in disorders characterized by marked left ventricular hypertrophy (such as aortic stenosis, severe hypertension, or hypertrophic obstructive cardiomyopathy). In this case, the ventricular septum bulges toward the right, making right ventricular filling more difficult (the Bernheim effect, from Hippolyte Bernheim, the French physician and hypnotist who described it in the nineteenth century).

2. **Cannon A waves** are the hallmark of atrioventricular dissociation (i.e., the atrium contracts against a closed tricuspid valve). They are different from giant A waves.

3. The **X descent** is quite prominent in a patient with vigorous ventricular contraction, as in tamponade or right ventricular overload states.

4. The **V wave** is classically increased in tricuspid regurgitation; it becomes the dominant deflection and is associated with a brisk Y collapse. A more gentle Y descent in the setting of a giant A wave usually indicates concomitant tricuspid regurgitation and stenosis. Abdominal compression may help to unmask more subtle and subclinical cases. Prominent V waves can become so large that they were dubbed by Paul Wood "the venous Corrigan." In fact, they may even cause bobbing of the earlobes. The CV merger responsible for the giant V wave entirely eliminates the X descent. Thus, a giant wave is quite easy to spot. It leaves the patient with only one ascent (the V wave) and one descent (the Y descent). The giant V wave is not highly sensitive; it is present in only 40% of patients with tricuspid regurgitation.

5. The **Y descent** is exaggerated in patients with increased venous pressure, regardless of the etiology. The striking descent of the Y wave is often referred to as Friedreich's sign from the German physician, Nikolaus Friedreich, who described it in 1864. It often is associated with an S3. It often is seen in restrictive right ventricular disease or constrictive pericarditis (in approximately one-third of patients). The finding is not highly sensitive for constrictive pericarditis but usually quite specific. Conversely, the Y descent may be diminished in pericardial tamponade or tricuspid stenosis. (See figure at top of following page.)

6. **Equally prominent A and V waves** can be seen in patients with atrial septal defect. The V wave in the higher-pressure left atrium is transmitted through the perforated septum into the right atrium and from there to the jugular veins. This pattern, however, is seen more commonly in patients with simple right ventricular failure.

7. **Prominent X and Y descents** are typical of constrictive pericarditis and restrictive cardiomyopathy and result from high venous pressure.

69. How do you estimate the CVP?

1. First position the patient to get a good view of the internal jugular vein and its oscillations.

2. Identify the highest point of pulsation in the internal jugular vein, which usually occurs during exhalation and coincides with the peak of the A and V waves.

3. Find the sternal angle of Louis (junction of the manubrium with the body of the sternum).

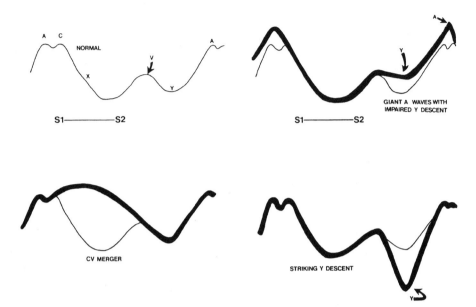

Jugular venous pulsations. Normal tracing *(top left)* and abnormal tracings superimposed on the normal. See text. (From Sapira JD: The Art and Science of Bedside Diagnosis. Baltimore, Urban & Schwarzenberg, 1990, with permission.)

4. Measure the vertical distance from the sternal angle to the top of the jugular pulsations in centimeters. This distance represents the jugular venous pressure (JVP).

This method relies on the fact that the center of the right atrium (in which venous pressure is, by convention, zero) is approximately 5 cm below the sternal angle of Louis. This relationship occurs in people of normal size and shape, regardless of body position. Thus, using the sternal angle as the reference point, the vertical distance (in centimeters) to the top of the column of blood in the jugular vein provides an adequate measurement of the JVP. JVP, in turn, is 5 cm lower than CVP. Thus, CVP = JVP + 5. (See figure at top of facing page.)

70. Are there any special caveats to this method?

Yes. They are related primarily to positioning:

1. Because the clavicle lies at a vertical distance of about 2 cm above the sternal angle, only CVPs of at least 7 cm are observable in patients positioned at 45° above the horizontal. Because the normal CVP is 7 cmH_2O or less, the top of the venous pressure column may become visible only as the patient reclines toward the horizontal, usually at an angle of 15–30°.

2. Conversely, because the upper limit of normal for CVP is 9 cmH_2O, JVP may well extend 4 cm above the sternal angle even in patients at 45°. Thus, you may have to modify the reclining angle as much as necessary.

3. Jugular veins may be visible to a height of 30 cm above the sternal angle (25 cm above the right atrium) before they disappear behind the angle of the jaw. Thus, you may need to position the patient accordingly to get an unimpeded view of venous pulsations.

71. Are there alternative methods to assess CVP?

Alternative methods of assessing CVP have not been validated:

1. **Von Recklinghausen's maneuver** consists of asking the patient to lie supine with one palm over the thigh and the other palm over the bed (thereby lying 5–10 cm below the first hand). If the veins in both hands are engorged, the patient has high CVP. If, on the other hand, veins are engorged only in the lower hand, CVP is normal.

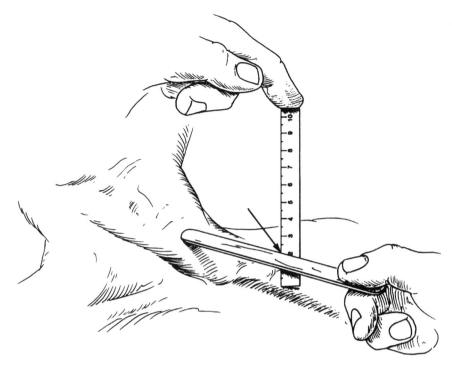

Measurement of central venous pressure. (From Adair OV, Havranek EP: Cardiology Secrets. Philadelphia, Hanley & Belfus, 1995, with permission.)

2. An alternative but similar maneuver consists of inspecting the veins of the back of the hand in a reclining patient as the arm is slowly, passively raised. The level at which the veins collapse can then be related to the angle of Louis and the CVP measured.

Both methods may give falsely high readings because of local obstruction or peripheral venous constriction. Thus, they are not recommended for general use.

72. How precise is the clinical assessment of CVP?

Interobserver and intraobserver variability may be as high as 7 cm. In a study of fourth-year medical students, medical residents, and attending physicians, agreement concerning CVP of 50 intensive care patients was quite substantial between students and residents, moderate between students and attendings, and modest between residents and staff. Variations in patients' positioning, poor ambient lighting, confusion between carotid and venous pulsations, and changes in CVP with respiration interfered with the precision of measurement.

73. How accurate is the clinical assessment of CVP?

Compared with the gold standard of a central venous catheter, clinical assessment of CVP is poor. Three studies address this question:

1. In the above study of 50 critically ill patients, the pooled overall accuracy of the test was 56%. All groups (students, residents, and attendings) tended to underestimate CVP. Residents' underestimation even reached statistical significance. The correlation coefficient between clinical assessment and central venous catheter recording was highest for medical students (0.74), slightly lower for residents (0.71), and lowest for staff physicians (0.65). These correlations improved slightly when patients receiving mechanical ventilation were excluded, suggesting that CVP assessment is more accurate when carried out among patients who breathe spontaneously. From this study, the following conclusions can be drawn:

- A clinically assessed low CVP increases the likelihood by about threefold that the measured CVP also will be low. Conversely, a clinically assessed low CVP makes the probability of a high measured CVP extremely unlikely.
- A clinically assessed high CVP increases the likelihood by about fourfold that the measured CVP also will be high. In fact, no patient with a high CVP by clinical assessment had a low measured CVP.
- Clinical assessment of a normal CVP is truly indeterminate (with likelihood ratios approaching 1). Thus, clinical estimates of normal CVP provide no information because they neither increase nor decrease the probability of an abnormal CVP.

2. In a second study, an attending physician, a critical care fellow, a medical resident, an intern, and a student were asked to predict whether the CVP of 62 patients was low, normal, high, or very high. Right-heart catheterization provided the gold standard. The sensitivity values of clinical examination were 0.33, 0.33, and 0.49, respectively, for the identification of low (< 0 mmHg), normal (0–7 mmHg), or high (> 7 mmHg) CVP. The specificity values of the clinical examination were 0.73, 0.62, and 0.76, respectively. Accuracy was greater in patients with low cardiac indexes (< 2.2 L/min) and high pulmonary wedge pressures (> 18 mmHg). It was lower in comatose patients or patients on mechanical ventilation. Higher precision (interobserver agreement) did not translate into greater accuracy.

3. In a third study, Eisenberg and colleagues compared bedside assessment of 97 critically ill patients with pulmonary artery catheter readings. They compared various hemodynamic variables, including CVP. Based on clinical assessment, physicians were asked to predict whether CVP was < 2, 2–6, or > 6 mmHg. Predictions were correct only 55% of the time. CVP was underestimated more frequently than overestimated (27% and 17%, respectively).

74. What is the significance of an abnormal JVP?

1. An **elevated JVP** reflects a high CVP, which may be due to either hypervolemia or problems with right-sided filling, including (1) decreased right ventricular compliance with increased diastolic pressure (as in right ventricular failure or infarction, pulmonary hypertension, or pulmonic stenosis); (2) obstruction to right ventricular inflow (as in tricuspid stenosis, right atrial myxoma, constrictive pericarditis, or pericardial tamponade); (3) tricuspid regurgitation; and (4) superior vena cava obstruction (no jugular venous pulse is present, and the abdominojugular reflux test is negative).

2. A **decreased JVP** reflects a low CVP, which is due to depletion of intravascular volume caused by gastrointestinal losses (vomiting or diarrhea), urinary losses (diuretics, uncontrolled diabetes mellitus, or diabetes insipidus), or third-space losses.

75. What are the jugular findings of a right ventricular infarction?

The right ventricular filling pressure is increased as a result of a stiffer and ischemic ventricle. Moreover, the ventricle cannot handle incoming venous flow. Thus, the mean JVP is increased, the A wave is increased, and the X and Y descents at times may be so prominent that they mimic constrictive pericarditis. The abdominojugular reflux test is positive. Concomitant tricuspid regurgitation gives additional findings (such as giant V waves, pulsatile liver, right earlobe bobbing; see chapters 11 and 12).

76. What is the abdominojugular (hepatojugular) reflux?

It is a maneuver first described by Louis Pasteur in 1885 as a sign of tricuspid regurgitation. Interest was rekindled in 1898 by Rondot, who coined the term hepatojugular reflux. Rondot was also the first to suggest that a positive hepatojugular reflux was not pathognomonic of tricuspid regurgitation but also occurred in other cardiac disorders. Currently the Pasteur-Rondot maneuver is a useful test in patients whose jugular venous pulse is borderline elevated. In fact, the maneuver can unmask subclinical right ventricular failure or silent tricuspid regurgitation.

77. How is the Pasteur-Rondot maneuver carried out?

By observing the JVP before, during, and after compression of the abdomen.

78. What is the mechanism behind the abdominojugular reflux?

The pressure applied over the abdomen shifts blood into the thorax and right atrium. If the right ventricle is unable to handle this increased load, the result is a sustained increase in JVP. Compression of the liver (as originally recommended by Pasteur) is unnecessary. In fact, in patients with passive hepatic congestion compression of the right upper quadrant may elicit pain and therefore be detrimental. Thus, compression of the periumbilical area or any other area of the abdomen has become the preferred method. For this reason the original term (hepatojugular reflux) has been replaced with the more correct term, abdominojugular reflux test.

79. How do you perform an abdominojugular reflux test?

1. The patient should be well positioned so that the jugular venous pulsations are properly monitored. An angle of 45° for the patient's trunk usually suffices. The patient should be instructed to relax and breathe normally through an open mouth. This technique avoids the false-positive increase in jugular pressure due to a Valsalva maneuver inadvertently triggered by abdominal discomfort.

2. Your hand should be applied over the patient's mid-abdomen (periumbilical area), with fingers widely spread and palm gently rested. Once the patient is well relaxed, gradual and progressive pressure should be applied for 15–30 seconds. Compression should be firm and soon reach a steady level of 20–35 mmHg. The level can be confirmed by placing an unrolled bladder of a standard adult blood pressure cuff between the examiner's hand and the patient's abdomen. The cuff should be partially inflated with six full-bulb compressions.

3. The precision of the abdominojugular reflux test may vary, depending on the force of abdominal compression. Different investigators, in fact, have suggested different forces. Ducas and colleagues recommend 35 mmHg (equivalent to a weight of approximately 8 kg), whereas Ewy recommends 20 mmHg.

4. Throughout the maneuver (i.e., before, during, and after compression), observe the column of blood in the internal and external jugular veins.

5. Either pain or the Valsalva maneuver creates a false-positive outcome. To avoid this risk, describe the test to the patient in advance and ask him or her to avoid any breath-holding or "bearing down." Consider a trial run, which is useful to demonstrate in advance the force that will be applied over the abdomen.

80. When is an abdominojugular test considered positive?

When the *sustained* increase in JVP is ≥ 4 cm. Conversely, an abdominojugular test is considered negative (normal) when any of the following occurs:

1. No change in JVP.
2. A sustained increase ≤ 3 cm during abdominal compression.
3. At the beginning of abdominal compression there may be an initial increase in the prominence of the external jugular vein and the peaks and troughs of the internal jugular vein. The JVP may even increase by 4 cm or more, but the increase is *transient*. JVP returns to normal (or near-normal) during the remaining 10 seconds of abdominal compression.

81. What is the value of the abdominojugular reflux test?

It reflects the inability of the right heart chambers to handle an increased venous return. It is particularly useful in the most subtle and difficult cases. Thus, the abdominojugular reflux test is positive in patients with (1) subclinical right ventricular failure or reduced right ventricular compliance, (2) tricuspid regurgitation, (3) tricuspid stenosis, (4) constrictive pericarditis, (5) pericardial tamponade, (6) inferior vena caval obstruction, and (6) hypervolemia. The abdominojugular test is *not* positive in patients with left ventricular failure.

82. How good is the abdominojugular reflux test?

It is a useful bedside test with positive likelihood ratios. The maneuver has a 66% sensitivity and a 100% specificity for distinguishing tricuspid from mitral insufficiency. It also has low sensitivity but high specificity for recognition of congestive heart failure.

83. Should abdominal pressure be applied for at least 1 minute?

No. One minute was recommended in the past, but application of pressure for 15–30 seconds is enough.

84. What is Kussmaul's sign?

It is the paradoxical increase in JVP that occurs during inspiration. JVP normally decreases during inspiration because of the inspiratory fall in intrathoracic pressure and its sucking effect on venous return. Thus, Kussmaul's sign is a true physiologic paradox.

85. Which disease processes are associated with a positive Kussmaul's sign?

Mostly diseases that interfere with right ventricular filling. The original description by Kussmaul was in a patient with constrictive pericarditis (Kussmaul's sign is still seen in one-third of patients with severe and advanced disease). Now, however, the most common cause of Kussmaul's sign is severe right-sided heart failure, independent of etiology. Working backward from the heart to the superior vena cava, other common causes of Kussmaul's sign include (1) restrictive cardiomyopathy (such as sarcoidosis, hemochromatosis, and amyloidosis), (2) tricuspid stenosis, and (3) superior vena cava syndrome. Kussmaul's sign is also present in 33–100% of patients with right ventricular infarction. Therefore, in the setting of an acute myocardial infarction, Kussmaul's sign should *not* be interpreted as a sign of tamponade but as a sign of right ventricular infarction. In other words:

1. Kussmaul's sign does not occur in pure tamponade (if it does, concomitant epimyocardial fibrosis is present), but it occurs in one-third of patients with pure constrictive pericarditis.

2. Pulsus paradoxus, on the other hand, does not occur in pure, totally dry constrictive pericarditis (if it does, a concomitant amount of pericardial effusion is present), but it occurs in almost all patients with tamponade.

3. Pulsus paradoxus occurs in two-thirds of patients with right ventricular infarction, whereas Kussmaul's sign occurs in 33–100% of right ventricular infarctions.

4. Both signs were first described by Kussmaul.

86. How can you improve the clinical examination of the jugular veins?

Blind examination of patients with indwelling central venous catheters may provide valuable feedback. Pocket cards displaying the normal jugular pulse also may be helpful. Finally, evaluation of patients with tachycardia, irregular cardiac rhythms, rapid and deep respirations, or need for mechanical ventilation may provide useful challenges and hone one's skill.

87. What is venous hum?

It is an innocent murmur (see chapter 12) that often can be confused with a murmur of arteriovenous fistula (including patent ductus arteriosus), aortic regurgitation, or carotid disease. The murmur is in fact continuous (although louder in diastole), typically elicited by a 30–60° leftward rotation of the head and best heard at the base of the neck or right supraclavicular area. It is heard only in the sitting position, vanishes upon reclining, and fades (or altogether disappears) with a Valsalva maneuver or jugular compression distal to the hum.

Its mechanism is mild compression of the internal jugular vein by the transverse process of the atlas in people with strong cardiac output and increased venous flow (usually young adults or patients in a high-output state, such as anemia, fever, thyrotoxicosis, Paget's disease, arteriovenous fistulas, pregnancy, cirrhosis, anxiety, or beriberi). A cervical hum can be heard in 31–66% of normal children and 2.3–27% of adult outpatients. This finding also is quite common among hemodialysis patients: a cervical hum has been reported in 56–88% of patients undergoing hemodialysis and in 34% of patients between dialysis sessions.

Pearl. Various right-sided cardiac sounds (such as S3 and S4 gallops) also may be audible over the neck, usually in patients with right ventricular failure and elevated right-sided pressure. Similarly, even the murmur of tricuspid regurgitation at times may be heard over the neck.

PRECORDIAL MOVEMENT AND IMPULSE

In the first place, then, when the chest of a living animal is laid open and the capsule that immediately surrounds the heart is slit up or removed, the organ is seen now to move, now to be at rest; there is a time when it moves, and a time when it is motionless.
William Harvey, *Exercitatio Anatomica de Motu Cordis et Sanguinis in Animalibus*. London, 1628

In the natural condition of the organ, the heart, examined between the cartilages of the fifth and sixth ribs, at the lower end of the sternum, communicates, by its motions, a sensation as if it corresponded evidently with a small point of the thoracic parietes, not larger than that occupied by the end of the stethoscope.
René T.H. Laennec, *Treatise on Mediate Auscultation*, Paris, 1819

CONVENTIONAL TEACHING WATCH

Inspection and palpation of precordial impulse and movements completes the preauscultatory evaluation of the cardiovascular system. In fact, percussion of the cardiac area (although still quite accurate when competently performed) has become more a memory of the past than a standard of current practice. Evaluation of the precordial impulse, on the other hand, remains an important part of cardiac examination, even in our electronic age. In fact, it provides valuable information about intracardiac size and function and may even provide the first clue to ventricular enlargement, well before the electrocardiogram or chest radiograph shows any change.

FINDING/MANEUVER		CONVENTIONAL TEACHING REVISITED
Precordial impulse	⇑	Analysis of the characteristics of the precordial impulse(s) requires sequential assessment of location, duration, size, force, and contour. The information provided can be essential.
Precordial percussion	⇓	Still provides valuable information (if well performed) but probably should become part of the history rather than the practice of medicine.

88. What is the history behind the palpation and percussion of the precordial area?

Precordial palpation goes back 3,500 years to the Ebers Papyrus of 1550 B.C., which was the principal medical document of ancient Egypt. The papyrus covers 15 diseases of the abdomen, 29 of the eyes, and 18 of the skin and lists no fewer than 21 cough treatments. In a section titled "Beginning of the Secret of the Physicians: Knowledge of Heart's Movement and Knowledge of the Heart," palpation of the cardiac impulse is clearly described. Palpation of the chest was carried out by physicians up to medieval times. Only with William Harvey, however, did the motions of the heart again become a specific topic of scientific discussion. In his 1628 book *De Motu Cordis*, Harvey wrote: "[T]he heart is erected and rises upward to a point so that at this time it strikes against the breast and the pulse is felt externally." Subsequently, important contributions to the art of precordial palpation came from R.T.H. Laennec and Sir James MacKenzie.

89. Which precordial impulse can be appreciated on physical exam?

The only precordial impulse that can be seen and palpated in the normal person is the apical impulse, which is produced by contraction of the left ventricular wall and septum. In disease states, however, several abnormal precordial or chest wall impulses may be present. These impulses correspond to contraction of either ventricle and sometimes to contraction of the atria.

90. Can the right ventricle be appreciated in a normal person?

No. The contraction of the right ventricle produces neither visible nor palpable chest wall movements. Occasionally in children or young people with a narrow anteroposterior diameter it may be possible to feel a gentle right ventricular activity.

91. Can atrial events be appreciated on the precordium?

Only when altered by the presence of an abnormal ventricular compliance. In this case precordial impulses may become the palpable equivalent of an S3 or an S4.

92. How do you assess the precordial impulse?

1. First by inspection, which may be even more useful than palpation. As for the jugular veins, tangential light may be essential to help identify the retraction (and occasionally the outward motion) of the precordial movement(s).

2. After inspection, the examiner should palpate the precordium, looking for impulses and thrills. Stand comfortably at the patient's right side, and use both the palm of the hand and the proximal metacarpals. The fingerpads are usually best suited for localizing the various abnormalities, whereas the palm is better adapted to detect heaves or lifts. Finally, the proximal metacarpals are usually the best site for the identification of thrills.

93. How do you time precordial events?

By either simultaneous palpation of the carotid pulse (using the left hand) or by concomitant auscultation of S1 and S2.

94. Which characteristics of the apical impulse should be analyzed?

1. The normal **location** of the apical impulse is in the midclavicular line at the fifth left intercostal space. Correlation with other anatomic landmarks (such as the left anterior axillary line or parasternal area) should be used to identify displaced or abnormal impulses.

2. The **duration** of the apical impulse is probably one of the most important characteristics. In fact, a sustained impulse is always abnormal and usually suggests a pressure-overloaded left ventricle (as in patients with aortic stenosis or severe and protracted hypertension).

3. The normal **size** of the apical impulse is 1 cm in diameter. An area greater than 2–2.5 cm in diameter in the supine patient or greater than 3 cm in a left lateral decubitus position should be considered pathologic. It usually reflects ventricular enlargement.

4. The **force** of the impulse is also important. A hyperdynamic impulse that lifts the examiner's finger is clearly pathologic and reflects left ventricular hypertrophy with good systolic function.

5. The normal **contour** of the apical impulse consists of a brief, early-systolic, nonsustained impulse.

95. What are the most common abnormal precordial movements?

1. A **double systolic apical impulse** is seen in some patients with hypertrophic obstructive cardiomyopathy. Such patients may even have a triple apical impulse (tripple ripple). One of these impulses is presystolic and corresponds to a strong atrial contraction, whereas the other two are systolic and correspond to ventricular contraction. A thrill is often present. A double systolic impulse also may be seen in patients with left ventricular diskinesia due to either ischemia or ventricular aneurysm (see below).

2. A **sustained apical impulse** usually reflects a pressure-overloaded left ventricle. It typically is seen in longstanding systemic hypertension.

3. A **presystolic impulse** represents the palpable equivalent of a fourth heart sound. It is an important finding because it provides a clue to reduced left ventricular compliance, as in aortic stenosis or hypertension. In aortic stenosis, a palpable S4 usually correlates with a significant gradient between the left ventricle and the aorta. It often is associated with a palpable thrill over the second right interspace.

4. An **early diastolic impulse** represents the palpable equivalent of a third heart sound. It may be felt in patients with a dilated left ventricle due to volume overload and/or left ventricular failure. In this case, the early-diastolic impulse may be associated with a sustained apical impulse.

5. A **hyperdynamic impulse**—larger, nonsustained, and, at least initially, nondisplaced— may be seen in patients with a volume-overloaded left ventricle (as in mitral or aortic regurgitation).

Progression of the disease leads to lateral and downward displacement of the precordial impulse (for example, toward the sixth intercostal space at the anterior axillary line).

6. A **hypokinetic and hypodynamic impulse** is typical of patients with congestive cardiomyopathy. In addition to being hypodynamic, the precordial impulse is also quite diffuse, somewhat sustained, and usually displaced downward and laterally.

7. A **parasternal or epigastric impulse** is usually a clue to the presence of right ventricular hypertrophy. It may be associated with a palpable P2 and/or a pulmonary artery impulse in the second or third left interspace.

96. What precordial evidence suggests mitral stenosis?

In patients with mitral stenosis both S1 and S2 (primarily its P2 component) may be palpable. The opening snap is often palpable too, and a diastolic thrill may be felt in the left lateral decubitus position over the apex.

97. What precordial evidence suggests tricuspid regurgitation?

Adult patients with tricuspid regurgitation almost always have precordial evidence of pulmonary hypertension and right ventricular hypertrophy, such as a palpable P2 over the pulmonic area and a right ventricular parasternal impulse. At times the right ventricular impulse may even be palpable over the epigastric or subxiphoid area. A pulsatile liver in synchrony with each cardiac systole also is appreciated.

98. What precordial evidence suggests angina? Previous infarction?

In patients with angina, the apical impulse is usually normal, but there may be a palpable S4 (presystolic impulse). Conversely, in patients with preexisting infarctions, the apical impulse may be felt superior and medial to the normal apical location. Such an ectopic impulse usually suggests a left ventricular aneurysm or a left ventricular diskinesia.

99. What does a dilated aorta or pulmonary artery suggest?

In patients with pulmonary hypertension a dilated pulmonary artery may be felt at the upper left parasternal area. Conversely, in patients with aortic aneurysm a dilated aorta may be felt at the right parasternal area.

100. What is a thrill?

A thrill is a palpable vibration associated with an audible murmur. It is a sign of pathology. In fact, innocent murmurs never present with a thrill. Moreover, the presence of a thrill automatically qualifies a murmur as having an intensity equal to or greater than 4/6.

101. What is the value of precordial percussion?

When properly carried out, precordial percussion retains some clinical value. In fact, competently performed, percussion can outline the cardiac area with errors of only 1 cm. But given the difficulty in mastering this skill and the ubiquity of chest radiography, cardiac percussion may be one of those areas of physical examination in which the baton has been passed to technology-based diagnosis.

BIBLIOGRAPHY

1. Abrams J: Essentials of Cardiac Physical Diagnosis. Philadelphia, Lea & Febiger, 1987.
2. Connors AF, McCaffree DR, Gray BA: Evaluation of right heart catheterization in the critically ill patient without acute myocardial infarction. N Engl J Med 308:263–267, 1983.
3. Cook DJ: The clinical assessment of central venous pressure. Am J Med Sci 299:175–178, 1990.
4. Cook and Simel: Does this patient have abnormal central venous pressure? JAMA 275:630–634, 1996.
5. Davision R, Cannon R: Estimation of central venous pressure by examination of the jugular veins. Am Heart J 87:279–282, 1974.
6. Ducas J, Magder S, McGregor M: Validity of the hepatojugular reflux as a clinical test for congestive heart failure. Am J Cardiol 52:1299–1303, 1983.

 7. Ewy GA: The abdominojugular test: Technique and hemodynamic correlates. Ann Intern Med 109: 456–460, 1988.
 8. Heckerling PS, Wiener S, Moses VK, et al: Accuracy of precordial percussion in detecting cardiomyopathy. Am J Med 91:327–334, 1991.
 9. Maisel AS, Atwood JE, Goldberger AL: Hepatojugular reflux: Useful in the bedside diagnosis of tricuspid regurgitation. Ann Intern Med 101:781–782, 1984.
10. Marantz PR, Kaplan MC, Alderman MH: Clinical diagnosis of congestive heart failure in patients with acute dyspnea. Chest 97:776–781, 1990.
11. Pasteur W: Note on a new physical sign of tricuspid regurgitation. Lancet 2:524, 1885.
12. Perloff JK: Physical Examination of the Heart and Circulation, 2nd ed.. Philadelphia, W.B. Saunders, 1990.
13. Sapira JD: The Art and Science of Bedside Diagnosis. Baltimore, Urban & Schwarzenberg, 1990.
14. Sauve JS, Laupacis A, Ostbye T, et al: Does this patient have a clinically important carotid bruit? JAMA 270:2843–2845, 1993.
15. Upshaw CN, Silverman ME: The Wenckebach phenomenon: A salute and comment on the centennial of its original description. Ann Intern Med 130:58–63, 1999.

11. CARDIAC AUSCULTATION—HEART SOUNDS

Salvatore Mangione, M.D.

. . . I rolled a quire of paper into a sort of cylinder and applied one end of it to the region of the heart and the other to my ear, and was not a little surprised and pleased, to find that I could thereby perceive the action of the heart in a manner much more clear and distinct than I had ever been able to do by the immediate application of the ear. From this moment, I imagined that the circumstance might furnish means for enabling us to ascertain the character, not only of the action of the heart, but of every species of sound produced by the motion of all thoracic viscera.

Laennec RTH: *A Treatise on the Diseases of the Chest.* Philadelphia, James Webster, 1823 [translated by John Forbes].

The gallop stroke is diastolic and is due to the beginning of sudden tension in the ventricular wall as a result of the blood flow into the cavity. It is more pronounced if the wall is not distensible and the failure of distensibility may depend on either a sclerotic thickening of the heart wall (hypertrophy) or to a decrease in muscular tonicity.

Potain PC: Note sur les dedoublements normaux des bruits du coeur. Bull Mem Soc Med Hop Paris 3:138, 1866.

CONVENTIONAL TEACHING WATCH

Conventional teaching has long recognized auscultation of the heart as the centerpiece of physical diagnosis. Indeed, proper identification of the various auscultatory findings can still allow the prompt recognition of many important cardiac diseases, particularly in the area of sounds and extra sounds, a field that has fascinated physicians since the introduction of stethoscopy. A plethora of gallops, clicks, snaps, knocks, and plops has since entered everyday vocabulary. Accordingly, we have granted all but a few of these sounds a "high pass" in our conventional teaching test. The few that failed did so not because of the paucity of information that they deliver but because of the rarity of the disease processes that they represent.

SOUNDS AND EXTRA SOUNDS		CONVENTIONAL TEACHING REVISITED
S1	⇔	Still informative and valuable, albeit not as much as S2.
S2	⇑	One of the most valuable sounds, particularly in its variations of intensity and splitting.
S3	⇑	The most clinically valuable cardiac extra sound.
S4	⇔	Most important for what it sounds like without being it (e.g., an S4 is important for *not* being an S3).
Pericardial friction rub	⇑	One of the most valuable extra sounds (probably at the top of the list with S3).
Early systolic (ejection) click	⇑	Valuable and not too uncommon; should not be missed.
Mid-to-late systolic click	⇑	As above.
Opening snap	⇔	Important, but its prevalence is rapidly fading.
Pericardial knock	⇓	Neat to think of it, but it is more zebra than horse.
Tumor plop	⇓	As above

NORMAL HEART SOUNDS

First Heart Sound (S1)

1. Where is S1 best heard?
At the apex (for its mitral component) and over the epigastric or subxiphoid area (for its tricuspid component). In these locations S1 (detected through the diaphragm of the stethoscope) should be clearly louder than S2.

2. How is S1 generated?
The first sound is generated by two major events:
1. The **closure** of the atrioventricular valves.
2. The **opening** of the semilunar valves, which in itself is a combination of two separate sounds: (1) the sound directly produced by the opening of the semilunar valves and (2) the sound produced by the ejection of blood into the large vessels.
Pearl. *The closure of the atrioventricular valves (and their mitral and tricuspid component) is usually quite loud, whereas the opening of the semilunar valves is usually inaudible.*

3. Which characteristics of S1 are clinically valuable and therefore should be recognized?
The most valuable is **intensity** (and variations thereof). The second most valuable is **splitting** (and variations thereof).

4. What is the significance of an S2 louder than S1 at the apex?
This finding indicates two possibilities: (1) S2 is indeed louder than S1 (usually the result of either pulmonary or systemic hypertension) or (2) S2 is normal in intensity, and S1 is softer.

5. What hemodynamic factors are responsible for the loudness of S1?
If the chest wall shape and thickness are constant, three major factors influence the loudness of S1. All three apply to both the mitral and the tricuspid component of S1:

1. **Thickness of the atrioventricular (AV) leaflets.** The thicker the leaflets, the louder the S1. This principle is intuitive; for example, banging two hardback books against each other generates much more noise than banging two thin paperbacks. If the AV leaflets become too thick and rigid, however, the loudness of S1 is decreased. For example, a thickened and stenotic mitral valve generates a booming S1 early in the course of the disease, but as soon as the leaflets become rigid and fixed, the same valve generates a softer or even absent S1.

2. **Separation between the mitral leaflets at onset of ventricular systole.** The closer the leaflets, the softer the sound; the more separated the leaflets, the louder the sound. This mechanism feeds into two other factors:

   • **Duration of the P-R interval.** A short P-R causes the ventricle to start contracting while the leaflets are still widely separated. Because the leaflets must close from far away, they generate a loud S1. The opposite occurs in first-degree AV block, in which a long P-R allows enough time for the leaflets to get close to each other. A muffled S1, for example, is quite common in patients with rheumatic fever and first-degree AV block. The leaflets travel a shorter distance before being shut by the ventricles. This, in turn, generates a softer S1. A progressive increase in the duration of the P-R interval, as may be encountered in patients with the Wenckebach phenomenon, also may increasingly soften the intensity of S1 (see below).

   • **Atrioventricular pressure gradient.** A large pressure gradient between atrium and ventricle (as in patients with mitral stenosis) keeps the AV leaflets wide open until the ventricular pressure eventually rises high enough to close them. The long distance traveled by the leaflets is responsible for the loudness of the S1. Thus, the longer the left ventricle must contract to close the mitral valve, the louder S1 will be. This mechanism is quite common in mitral stenosis, in which it is partially responsible for the loudness of S1 (together with the thickening of the AV leaflets).

3. **Rate of rise in left ventricular pressure.** The faster the rise, the louder the S1. Thus, a loud S1 is typically heard in hyperkinetic hearts (as in patients with thyrotoxicosis, pregnancy, fever, arteriovenous fistulas, patent ductus arteriosus, aortic regurgitation). Conversely, a soft (muffled) S1 is commonly heard in patients with congestive heart failure, whose failing ventricles can generate only a slow rise in pressure.

6. What factors influence the rate of rise of ventricular pressure?

Contractility and all of its determining variables are the most important factors that influence the rate of rise of ventricular pressure. Thus, an increase in contractility (by either exogenous or endogenous inotropic agents) augments the intensity of the mitral component of S1. Conversely, a decrease in contractility, as may be seen in patients with congestive heart failure, softens the mitral component of S1.

7. What disease processes are associated with a variable intensity of S1?

Heart blocks. A variable S1 is typical of (1) second-degree AV block (Mobitz type I, also called Wenckebach phenomenon) and (2) third-degree (complete) AV block.

The **Wenckebach phenomenon** is associated with progressive softening of S1, whereas the intensity of S2 remains constant. This finding is due to the gradual lengthening of the P-R interval until eventually a beat is dropped. Such progressive softening of S1 is so typical that Wenckebach was able to describe the phenomenon even before the EKG was invented.

In third-degree AV block, on the other hand, the rates of atrial and ventricular contraction are totally independent. Thus, whenever ventricular systole catches the AV valves wide open, S1 is booming. Conversely, whenever the ventricular contraction catches the AV valves partially closed, S1 is soft. This variable intensity of S1 (in association with bradycardia, which represents either a nodal or a ventricular escape rhythm) is so random and chaotic that complete AV block can be recognized on the basis of auscultation alone.

Pearl. Second-degree AV block is associated with progressive softening of S1, whereas in third-degree A-V block the change in intensity of S1 is random and chaotic.

Intensity of S1

LOUD	VARIABLE	SOFT
Short P-R interval (< 160 msec)	Atrial fibrillation	Long P-R interval (> 200 msec)
Increased contractility (hyper-kinetic states)	Atrioventricular block (Wenckebach and third-degree block)	Decreased contractility (left ventricular dysfunction)
Thickening of mitral (or tricuspid) leaflets	Ventricular tachycardia (due to atrioventricular dissociation)	Left bundle-branch block
Increased atrioventricular pressure gradient (stenosis of AV valves)		Calcification of AV valve(s)
		Premature closure of mitral valve (acute aortic regurgitation)
	Pulsus alternans	Mitral (or tricuspid) regurgitation

8. Who were Mobitz and Wenckebach?

Karel F. Wenckebach (1864–1940) was a Dutch physician who taught at the University of Vienna between 1914 and 1929. A modest man with a passion for the arts and the English countryside, Wenckebach linked his name not only to the famous phenomenon that he described but also to one of the first reports of the beneficial use of quinine for the treatment of atrial fibrillation. Woldemar Mobitz was a German cardiologist, born at the end of the nineteenth century, who during the first half of the twentieth century linked his name to various arrhythmias and second-degree AV block.

9. What is the intensity of S1 in atrial fibrillation?

The intensity is variable because of the irregular ventricular rate, which may catch the AV valves widely open, partially closed, or in between.

10. How can one distinguish the variable S1 of atrial fibrillation from the variable S1 of third-degree AV block?

In atrial fibrillation the rhythm is irregularly irregular, whereas in third-degree AV block the rhythm is a regular bradycardia (due to either nodal or ventricular escape).

11. Describe S1 in mitral stenosis.

S1 tends to be loud in mitral stenosis, usually because of the following factors:

1. **High-pressure gradient between the atrium and the ventricle**, which is produced by stenosis of the mitral valve and keeps the AV leaflets maximally separated at onset of ventricular contraction.

2. **Thickening of the AV leaflets**, which makes the leaflets more rigid and more likely to produce a loud sound when banging against each other at onset of ventricular systole. In the late stages of the disease, however, the mitral leaflets become stiff and poorly mobile. At that point S1 softens and eventually disappears.

12. What other conditions may be associated with a loud S1?

Other than mitral stenosis or hyperkinetic heart syndrome, a loud S1 is usually encountered in (1) hypertrophic ventricles, (2) holosystolic mitral valve prolapse with regurgitation, (3) short P-R intervals (such as preexcitation syndromes [e.g., Wolff-Parkinson-White and Ganong-Levine syndromes]), and (4) left-atrial myxoma.

13. What conditions may be associated with a soft S1?

Other than calcific mitral stenosis, a soft S1 should suggest the presence of (1) prolonged P-R interval, (2) impaired left ventricular contraction (as in patients with congestive heart failure, severe aortic and mitral regurgitation, or myocardial infarction), or (3) left bundle-branch block, in which the left ventricle contracts late and M1 follows T1 (M = mitral, T = tricuspid).

14. Which atrioventricular valve closes first?

The mitral valve, followed by the tricuspid valve. Because mitral closure is much louder than tricuspid closure, the first component of S1 is usually referred to as M1 and predominates in the formation of S1.

15. Which semilunar valve opens first?

The pulmonic valve, followed by the aortic valve. The aortic ejection sound is usually louder than the pulmonic sound but still not loud enough to be audible in normal patients.

16. Summarize the sequence of closure and opening of the various valves at the time of S1.

1. Mitral closure (M1)   3. Pulmonic opening
2. Tricuspid closure (T1)   4. Aortic opening

The first two events are the real contributors to S1. The last two events may become important (and audible) only in pathologic settings, such as patients with ejection clicks (sounds).

17. What is the significance of a narrowly split first sound?

It usually reflects the audible separation of M1 and T1 components. This narrow split is normal and may be detected in many people by listening over the lower left sternal border or epigastric area (where the tricuspid component is louder and therefore more readily separable from the mitral component).

18. Is the tricuspid component of S1 (T1) audible at the apex?

No. It is audible only at the lower left sternal border. T1, however, may become audible at the apex in patients with (1) thickening of the tricuspid valve leaflets (i.e., early tricuspid stenosis) or (2) right ventricular pressure overload, as in pulmonary hypertension or atrial septal defect.

19. What is the significance of a split S1 at the base?

It does *not* indicate the audible separation of M1 and T1; it indicates instead the presence of an early ejection sound of either pulmonic or aortic origin (see below).

20. What is the significance of a widely split first sound?

It usually indicates delayed closure of the tricuspid valve, most commonly due to right bundle-branch block. A bundle-branch block also may cause a split S2 (see below).

21. What other processes may present with an apparently split S1?

An apparently split S1 may represent a normal S1 that happens to be either preceded by an S4 or followed by an early systolic (ejection) click (see below). This is an important differential diagnosis to keep in mind.

22. How can one separate a truly split S1 from a pseudosplit S1?

A truly split S1 is usually heard over the lower left sternal border. An S4 of left atrial origin, on the other hand, is audible only at the apex, whereas an early systolic click usually is louder over the base. To separate the S4 from the early systolic click, remember that the S4 is lower-pitched, softer, located before the true S1, and heard at the apex. An early ejection click, on the other hand, is higher-pitched, louder, located *after* the true S1, and heard at the base.

Finally, the lower-pitched S4 is best heard with the bell of the stethoscope (while applying light pressure on the instrument); conversely, the higher-pitched early systolic click is best heard with the diaphragm or by applying strong pressure on the bell (thereby converting it into a diaphragm).

Second Heart Sound (S2)

23. Where is S2 best heard?

At the base. More specifically, S2 is best heard over the second or third *left* parasternal interspace (pulmonic component) and over the second or third *right* parasternal interspace (aortic component). Because of its medium-to-high pitch, S2 can be recognized quite easily through the diaphragm of the stethoscope.

24. How is S2 generated?

Primarily by the closing of the aortic (A2) and pulmonic (P2) valves (more precisely, by the sudden deceleration of blood after closure of the semilunar valves).

25. Which of the two semilunar valves closes earlier?

The aortic valve. The pressure is usually higher in the systemic circulation than in the pulmonic circulation.

26. How clinically useful is S2?

Very useful. Indeed, it has been suggested that careful clinical evaluation of the second heart sound ranks with electrocardiography and roentgenography as one of the most valuable routine screening tests for heart disease. Leatham referred to S2 as "the key to auscultation of the heart."

27. What characteristics of S2 are more clinically valuable and therefore should be examined carefully?

Sound intensity and sound splitting. Splitting (and its variations) is the most informative. In SI, on the other hand, intensity (and its variations) is the most informative feature.

28. Which is louder—A2 or P2?

A2 is consistently louder throughout the precordium. In fact, P2 is loud enough to be audible in only one area—a few centimeters to the left of the upper sternal border. This site is called the **pulmonic area** (second or third left interspace next to the sternum). Thus, if P2 is heard anywhere else (such as the apex or second right interspace), it probably is louder than normal.

Pearl. Because the pulmonic area is the only site at which the pulmonic component of S2 can be appreciated, the splitting of the second sound also is heard best over the pulmonic area.

29. How can the two components of S2 be differentiated?

By remembering that only A2 is heard at the apex. Indeed, in the absence of pulmonary hypertension P2 is too soft to be transmitted to the apex. Thus, to tell A2 from P2, one should move the stethoscope from the base to the apex and then pay attention to which component of S2 becomes softer. If it is the first component, P2 precedes A2. If, on the other hand, the second component disappears, A2 precedes P2. This maneuver may be helpful in differentiating a right bundle-branch block (in which A2 precedes P2) from a left bundle-branch block (in which P2 precedes A2).

30. What is the significance of a split S2 at the apex?

A split S2 cannot be heard at the apex, unless the patient has pulmonary hypertension (P2 is normally heard only over the pulmonic area). Thus, a split S2 at the apex suggests the presence of pulmonary hypertension until proved otherwise.

31. Which conditions cause a loud P2 or a loud A2?

Increased pressure in either the pulmonary or systemic circulation leads to a louder P2 or A2, respectively. Such conditions include (1) pulmonary hypertension, (2) systemic hypertension, and (3) coarctation of the aorta. High-output states, which may cause a loud S1, also may be associated with a loud S2. Examples of hyperdynamic conditions include (1) atrial septal defects, (2) ventricular septal defects, (3) thyrotoxicosis, and (4) aortic regurgitation.

32. What is a tambour S2?

It is a loud and ringing S2, rich in overtones. *Tambour* in French means "drum." The word conveys the peculiar character of this sound (which is drum-like). A tambour S2 usually indicates a dilatation of the aortic root. In patients with a murmur of aortic regurgitation, a tambour S2 suggests Marfan syndrome, syphilis, or a dissecting aneurysm of the ascending aorta (Harvey's sign).

33. Which conditions cause a P2 louder than A2?

Pulmonary hypertension (in which P2 is indeed louder than A2) or aortic stenosis with reduced valve mobility (in which A2 is actually softer than P2).

34. What are the other precordial findings of pulmonary hypertension?

In addition to a loud and palpable P2 over the pulmonic area, pulmonary hypertension may be associated with a right-sided S4, a pulmonic ejection sound, and a murmur of tricuspid regurgitation.

35. What conditions may cause a soft A2 or P2?

Low cardiac output or lower systolic pressure in the pulmonary or systemic circulation. A soft A2 or P2 also may occur in settings of reduced mobility of the semilunar valves due to either calcification or sclerosis. For example, in aortic or pulmonic valvular stenosis soft or absent A2 or P2 indicates severe stenosis and a poorly mobile valve.

36. What is the significance of an S2 that is louder than S1 at the apex?

Either pulmonary or systemic hypertension. Otherwise S2 at the apex should be softer than S1.

Pearl. *P2 normally cannot be heard at the apex. Thus, a physiologic splitting of S2 over the apex (produced by a now audible P2) suggests pulmonary hypertension until proved otherwise.*

37. What is the significance of an S2 that is softer than S1 at the base?

It depends on which part of the base is involved and therefore on which of the S2 components is softer. If S2 is softer than S1 over the aortic area, A2 is diminished, usually because of fibrosis or calcification of the aortic valve, as in patients with aortic stenosis. If, on the other hand, S2 is softer than S1 over the pulmonic area, P2 is decreased, usually because of pulmonic stenosis.

38. What is a physiologic splitting of S2?

Physiologic splitting of S2 refers to an inspiratory widening in the normal interval between the closure of the aortic and pulmonic valves (see figure on facing page). This finding results from two phenomena during inspiration:

1. Greater venous return to the right ventricle (due to the increasingly negative intrathoracic pressure) delays closure of the pulmonic valve.

2. Decreased venous return to the left ventricle (due to pooling of blood in the lungs) accelerates closure of the aortic valve.

Pearl. *The widening between A2 and P2 becomes large enough in inspiration to be easily detectable by the human ear. For most ears, a large enough widening tends to be 30–40 msec. The reverse occurs in exhalation to the point that, although aortic closure still precedes pulmonic closure, the interval between the two components is too narrow for the ear to identify them separately.*

39. How common is a physiologic splitting of S2?

In a study of 196 normal adults examined in supine position, only 52.1% had an audible inspiratory split of S2. Physiologic splitting was much more common among younger adults (60% between 21 to 30 and 34.6% older than 50). Indeed, after age 50, S2 appeared single in both inspiration and expiration in most subjects (61.6% vs. 36.7% for all ages).

Pearl. *In older patients a single S2 should not be considered evidence for a delayed A2 and therefore does* not *suggest underlying aortic stenosis or left bundle-branch block.*

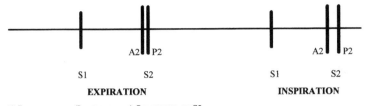

A) Physiologic (Inspiratory) Splitting of S2

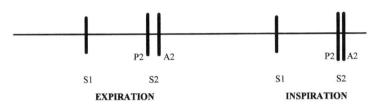

B) Paradoxical or Reversed (Expiratory) Splitting of S2

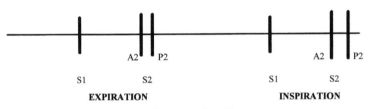

C) Wide Splitting (Inspiratory > Expiratory) of S2

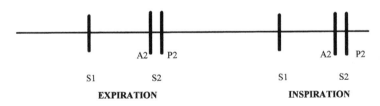

D) Fixed Splitting (Inspiratory = Expiratory) of S2

Splitting of S2.

40. What is the effect of patient position on the splitting of S2?

Very important. A supine position increases venous return, lengthens the right ventricular systole, and thus widens the physiologic split of S2. Conversely, a sitting or standing position decreases venous return, shortens right ventricular systole, and thus narrows the physiologic split. This difference is particularly important for the analysis of an expiratory splitting. Indeed, in the study by Adolph and Fowler, an expiratory splitting was found in 22 normal subjects in the recumbent position (11% of total). Yet 21 of the 22 lost the expiratory splitting on assuming an upright position. Thus, before diagnosing an expiratory splitting of S2 (which is an important clue to underlying pathology), make sure that the splitting is present not only in the recumbent position but also in the upright position (either sitting or standing).

Pearl. *As a corollary, audible splitting that persists during expiration in the standing position should be considered pathologic until proved otherwise.*

Use of Sitting Position to Assess Audible Expiratory Splitting

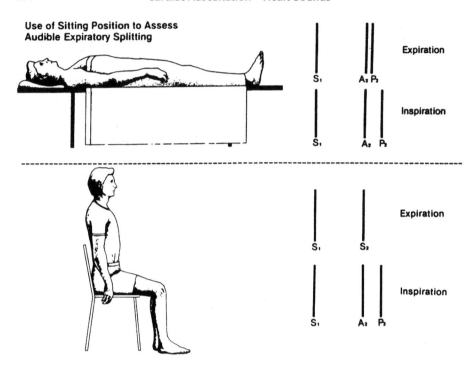

Evaluation of audible expiratory splitting of S2. The presence of expiratory splitting in the supine position is usually abnormal. Sometimes expiratory splitting of S2 in the supine position disappears when the patient is upright and the S2 becomes single on expiration. This response is normal. Patients should be examined carefully in the sitting and standing positions whenever S2 appears to be abnormally split during expiration. (From Abrams J: Prim Cardiol, 1982, with permission.)

41. What is the significance of an expiratory splitting of S2?

If persistent in the upright position, an expiratory splitting of S2 may represent one of three conditions: (1) wide splitting of S2, (2) fixed splitting of S2, or (3) paradoxical splitting of S2. Wide splitting of S2 may be normal in young people, albeit abnormal in patients above the age of 50, whereas both fixed splitting and paradoxical splitting reflect important underlying cardiovascular pathology.

42. What is the significance of a wide splitting of S2?

A widening of the physiologic splitting of S2 (to the point that S2 appears split throughout respiration, although more markedly so during inspiration) occurs in (1) delayed closure of the pulmonic valve (= delayed P2), (2) premature closure of the aortic valve (= premature A2), or (3) a combination of both.

43. In which conditions is wide splitting of S2 due to delayed closure of the pulmonic valve?

The classic condition is complete right bundle-branch block (RBBB). RBBB delays both depolarization of the right ventricle and closure of the pulmonic valve; as a result, it widens the physiologic splitting of S2 to the point of making it audible not only in inspiration but also in expiration. Loss of elastic recoil of the pulmonary artery (as in idiopathic dilatation of the pulmonary artery) or severe impedance to right ventricular emptying also may cause delayed closure of the pulmonic valve. Severe impedance may be seen in (1) pulmonic stenosis, (2) cor pulmonale with right ventricular failure, (3) atrial septal defect, and (4) massive pulmonary embolism. In pulmonary embolism an audible expiratory splitting of S2 (with a loud pulmonic component) has diagnostic and prognostic significance, usually reflecting acute cor pulmonale.

44. In which conditions is wide splitting of S2 due to premature closure of the aortic valve?
The most common conditions are characterized by rapid emptying of the left ventricle (e.g., ventricular septal defect or severe mitral regurgitation). Premature closure also may be found in patients with severe congestive heart failure, usually because of a reduction in left ventricular stroke volume. Finally, a widely split S2 also may be encountered in pericardial tamponade. In this setting the heart is literally sitting in a water bag. Thus, the room available for expansion of the two ventricles is limited and fixed. Because the right ventricle fills relatively more during inspiration, the septum protrudes into the left ventricular chamber. This protrusion, in turn, reduces the room available for filling of the left ventricle. As a result, the decrease in left ventricular size during inspiration is dramatic. The resulting decrease in left ventricular stroke volume causes early closure of A2 and a wide inspiratory splitting of S2. The opposite occurs in exhalation.

45. What is the significance of a fixed splitting of S2?
A fixed splitting of S2 (which, by definition, should be present in both upright and supine positions) refers to a second sound that remains audibly and consistently split throughout respiration. Although this phenomenon may be encountered in patients with severe heart failure, a fixed splitting of S2 is seen most commonly in patients with a septal defect (usually atrial, but occasionally ventricular, particularly if associated with pulmonary hypertension). The septal defects and their resulting shunt equalize the changes in right and left ventricular stroke volume that are secondary to respiration. Thus, the septal defects are responsible for fixing the widening of S2.
More rarely, a fixed splitting of S2 is heard in patients with severe impedance to right ventricular emptying, such as those with pulmonary stenosis, pulmonary hypertension, or massive pulmonary embolism. Such patients are unable to cope with the increased venous return of inspiration. Accordingly, they are not able to increase right ventricular stroke volume and therefore keep the S2 widely and persistently split throughout respiration.

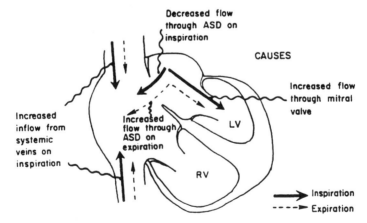

The increased inflow into the right atrium on inspiration (vertical solid arrows) causes a decreased flow through the atrial septal defect (ASD) and thus increased flow through the mitral valve. (From Constant J: Bedside Cardiology. Boston, Little, Brown, 1976, with permission.)

46. What is the differential diagnosis of a fixed splitting of S2?
The differential diagnosis includes a late systolic click (which precedes S2) and an early diastolic extra sound (which follows S2). The most common early diastolic extra sounds are S3 and the opening snap of mitral (or tricuspid) stenosis (to differentiate an opening snap from a wide

splitting of S2 or an S3, see below). Two other (albeit less common) early diastolic sounds also should be included in the differential diagnosis: (1) pericardial knock and (2) the opening sound of an atrial myxoma (i.e., tumor plop, see below).

47. What is the significance of a paradoxical splitting of S2?

Paradoxical splitting of S2 means pathology until proved otherwise. A paradoxical (or reversed) splitting of S2 indicates a second sound that becomes audibly split only in exhalation; it remains single in inspiration. This paradoxical behavior (opposite to normal physiologic splitting) results from a delay in the aortic component of S2. Because of this delay, A2 follows instead of precedes P2, and the pulmonic valve closes earlier than the aortic valve. The respiratory behavior of the two valves, however, remains unchanged. For example, in inspiration venous return to the right ventricle is increased (because of the increasingly negative intrathoracic pressure), and venous return to the left ventricle is decreased (because of lung pooling). These phenomena delay pulmonic closure and anticipate aortic closure. Because of the reversed closure of the two valves, the two components become so close during inspiration that they are perceived as a single sound. The opposite occurs in exhalation, explaining the expiratory (and therefore paradoxical) split of S2.

48. Which disease processes cause a paradoxical splitting of S2?

Conditions that delay the aortic closure. The most common is delayed depolarization of the left ventricle, as in complete left bundle-branch block (LBBB). A reversed splitting of S2 may be present in as many as 84% of patients with LBBB. Two other mechanisms may delay aortic closure, thereby causing a paradoxical or reversed splitting of S2: (1) increased impedance on left ventricular emptying (e.g., in systemic hypertension, aortic stenosis, and coarctation of the aorta) or (2) weakening of left ventricular function, which may be seen in acute ischemia (infarction and/or angina) and various cardiomyopathies. More rarely, a paradoxical splitting of S2 may be due to premature closure of P2, which usually results from decreased filling of the right ventricle, as may be seen in tricuspid regurgitation or right atrial myxoma.

49. Is the detection of a paradoxical splitting of S2 a sign of myocardial ischemia?

Yes. Although paradoxical splitting of S2 rarely occurs with stable coronary artery disease, it often may be heard during acute decompensation, such as after exercise or during angina. It also may be heard during the first three days after an acute myocardial infarction in as many as 15% of patients. Finally, it is commonly heard in elderly hypertensive patients with underlying coronary artery disease and evidence of heart failure.

50. What is the significance of a single splitting of S2?

Single splitting refers to either a single S2 or an S2 too narrowly split for its two components to be heard. A single S2 usually results from one of the following:

1. **Aging.** The audible splitting of S2 decreases in prevalence with age to the point of becoming absent in as many as half of all people over the age of 60.

2. **Reversed or paradoxical splitting.** The split occurs not in inspiration but in expiration (see above).

3. **Pulmonary hypertension.** The increased impedance on right ventricular emptying makes the ventricle unable to cope with the increased venous return of inspiration. As a result, there is no inspiratory lengthening of right ventricular systole and therefore no inspiratory splitting of S2.

4. **Emphysema.** The aerated and hyperinflated lungs muffle P2 during inspiration, making A2 the only audible sound. Because this phenomenon is less pronounced in exhalation, patients may be misdiagnosed with paradoxical splitting of S2 when, in fact, they have pseudoparadoxical splitting, which becomes evident only in expiration.

5. **Semilunar valvular disease.** Stiffening and reduced mobility of the semilunar valves lead to disappearance of either A2 or P2, thus making S2 a single sound.

EXTRA SOUNDS

51. What are extra heart sounds?

Pathologic sounds that occur in addition to normal cardiac sounds (i.e., S1, S2). They may originate in either systole or diastole. Based on their place in the cardiac cycle, extra sounds are therefore divided into systolic (usually referred to as early, mid, or late systolic clicks) and diastolic (usually referred to as snaps, knocks, or plops).

Pearl. *All extra sounds should be considered pathologic until proved otherwise.*

Extra Sounds

SYSTOLIC		DIASTOLIC	
TIMING	NAME	TIMING	NAME
Early systolic	Ejection sounds (aortic or pulmonary) Click (mitral or tricuspid) Aortic prosthetic valve sounds	Early diastolic	Opening snap (mitral or tricuspid) Early S3 Pericardial knock Tumor plop
Mid-to-late systolic	Click (mitral or tricuspid)	Mid diastolic	S3 Summation sound (S3 + S4)
		Late diastolic (presystolic)	S4 Pacemaker sound

ES = early systolic (ejection sound), MS = mid systolic, LS = late systolic, ED = early diastolic, MD = mid diastolic, LD = late diastolic, S1 = first sound, S2 = second sound.

52. Should S3 and S4 be considered extra sounds?

S3 and S4 should be considered more like heart sounds than extra sounds. They are, however, indicative of pathology (S4 almost always, S3 in most cases). Thus, their clinical significance is much closer to that of extra sounds, and they are included in this section.

53. Where are extra sounds best heard?

It depends on the type. Snaps, knocks, and plops usually are heard best at the apex, whereas clicks (particularly ejection clicks) can be heard both at the base and at the apex.

54. Where are S3 and S4 best heard?

Both are heard best at the apex. Both also are palpable (although S4 is more so). The bell is essential for the detection of these sounds because of their extremely low frequency (a mere 20–60 Hz), which puts them almost at the threshold of audibility.

55. Which bedside maneuvers can intensify S3 or S4?

Both S3 and S4 are increased by exercise, even as little as a change in position (for example, assuming the left lateral decubitus position). Similarly, both S3 and S4 are intensified by maneuvers that increase venous return and intracardiac blood volume (such as leg elevation, abdominal compression, hand grip, and the release of Valsalva's maneuver). Because expiration increases the venous return to the left ventricle, both left-sided S3 and S4 increase in exhalation (although S4 increases in early exhalation, whereas S3 increases in end exhalation). Right-sided S3 and S4 increase in inspiration (Rivera-Carvallo maneuver).

Maneuvers that decrease venous return and intracardiac blood volume, on the other hand, soften a pathologic S3 or S4 and totally eliminate a physiologic S3. A simple maneuver is to ask a supine patient to sit or stand. In addition, the strain phase of Valsalva's maneuver also decreases venous return, thereby softening (or obliterating) S3 and S4.

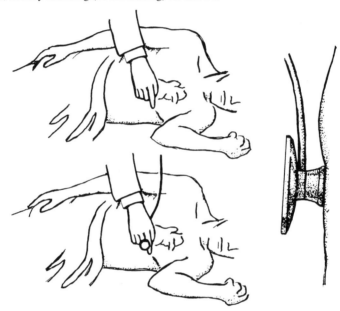

Use of the left lateral decubitus position in detection of S3 and S4. *Upper,* The left ventricular apex is identified first by careful palpation. *Lower,* The bell of the stethoscope is then applied directly over the apical impulse, using the lightest pressure possible to create a skin seal. This technique enhances audibility of low-frequency cardiac sounds (e.g., S3, S4, mitral diastolic murmurs). (Adapted from Abrams J: Prim Cardiol, 1982)

Diastolic Extra Sounds

56. How many diastolic extra sounds may be encountered?

Of the five diastolic extra sounds, two are quite common (S3 and S4); one is less common (the opening snap of mitral or tricuspid stenosis), and two are rare (the opening plop of a mitral or tricuspid valve myxoma and pericardial knock). Only S4 occurs late in diastole (or presystole); all others occur early in diastole. Two of the five extra sounds are low-pitched and soft (S3 and S4), two are high-pitched and loud (opening snap and pericardial knock), and one is medium-pitched and of varying intensity (tumor plop).

Third Heart Sound (S3)

57. What is a third heart sound?

S3 is a low-pitched, soft, early diastolic extra sound of great clinical importance. It was described in the nineteenth century by Potain and has since been recognized as an important sign of ventricular disease. In a nationwide survey of internal medicine and cardiology program directors, it was ranked as the most important extra sound for clinical value (together with the pericardial friction rub).

58. How easy is detection of an S3?

Not that easy. Because of its low frequency (40–50 Hz), S3 is literally at the threshold of audibility. Moreover, because its intensity may vary greatly as a result of many variables, an S3 may be fleeting. It should be sought quite aggressively in any patient with suspected heart failure.

59. Which factors modify the loudness of S3?

The loudness of S3 (i.e., the subjective perception of its sound intensity) may be increased by using the bell of the stethoscope. The bell filters out all extraneous high-frequency sounds, making it easier to hear the low-pitched S3. Because of its low frequency, the S3 may not be audible through the diaphragm of the stethoscope. It may not even be audible if too much pressure is applied on the bell (thereby transforming it into a diaphragm). In fact, the disappearance of the S3 upon application of firm pressure on the bell may be used as a maneuver to confirm that the sound is indeed an S3 and not, for example, a higher-pitched extra sound such as an opening snap.

Pearl.   The examiner must listen for the S3 by holding the bell gently over the patient's chest.

60. How is S3 best detected?

At the apex and in the left lateral decubitus position, which brings the left ventricle closer to the chest wall, thus allowing better transmission of the S3. Of course, the physician must have enough suspicion to turn the patient into left lateral decubitus position after a negative initial examination in the supine position. A high index of suspicion is also necessary for the performance of various other bedside maneuvers.

61. Can an S3 be palpable?

Yes. In fact, in patients with left ventricular hypertrophy, an S3 may be more easily palpated than heard (particularly in the left lateral decubitus position).

62. What is the interobserver agreement by auscultation about the presence of an S3 in patients with congestive heart failure?

Moderate at best and slight at worst. Ishmail et al. showed that agreement among four trained observers examining 81 hospitalized patients was indeed poor (ranging between 48% and 73% for pairs of observers). Thus, although the S3 is a valuable sign, it is difficult to detect.

63. Which is easier to detect: an S3 or an S4?

An S4 is higher-pitched and louder than an S3, although not as long in duration, because the S4 is usually produced by healthier and more forceful hearts. The S3 is often prolonged by a series of low-pitched and humming vibrations that follow the S3 per se (see below).

64. Which bedside maneuvers intensify an otherwise soft or absent S3?

Maneuvers that increase the volume and flow of blood across the mitral valve, even minor exercise (such as passive leg raising, squatting, or even coughing). Standing or sitting causes a decrease in the volume and flow of blood across the mitral valve and thus softens the pathologic S3 and even eliminates the physiologic S3. Finally, either inspiration or exhalation increases the loudness of the S3 (exhalation by increasing venous return to the left ventricle, inspiration by increasing the sympathetic tone to the heart, which, in turn, increases circulation time, heart rate, and blood flow across the mitral valve). In general, held exhalation tends to intensify the left-sided S3, whereas held inspiration tends to intensify the right-sided S3.

65. Describe the intensity of S3 after an extrasystole.

The intensity is greater. The mechanism is the same: increased ventricular filling after the premature beat.

66. Should the S3 be pursued over the point of maximal apical impulse (PMI)?

Yes, if it is possible to identify the PMI. In fact, there are times when the S3 is too soft to be heard anywhere else. That the PMI is the best area of auscultation derives directly from the site of origin of S3 (over the left ventricular wall).

67. How is S3 produced?

The S3 is not produced by the left ventricle hitting against the chest wall. Instead, the S3 reflects the transition between the rapid and slow phase of left ventricular filling. An increase in left-ventricular preload and/or a subnormal left-ventricular compliance causes a sudden slowing of flow into the left ventricle. This deceleration, in turn, distends the ventricle and the AV valve apparatus, thereby generating the S3.

Pearl. *S3 is due to a sudden and abnormal deceleration in left ventricular flow at the end of its rapid filling phase.*

68. Why is the S3 located in early diastole?

S3 reflects the phase of rapid left (and right) ventricular filling. This phase follows the opening of the atrioventricular valves and occurs in early diastole. It accounts for the majority of ventricular filling (approximately 80%); the remaining 20% occurs much later in diastole (primarily at the time of atrial contraction, which is the phase of active ventricular filling). This later phase of atrial kick is heralded not by S3 but also by S4.

Pearl. *S3 signals the phase of early (or passive) ventricular filling, whereas S4 signals the phase of late (or active) ventricular filling. Both sounds occur within the ventricle.*

69. Is an S3 always a gallop?

Not necessarily. A gallop is any triple lilt at a rate so fast that it mimics the gait of a horse. A ventricular gallop (i.e., a gallop produced by an S3) is only one of three forms (see below). Thus, the term gallop usually implies a faster heart rate (often in association with a softer S1 and S2) and a typical cadence. It is also a more ominous clinical connotation than a simple S3.

Pearl. *A third heart sound may be physiologic and not a gallop. An S3 gallop, on the other hand, is almost always pathologic.*

70. What are the most important gallops?

The two most important are (1) the **ventricular gallop** (in which the third heart sound, together with a soft S1 and S2, is responsible for the galloping lilt) and (2) the **atrial gallop** (in which the fourth heart sound, together with S1 and S2, is responsible for the galloping lilt). Traditionally, we mimic these gallops by saying, in a cadenced fashion, *Ken-tú-cky* (for an early diastolic or S3 gallop) and *Ten-ne-ssée* (for a late diastolic or S4 gallop). In addition, a third and less common form is called the **summation gallop**.

71. What is a summation gallop?

A summation gallop (sometimes called S7 from the sum of S3 and S4) is the peculiar lilt of highly tachycardic patients with both S3 and S4. Usually such patients are prone to both an atrial and a ventricular gallop (for example, patients with hypertensive heart failure). The tachycardia reduces diastole, thus leading to the fusion and S3 and S4 into a loud S7. A summation gallop also may occur in first-degree AV block, in which the prolonged P-R interval causes S4 to move backward in diastole, thereby merging with S3.

72. What are the acoustic characteristics of a summation gallop?

A summation gallop is a higher-pitched, longer, and louder extra sound than an isolated S3 or S4. It is also easily palpated. Given its location (in early-to-mid diastole) and longer duration, a summation gallop often is mistaken for a mid diastolic rumble. It is easily unmasked into its two components, however, by slowing the heart rate (for example, by cautious carotid massage).

73. Is a quadruple rhythm the same as a summation gallop?

No. A quadruple rhythm is a gallop lilt characterized by the presence of both S3 and S4, each separately audible.

74. What is a physiologic S3?

The S3 encountered in normal children and young adults (usually in association with a venous hum or innocent systolic murmur). It also may be encountered in athletes, especially young athletes. A physiologic S3 reflects a more energetic expansion and filling of the left ventricle, probably due to higher cardiac output. It typically softens or disappears whenever the person assumes an upright posture (because of the decreased venous return). Although it may be found in normal men in their late 30s and normal women in their early 40s, a physiologic S3 is usually not heard after the age of 45.

75. Can a physiologic S3 be present in any setting other than young and healthy people?

Yes. A physiologic S3 may occur whenever sympathetic tone is increased or levels of catecholamines are high, such as during tachycardia, thyrotoxicosis, fever, exercise, anemia, pregnancy, and anxiety. All of these high-output states have rapid circulation time, tachycardia, and a frequent venous hum in the neck. The S3 associated with such conditions is usually louder and higher-pitched than a pathologic S3.

76. What is the significance of a pathologic S3?

A pathologic S3 reflects either increased left ventricular preload (i.e., diastolic overload) or poor ventricular function (with decreased myocardial contractility and low ejection fraction). The first (and less common) mechanism plays a role in conditions of high-output failure; the second (and more common) mechanism plays a role in situations of low-output failure, such as dilated cardiomyopathies (hypertrophic cardiomyopathies are usually associated with S4, not S3).

77. What are the acoustic characteristics of a pathologic S3 as opposed to a physiologic S3?

A pathologic S3 tends to be softer, lower-pitched, and more likely to have a gallop lilt. In addition, it tends to have longer duration. At times, however, a pathologic S3 may sound much like a physiologic S3. The lower intensity of the pathologic S3 is due to reduced ventricular contractility, which is also responsible for the tachycardia and softer S1 and S2. Altogether, these findings make the pathologic S3 a much more subtle and difficult sound to detect.

Pearl. The most important feature in differentiating these sounds is the company they keep: a pathologic S3 keeps bad company (symptoms or other abnormal physical findings), whereas a physiologic S3 keeps no bad company.

78. What is the low-pitched diastolic murmur often heard in patients with a pathologic S3?

It is a sound produced by the sudden rush of blood across the mitral valve and into a flaccid left ventricle. This short rumble is often seen in settings of increased mitral flow (as in patients with mitral regurgitation) or ventricular dysfunction. It may even be present by itself (in the absence of an S3). This low-pitched, early diastolic rumble is rarely encountered in patients with a physiologic S3.

Pearl. The association between an early diastolic rumble and an S3 suggests a pathologic S3 until proved otherwise.

79. What are the hemodynamic implications of an S3?

They depend on the mechanism responsible for the generation of S3:

1. In patients with **increased left ventricular preload** (i.e., diastolic overload), cardiac index and ejection fraction are normal (or even increased), whereas atrial pressure is elevated.

2. In patients with **ventricular dysfunction** and **abnormal ventricular compliance**, both cardiac index and ejection fraction are decreased, whereas the left atrial, pulmonary artery diastolic, pulmonary capillary wedge, and left ventricular pressures are increased. As a result, the left ventricle is dilated, and the end-diastolic volume is increased.

Pearl. As a rule of thumb, in patients with ventricular dysfunction the presence of a third sound usually reflects a filling pressure of 25 mmHg or greater.

80. What are the clinical implications of an S3?

Quite a few. An S3 is the best predictor for response to digoxin in patients with congestive heart failure. It also is the most significant predictor of cardiac risk during noncardiac surgery. Finally, even in the absence of other signs of decompensation, an S3 can identify patients prone to develop congestive failure after a surgical procedure.

81. Which conditions are most commonly responsible for an S3 secondary to diastolic overload?

1. **Intracardiac or intravascular shunts**, such as a ventricular septal defect (VSD) or patent ductus arteriosus (PDA). An atrial septal defect, on the other hand, is not responsible for diastolic overload of the left ventricle because the right-to-left atrial shunt actually decreases the flow over the mitral valve, whereas increased flow over the tricuspid valve is much less likely to cause a right-sided S3.

2. **Mitral regurgitation** with increased diastolic flow across the mitral valve. The S3 is louder and higher-pitched than the more typical S3, almost resembling an opening snap. In patients with mitral regurgitation, the presence of an S3 does not indicate heart failure, but it does signify a large degree of regurgitation.

82. What is the effect of pulmonary hypertension on the intensity of S3 secondary to diastolic overload?

If the diastolic overload is due to left-to-right shunt (such as a VSD or PDA), the development of pulmonary hypertension gradually decreases the shunt into the left ventricle and flow across the mitral valve. As a result, the S3 progressively softens and eventually disappears. This finding, for example, may herald the development of Eisenmenger's syndrome. In such patients, the return of an audible S3 usually indicates development of a new right-sided (not left-sided) failure.

83. What is Eisenmenger's syndrome?

Any left-to-right shunt complicated by pulmonary hypertension, reversal of the shunt, and cyanosis. Eisenmenger's syndrome usually is more common with PDA or VSDs and less common with atrial septal defects. The syndrome was first described by the German physician Eisenmenger (1864–1932).

84. Is an S3 always generated by the left ventricle?

No. It also may be generated by the right ventricle through the same mechanisms of either right ventricular dysfunction and flaccidity or increased filling over the tricuspid valve (i.e., tricuspid regurgitation). The right-sided S3 is usually best heard on inspiration and over the epigastric/subxiphoid area instead of the apex.

85. Can a right ventricular S3 be differentiated from a left ventricular S3?

A right ventricular S3 is best heard over the right ventricular area (left parasternal and epigastric area). Like all right-sided findings, it tends to be louder in inspiration. A left ventricular S3, on the other hand, is best heard over the apex (usually over the PMI) and tends to be louder in exhalation (see figure at top of facing page).

86. Which disease processes are associated with a right ventricular S3?

A right ventricular S3 is commonly encountered in settings of either increased blood flow across the tricuspid valve (such as severe tricuspid regurgitation) or increased impedance to right ventricular emptying (such as massive pulmonary embolism or cor pulmonale).

87. What is the differential diagnosis of an S3?

1. **Split S2.** In contrast to the S3, a split S2 is higher-pitched and best heard with the diaphragm over the base of the heart. It does not soften on assuming the sitting or standing position and has respiratory variations.

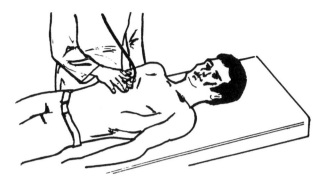

Where to listen for right-sided S3 or S4. Note the use of the bell of the stethoscope. (Adapted from Tilkian AG, Conover MB: Understanding Heart Sounds, 3rd ed. Philadelphia, W.B. Saunders, 1993.)

2. **Tumor (plop).** The hallmark of this sound is its variability from cycle to cycle, which is not usually a feature of S3 (see below).

3. **Pericardial knock and opening snap.** In contrast to S4, both the pericardial knock and the opening snap are medium- to high-pitched sounds and thus are best detected with the diaphragm.

88. How can S3 be differentiated from an opening snap?

S3 tends to occur later than the opening snap and much later than a split S2. The opening snap occurs 100 msec after the second sound (A2), whereas S3 usually occurs at least 120 msec after A2 (often even later). Although this difference appears trifling to the untrained ear, it helps quite a bit in differentiating the two sounds. In addition, S3 is a faint, low-pitched sound, whereas the opening snap is a short, snapping, high-pitched, and loud sound. Finally, because the left ventricle is usually small in mitral stenosis, the opening snap tends to be closer to the left sternal border than the S3, which is loudest at the apex.

89. How common is the S3 in patients with mitral stenosis?

Not common at all. As a matter of fact, the presence of an S3 usually should rule out concomitant mitral stenosis of significant degree because the valvular obstruction of mitral stenosis prevents the rapid left ventricular early diastolic filling that is responsible for the genesis of the S3.

Pearl.   A pathologic S3 is usually absent in mitral stenosis and vice versa.

Fourth Heart Sound (S4)

90. What is a fourth heart sound?

S4 is a low-pitched, soft, late diastolic extra sound. It is much more common than the S3. In fact, some authors consider S4 a sound of aging due to the progressive loss of compliance of the ventricles.

91. How is the fourth sound best detected?

Like S3, S4 is best heard at the apex through the bell of the stethoscope. Firmer pressure on the bell softens and eliminates S4, just as it softens or eliminates S3.

Pearl.   Both S3 and S4 are often inaudible in the supine position and become transiently evident only when the patient assumes a left lateral decubitus position.

92. What are the auscultatory differences between a third and a fourth heart sound?

The fourth sound is higher-pitched, louder, and shorter and, of course, has a different timing. In addition, S4 is late diastolic (or presystolic) and precedes S1. S3, on the other hand, is

early diastolic and follows S2. Both sounds vary with respiration (although S3 much more prominently), and both are louder in exhalation.

93. Why is S4 located late in diastole?

S4 relates to atrial contraction (primarily left-sided, but also right-sided); thus, it is generated
late in diastole and immediately before ventricular systole (and before S1, which signals its
onset). For this reason, S4 is often referred to as a late diastolic or presystolic extra sound.

94. How is S4 produced?

S4 corresponds to atrial systole, but the sound is not generated by atrial contraction per se. It
is produced instead by the sudden tension of the ventricle/AV valve apparatus as a result of forceful atrial contraction.

Pearl.   *S4 is classically absent in patients with atrial fibrillation or atrial flutter.*

95. What are the clinical implications of S4?

An S4 usually indicates a hypertrophic, thickened, and poorly compliant ventricle (either left
or right); usually it does not indicate a dilated ventricle. S4 is the result of a reduction in ventricular distensibility and a decrease in the passive filling of early-to-mid diastole (which is responsible
for 80% of ventricular filling). The decrease in ventricular compliance places greater demand on
the atrial booster. As a result, the atrium is required to handle as much as 30–40% of the entire
ventricular filling instead of the usual 20%. The stronger atrial kick rushes into the noncompliant
ventricle and produces the S4. In tachycardic patients this S4 assumes a gallop cadence.

96. What is the hemodynamic significance of an S4?

Hemodynamically, the S4 corresponds to an increase in late ventricular diastolic pressure.

97. How common is an S4?

It depends on the method of detection. By phonocardiography an S4 is so common that it may
reflect no true pathology. In fact, an S4 can be recorded in as many as 75% of normal middle-aged
adults. On the other hand, an audible, loud, and even palpable S4 almost certainly reflects an underlying pathology. Even in older adults (in whom S4 is extremely common in the absence of
clearcut pathology), the presence of a distinctly audible S4 may reflect underlying disease. Indeed,
follow-up of such "normal" patients over time usually reveals underlying coronary artery disease.

Pearl.   *An audible S4 (particularly if palpable) indicates underlying pathology, independently of the age of the patient.*

98. Is there such a thing as a normal (or physiologic) S4?

Probably not, although an S4 may be common in older patients, in whom it may reflect the
effect of aging on ventricular compliance. Yet it is not entirely clear whether such S4s reflect subclinical pathology (see below). An S4 also may be heard in young adults with no clear evidence of ventricular dysfunction or anatomic abnormalities; usually they have only an increase in blood flow.

99. Which conditions may cause a pathologic S4?

Conditions in which ventricular filling requires substantial contribution from atrial contraction. Approximately 80% of ventricular filling occurs in early-to-mid diastole, whereas only 20%
occurs in late diastole (as a result of atrial contraction). In patients with thickened and stiffened
ventricles, however, the atrial contribution may increase by as much as 40%. Among the conditions responsible for ventricular stiffening are (1) hypertension, either systemic pulmonary (S4
may precede electrocardiographic signs of ventricular hypertrophy); (2) aortic stenosis (S4 is
usually associated with a gradient of over 70 mmHg); (3) coarctation of the aorta; (4) hypertrophic cardiomyopathy (an audible and palpable S4 is almost a sine qua non); (5) coronary heart
disease (S4 can be heard in as many as 90% of patients experiencing myocardial infarction); and
(6) prolonged P-R interval. In all of the above settings there often is a prominent P wave on EKG.

Once ventricular hypertrophy evolves into ventricular failure (with a dilated and more flaccid ventricle), S4 gradually softens and disappears, leaving in its place an S3.

Pearl. An S4 implies an earlier, more compensated, and less severe condition than an S3. It is, therefore, a less ominous sign.

100. What maneuvers can be used to detect an S4?

All maneuvers that increase venous return (the same maneuvers that increase the intensity of S3). Examples include (1) leg raising, (2) mild exercise, (3) abdominal compression, (4) release phase of Valsalva's maneuver, and (5) exhalation. Conversely, maneuvers that decrease venous return (such as sitting, standing, and the strain phase of Valsalva's maneuver) soften both S3 and S4. All of the above maneuvers increase (or decrease) the intensity of both S4 and S3, but they do so much more dramatically for S3.

Pearl. Physiologic S3 and S4 disappear when the patient assumes a standing position, whereas pathologic gallops usually soften but remain.

101. Can an S4 be palpable?

Yes, usually in the left lateral decubitus position and over many cardiac cycles (because of its respiratory variations). In fact, an S4 is much more likely to be palpable than an S3, thus allowing differentiation between the two diastolic extra sounds.

Pearl. A palpable S4 should be considered pathologic, whereas an S4 that is audible but not palpable may be a normal physiologic finding.

102. Can a right-sided S4 be differentiated from a left-sided S4?

A right-sided S4 is best heard over the lower left sternal border or subxiphoid areas. At times it may be heard over the neck veins. A right-sided S4 is commonly associated with other signs of right ventricular strain, such as distended neck veins with large A or V waves, loud P2, and right-ventricular heave. Finally, like all right-sided findings, a right-sided S4 is louder in inspiration.

103. What is the differential diagnosis of an S4?

1. **Split S1.** In contrast to S4, a split S1 is best heard with the diaphragm over the lower left sternal border. It does not soften when the patients assumes a sitting or standing position.

2. **S1-ejection click (sound) complex.** This complex may easily simulate an S4–S1 complex and thus presents a difficult challenge. In contrast to S4, both S1 and ejection sounds are medium- to high-pitched and thus are best detected with the diaphragm; in addition, neither S1 nor the ejection sound softens in the upright position (as does S4).

Opening Snap

104. What is an opening snap?

It is a loud, snapping, and high-pitched early diastolic extra sound. It is louder at the lower left sternal border and softer at the apex; it is best heard by using the diaphragm of the stethoscope or by applying firm pressure over the bell (see figure at top of next page). The snap is produced by the opening and stretching of a stenotic mitral (or tricuspid) valve and should be considered abnormal until proved otherwise.

105. Why are these sounds called snaps?

Extra sounds produced by the atrioventricular valves are conventionally called (1) snaps (if they occur in diastole and are caused by the abnormal opening of the leaflets) or (2) clicks (if they occur in systole and are caused by the prolapse and backward ballooning of the leaflet[s]). Clicks due to atrioventricular valve prolapse are usually mid or late systolic in timing. They also may be early systolic, but early systolic clicks are more commonly due to abnormal ejection of blood across the semilunar valves. Thus, to avoid confusion with the AV clicks of prolapse, these ejection clicks are usually referred to as ejection sounds. In addition to this semantic differentiation, the term *snap* conveys quite well the typically high-pitched, short, and snapping quality of the sounds.

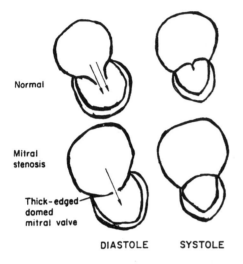

Normal

Mitral
stenosis

Thick-edged
domed
mitral valve

DIASTOLE   SYSTOLE

Cause of the opening snap. The belly of the stenotic mitral valve (mostly the anterior leaflet) bulges downward with a jerk to produce a clicking or snapping sound as it opens. Therefore, it also must close with a snap as it domes upward. (Adapted from Constant J: Bedside Cardiology. Boston, Little, Brown, 1996.)

106. Is the opening of a normal atrioventricular valve audible?

Usually not. In patients with hyperkinetic heart syndrome the increased blood flow may make audible the opening of a normal AV valve. This finding, however, is the exception rather than the rule. In all other patients, an audible opening of the AV valves indicates thickening and stiffening of the valve leaflets or commissures. As a result, the leaflets behave much like a sail suddenly filling under wind, with ballooning and bellowing and a final snap due to the tight grip of the chordae tendinae. In patients with mitral stenosis, much of the snapping is produced by the filling of the anterior leaflet, which is larger and more mobile than the posterior leaflet.

107. How can one differentiate the closing of the second sound from an opening snap?

From the difference in timing. There is usually enough separation between the closing of the semilunar valve (A2) and the opening of the mitral valve (OS) for the human ear to perceive them as two separate acoustic events. This interval, usually around 10 ms, is commonly called the **A2–OS interval**.

108. What does the A2–OS interval reflect?

The A2–OS interval reflects the length of the isometric relaxation of the ventricle (also called isovolumic relaxation). In this phase of diastole all four valves are closed and the ventricular size remains constant.

Pearl. A shorter isometric (isovolumic) relaxation leads to a shorter A2–OS interval and an earlier opening snap. Conversely, a longer isometric (isovolumic) relaxation leads to a longer A2–OS interval and a delayed opening snap.

109. What factors control the A2–OS interval and therefore the timing of the opening snap?

1. **Pressure in the left atrium at the time of mitral valve opening.** For example, a high left atrial pressure (with a high atrioventricular pressure gradient) shortens the A2–OS interval because the pressure in the left ventricle does not have to fall much for the mitral valve to open. Conversely, a low left atrial pressure (due to a milder degree of mitral stenosis or, paradoxically, to a large left atrium with heart failure and low flow) prolongs the isometric relaxation time, lengthens the A2–OS interval, and delays the opening snap.

Pearl. The timing of the opening snap accurately reflects the severity of stenosis: the earlier the timing, the worse the stenosis.

2. **Heart rate.** Bradycardia lengthens the A2–OS interval and delays the opening snap; tachycardia anticipates the opening snap.

3. **Rigidity or stiffness of the mitral valve.** The stiffer the valve, the longer the A2–OS interval and the more delayed the opening snap. A stiffer valve requires a higher left atrial pressure to open. The degree of stiffness of a valve does not necessarily reflect its degree of stenosis. Stenosis is related to the degree of opening of the valve, whereas stiffness reflects the mobility of its leaflets.

4. **Myocardial contractility.** Myocardial dysfunction prolongs the isometric relaxation time, lengthens the A2–OS interval, and delays the opening snap.

5. **Closing pressure for the aortic valve.** The higher the aortic pressure, the longer the isometric relaxation time and the more delayed the opening snap. A high aortic pressure requires a much larger drop in ventricular pressure before the mitral valve can open.

110. Is the timing of the opening snap valuable in assessing the degree of stenosis of the mitral valve?

Quite valuable. Indeed, both the timing of the snap and the length of the A2–OS interval are strong and reliable indicators of severe mitral stenosis; only severe stenosis or tachycardia can shorten the A2–OS interval and anticipate the opening snap. Conversely, many factors other than a mild degree of mitral stenosis can lengthen the A2–OS interval and delay the opening snap. Examples include (1) bradycardia, (2) poor myocardial function, (3) high aortic pressure, (4) aortic regurgitation, (5) reduced left atrial flow (as in patients with pulmonary hypertension or an enlarged atrium), and (6) degree of stiffening of the mitral leaflets.

Pearl.   *The earlier the opening snap, the more severe the mitral stenosis.*

111. Is the intensity of the opening snap valuable in assessing the degree of stenosis of the mitral valve?

Yes. A soft or absent opening snap indicates a stiff and poorly mobile mitral valve (usually a calcific mitral valve). A softer opening snap also may reflect the thickness of the chest wall or the degree of emphysema (the thicker the chest wall and/or the greater the degree of emphysema, the softer the opening snap). In addition to severe mitral stenosis, other conditions may soften the opening snap:

1. **Heart failure.** The softening of the snap is due to the low blood flow of heart failure.

2. **Very large right ventricle** (as a result, for example, of pulmonary hypertension). A large ventricle may push the left ventricular wall away from the chest surface and therefore soften the opening snap.

3. **Pulmonary hypertension.** Noncalcific mitral stenosis and pulmonary hypertension may soften the opening snap as a result of low flow at both the mitral and pulmonary artery levels.

Conversely, an increase in venous return and left atrial pressure increases the intensity of the snap—for example, after exercise (as mild as turning from supine to left decubitus position) or leg-raising maneuvers.

112. How common is an opening snap in patients with mitral stenosis?

In the absence of calcification, an opening snap is present in 75–90% of all patients with mitral stenosis. It reflects a milder form of disease and therefore is absent in more advanced (and calcific) cases.

113. How can one distinguish the pulmonary sound of a split S2 from an opening snap?

This distinction may not be easy. P2 and an opening snap share many characteristics: (1) the interval between A2 and P2 is similar to the interval between A2 and opening snap (both are between 30 and 100 msec); (2) both P2 and opening snap are high-pitched and short; and (3) both can be heard at the left lower sternal border. However, the opening snap is louder at the apex than the base, whereas P2 is louder at the base and almost inaudible at the apex, unless the patient has pulmonary hypertension.

Pearl.   *A split S2 that is louder at the apex than at any other site is much more likely to represent an opening snap than a true P2.*

A good maneuver to differentiate the two sounds is to ask the patient to inspire and exhale. This maneuver is based on the physiologic principle that an opening snap occurs earlier during inspiration (as a result of decreased venous return to the left side), whereas the P2 of a widely split S2 occurs much later in inspiration (unless, of course, the patient has a complete left bundle-branch block).

Pearl. *A split S2 that becomes wider and louder on exhalation usually represents an opening snap and not an A2–P2 complex.*

A loud S1 is another important clue that an early diastolic extra sound represents an opening snap rather than a P2. A loud S1 is common in mitral stenosis, particularly in patients whose valve leaflets are thickened, stiff, and yet quite mobile. Conversely, a soft S1 is so rare in patients with an opening snap that it almost always rules out the diagnosis.

In summary, to differentiate a P2 from an opening snap one should rely on (1) the **area of maximum intensity** of the sound (a sound that is loudest at the apex rather than at the base is more likely to be an opening snap than a P2); (2) the **respiratory changes** of the sound (an expiratory widening of a split S2 in a patient without a left bundle-branch block is much more suggestive of an opening snap than an A2–P2 complex); and (3) the **intensity of S1** (a soft S1 tends to exclude an opening snap).

Pearl. *In patients with pulmonary hypertension, the best way to differentiate P2 from an opening snap is to rely not on the apical intensity of the sound (which may be quite loud) but on its respiratory variations.*

114. How can one distinguish an S3 from an opening snap?

Although both are well heard at the apex, the S3 is softer, lower-pitched, and best detected with the bell. The opening snap is louder, higher-pitched, and best detected with the diaphragm.

115. What is a tricuspid opening snap?

A tricuspid opening snap is an opening sound produced by a stenotic tricuspid valve. It may be present in 5% of all patients with mitral stenosis.

116. How can one differentiate a mitral from a tricuspid opening snap?

Like all right-sided findings, a tricuspid opening snap is louder in inspiration because the increased venous return of inspiration creates a greater flow across the stenotic tricuspid valve and, in turn, a louder snap. The opening snap of mitral stenosis is louder in exhalation (because of the increased venous return to the left side during exhalation).

Pericardial Knock

117. What is a pericardial knock?

A pericardial knock is a sharp, loud, and high-pitched early diastolic extra sound corresponding to the phase of early ventricular filling. From this standpoint, the knock represents a particular form of S3. It is, however, much louder and higher-pitched.

118. What is the cause of a pericardial knock?

It is due to the sudden distention of the left ventricle against a thick and calcific pericardium.

119. Is acute pericarditis commonly associated with a pericardial knock?

No. The pericardial knock is always absent in acute or subacute pericarditis, in which a rub is a much more typical feature (see below) and even in tamponade. It is often encountered in chronic calcific and constrictive pericarditis, which usually is the sequela of an old tuberculous process.

120. What are the other physical findings in patients with a pericardial knock due to constrictive pericarditis?

1. **Right-sided heart failure:** distended neck veins (with deep x and y descents), hepatomegaly, ascites, leg edema, often anasarca
2. **Kussmaul's sign:** inspiratory distention (not collapse) of the neck veins
3. **Pulsus paradoxus** (see above)

121. What is the differential diagnosis of a pericardial knock?

S3 and opening snap. The knock can be differentiated from the opening snap because of its timing (it occurs later than the opening snap) and from S3 because of its acoustic characteristics (it is much louder and higher-pitched than S3). Because it can be well heard over the pulmonic area, the knock also may have to be differentiated from a split S2. Respiratory variations and lack of transmission to the apex aid the recognition of a split S2.

Mitral (or Tricuspid) Valve Myxoma

122. What is a tumor plop?

A tumor plop represents the diastolic prolapse of a left (or right) atrial myxoma through an opened mitral (or tricuspid) valve. Such tumors are typically pedunculated and attached to a stalk. The plop belongs in the differential diagnosis of an early diastolic extra sound (together with S3, opening snap, pericardial knock, and split S2). Some patients may have a sudden drop in blood pressure and syncope after a change in body position because of transient obstruction of diastolic ventricular flow by the tumor.

Pearl. The hallmark of tumor plops is that they are intermittent sounds, varying in intensity and quality from cycle to cycle.

Systolic Extra Sounds

123. What are ejection sounds?

They are high-pitched, loud, and clicky early systolic extra sounds that are best detected through the diaphragm. They used to be called ejection clicks or early systolic clicks, but recently the term ejection sounds has become more commonly used to avoid confusion with the mid-to-late systolic clicks of atrioventricular valve prolapse. Ejection sounds are produced by blood flowing across the semilunar valves and into the large vessels. They are a normal but usually inaudible component of S1. They may become loud enough to be identifiable as distinct acoustic events in patients with either hyperkinetic heart syndrome or underlying pathology of the semilunar valves and/or large vessels.

Early Systolic Clicks (Ejection Sounds)

124. What is the mechanism of production of an ejection sound?

In patients with no cardiovascular pathology, an ejection sound usually results from a hyperkinetic heart syndrome (e.g., anemia, fever, thyrotoxicosis, pregnancy). In patients with cardiovascular pathology, an ejection sound may be produced by two different mechanisms:

1. The opening or doming of a congenitally bicuspid or stenotic semilunar valve (in this case, purists refer to the sound as an ejection click).
2. The sudden distention of the root of a great vessel (either aorta or pulmonary artery) during the early part of ventricular systole. The tensing of the proximal portion of the great vessel occurs almost invariably in association with either a dilatation of the vessel itself or the stiffening and high pressure of the corresponding vascular bed (pulmonary or systemic hypertension).

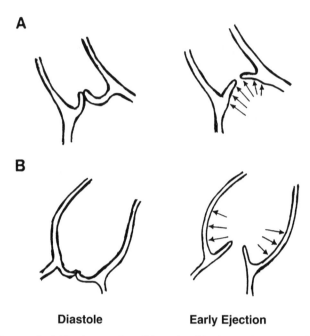

Diastole   **Early Ejection**

Origin of ejection sounds. *A,* Ejection sound or click produced by the opening motion of a thickened, often stenotic aortic or pulmonary valve. *B,* Ejection sound produced by sudden tensing of the proximal aorta or pulmonary artery during early ejection. This is usually associated with a dilated and/or hypertensive great vessel. (Adapted from Abrams J: Essentials of Cardiac Physical Diagnosis. Philadelphia, Lea & Febiger, 1987.)

125. What is the clinical significance of an ejection sound?

In the absence of a hyperkinetic heart, it should be considered a sign of either semilunar valve or great vessel disease. More specifically, (1) a congenitally bicuspid semilunar valve (with or without stenosis) or (2) a dilation of the aortic (or pulmonary) root with or without systemic or pulmonary hypertension.

Pearl.   *An ejection sound should be considered indicative of valvular or vascular pathology until proved otherwise.*

126. Can an ejection sound be accompanied by a systolic murmur?

Yes. In fact an ejection sound due to a bicuspid valve is often accompanied by an ejection murmur. The murmur is caused by relative stenosis of the semilunar bicuspid valve, which, in turn, leads to poststenotic dilatation of the aortic or pulmonary root. This dilatation further enhances the ejection sound, and the cycle continues.

Pearl.   *The presence of an early systolic click (ejection sound) is an important clue for the identification of a concomitant systolic murmur as organic in origin.*

127. What causes an aortic ejection sound?

1. The forceful ejection of blood into a normal aortic root (as in high-output states such as thyrotoxicosis, anemia, exercise, or pregnancy) or the normal ejection of blood into a stiffened and dilated aortic root (as in patients with hypertension, atherosclerosis, aortic aneurysm, or aortic regurgitation).

2. The normal ejection of blood through an abnormal aortic valve—either a semilunar valve stiffened and fused by a rheumatic process or (more commonly) a congenitally bicuspid valve.

128. Where is the aortic ejection sound best heard?

In patients with semilunar valve disease, the ejection sound is heard well at the base but even better at the apex. In some cases, the apex may be the only area where the click is detected. This is also true in patients with emphysema. When it originates from the aortic root (not from a semilunar bicuspid valve), the ejection sound is best heard throughout the sash area of aortic projection (from the apex to the right shoulder), with the area of highest intensity at the base. Finally, the aortic ejection sound is best heard on full expiration with the patient in a sitting position.

129. What are the implications of detecting an aortic ejection sound in patients with aortic stenosis?

An aortic ejection sound indicates the presence of valvular aortic stenosis (in this case, a valvular ejection sound is still often called a click). A click is in fact absent in both the subvalvular and the supravalvular forms of aortic stenosis. Even more importantly, a click should indicate the presence of a bicuspid aortic valve, one of the most common (if not the most common) congenital abnormalities of the heart, and medication for endocarditis prophylaxis.

130. What is the clinical significance of the intensity of the aortic click?

Intensity reflects the mobility of the valve: it decreases with fibrosis and disappears with calcification. Thus, a softening of the click over time indicates progressive fibrosis and stiffening of the valve, whereas the absence of an aortic ejection click usually reflects a calcific aortic stenosis with a transvalvular gradient greater than 50 mmHg.

131. Can the opening of the pulmonary semilunar valve be responsible for an ejection sound?

Yes. In patients with pulmonic stenosis, the sudden upward movement and opening of a dome-shaped pulmonary valve can generate an ejection sound.

132. How can one distinguish the ejection sound of a pulmonary semilunar valve from that of an aortic semilunar valve?

An aortic ejection sound has constant intensity throughout the respiratory cycle, whereas a pulmonary ejection sound is louder in expiration and softer in inspiration. The ballooning of the pulmonic valve (which is responsible for the click) tends to be less during inspiration as a result of the stronger right atrial contraction (which, in turn, is triggered by the inspiratory increase in venous return).

Pearl.   The softening or even disappearance of the pulmonary ejection sound during inspiration contrasts strongly with the normal behavior of all other right-sided findings, the intensity of which increases during inspiration (Rivera-Carvallo maneuver).

133. Does the presence of a pulmonic ejection sound correlate with the severity of pulmonary stenosis?

Usually it tends to correlate more with mild-to-moderate pulmonic stenosis. Rarely it correlates with right ventricular pressures exceeding 70 mmHg. In more severe cases of pulmonic stenosis the pulmonic ejection sound tends to occur quite early, either merging with S1 or even preceding it.

134. What is the clinical significance of the intensity of the pulmonary ejection sound?

Not much. In patients with valvular pulmonic stenosis, a softer click may be present in both mild and severe disease. In both cases the intensity of the click correlates with respiration (louder in exhalation and softer in inspiration).

135. Where is the pulmonic ejection sound best heard?

The pulmonic ejection sound is usually best heard with the diaphragm placed over the pulmonic area (i.e., along the left sternal border in either the second or third interspace).

136. What causes a nonvalvular pulmonic ejection sound?

1. **Pulmonary hypertension.** This sound is generated by ejection of blood into a stiffened pulmonary artery. The timing of the pulmonary ejection sound correlates with pulmonary artery diastolic pressure: the higher the pressure, the later the sound occurs in systole.

2. **Dilatation of the pulmonary artery.** This ejection sound also is generated in the pulmonary artery.

Pearl.   Unlike valvular sounds, both of these ejection sounds remain constant in intensity throughout respiration.

137. What is the Means-Lerman scratch of hyperthyroidism?

It is a combination ejection sound and ejection murmur heard over the pulmonic artery of patients with hyperthyroidism. Described in 1932 by Lerman and Means, this raspy sound is due to hyperkinetic heart syndrome, which is typical of patients with hyperthyroidism. Thus, a Means-Lerman scratch also may be heard in patients without hyperthyroidism who have a similar hyperdynamic condition, such as anemia or fever.

138. What is the differential diagnosis of an ejection click?

The most difficult differentiation is between an ejection click and a split S1. Less difficult is separation from either an S4 (which is softer, lower-pitched, located before S1, and detected better by the bell than by the diaphragm) or a mid-to-late systolic click (which is as high-pitched and loud as the ejection sound but located a bit later in systole).

Mid-to-Late Systolic Clicks

139. What are mid-to-late systolic clicks?

They are short, high-pitched, and snapping but relatively faint extra sounds. They are best heard at the apex or left lower parasternal area, ideally in left decubitus position (although dynamic bedside maneuvers may be necessary; see below) while applying firm pressure on the diaphragm.

140. What is the clinical significance of a single or multiple mid-to-late systolic clicks?

They indicate the presence of mitral (or tricuspid) valve prolapse (MVP).

141. What are the auscultatory characteristics of a systolic click due to MVP?

The major characteristic is the variability of this high-frequency and short extra sound. From cycle to cycle clicks may vary in intensity, number, and timing. They often become faint enough to elude detection by an unskilled clinician. At times they may even be multiple, thus adding to the confusion of an inexperienced observer.

142. How are the clicks generated?

They are probably generated by the combined backward snapping of a prolapsing mitral leaflet and sudden distention of its chordal apparatus (chordal snap). These different acoustic events may explain the occasional presence of multiple systolic clicks in the same patient.

143. Why do clicks of MVP not occur in early systole?

Most prolapse clicks occur in mid-to-late systole (not early systole) because of their mode of generation. Early systolic clicks are caused by the ejection of blood across the semilunar valves and into the arterial root, aortic or pulmonic. Thus, they necessarily take place at the onset of ventricular ejection (i.e., early systole). Mid-to-late systolic clicks, on the other hand, are nonejection sounds caused by prolapsing of the mitral apparatus. This, in turn, usually requires a significant decrease in left ventricular size. Thus, it usually takes place during the mid-to-late portion of systole. There are, however, exceptions that confirm the rule. Some patients may have a prolapse click that either follows or is superimposed on S1, thus creating a loud summation sound. Such patients have prolapse of sufficient severity that it occurs even in the large and distended ventricle of early systole.

144. How can one identify MVP when the click occurs so early in systole that it is superimposed on S1?

By the presence of a holosystolic murmur in association with a loud S1, which is actually a merged S1 + click complex. These two findings are due to the severity of the prolapse, which leads to holosystolic regurgitation and holosystolic murmur and superimposition of the mitral click on S1 with a resulting increase in the intensity of S1 (otherwise uncommon in patients with simple mitral regurgitation).

145. Which bedside maneuvers can be used to change the timing of an MVP click or murmur?

All maneuvers that modify left ventricular size. The most common examples are Valsalva's maneuver, squatting or standing, and passive leg raising, all of which either increase or decrease preload and afterload. For example, an increase in preload/afterload results from squatting or passive leg raising. This, in turn, increases the size of the left ventricular cavity and thus pulls tight the chordae tendinae. As a result, prolapse of the valve is delayed, the click is delayed, and the murmur is shortened. Conversely, a decrease in preload/afterload (as typically occurs in a standing position) shrinks left ventricular size and leads to earlier prolapse, earlier click (i.e., closer to S1), and longer murmur.

Pearl. By decreasing left ventricular size, the strain phase of Valsalva's maneuver also anticipates the click and lengthens the murmur. In contrast, by increasing left ventricular size, the release phase of Valsalva's maneuver delays the click and shortens the murmur. Only two murmurs are enhanced by Valsalva's maneuver: (1) MVP and (2) idiopathic hypertrophic subaortic stenosis.

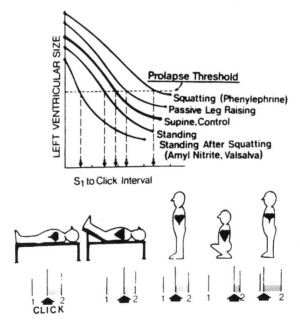

Variation of the timing of the click and systolic murmur in mitral valve prolapse with changes in body position. The diagram indicates the presence of an arbitrary "prolapse threshold" and suggests a relationship between left ventricular size and the mitral valve that affects the timing and extent of leaflet prolapse. Whenever the prolapse threshold is reached during left ventricular systole, the leaflets prolapse, resulting in a click and systolic murmur. If the threshold is achieved in early systole as a result of reduced preload and/or afterload (e.g., standing position), the click moves closer to S1 and the murmur becomes longer and louder. Conversely, an increase in preload and afterload, such as occurs during squatting, results in the click and murmur appearing later in systole because the prolapse threshold is not reached until later during ejection. Pharmacologic agents also may affect left ventricular filling and outflow resistance and alter ventricular geometry to produce predictable changes in the timing of the click and murmur. (From Criley JM, Heger J: Prolapsed mitral leaflet syndrome. In Roberts WC (ed): Congenital Heart Disease in Adults. Philadelphia, F.A. Davis, 1979, with permission.)

146. Are mid-to-late systolic clicks always associated with a late systolic murmur?

No. If associated, however, they suggest MVP with regurgitation. Many patients with MVP have only the click (or clicks). Because the presence of a murmur (and therefore regurgitation) varies from day to day and from cycle to cycle, prophylaxis becomes very important.

Pearl.   Many cases of endocarditis have been documented in patients with only a mid systolic click, suggesting that regurgitation may not occur all of the time.

147. Can patients with MVP present with a diastolic click?

Yes. About 5–15% of all patients with MVP may have an early diastolic click. The click is still caused by ballooning of the mitral leaflet, although in a reversed direction.

148. What is the differential diagnosis of a mid systolic click?

It depends on timing. Earlier clicks tend to be confused with ejection sounds, split S1, or even S4 (in this case, the high frequency of clicks makes it easy to separate them from the softer and lower-pitched S4). Mid-to-late clicks, on the other hand, may be misinterpreted for a split S2 or even for an S2/opening snap complex. At times the presence of a late systolic murmur following a late systolic click adds to the confusion and leads to a misdiagnosis of an opening snap/diastolic murmur complex. Finally, multiple clicks are often mistaken for pericardial friction rubs.

Pericardial Friction Rub

149. What is a pericardial friction rub?

It is a scratching, scraping, crackling, and typically fleeting, high-pitched extra sound heard in patients with inflammation of the two pericardial layers. Because of their high frequency, rubs are best heard using the diaphragm. Applying firm pressure on the stethoscope head also increases the loudness of a rub.

150. What are the auscultatory characteristics of a pericardial friction rub?

A rub is usually characterized by as many as three components, all scratchy and leathery: (1) one in systole (corresponding to ventricular contraction and occurring anywhere in systole, although most commonly in mid systole) and (2) two in diastole (corresponding, respectively, to atrial contraction and early ventricular filling). Although the systolic component is always present, the two diastolic components may be absent. The atrial (or early diastolic) component is more frequently present than the ventricular (or late diastolic) component. In a review of 100 patients with pericardial friction rubs, Spodick found that 55% had three components and 33% only two components.

151. Where are rubs best heard?

They can be heard throughout the precordium, although more than 80% tend to be louder along the left parasternal area and lower left sternal border (third and fourth interspaces). Rubs also vary tremendously in intensity from area to area; at times they are audible only in a highly circumscribed focus.

152. What bedside maneuvers can be used to increase the intensity of a pericardial friction rub?

The most common is inspiration. In approximately one-third of patients, rubs become louder in deep and held inspiration because the inspiratory descent of the diaphragm stretches the pericardium, thus making more likely and more intense the rubbing of the two pericardial layers against each other. Contact between the visceral and parietal pleura (and hence their rubbing) also can be increased by having the patient rest on elbows and knees during examination of the precordium.

Pearl.   A new change in rub intensity during inspiration also may be a clue to pericardial fluid accumulation. Fluid accumulation also may be suggested by the softening over time (or even disappearance) of a previously loud rub.

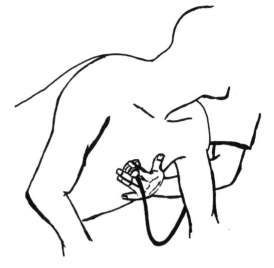

Alternate position for hearing the pericardial friction rub. (Adapted from Tilkian AG, Conover MB: Understanding Heart Sounds, 3rd ed. Philadelphia, W.B. Saunders, 1993.)

153. Does the presence of a rub exclude a pericardial effusion?

No. Ten percent of patients with a rub have a pericardial effusion.

154. Can rubs be palpated?

Yes. A particularly loud rub may become palpable (the same is true for a pleural friction rub). Approximately one-fourth of all rubs are palpable.

155. What is the differential diagnosis of a pericardial friction rub?

A three-component rub at times may resemble a ventricular gallop because the early diastolic component coincides in timing with S3. Thus, in patients with a rapid heart rate (i.e., most patients with pericarditis), the fast triple lilt of a pericardial rub may easily be mistaken for a gallop. To separate the rub from S3, one should rely on the loudness, high frequency, and typically scratchy quality of the rub. In patients with only a two-component rub, the diagnosis remains relatively easy. Diagnosis may be more difficult in patients with only a one-component systolic rub. Such patients may be misdiagnosed as having a systolic ejection murmur. To sort these diagnoses, it is important to monitor the sound over time. A systolic rub most likely changes in quality and intensity, often acquiring one or two more diastolic components.

156. How can one distinguish a pericardial from a pleural friction rub?

By asking the patient to hold his or her breath, first in inspiration and then in exhalation. A pericardial rub should persist in at least one of the two situations (usually in both), whereas a pleural rub disappears. Some patients (with either viral pleuropericarditis or Dressler's syndrome) may have both a pleural and a pericardial friction rub.

157. What disease processes are associated with rubs?

Pericarditis, of course, usually acute or or subacute. A rub is usually not present in the more chronic and constrictive forms of pericarditis, in which a pericardial knock may be more typical (see above). A rub is one of the three key diagnostic features of acute pericarditis (together with chest pain and EKG changes). Pericarditis may be diffuse (as in viral or bacterial infections, postradiation pericarditis, uremia, and collagen vascular diseases, such as systemic lupus erythematosus or rheumatoid arthritis). For example, a rub can be heard in 14–83% of patients with uremic pericarditis. Localized pericarditis, on the other hand, is usually the result of either trauma or myocardial ischemia. Rubs can be heard in as many as 20% of patients with an acute myocardial infarction, usually a few days into the course of the disease (they are usually absent in the first 24 hours). In simple postinfarction pericarditis the rub is usually quite fleeting. On the contrary, it may last much longer in patients with postmyocardial infarction (Dressler's) syndrome. A pericardial rub also may be heard (albeit rarely) in patients with pulmonary embolism. Finally, a localized rub is often heard in patients with metastatic involvement of the pericardium, even though only 7% of all neoplastic effusions are associated with a rub.

BIBLIOGRAPHY

1. Adolph RJ, Fowler NO: The second heart sound: A screening test for heart disease. Mod Concept Cardiovasc Dis 39(4):91–96, 1970.
2. Benchimol A, Desser KB: The fourth heart sound in patients without demonstrable heart disease. Chest 93:298–301, 1977.
3. Cheng TO: Mitral valve prolapse. Dis Mon 33:481–534, 1987.
4. Goldman L, Caldera DL, Nussbaum SR, et al: Multifactorial index of cardiac risk in noncardiac surgical procedures. N Engl J Med 297:845–850, 1977.
5. Harvey WP, Stapleton J: Clinical aspects of gallop rhythm with particular reference to diastolic gallop. Circulation 18:1017–1024, 1958.
6. Ishmail AA, Wing S, Ferguson J, et al: Interobserver agreement by auscultation in the presence of a third heart sound in patients with congestive heart failure. Chest 91:870–873, 1987.
7. Leathma A: The second heart sound: Key to auscultation of the heart. Acta Cardiol 19:395, 1964.
8. Lee DC-S, Johnson RA, Bingham JB, et al: Heart failure in outpatients: A randomized trail of digoxin versus placebo. N Engl J Med 306:699–705, 1982.
9. Mangione S, Nieman LZ, Gracely E, Kaye D: The teaching and practice of cardiac auscultation during internal medicine and cardiology training. Ann Intern Med 119:47–54, 1993.
10. Potain PC: Du rhythme cardiaque appelee bruit de gallop: De son mechanisme et de sa valeur semeiologique. Bull Soc Med Hop Paris 12:137, 1875.
11. Reddy PS, Salemi R, Shaver JA: Normal and abnormal heart sounds in cardiac diagnosis. Part II: Diastolic sounds. Curr Probl Cardiol 10(4):8–55, 1985.
12. Shah PM, Gramiak R, Kramer DH, Yu PN: Determinants of atrial (S4) and ventricular (S3) gallop sounds in primary myocardial disease. N Engl J Med 278:845–850, 1968.
13. Shah PM, Jackson D: Third Heart Sound and Summation Gallop. Monograph 46. New York, American Heart Association, 1975.
14. Spodick DH: Pericardial rub: Prospective, multiple observer investigation of pericardial friction in 100 patients. Am J Cardiol 35:357–362, 1975.
15. Surawicz B, Mercer C, Chlebus H, et al: Role of the phonocardiogram in evaluation of the severity of mitral stenosis and detection of associated valvular lesions. Circulation 34:795–806, 1966.

12. CARDIAC AUSCULTATION— HEART MURMURS

Salvatore Mangione, M.D.

That the stethoscope will come in general use notwithstanding its value I am extremely doubtful, because its beneficial application requires much time and gives a great deal of trouble both to the patient and the practitioner, and because its whole hue and character is foreign and opposed to our habits and associations.

It must be confessed that there is something even ludicrous in the picture of a grave physician acutally listening through a long tube to the patient's thorax as if the disease within were a living being that could communicate its conditions to the sense without.

Besides, there is in this method a sort of bold claim and pretension to certainty, which cannot, at first sight, but be somewhat startling to a mind deeply versed in the knowledge and uncertainties of our art, and to the calm and cautious habits of philosophizing to which the physician is accustomed. On all these accounts and others that might be mentioned, I conclude that the new method will only in a few cases be speedily adopted, and never generally.

John Forbes, preface to his translation of R.T.H. Laennec,
De L'Auscultatione Mediate. London, T. & J. Underwood, 1821

TOPICS COVERED IN THIS CHAPTER

General Issues
Areas of auscultation
Mechanisms of production of murmurs
Significance of murmurs
Classification of murmurs
Characteristics of murmurs
Bedside maneuvers to elicit murmurs
Functional and pathologic murmurs—
criteria of differentiation
Innocent (Functional) Murmur
Definition
Mechanisms of production
Classification
Characteristics of innocent murmur
Innocent murmurs in children
Innocent murmurs in adolescents
Innocent murmurs in the elderly
Systolic Murmurs
Systolic ejection murmurs
General characteristics
Ejection vs. regurgitant murmurs
Aortic stenosis
Classification
Characteristics
Effect of bedside maneuvers
Etiology
Aortic vs. pulmonic stenosis

Systolic regurgitant murmurs
General characteristics
Mitral regurgitation
Classification
Characteristics
Mitral valve prolapse
Effect of bedside maneuvers
Mitral vs. tricuspid regurgitation
Tricuspid regurgitation
Characteristics
Peripheral findings
Effect of bedside maneuvers
Etiology
Miscellaneous Ejection Murmurs
Ventricular septal defect
Continuous murmurs
Diastolic Murmurs
Atrioventricular valves
Mitral stenosis
Etiology
Characteristics
Reponse to bedside maneuvers
Austin Flint murmur
Mitral diastolic flow murmurs
Definition
Pathogenesis
Characteristics

Diastolic Murmurs *(Continued)*
  Atrioventricular valves *(continued)*
    Mitral diastolic flow murmurs *(continued)*
      Response to bedside maneuvers
      Carey Coombs murmur
    Tricuspid stenosis
    Tricuspid diastolic murmurs

Semilunar valves
  Aortic regurgitation
    Definition
    Pathogenesis
    Characteristics
    Response to bedside maneuvers
    Graham-Steell murmur

CONVENTIONAL TEACHING WATCH

Cardiac auscultation is the centerpiece of physical diagnosis—and the recognition of cardiac murmurs is the most challenging of all its components. It requires the identification of several sounds, jam-packed in less than 0.8 seconds, often overlapping, and not infrequently at the threshold of audibility. Learning how to use the stethoscope, therefore, is a bit like learning how to play a musical instrument. It is also as rewarding. Although the stethoscope was born just 1 year after the battle of Waterloo, this tool and this skill still occupy an important role in 21st century medicine.

FINDING/MANEUVER		CONVENTIONAL TEACHING REVISITED
Innocent murmur	⇑	Common and important problem that challenges pediatricians, obstetricians, internists, and family physicians alike.
Aortic stenosis	⇑	Important and often difficult to recognize in elderly people.
Aortic regurgitation	⇑	Still quite prevalent. Some of classic findings, however, are much less frequent now that patients present earlier to medical care.
Pulmonic regurgitation	⇔	Subtle at times but clinically important.
Mitral regurgitation	⇑	Most common valvular disease.
Mitral stenosis	⇓	Becoming too rare (at least in western world) to achieve high rating.
Tricuspid stenosis	⇓	As above.
Tricuspid regurgitation	⇑	More common and therefore important for differential diagnosis of mitral regurgitation.
Patent ductus arteriosus	⇔	Importance depends on age of patient population.

GENERAL ISSUES

1. Which are the cardiac areas of auscultation?
The classic areas of auscultation are shown in the figure and table on the facing page. Auscultation is typically started over the aortic area. Then the stethoscope is moved sequentially over the pulmonic, tricuspid, and mitral areas. Because murmurs may radiate widely, they may become audible in areas outside those to which they normally are assigned. Inching the stethoscope (i.e., slowly dragging it from area to area) is a good technique to avoid missing important findings.

2. What is the clinical significance of a heart murmur?
It depends on the type of murmur. For example, whereas almost all diastolic and continuous murmurs are pathologic (and therefore reflect an organic abnormality of the heart), most systolic murmurs are benign and occur in the absence of any structural lesion. Such murmurs are often called functional or innocent.

3. What should be the approach to a newly detected murmur?
The physician should use the cardiovascular exam to differentiate an **organic** from a **functional** murmur. This essential step avoids expensive and possibly dangerous laboratory evaluations; therefore, it should be the initial step in the assessment. If the murmur is identified as organic, the physical examination should provide clues to its site of origin, hemodynamic cause, and possibly, severity.

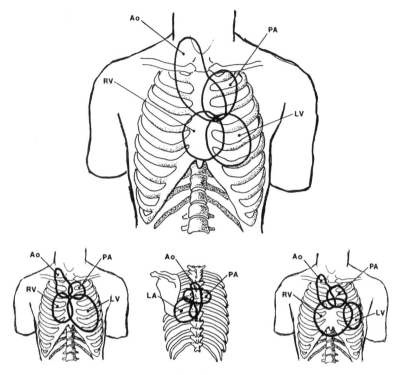

Top, Classic precordial sites for auscultation. *Lower left,* Projection of auscultatory areas when the left ventricle is enlarged. *Lower middle,* Radiation sites in the back. *Lower right,* Projection of auscultatory areas when the right ventricle is enlarged. AO = aorta, PA = pulmonary artery, RV = right ventricle, LV = left ventricle, LA = left atrium. (Adapted from Abrams J: Essentials of Cardiac Physical Diagnosis. Baltimore, Williams & Wilkins, 1987.)

Locations of Aucultatory Sites

AREA	PRIOR DESIGNATION	LOCATION	MURMURS HEARD BEST	SOUNDS HEARD
Left ventricular	Mitral area	At apex impulse: extends to 3–5 LICS, 2 cm medially and laterally to left anterior axillary line. Isolated LVE: extends medially; isolated RVE: may be displaced to left axilla	Mitral stenosis Mitral regurgitation Aortic stenosis Aortic insufficiency IHSS Functional middiastolic rumble	LV S3 LV S4 A2
Right ventricular	Tricuspid area	Lower sternum and 3–5 LICS 2 cm to left and right. Isolated RVE: can extend laterally and occupy the apex	Tricuspid stenosis Tricuspid regurgitation- Pulmonary regurgitation Ventricular septal defect	RV S3 RV S4 TV opening snap
Left atrial		Left posterior thorax between axillary line and spine at level of scapular tip	Mitral regurgitation	

Table continued on following page

Locations of Aucultatory Sites (Continued)

AREA	PRIOR DESIGNATION	LOCATION	MURMURS HEARD BEST	SOUNDS HEARD
Right atrial		Lower sternum and 4–5 RICS, 2 cm to right of sternum	Triscuspid regurgitation	
Aortic area	Erbs' point (3rd left interspace)	3 LICS near sternal edge across manubrium to 1–3 RICS, may include 2 LICS, suprasternal notch, right sternoclavicular joint	Aortic stenosis Aortic insufficiency Aortic flow murmurs	A2 Aortic ejection click
Pulmonary area		1–3 LICS adjacent to sternum, medial left intraclavicular area; posterior thorax: T4,5 2–3 cm to either side of spine	Pulmonary stenosis Pulmonary regurgitation Pulmonary flow murmurs PDA murmur	Pulmonay ejection click P2
Descending thoracic area		Posterior thorax: T2–T16, 2–3 cm to either side of the spine	Coarctation of aorta Aortic aneurysms Aortic stenosis	

LICS = left intercostal space, LVE = left ventricular enlargement, RVE = right ventricular englargement, RICS = right intercostal space, IHSS = idiopathic hypertrophic subaortic stenosis, PDA = patent ductus arteriosus, LV = left ventricular, RV = right ventricular, TV = tricuspid valves.
Adapted from Abrams J: Essentials of Cardiac Physical Diagnosis. Baltimore, Williams & Wilkins, 1987.

4. What physical examination criteria differentiate a functional from a pathologic murmur?

There are two golden and three silver rules.

Golden rules

1. Always judge murmurs like people—by the company they keep. Thus, a murmur that keeps bad company (such as an extra sound, an abnormal arterial or venous pulse, an abnormal electrocardiogram, an abnormal chest radiograph, or any cardiovascular symptom) should be considered suspicious until proved otherwise. Murmurs of this type must receive careful attention, including technology-based evaluation.

2. A diminished or absent second sound usually indicates a poorly moving and abnormal semilunar valve. This finding is the hallmark of pathology. As a flip side to this rule, functional systolic murmurs are always accompanied by well-preserved second sounds with a normal intensity and normal split.

Silver rules

1. All diastolic murmurs are pathologic.
2. All holosystolic or late systolic murmurs are pathologic.
3. All continuous murmurs are pathologic.

The silver rules are rooted in the pathogenesis of cardiac murmurs, which, in turn, relates to **intracardiac pressure gradients and velocity of blood flow**. Both variables are maximal in early systole and taper during late systole and diastole. Thus, sounds and murmurs should not be generated during late systole or diastole. If they are, they reflect high pressure gradients and, therefore a structural cardiac abnormality. For the same reason, benign systolic murmurs should always be ejection (i.e., they should have a crescendo-decrescendo shape) and not holosystolic (i.e., they should not start with S1 and end with S2 in a plateau pattern).

All of these rules, as often is the case in medicine, have exceptions. Yet they remain valid and useful for the practicing physician. They should be kept in mind at the bedside. For example, although a few benign murmurs happen to be diastolic (due to rapid ventricular filling), they are extremely rare. In fact, they are encountered in less than 0.3% of all schoolchildren between the ages of 2 and 18 years. When encountered, they are always associated with either a physiologic S3 or some other benign murmur (such as Still's murmur). They never present as an isolated finding. The same is true for continuous murmurs: although both a venous hum and a supraclavicular carotid bruit may resemble a murmur of patent ductus arteriosus, they are usually easy to differentiate at the bedside from their pathologic counterpart.

5. Do the acoustic characteristics of the sound wave help to differentiate a benign from an organic murmur?

No. As indicated before, acoustic characteristics per se (such as frequency or shape) and even the radiation pattern of a murmur are usually nonspecific. Therefore they are not clinically helpful. Only one acoustic characteristic is valuable enough to help at the bedside: the intensity of the murmur. In general, benign murmurs tend to be softer than pathologic murmurs and are never louder than grade III/VI. Therefore, they are never associated with a palpable thrill (which is indicative of a grade IV/VI intensity or higher).

MECHANISMS OF PRODUCTION

6. How are murmurs produced?

All murmurs (whether organic or functional) are produced whenever blood flow becomes turbulent enough to cause auditory vibrations in the various cardiac structures. The intensity of a murmur depends on various other factors, including blood flow velocity. Two major mechanisms can increase blood velocity and thus lead to turbulent and audible flow: (1) local or concentric narrowing of a vessel or valve (causing a pressure gradient) and (2) sudden change in the diameter of a vessel.

7. Give specific examples of structural cardiac abnormalities that can produce turbulent flow.

1. **Abnormal size** of the area through which the flow is passing (the smaller the area, the greater the turbulence).

2. **Irregular shape** of the orifice through which the flow is passing (such as an irregular valve orifice).

3. **Irregular edge** of the orifice through which the flow is passing (the sharper the edge, the higher the turbulence).

In addition to structural abnormalities, an **abnormal blood viscosity** also may lead to turbulence and murmurs (the lower the viscosity, the higher the turbulence and the more likely the murmur).

CLASSIFICATION

8. How are murmurs usually classified?

1. The first and most important distinction is pathologic vs. functional. The primary classification, however, is based on the phase of the cardiac cycle in which the murmur is located. Accordingly, murmurs are divided into **systolic, diastolic,** and **continuous.**

2. Systolic murmurs are further classified into **ejection** and **regurgitant.** The two subtypes are identified by systolic length: ejection murmurs tend to be early or mid systolic, whereas regurgitant murmurs are more likely to span throughout systole (i.e., they start with S1 and end with S2). Regurgitant murmurs, however, also may occur in late systole only. In either case, the hallmark of regurgitant murmurs is that they extend into and touch the S2.

Pearl. Holosystolic (and late systolic) murmurs tend to be pathologic, whereas early or mid-systolic murmurs tend to be functional.

9. What are continuous murmurs?

Continuous murmurs are not murmurs that occur in both systole and diastole (such as a murmur of combined aortic stenosis and regurgitation); rather, they span uninterruptedly throughout the entire cardiac cycle. Because continuous murmurs are due to pressure gradients that persist during the entire cardiac cycle, they do not have a silent pause in either systole or diastole. The most common cardiac abnormality responsible for a to-and-fro, machine-like, continuous murmur is patent ductus arteriosus.

10. Why are systolic murmurs much more common than diastolic murmurs?

Because the pressure gradients generated in systole are much higher than those generated in diastole. Thus systolic murmurs are more common than diastolic murmurs simply because hemodynamically they are more likely to occur. For the same reason, a diastolic murmur (at rest or after exercise) should be considered pathologic until proved otherwise. Diastolic pressure gradients are usually so small that the presence of a murmur in diastole indicates an abnormal pressure gradient.

11. Can exercise increase the intensity of a diastolic murmur?

Yes and no. An increase in cardiac output (such as after exercise) may enhance the hemodynamic likelihood of any murmur. But this increased likelihood is still much greater during systole than during diastole.

12. Which characteristics of a murmur should be analyzed and described?

1. The **phase of the cardiac cycle** during which the murmur occurs (systole, diastole, or the entire length of the cycle, like a continuous murmur). Again: systolic murmurs may be benign, whereas diastolic and continuous murmurs should be considered pathologic until proved otherwise.

2. Once the phase has been identified, the **timing of the murmur** should be recognized. A murmur may span throughout systole or diastole (such as a holosystolic or holodiastolic murmur, respectively) or it may occur only in the early, mid, or late phases.

- **Holosystolic and late systolic murmurs** are clinically more important than early or mid systolic murmurs because usually they are pathologic. Benign systolic murmurs are flow-generated. Because flow is maximal during the early part of ventricular systole, all benign systolic murmurs tend to have a short duration and an early systolic peak. Because systolic pressure gradients reach their peak during the early part of systole, innocent murmurs (i.e., murmurs related to flow) typically are located during the first half of systole and should not extend into S2.

Pearl. A murmur that extends into S2 (whether holosystolic or late systolic) is usually pathologic and due to atrioventricular regurgitation. Conversely, a murmur that occurs during the first half of systole (whether early or mid systolic) is usually benign and due to ejection through the semilunar valves.

- **Early diastolic murmurs** (starting immediately after S2) reflect regurgitation through the semilunar valves, whereas mid-to-late diastolic murmurs (starting slightly after S2) reflect stenosis of the atrioventricular valves. Mid-to-late diastolic murmurs may extend into S1 as a result of a pre systolic accentuation (due to a strong atrial contraction), but are never truly holodiastolic. Murmurs of severe regurgitation through the semilunar valves, on the other hand, may cover the entire length of diastole and be truly holodiastolic. This may provide a useful distinguishing feature. Remember, however, that holodiastolic murmurs can be so faint in late diastole to become almost inaudible.

3. The last characteristic to assess is the **intensity** or **loudness** of the murmur, which traditionally is graded from I/VI to VI/VI:

- I/VI: a murmur so soft that it can be heard only with concentration and effort—and not immediately.
- II/VI: a murmur loud enough to be immediately audible.
- III/VI: an easily audible murmur.
- IV/VI: a murmur relatively loud and associated with a palpable thrill.
- V/VI: a murmur loud enough that it can be heard even by placing the edge of the diaphragm of the stethoscope over the patient's chest.
- VI/VI: a murmur so loud that it can be heard even when the stethoscope is not in contact with the chest but held slightly above its surface.

Pearl. *All other factors being equal, increased intensity usually reflects increased turbulence of flow. Thus, a louder murmur is much more likely to be pathologic than a softer murmur.*

13. Are the shape and frequency of a murmur clinically useful?

Not as much as the intensity. For example, although ejection murmurs tend to have a crescendo-decrescendo shape (diamond-shaped), even regurgitant murmurs (such as the plateau-shaped murmur of mitral regurgitation) at times may exhibit a late systolic accentuation. Frequency, on the other hand, is more useful and tends to correlate with flow velocities and pressure gradients. Thus, murmurs generated by high-pressure gradients (such as aortic regurgitation) tend to be higher-pitched (>300 Hz), whereas murmurs generated by low-pressure gradients (such as mitral stenosis) tend to be lower-pitched (30–100 Hz). Because the human ear does not perceive low frequencies well, low-pitched murmurs are faint and therefore difficult to detect.

14. What about the radiation of a murmur?

This can be quite helpful in identifying the murmur (such as the radiation to the axilla of a mitral regurgitant murmur, or the radiation to the neck of an aortic stenosis murmur), and yet not all murmurs always present with a typical radiation.

15. Which maneuvers can be used at the bedside to modify the intensity and characteristics of a murmur and make it easier to recognize?

Quite a few, all time-honored and often linked to the name of the physician who first described them:

1. The **Valsalva maneuver** was first described by the Italian Antonio Valsalva (1666–1723), professor of anatomy in Bologna, a student of Malpighi, and the teacher of Morgagni. Valsalva developed this maneuver as a bedside trick to inflate and clean the eustachian tube. He reported it in 1704 in a book about the ear. The Valsalva maneuver is an exaggeration of inspiration and expiration and the resulting swings in intrathoracic pressures and venous return. It is a little tricky to perform and should be well explained to the patient in advance. It is particularly important that the patient be instructed to continue straining until told to stop and to breathe as quietly as possible after stopping straining. The maneuver consists of two phases:

- The **held (or strain) phase** is carried out by asking the patient to bear down as if having a bowel movement. Alternatively, a supine patient can be asked to strain against the examiner's hand applied to the mid abdomen. Either technique leads to an increase in intrathoracic pressure, a decrease in venous return, and a smaller left ventricular volume. The strain phase, therefore, increases the left ventricular gradient in hypertrophic obstructive cardiomyopathy (HOCM) and makes its systolic murmur much louder. This is clinically useful because it is the opposite of how left ventricular outflow murmurs usually react with the Valsalva maneuver (see below). The strain phase also favors the prolapse of a floppy mitral valve, making its murmur longer and its click earlier. Finally, straining fuses a widely split (but still normal) S2 but has no effect on the fixed S2 splitting of atrial septal defect.
- The **release phase** is carried out by asking the patient to stop bearing down or by releasing the pressure of the fist over the abdomen. This phase has an opposite effect that depends on the site of origin of the acoustic event: murmurs of the right heart generally return to baseline intensity within 2–3 cardiac cycles, whereas murmurs of the left heart take a little longer (5–10 cardiac cycles).

Pearl. *Murmurs become louder during the strain phase of the Valsalva maneuver in only two diseases: HOCM and mitral valve prolapse. Conversely, most heart sounds and murmurs will become softer during the strain phase, especially in patients with aortic stenosis and pulmonic stenosis (because of the decreased venous return to both ventricles, and the resulting decrease in cross-valvular gradients).*

2. The **effects of respiration** were noted first by Pierre Potain in 1866 and rediscovered in 1954 by Leatham. Respiration has important effects on the intensity and characteristics of a murmur (not to mention the splitting of S2) because of the extreme swings in intrathoracic pressures caused by respiration and the resulting variations in venous return. The general rule is that all right-sided findings (with the exception of the pulmonary ejection sound) become louder on inspiration because of greater venous return to the right ventricle. Conversely, all left-sided findings become louder on expiration because of greater venous return to the left ventricle. This principle is also the basis for Carvallo's sign (an increase in the intensity of the holosystolic murmur of tricuspid regurgitation during *or* at the end of inspiration). This sign is a useful bedside maneuver to distinguish tricuspid from mitral regurgitation (see below), quite specific but not extremely sensitive (only 61%). Carvallo's maneuver is carried out by asking the patient to breathe in and hold inspiration for 3–5 seconds. Conversely, held exhalation is particularly useful in searching for a pericardial rub, the soft murmurs of aortic regurgitation, or the faint pulmonic mid-systolic murmur associated with loss of thoracic kyphosis (murmur of straight back syndrome).

3. **Effects of posture.** Sitting, squatting, and standing may have a profound effect on the characteristics of murmurs. Particularly important is the squatting-standing maneuver. The click and murmur of mitral valve prolapse transiently accentuate upon standing.

4. **Alterations in cardiac cycle.** The murmur of aortic stenosis becomes accentuated after a premature ventricular beat. Conversely, a murmur of mitral regurgitation does not change.

5. An **isometric handgrip** increases peripheral vascular resistances and, therefore, makes the murmur of mitral regurgitation louder and the murmur of aortic stenosis softer.

6. **Pharmacologic maneuvers.** Vasoactive drugs, such as amyl nitrite or phenylephrine, can induce profound changes in the characteristics of a murmur and therefore were used quite often before the advent of echocardiography. Such techniques now belong more to the folklore than to the science of medicine. They are also possibly dangerous and therefore should be abandoned.

16. Who was Carvallo?

J.M.R. Carvallo was a Mexican physician who worked at the National Cardiological Institute of Mexico City. He reported his sign in 1946. In medical folklore he has even acquired a partner (Dr. Rivera). As a result, his sign is often called the Rivera-Carvallo sign. In fact, Rivera was one of Carvallo's middle names.

BENIGN MURMURS

17. What are functional (innocent) murmurs?

Functional murmurs are usually (but not only) related to the ejection of blood across the semilunar valves. They are therefore systolic ejection murmurs produced by increased flow across a normal semilunar valve, most commonly the aorta. Unlike pathologic murmurs (which are caused by structural abnormalities of valves, chambers, or great vessels), functional murmurs are purely flow-related. Thus they have little or no clinical relevance other than inclusion in the differential diagnosis of a systolic murmur.

18. Can functional murmurs occur outside systole?

Rarely. Some innocent murmurs in fact may be continuous and fewer still may even be diastolic (in a survey of 12,000 South African children innocent mid-diastolic murmurs had a prevalence of 0.3%). These, however, are exceptions that confirm the general rule: a murmur that is either continuous or diastolic should be considered pathologic until proved otherwise.

19. What are the clinical implications of a functional murmur?

1. Functional murmurs are not related to structural abnormalities.
2. Functional murmurs do not require antistreptococcal prophylaxis.

3. Functional murmurs do not require prophylaxis for bacterial endocarditis.

4. Functional murmurs do not require any further work-up.

5. Functional murmurs carry an excellent long-term prognosis (cohorts of children with functional murmurs who have been followed over time had no greater incidence of cardiac disease than a similar cohort of children with no murmurs).

20. Do the terms functional, innocent, physiologic, benign, and systolic flow murmurs refer to different acoustic events?

No. They are among the several names given over the years to nonpathologic murmurs. All of these terms define murmurs that are *not* generated by a structural abnormality of the heart or great vessels but by abnormalities of flow. Because the terminology may lead to confusion, it is important to review a few of these terms:

- Murmurs are said to be *functional* or *innocent* when the disturbance in flow is generated by a heart with normal resting output.
- Murmurs are said to be *physiologic* if the disturbance in flow is generated only by a hyperkinetic heart, such as a heart with increased output and stroke volume (as during exercise).
- The term *functional*, although criticized by some authorities as too vague, is still commonly used to indicate this entire class of murmurs. It is preferable to *innocent*, which seems to convey a sense of clinical unimportance, or *benign*, which indicates an abnormality of little clinical relevance. The following discussion uses the term functional.
- The term *systolic flow murmurs of relative stenosis* also may be encountered. It is not entirely correct because stenosis requires a pressure gradient across the valve, whereas benign murmurs occur not because of a pressure gradient but because of an increase in flow velocity.

21. How common are functional murmurs?

Extremely common, in both children and adults. Because they are heard more easily in thin people, functional murmurs tend to be extremely prevalent in children (who have not only thin chests but also high flow velocity due to a rapid circulatory time). Functional murmurs can be encountered in 40–50% of children between the ages of 2 and 14. In fact, in a study of more than 12,000 South African schoolchildren, innocent murmurs had a prevalence of 72%. Functional murmurs, on the other hand, are rare before 2 years of age. Thus, a murmur in a very small child should be considered pathologic until proved otherwise. Functional murmurs are also extremely common during pregnancy (as many as 80% of pregnant women may have a benign ejection murmur). Finally, functional murmurs are frequent even in the elderly: as many as 50% of patients above the age of 50 may have the systolic ejection murmur of aortic sclerosis. Thus, functional murmurs are the most common type of heart murmur encountered by the generalist. Indeed, each of us probably had an innocent murmur at some point in his or her life.

22. How significant is a murmur that appears only after exercise or in anemic and febrile patients?

It may be quite significant. Exercise may function as a trigger of both functional and pathologic murmurs that otherwise are inaudible because of the increased flow velocity associated with physical activity. Anemia also may trigger a murmur through an increase in circulatory time. This increase may elicit murmurs that are either totally innocent (such as the hemic murmurs heard in patients with normal valves and no pressure gradient) or possibly pathologic (as in patients in whom a valvular pressure gradient may not be significant enough to create turbulence unless enhanced by the rapid circulation time of anemia). Fever behaves similarly to exercise and anemia. Patients with mild aortic stenosis or mild mitral regurgitation may have murmurs that are audible only when the circulatory time is increased by one of these cofactors. Such murmurs disappear with resolution of the triggering condition.

23. Is a benign murmur always caused by an increase in flow velocity?

Not necessarily. A decrease in flow velocity also may be responsible for the murmur. The decrease may be caused by a dilated aortic or pulmonic root or by the sudden slowing of blood upon entering the enlarged arterial root. Rapid change in flow velocity (a decrease as well as an increase) produces the murmur. Such murmurs are encountered in patients with aortic sclerosis and a dilated and tortuous aortic root. As a rule of thumb, however, benign flow murmurs are heard much more commonly when flow velocity is increased (e.g., childhood, tachycardia, pregnancy, or, quite simply, during and after exercise).

24. What is the significance of a systolic ejection murmur in patients with semilunar valve regurgitation?

It may indicate concomitant semilunar valve stenosis but most commonly indicates severe regurgitation. These benign flow murmurs accompany severe aortic or pulmonic regurgitation because of the increased systolic flow across the semilunar valves. A similar increase in stroke volume also may be seen in patients with atrial septal defect, ventricular septal defect, or patent ductus arteriosus. In all of these conditions benign systolic ejection murmurs are relatively common. Finally, a bicuspid aortic valve (one of the most common congenital valvular abnormalities) also may be responsible for a benign ejection murmur. Such murmurs usually are best heard over the second right interspace and are also caused by increased flow, not by a pressure gradient.

25. How many types of innocent murmurs are known?

There are four innocent systolic murmurs and three innocent continuous murmurs. There is also a rare innocent diastolic murmur, usually encountered in children and always associated with either a physiologic S3 or Still's murmur.

The four innocent systolic murmurs are (1) the precordial vibratory murmur (Still's murmur), (2) the pulmonary ejection systolic murmur, (3) the carotid (supraclavicular) arterial bruit, and (4) the aortic sclerosis murmur. The first three are encountered in children and adolescents, whereas the fourth is encountered in the elderly.

The three innocent continuous murmurs are (1) the venous hum (see chapter 12), (2) the mammary souffle, and (3) straight back syndrome murmur.

Precordial Vibratory Murmur (Still's Murmur)

- Short, soft (I–II/VI) mid-systolic murmur
- Low-frequency musical, buzzing, or vibratory intonation; like "twanging a piece of string" (Still, 1918)
- Loudest at the apex or over left sternal border
- Also can be heard over the entire precordium
- May radiate to the neck (rarely)
- Softens or disappears on standing, reappears on squatting
- Most commonly heard between the ages of 2 and 6 years

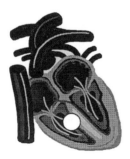

1. Location - left lower sternal border
2. Low frequency, coarse, *twangy*
3. Starts after the first heart sound
4. Changes with position
5. Differentiate from VSD

1st   2nd

Pulmonary Ejection Systolic Murmur

- Short, crescendo-decrescendo systolic murmur

- Early- to mid-systolic

- High-frequency, blowing intonation

- Loudest at the second or third left interspace

- Also can be heard over the aortic area, left sternal border, apex, neck (left)

- S2 normally split

- S2 components of normal intensity

- Most commonly heard in thin adolescents

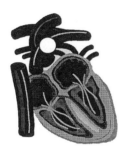

1. Location - pulmonary area
2. Early systolic ejection murmur
3. Soft in quality, localized
4. Increased in supine position
5. Normal P2, no diastolic murmur, no clicks,   heaves or thrills
6. Differentiate from ASD and Pulmonic Stenosis

1st   2nd

Carotid (Supraclavicular) Arterial Bruit

- Harsh, crescendo-decrescendo, ejection systolic murmur

- Loudest at the base of the heart or right supraclavicular area (opposite to aortic stenosis, which is loudest over the second right intercostal space)

- Becomes louder as one gets closer to neck/carotid artery

- Hyperextension of the shoulders toward the back may diminish it

- Compression of the subclavian artery may abolish or diminish it

- Unaffected by Valsalva maneuver

- Most common in children and adolescents

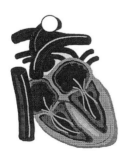

1. Location - loudest in neck over carotid artery
2. Heard faintly at the base
3. Systolic ejection murmur
4. No precordial or supra-sternal notch thrill
5. Differentiate from Aortic Stenosis

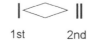

1st   2nd

Venous Hum

- Continuous murmur unrelated to the cardiac cycle
- Loudest at the right supraclavicular area or right upper sternal border
- Intensity changes with rotation of the head
- Loudest when patient is upright with neck extended and rotated contralaterally
- Softens or disappears in supine position
- Compresison of the jugular veins diminishes but does not abolish it
- Sudden release of the jugular veins increases the murmur
- Thrill palpable over the jugular veins
- Most common in children, but frequently heard in young adults

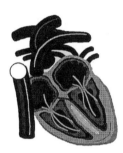

1. Location - infraclavicular
2. Maximal in early diastole
3. Loudest in upright position
4. Disappears when jugular occluded
5. Disappears when lying down
6. Differentiate from PDA

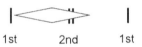

1st   2nd   1st

Mammary Souffle

- Continuous murmur related to the cardiac cycle
- In some patients may be primarily systolic
- Much less prevalent than the venous hum
- Usually present in late pregnancy or early lactation
- Loudest at the third or fourth interspace (either side or bilateral)
- Unaffected by Valsalva maneuver
- Firm compression may abolish it
- Varies from day to day; disappears after lactation period

Straight Back/Pecuts Excavatum

- Short, crescendo-decrescendo, mid-systolic ejection murmur
- Loudest at the left upper sternal border, louder in held exhalation
- Grade I–III/VI
- S2 usually widely split
- P2 (less commonly A2) can be loud
- Resembles atrial septal defect or pulmonic stenosis, but chest radiograph is diagnostic
- Due to narrow anteroposterior diameter with close proximity of pulmonary artery

Innocent Mid-Diastolic Murmur

- Very short and soft mid-diastolic murmur
- Loudest at the apex or left sternal border
- Follows immediately after a physiologic S3
- Heard in normal young people
- No supportive evidence of organic heart disease
- Almost always associated with Still's murmur (a purely diastolic murmur should be considered organic until proved otherwise)
- Due to rapid flow across the mitral or tricuspid valve or to distention of the left ventricular wall

26. Who was Still?

Sir Frederick Still (1868–1941) was an English pediatrician who graduated and subsequently trained at Guy's Hospital in London. He became house physician at the Hospital for Sick Children, where he remained for the rest of his career. A popular London figure, with a waiting room full of toys for his young patients, Still was a good-looking, shy man, a workaholic with a penchant for the classics, and a bachelor all his life. He lived with his widowed mother until she died, taking her to church every Sunday. Four years before his death he was knighted by King George VI. Still's name is linked not only to the innocent murmur but also to a form of juvenile rheumatoid arthritis presenting with lymphadenopathy and hepatosplenomegaly, which he described in his 1896 Cambridge M.D. thesis.

27. What mechanism is responsible for the generation of innocent murmurs?

It depends on the phase of the cardiac cycle in which the murmurs are located:

- Functional *continuous* murmurs are caused by turbulent blood flow in either the great veins or the great arteries.
- Functional *diastolic* murmurs are never an isolated finding. They reflect a rapid and vigorous ventricular filling with no intracardiac pressure gradient and no structural abnormalities. They are so rare that, once again, every diastolic murmur should be considered pathologic until proved otherwise.
- Functional *systolic* murmurs are due to rapid and vigorous ejection of blood across normal semilunar valves and into the large vessels. Because their site of origin is probably in the large vessels themselves, they are loudest at the base of the heart, either over the pulmonic (second-to-third left interspace) or aortic area (second-to-third right interspace). Because the left ventricle can generate pressures that are much higher than those generated by the right ventricle, most functional murmurs occur over the aortic area.

28. What clinical information helps to distinguish benign systolic murmurs from pathologic murmurs?

1. **History**
   - Family history (other family members with heart disease)
   - Past medical history (antenatal and perinatal history, postnatal, infancy, and childhood history)
   - Personal history (age at which murmur first was heard, history of central cyanosis, feeding difficulties, poor weight gain)
2. **Physical examination**, more specifically the cardiovascular exam:
   - General physical examination
   - Blood pressure
   - Peripheral pulses
   - Respiratory pattern
   - Neck veins exam

- Palpation of liver edge
- Palpation of precordium
- Auscultation of heart sounds
- Assessment of second heart sound

3. **Characteristics of the murmur**
   - Area of maximal intensity
   - Timing of the murmur
   - Murmur intensity
   - Murmur quality
   - Murmur transmission
   - Variations with respiration
   - Variations with exercise
   - Variations with Valsalva maneuver (both pulmonary ejection and Still's murmur disappear with the onset of Valsalva)
   - Postural changes
   - Response to pharmacologic agents

4. **Simple laboratory tests** (e.g., electrocardiogram, chest radiograph) to look for "bad company"

29. Summarize the important clues to the presence of a functional murmur.
- Innocent murmurs do not keep "bad company."
- Innocent murmurs do not radiate.
- Innocent murmurs disappear with inspiration.
- Innocent murmurs vary with the position of the patient.
- Innocent murmurs are usually grade III/VI or less.

30. What are the clues to the presence of a pathologic murmur?
1. **On palpation**
   - Systolic thrill
       Location over the suprasternal area
       Precordial/basilar
   - Abnormal apical impulse
2. **On auscultation**
   - Holosystolic murmurs
   - Diastolic murmurs
   - Presence of ejection clicks/sounds
   - Fixed splitting of second heart sound

(See figure on facing page.)

31. What is the most common cause of a systolic ejection murmur in the elderly?
Aortic sclerosis. As many as 50% of patients around the age of 50 may have this systolic murmur and still exhibit no evidence of valvular stenosis. The murmur of aortic stenosis is so closely related to age that almost 70% of nonagenarians have it.

32. What causes the murmur of aortic sclerosis?
It is *not* a pressure gradient at the level of the valvular orifice but abnormalities in the aortic root. These abnormalities may be (1) localized (such as calcific spurs or atherosclerotic plaques that, by protruding into the lumen of the aorta, create turbulence in the blood stream) or (2) diffuse (such as a dilatation of a tortuous aortic root). The murmur of aortic sclerosis also may be due to fibrotic changes in the valve per se. Such changes may make the valve stiffer and more sclerotic, yet not stiff enough to create a pressure gradient. This form of aortic sclerosis is called **aortic valve sclerosis**, whereas the first two mechanisms are called **true aortic sclerosis** (indicating that the valve is not involved, but the dilatation of the aortic root and its irregularities cause the murmur).

Phonocardiogram (inspiration unless noted)   Description

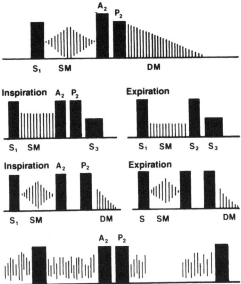

Mitral Stenosis

Precordium - Tapping apex beat; diastolic thrill at apex; parasternal lift. Auscultation - Loud S_1, P_2; diastolic opening snap followed by rumble with presystolic accentuation. Atrial fibrillation may be pulse pattern. Cold extremities.

Mitral Regurgitation

Precordium - Apical systolic thrill; apex displaced to left
Auscultation - Apical systolic regurgitant murmur following a decreased s_1; radiating to axilla; often hear S_3 due to increased left ventricular end diastolic volume.

Mitral Valve Prolapse

Most common in women younger than 30
Auscultation - A mid or late systolic click 0.14 seconds or more after S_1. Often followed by a high pitched systolic murmur; squatting may cause murmur to decrease.

Aortic Stenosis

Precordium - Basal systolic thrill; apex displaced anteriorly and laterally.
Carotids - Slow upstroke to a delayed peak.
Auscultation - A_2 diminished or paradoxically ejection systolic murmur radiating to carotids. Cold extremities.

Aortic Regurgitation

Often associated with Marfan's syndrome, rheumatoid spondylitis.
Precordium - Apex displaced laterally and anteriorly; thrill often palpable along left sternal border and in the jugular notch.
Carotids - Double systolic wave.
Auscultation - Decrescendo diastolic murmur along left sternal border; M_1 and A_2 are increased.

Tricuspid Regurgitation

Usually secondary to pathology elsewhere in heart.
Precordium - Right ventricular parasternal lift; systolic thrill at tricuspid area.
Auscultation - Holosystolic murmur increasing with inspiration; other: V wave in jugular venous pulse; systolic liver pulsation.

Atrial Septal Defect

Normal pulse; break parasternal life; lift over pulmonary artery; normal jugular pulse; systolic ejection murmur in pulmonic area; low pitched diastolic rumble over tricuspid area (at times); persistent wide splitting of S_2.

Pericarditis

Tachycardia; friction rub; diminished heart sounds and enlarged heart to percussin (with effusion); pulsus paradoxicus; neck vein distention, narrow pulse pressure and hypotension (with tamponade).

Phonocardiographic description of pathologic cardiac murmurs. (From James EC, Corry RJ, Perry JF: Principles of Basic Surgical Practice. Philadelphia, Hanley & Belfus, 1987, with permission.)

33. What other factors increase the prevalence of an aortic sclerosis murmur?

Both hypertension and female sex are predisposing factors. The female-to-male ratio is 2:1.

34. How can the murmur of aortic sclerosis be differentiated from the murmur of aortic stenosis?

By the same rules previously outlined for the differentiation of organic from functional murmurs. The golden rule is to judge a murmur by the company it keeps. Accordingly, a systolic ejection murmur associated with peripheral findings of aortic stenosis (slow, small pulse and palpable precordial thrill), electrocardiographic findings of left ventricular hypertrophy and symptoms of left ventricular outflow obstruction (exertional dizziness or syncope, chest pain, and dyspnea) are much more likely to be aortic stenosis than a similar murmur heard in a patient with none of these associations.

The auscultatory characteristics of the murmur also help in the differentiation. For example, a murmur of aortic stenosis lasts longer, peaks late in systole, and is associated with a soft or absent second sound (or at least softer in its aortic component). Conversely, a benign murmur of aortic sclerosis is more likely to be short, to peak during the first half of systole, and to be associated with a well-preserved, even loud second sound. Most patients with aortic sclerosis have hypertension; hence the louder A2.

The early peak in intensity of aortic sclerosis is based on hemodynamic principles. Because the greatest fraction of ventricular ejection occurs during the first half of systole, a murmur like that of aortic sclerosis (which is due to flow and velocity but not to a pressure gradient) tends to occur whenever flow and velocity are indeed higher: early systole. In addition, because the integrity of the valve is well preserved in aortic sclerosis, the intensity of the second sound is well maintained. Finally, all other factors being equal, a murmur of aortic sclerosis is more likely to be softer than a murmur of aortic stenosis. Indeed, only 2% of aortic sclerosis murmurs are louder than grade IV. For the same reasons they are almost never accompanied by a palpable thrill.

35. Should echocardiograms be ordered for the evaluation of a systolic murmur?

Not necessarily. In fact, a well-performed cardiovascular exam may be enough for ruling out an organic murmur. In this case an echocardiogram is not only superfluous but also expensive and possibly even dangerous (because of the risks of tests begetting more tests). A well-performed examination is highly sensitive and highly specific in the evaluation of such murmurs. A recent study showed that the most cost-effective strategy in the evaluation of a pediatric murmur is referral to a cardiology specialist, leaving to his or her bedside skills the decision to order an echocardiogram.

SYSTOLIC MURMURS

36. How common are systolic murmurs?

Very common. Systolic murmurs in fact are encountered in 5–52% of unreferred young adults and 29–60% of elderly medical outpatients or nursing home residents. Most of these murmurs are benign (echocardiography is normal in 86–100% of young adults and 44–100% of the elderly). Echocardiography also is normal in 90–94% of pregnant women referred for evaluation of a systolic murmur.

Pearl. *Benign systolic murmurs are so prevalent in the general population that the practicing physician must recognize and properly interpret them.*

Systolic Ejection Murmurs

General Characteristics

37. What is the definition of an ejection murmur?

It is a systolic murmur produced by the forward flowing of blood. Usually it results from blood moving across the semilunar valves and into one of the large vessels.

38. What are the physical characteristics of the soundwave of an ejection murmur?

Ejection murmurs tend to have a crescendo-decrescendo shape and are therefore shaped like a diamond or kite. They typically end before the second sound component corresponding to the cardiac side from which the murmur originated. Therefore, an ejection murmur produced by blood flowing across the aortic valve ends before the A2 component of the second sound, whereas an ejection murmur produced by blood flowing across the pulmonary valve ends before the P2 component of the second sound. In reality these murmurs extend to cover the second sound, but they usually become so faint that the human ear cannot perceive their late systolic phase.

39. Do all ejection murmurs have a crescendo-decrescendo shape?

All ejection murmurs *tend* to have a crescendo-decrescendo shape because the intensity of the murmur is regulated by the pressure gradient across the obstructing valve. The pressure gradient, in turn, is determined by the velocity and acceleration of the blood flow. Whenever the flow has high velocity and acceleration, the pressure gradient is high, and the resulting murmur is louder. In an ejection murmur such as the murmur of aortic stenosis, the pressure gradient builds during the first part of ventricular systole. The loudness of the murmur also gradually increases, reaching a peak around mid systole. By then the ventricle loses contractility, the velocity and acceleration of the flow decrease, the pressure gradient decreases, and the loudness of the murmur starts to diminish. The result is the decrescendo shape of the second half of the murmur. The peak of an aortic sclerosis murmur tends to occur much earlier in systole than the peak of aortic stenosis. This finding is another useful differentiating feature.

40. Summarize the physical characteristics of an ejection murmur.

An ejection murmur (1) starts immediately after S1 (or after an ejection sound associated with S1); (2) has a crescendo/decrescendo shape; and (3) ends before the ipsilateral component of the second sound.

41. What are the frequency characteristics of ejection murmurs?

An important characteristic of systolic ejection murmurs is the predominance of low-to-medium frequencies, whereas systolic regurgitant murmurs tend to be higher-pitched. This auscultatory characteristic is important in the differential diagnosis of ejection and regurgitant murmurs. Thus, although systolic regurgitant murmurs also may have a crescendo-decrescendo pattern, they characteristically exhibit higher-frequency components than systolic ejection murmurs and, unlike ejection murmurs, typically extend into S2.

42. Does any other auscultory characteristic help to distinguish *ejection* from *regurgitant* murmur?

Ejection murmurs (but not regurgitant murmurs) are usually louder after a long diastole (as in atrial fibrillation) or after a premature beat. Because a long diastole allows a larger volume of blood to collect in the ventricle, end-diastolic volume and ventricular contractility are increased. This, in turn, produces a higher pressure gradient and a louder murmur. Conversely, in cases of regurgitation the ventricle has two possible outlets to discharge its content: a normal (forward) outlet and an abnormal regurgitant (backward) outlet. Thus, even an increase in ventricular contractility is offset by the two possible outlets. As a result, the intensity of a regurgitant murmur after a long diastolic phase remains unchanged. In addition, there are differences in response to handgrip and transmission of the murmur (to the neck for an ejection murmur and to the axilla for a regurgitant murmur).

43. All other factors being equal, is the intensity of an ejection murmur related to the severity of the pressure gradient?

Yes. The louder the ejection murmur, the higher the pressure gradient across the valve. This rule of thumb requires, of course, that all other parameters determining the murmur intensity (e.g., thickness of the chest wall, degree of emphysema) remain equal. Therefore, a softer murmur (i.e., grade II or less) is much more likely to be associated with a lower pressure gradient than a louder murmur (grade 4 or higher). A major exception to this rule is the presence of congestive heart failure and the associated reduction in ventricular contractility. In this case the softness of the murmur is not necessarily an indication of a low-pressure gradient. Many other factors, on the other hand, may increase the loudness of a systolic ejection murmur without necessarily being associated with a higher pressure gradient. In addition to obvious conditions, such as a thin chest wall or a dilated pulmonary artery or aorta, all high-output states are associated with a higher flow velocity and therefore with louder murmurs even in the absence of a higher pressure gradient. High-output states can be encountered in conditions such as fever, exercise, anemia, thyrotoxicosis, pregnancy, beriberi, atrioventricular fistulas, aortic regurgitation, patent ductus arteriosus, and Paget's disease.

Aortic Stenosis

44. How many types of aortic stenosis are known?

There are three major types of aortic stenosis (AS): supravalvular, valvular, and subvalvular. Subvalvular AS is further divided into two subtypes: (1) hypertrophic idiopathic subaortic stenosis (also called HOCM) and (2) fixed, fibrotic subvalvular stenosis.

45. What are the causes of valvular AS?

There are three major causes of valvular AS: (1) congenital, (2) rheumatic, and (3) degenerative. Congenital causes are predominant in patients younger than 50 years of age, whereas a degenerative etiology predominates in the elderly (a normal semilunar valve becomes stiffened, thickened, and eventually calcified). Rheumatic valvular disease, although still a common problem worldwide, is becoming increasingly rare in the western world. It should be suspected in any patient with involvement of more than one valve, such as patients with combined mitral and aortic disease.

46. What is the most common congenital cause of valvular AS?

A bicuspid semilunar valve, which is one of the most common cardiac congenital abnormalities (1–2% of the general population). A bicuspid semilunar valve may be entirely silent throughout the patient's life or may simply manifest as an early systolic click. In most patients, however, bicuspid semilunar valves tend to stiffen over time, eventually becoming calcified and stenosed. A bicuspid semilunar valve is the most common degenerative etiology of valvular AS in the elderly.

47. How much reduction in valvular orifice is required for a murmur of AS to become audible?

Although a loud murmur may be present even in patients with mild disease, a reduction in valve orifice area of at least 50% is required to generate a pressure gradient in the resting state. Significant hemodynamic compromise and symptoms usually occur with a 60–70% reduction in valve orifice. Thus, early or mild aortic stenosis may be difficult to diagnose at rest. Exercise, on the other hand, may increase cardiac output and thus pressure gradient and murmur intensity.

48. What are the characteristics of a peripheral arterial pulse in a patient with AS?

In **valvular AS** the pulse is typically small in amplitude (parvus) with a slow upstroke (tardus). Occasionally it may be accompanied by a palpable thrill. These characteristics are best appreciated in the large central arteries, such as the carotid and brachial arteries, and can be easily missed in the small peripheral arteries, such as the radial arteries.

In **supravalvular AS** the amplitude of the pulse tends to be greater in right-sided vessels than in left-sided vessels. This finding is also typical of a special form of supravalvular AS: coarctation of the aorta.

In **subvalvular AS** of the hypertrophic variety (HOCM), the arterial pulse tends to be brisk with a palpable double systolic impulse (pulsus bisferiens).

49. What are the characteristics of the point of maximal apical impulse (PMI) in patients with aortic stenosis?

1. **Location of the PMI**. In the typical patient with concentric left ventricular hypertrophy, the apical impulse is usually well sustained and only mildly displaced to the left. Increased displacement usually indicates the development of left ventricular failure or the concomitant presence of aortic insufficiency.

2. **Precordial thrill**. A palpable thrill is common in patients with AS and does not reflect the severity of disease. The best way to palpate the thrill is to have the patient sit up, lean forward, and hold the breath in forced exhalation.

Valvular Aortic Stenosis

50. Where is the murmur of AS heard the loudest?

The murmur of AS is loudest in the area from the second right intercostal space (traditionally termed the aortic area) down to the fifth-to-sixth intercostal space at the midclavicular line (apex; usually termed the "sash area"). The sash area is much wider than the traditional aortic area. Although most murmurs of AS are best heard at the base (at least their medium-to-low pitch components) some higher-pitched murmurs may be best heard at the apex. These high-frequency components at times may be so prominent that they are mistaken for a separate "cooing" murmur.

51. What are the characteristics of an AS murmur?

It is crescendo-decrescendo in shape, usually medium-pitched, and harsh in quality with a rasping or coarse timber. Length of the murmur and timing of its peak reflect the severity of the stenosis. As a rule of thumb, the longer the murmur and the later its peak, the more severe the stenosis. Therefore, a murmur peaking in early or mid systole reflects milder disease more than a murmur that peaks in late systole.

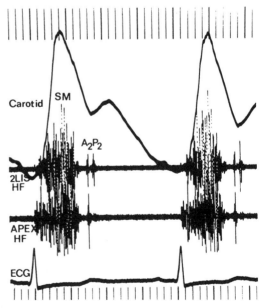

A loud, diamond-shaped murmur of aortic stenosis in a child. (From Fyler DC: Nadas' Pediatric Cardiology. Philadelphia, Hanley & Belfus, 1992, with permission.)

52. What other characteristics of an AS murmur may be associated with increased severity?

Loudness is also associated with severity, although this rule tends to apply primarily to children and young people. In the elderly, various other factors (such as obstructive lung disease or obesity) may soften the intensity of the murmur even in the presence of severe disease. In such patients, auscultation over the neck or clavicle (bone is a good conductor of sound) may help to restore adequate intensity.

Although a small number of patients with mild-to-moderate AS may have loud murmurs, loudness in association with a soft or absent second sound component (A2) almost always reflects severe AS. The transmission of the murmur to the neck does not reflect the severity of stenosis. Finally, a murmur of AS may become faint and almost disappear when the patient develops congestive heart failure. In this case, the failing ventricle becomes unable to overcome the high pressure gradient responsible for the generation of the murmur. Thus, severe AS may be associated with a soft or almost absent murmur.

53. What other acoustic event may indicate the presence of severe AS?

In younger patients, the presence of an audible S4 reflects severe left ventricular hypertrophy and a transvalvular pressure gradient usually greater than 70 mmHg. In children and in elderly adults this rule is not valid, because such patients may normally have an S4. A palpable S4, however, always reflects severe disease.

An early systolic click usually indicates valvular AS, usually due to a congenitally bicuspid valve. Because these abnormalities are less common in the elderly (in whom degeneration of a tricuspid valve is a more common event), early systolic clicks are rare in older patients and relatively common in younger patients.

54. Summarize the characteristics of a murmur of severe AS.

The murmur of severe AS is loud, long, peaking in the later part of systole, ending with a soft or absent A2 component of the second sound, preceded by an S4, and accompanied by a palpable precordial thrill.

Subvalvular Aortic Stenosis

55. What is the area of highest intensity for the murmur of HOCM?

When septal hypertrophy causes obstruction not only to left but also to right ventricular outflow, the murmur may become louder at the left lower sternal border. Most commonly, however, the HOCM murmur is loudest over the apex. This finding often causes a problem in the differential diagnosis of HOCM and the murmur of mitral regurgitation.

56. How can one differentiate the systolic ejection murmur of valvular AS from that of HOCM?

The timing of onset of the murmur usually helps in this differentiation. In valvular AS the murmur starts immediately after the first sound, whereas in HOCM the murmur usually starts in mid systole because the obstruction of HOCM is caused by the hypertrophic ventricular muscle, particularly its septal component. Therefore, the obstruction is much more likely to become critical whenever the lumen of the ventricle is reduced, such as during systole. In certain situations, however, the murmur may begin at the same time as the murmur of valvular AS (i.e., in early systole). Such situations usually are linked to moderate subaortic obstruction. The murmur is produced not by the pressure gradient linked to subaortic obstruction but by the rapid ejection that is characteristic of HOCM. In such patients, as much as 80% of the left ventricular volume is ejected during the first half of systole. This rapid flow, therefore, leads to the production of a flow murmur in early systole. By the time dynamic subaortic obstruction takes place, the murmur acquires the characteristic of the more typical mid-to-late systolic murmur of HOCM. When the systolic flow is not increased (because the obstruction is milder), the murmur is present only during the second part of systole. Thus, the presence of rapid ejection is usually signaled by a short ejection sound (ejection click), heard during the early part of systole immediately following S1.

57. What beside maneuvers can be used to modify the murmur of HOCM?

Factors that increase the diameter of the left ventricular cavity are associated with a reduction in the pressure gradient linked to subaortic obstruction and in the intensity of the murmur. Conversely, factors that decrease the diameter of the left ventricular cavity (such as a drop in systemic vascular resistances produced by vasodilators) are associated with an increase in the intensity of the murmur. Amyl nitrite, an inhaled short-acting dilator, was used for this purpose. Because of the risks related to its use, it is not currently used. Similarly the Valsalva maneuver also causes a reduction in the diameter of the left ventricular cavity because of a decrease in venous return and leads to a higher intensity in the murmur of HOCM. This response is different from the response of the murmur of valvular AS, in which the decrease in venous return leads to a reduction in stroke volume and therefore in the intensity of the murmur.

58. How does squatting affect the intensity of the murmur of HOCM?

Squatting softens the murmur of HOCM because it increases the left ventricular diameter (as a result of increased venous return and increased systemic vascular resistances). Conversely, squatting increases the intensity of the murmur of valvular AS because of the effects of both increased venous return and increased peripheral vascular resistance.

59. Can the murmur of HOCM be partially related to a murmur of mitral regurgitation?

Yes. Often the murmur of HOCM is associated with a murmur of mitral regurgitation because the thickened hypertrophic ventricular septum pulls the mitral valve (especially its anterior leaflet) open during systole, leading to mitral regurgitation. Evidence of regurgitation and ballooning of the mitral valve may be encountered in as many as 75% of patients with HOCM. The murmur of mitral regurgitation responds to various bedside maneuvers much like the murmur of HOCM. Thus, the murmur of mitral regurgitation due to HOCM is delayed in onset and ends before the A2 component of the second sound. If, on the other hand, the murmur does not behave in this fashion but spans throughout systole, it is much more likely to be related to primary mitral regurgitation.

60. What discrete narrowing is responsible for fixed subvalvular AS?

Subvalvular AS usually results from discrete and fixed obstructive fibrosis, which may be located either immediately below the aortic valve (as a thin membrane) or on the ventricular septum. In other patients the subvalvular obstruction is produced by a concentric fibrous ring coupled with muscular hypertrophy, located 2 cm below the aortic valve.

Supravalvular Aortic Stenosis

61. What are the characteristics of supravalvular AS?

Supravalvular AS usually is produced by a localized, discrete narrowing located above the sinuses of Valsalva. The area of highest intensity is either the suprasternal notch or the first right intercostal space (as opposed to the second right intercostal space for the murmur of valvular AS). Similarly, the murmur of supravalvular AS tends to radiate more toward the right carotid artery rather than toward the left carotid artery (as with the murmur of valvular aortic stenosis).

62. What other characteristics are typical of patients with supravalvular AS?

Male sex plus a number of congenital abnormalities, such as hypercalcemia, a peculiar elfin facies, patulous lip, and deep, husky voice. Such patients also tend to have a stronger pulse and a higher blood pressure in the right arm and right carotid artery compared with the left. Although this murmur occasionally may be accompanied by an aortic regurgitation murmur, it is almost never associated with an aortic ejection click.

Effect of Bedside Maneuvers on Ejection Murmurs

63. What are the effects of respiration on ejection murmurs?

Inspiration and expiration have different hemodynamic effects on the right and left ventricle. Inspiration increases the flow into the right-sided chambers because of the associated increase in venous return to the right side. Therefore, an ejection murmur across the pulmonic valve is louder during inspiration because of the increased flow across the right-sided valves (Rivera-Carvallo maneuver; see question 15). On the other hand, inspiration decreases the flow into the left-sided chambers; because of the associated decrease in venous return to the left side, blood pools in the lungs. The results are a decrease in flow across the aortic valve, a decrease in pressure gradient, and a reduction in the intensity of the murmur of aortic stenosis. The opposite takes place during exhalation.

The effect of inspiration on murmur intensity may be counterbalanced by an increase in lung aeration, which may act as a muffler, increasing the cushion of air between the heart and the stethoscope. This problem is common in the upper half of the chest, which corresponds to the base of the heart. Thus, the increase in loudness of a right-sided ejection murmur as a result of inspiration may be best heard in the *lower* instead of the upper chest.

64. What is the effect of standing on the intensity of ejection murmurs?

The respiratory variations in the intensity of ejection murmurs can be enhanced by having the patient stand. Although the right ventricular stroke volume is decreased during standing, the increase in pulmonary blood flow associated with inspiration will be proportionally higher. Thus, a right-sided ejection murmur is proportionally louder in inspiration than in expiration, whenever the patient is standing.

65. What is the effect of a Valsalva maneuver on a systolic ejection murmur?

It depends on the phase of the Valsalva maneuver (straining or releasing). As a rule of thumb, all ejection murmurs (with the exception of the murmur of HOCM) become softer during the straining phase because straining is associated with a decrease in venous return. As soon as the straining is released, there is a rebound increase in the intensity of all ejection murmurs; the peak is reached within 2–3 beats by the pulmonic ejection murmur and within 6–8 beats by the aortic ejection murmur. The delayed peak of the aortic ejection murmur is due to the longer time required by the left ventricle to be filled by the blood that was pooled during straining. During this time the blood flows from the right ventricle across the lungs into the left ventricle and finally into the aorta.

Aortic vs. Pulmonic Stenosis

66. What characteristics differentiate the murmur of pulmonic stenosis from the murmur of aortic stenosis?

1. The location is different. The area of maximal intensity for the murmur of aortic stenosis is the second right intercostal space or the apex, whereas the area of maximal intensity for the murmur of pulmonic stenosis is the left sternal border.

2. The murmur of aortic stenosis is louder in exhalation, whereas the murmur of pulmonic stenosis is louder in inspiration.

3. Standing makes the murmur of pulmonic stenosis proportionally louder, whereas the murmur of aortic stenosis becomes softer.

4. The straining phase of the Valsalva maneuver softens both murmurs. As soon as the straining is released, however, the murmur of pulmonic stenosis reaches its highest intensity within 2–3 beats, whereas the murmur of aortic stenosis takes significantly longer.

67. What other auscultatory features help to differentiate pulmonic from aortic stenosis?

1. An ejection click may be present in both pulmonic and aortic stenosis. Only the click associated with pulmonic stenosis, however, tends to decrease in intensity or totally disappear during inspiration.

2. A widening of the normal and physiologic splitting of the second sound tends to indicate the murmur of pulmonic stenosis. A paradoxical splitting of S2, on the other hand, tends to indicate the murmur or aortic stenosis.

3. Finally the presence of an S4 gallop during inspiration is more likely to be associated with pulmonic stenosis, whereas the presence of an S4 gallop during exhalation is more likely to be associated with aortic stenosis.

Systolic Regurgitant Murmurs

Definition

68. What is a systolic regurgitant murmur?

A systolic regurgitant murmur is produced by a pressure gradient that causes retrograde blood flow (i.e., from a high- to a low-pressure chamber) across an abnormal opening. This abnormal opening may be (1) a ventricular septal defect; (2) an incompetent mitral valve; (3) an incompetent tricuspid valve; and (4) a fistulous communication between a high-pressure and low-pressure vascular bed (such as patent ductus arteriosus). All of these murmurs should be called murmurs of regurgitation, not murmurs of *insufficiency* or *incompetence*. These last two terms define the anatomic or functional characteristics of the valve, whereas regurgitation more properly describes the blood flow derangement that is typical of these processes.

69. What are the auscultatory characteristics of a systolic regurgitant murmur?

Systolic regurgitant murmurs tend to start immediately after the first sound and often extend to cover the second sound. As opposed to systolic ejection murmurs, systolic regurgitant murmurs do not increase in intensity after a long diastole because the ejecting chamber has two outlets available: a higher-pressure and a lower-pressure bed. For example, in the case of mitral regurgitation, the left ventricle can discharge either into the atrium (low-pressure bed) or into the aorta (high-pressure bed). The percentage of blood ejected into each of the two beds depends on the resistance offered by the outlet. After a long diastole, such as that following a premature beat, the resistance offered by the aorta is decreased more than the resistance offered by the left atrium. The left atrium continues to fill during a long diastole, whereas the aorta continues to empty (thanks to the increased time available for its run-off into peripheral arteries). As a result, after a long diastole, proportionally more blood is ejected into the aorta than into the atrium. Thus, the intensity of a regurgitant murmur remains unchanged after a long diastole.

If the intensity of a systolic murmur after a long diastole is increased at the base but not at the apex, two murmurs usually are present: one of regurgitation and one of ejection. The ejection murmur becomes louder at the base after a long diastole, whereas the regurgitant murmur heard at the apex remains the same. In mitral valve prolapse this rule does not hold. Because the amount of regurgitation in mitral valve prolapse is dictated by the size of the left ventricle, a larger left ventricular volume (such as that seen after a long diastole) leads to reduced regurgitation and, therefore, to a softer murmur.

Mitral Regurgitation

70. What causes the murmur of mitral regurgitation?

The causes vary, depending on the age of the patient. In **adults** there are four major causes of mitral regurgitation: (1) rheumatic damage to the valve, (2) dysfunction of the papillary muscles, (3) rupture of the chordae tendinae, and (4) myxomatous degeneration of the mitral valve. The latter is commonly associated with mitral valve prolapse.

In **infants** the most common cause of mitral regurgitation is dysfunction of the papillary muscles, which usually is associated with either a congenital abnormality of the coronary artery (anomalous left coronary artery arising from the pulmonary artery) or endocardial fibroelastosis. Other congenital abnormalities that may lead to mitral regurgitation are endocardial cushion defect with a cleft mitral valve and myxomatous degeneration of the mitral valve (often associated with Marfan syndrome). Approximately 50% of all patients with Marfan syndrome have mitral regurgitation. Finally, acquired myocarditis also may lead to mitral regurgitation in infants.

71. Can the left ventricular dilatation encountered in congestive heart failure or cardiomyopathy lead to mitral regurgitation?

Contrary to popular belief, many patients with left ventricular dilatation do not have mitral regurgitation because the area of valvular orifice tends to remain constant while the left ventricle dilates. In addition, the mitral annulus is provided with a muscle ring that contracts during systole, thus behaving like a sphincter and preventing regurgitation. Calcification of the mitral annulus (which often can be visualized on chest radiograph) may lead to mitral valve regurgitation by disabling its sphincter function.

72. What is the cause of mitral regurgitation due to papillary muscle dysfunction?

Papillary muscle dysfunction is a common cause of mitral regurgitation in patients with an acute myocardial infarction. The incompetence and dysfunction of the papillary muscle are usually due to ischemia but also may be due to infarction of the ventricular muscle at the base of the papillary muscle itself. Such mitral regurgitant murmurs tend to be transient and may appear in as many as 10% of patients who present with a myocardial infarction.

Characteristics of the Murmur

73. Which is the area of maximal intensity for a murmur of mitral regurgitation?

The apex. In tall patients with long chests the area of maximal intensity may be close to the left sternal border.

74. Where is the murmur of mitral regurgitation best radiated?

Toward the left axilla or toward the left interscapular area. In addition, peculiar radiation patterns may be associated with rupture of the chordae tendinae. For example, rupture of the anterior chordae may lead to a regurgitant stream flowing posteriorly against the mid-thoracic spine or even, at times, toward the top of the head. On the other hand, rupture of the posterior chordae may lead to a regurgitant stream flowing toward the aorta and thus mimicking the murmur of aortic stenosis and its pattern of transmission (i.e., into the carotids).

75. Can a murmur of mitral regurgitation be soft and almost silent despite severe regurgitation?

Yes—usually as the result of a large right ventricle or a large and thick chest with lots of aerated lung tissue interposed between the ventricle and stethoscope. The alveolar air acts as a muffler, thereby softening the intensity of the murmur. In this case, even severe mitral regurgitation may be totally silent. Other patients may experience "flash pulmonary edema" as the only manifestation of an underlying mitral regurgitation worsened by ischemia. Most patients with this form of silent mitral regurgitation have a severe form of regurgitation, which presents as episodes of paroxysmal nocturnal dyspnea or nocturnal acute pulmonary edema. A large left ventricle, a large left atrium, and a widely split S2 often are the only clues to this diagnosis.

76. What is the typical shape of a murmur of mitral regurgitation?

The shape depends on whether the regurgitant murmur starts early or late in systole. When the murmur starts late, it usually extends to the second sound. On the other hand, when it starts early, it usually follows immediately the first sound. The shape of the murmur, therefore, may be a plateau throughout systole, a crescendo-decrescendo throughout systole, or a crescendo (starting at mid systole) or decrescendo (starting after S1 and ending toward mid systole). Usually the loudest murmurs of mitral regurgitation last throughout systole and have a crescendo-decrescendo pattern (although usually it is not as pronounced as the crescendo-decrescendo pattern of an aortic stenosis murmur). Often regurgitant murmurs, particularly those starting at mid systole, may extend slightly beyond the second sound because the left ventricular pressure remains higher than the left atrial pressure even after the aortic valve has closed, leading to continuing regurgitation after S2.

77. What is the usual pitch of a mitral regurgitant murmur?
The pitch depends on the flow and the pressure gradient. If the gradient is high and the flow is low, the murmur is high-pitched. On the other hand, if the gradient is low and the flow is high, the murmur is low-pitched. Murmurs in between tend to have a mixed frequency.

78. Can the shape of a mitral regurgitant murmur help to differentiate the various causes of mitral regurgitation?
Yes. Murmurs that are constant throughout systole (plateau) are more likely to be associated with rheumatic mitral regurgitation. On the other hand, murmurs that start in mid systole and have a crescendo pattern toward the second sound are more likely to be associated with either mitral valve prolapse or papillary muscle dysfunction. Because the papillary muscle does not contract well, its chordae tendinae become progressively longer as the ventricle becomes smaller. This leads to a murmur that increases in intensity throughout systole and has a crescendo pattern. Often this murmur has a cooing characteristic, almost like the cry of a seagull.

79. What is the difference between mitral regurgitation due to a dysfunctional papillary muscle and mitral regurgitation due to ruptured chordae tendinae?
Mitral regurgitation due to ruptured chordae tendinae is a much more serious clinical condition than mitral regurgitation due to a dysfunctional papillary muscle. Patients with ruptured chordae tendinae usually experience flash pulmonary edema, whereas patients with a dysfunctional papillary muscle tend to have a mild degree of congestive heart failure or may even be totally asymptomatic. Because the severity of mitral regurgitation is much higher in patients with ruptured papillary muscles or ruptured chordae tendinae, these regurgitant murmurs are quite intense (3/6 or more) and often associated with a loud third sound and dramatic symptoms of acute pulmonary edema. Moreover, the large amount of regurgitated blood rapidly increases the atrial pressure to the point of causing a decrease in regurgitation early during systole. Thus, the intensity of the murmur associated with ruptured chordae tendineae starts immediately after S1 and tends to decrease (or disappear) toward the mid-portion of systole. The opposite happens to the murmur of dysfunctional papillary muscle, which may start at mid systole and have a crescendo pattern ending at S2. Occasionally the radiation of a murmur or ruptured chordae tendineae may lead to a pattern of transmission that is similar to that of valvular aortic stenosis. This pattern usually is encountered whenever the posterior cusp is flail and the stream of regurgitation flows toward the atrial septum to produce a murmur that radiates into the carotids and has a crescendo pattern similar to that of aortic stenosis. Finally, the murmur of mitral regurgitation due to ruptured chordae tendineae is commonly associated with an S4 because of the Starling effect of a dilated atrium, which leads to a stronger and louder atrial contraction. S4 is almost never encountered in mitral regurgitation due to rheumatic diseases.

80. What is the most common cause of ruptured chordae tendineae?
Infective endocarditis. Often, however, there are no obvious causes, and the rupture is called idiopathic. In this case the valve or the chordae are abnormally constituted because of myxomatous degeneration, which makes them more prone to spontaneous rupture, particularly during unusual strains. This process is not uncommon in patients with mitral valve prolapse.

81. What are the other characteristics of severe mitral regurgitation?
1. In more severe mitral regurgitation the left ventricle is enlarged. This condition can be determined by palpation, noting the displacement and enlargement of the left-ventricular point of maximal impulse (PMI).

2. The length and intensity of the systolic regurgitant murmur are related directly to the severity of regurgitation. Therefore, the louder and longer the apical systolic murmur, the more severe the regurgitation.

3. An S3 is often present in severe mitral regurgitation, and the loudness of the S3 also is related directly to the severity of regurgitation. The more severe the regurgitation, the more likely the presence (and loudness) of the S3.

4. In addition to an S3, severe mitral regurgitation is often accompanied by an earlier diastolic flow murmur that follows the S3. The longer and louder this early diastolic murmur, the more severe the regurgitation.

5. Finally, the splitting of S2 may be widened in severe mitral regurgitation because of the early closure of the aortic component of S2. This effect may be offset by the development of pulmonary hypertension, which, in turn, narrows the S2 splitting.

Pearl.   *The severity of mitral regurgitation (a systolic murmur) is ironically assessed in diastole by looking for the presence of a diastolic flow murmur.*

Effect of Various Bedside Maneuvers on Murmur Intensity

82. Is the murmur of mitral regurgitation made louder or softer by respiration?

It depends on the phase of respiration. Usually murmurs of mitral regurgitation are louder during expiration because of the higher blood flow from the lungs into the left ventricle. This bedside maneuver can be used to differentiate a murmur of mitral from a murmur of tricuspid regurgitation (Rivera-Carvallo maneuver). The murmur of tricuspid regurgitation becomes louder in inspiration (because of the increased venous return to the right side of the heart), whereas the murmur of mitral regurgitation becomes softer (because of the decreased venous return to the left side of the heart).

83. What are the effects of various bedside maneuvers on mitral regurgitant murmurs?

To understand the effects of various bedside maneuvers (or drugs) on the intensity of a mitral regurgitant murmur, one must remember that in mitral regurgitation the left ventricle has two outlets for discharge: a high-resistance outlet (aorta), and a low-resistance outlet (left atrium). Therefore, by manipulating the resistances of the aorta (peripheral vascular resistances) one may influence the amount of blood that regurgitates into the left atrium (and therefore the intensity of the murmur). As a result, vasopressor agents and bedside maneuvers, such as handgrip or squatting, that increase peripheral vascular resistance also lead to more severe regurgitation and a louder murmur. All of these maneuvers, therefore, increase regurgitation and cause louder murmurs. Finally, passive leg-raising sometimes elicits the murmur of papillary muscle dysfunction by causing an increase in left ventricular volume. This maneuver may be used in dealing with the transient murmur of mitral regurgitation encountered during angina with left ventricular failure.

84. What is the effect of standing on the murmur of mitral regurgitation?

Standing increases peripheral vascular resistances, but its effect on the murmur of mitral regurgitation depends on the etiology. If mitral regurgitation is due primarily to a dilated left ventricle, the murmur becomes softer during standing because the decreased venous return leads to a reduction in ventricular size. If, on the other hand, the dilatation is not responsible for regurgitation, the murmur becomes louder during standing because the increased peripheral vascular resistance increases the amount of regurgitated blood. This effect, however, may be offset by the decrease in venous return caused by standing; therefore, the intensity of the murmur may remain unchanged. If mitral regurgitation is due to mitral valve prolapse, a smaller left ventricle (as may be seen during standing) causes more prolapse. Thus standing may accentuate the intensity and prolong the length of the murmur of mitral valve prolapse.

85. Which vasoactive drugs can be used to modify the intensity of the murmur of mitral regurgitation?

Drugs used to manipulate peripheral vascular resistances (PVR) are (1) **vasopressor agents** (that increase PVR and therefore lead to more severe regurgitation and more intense murmurs) or

(2) **vasodilators**, such as amyl nitrite, that decreases PVR and therefore lead to an immediate and marked drop in blood pressure. Amyl nitrite was used to separate an apical murmur due to mitral regurgitation from an apical murmur due to aortic stenosis. The first murmur became softer, whereas the second became louder. Amyl nitrite had to be administered to a supine patient (in a standing patient the drop in PVR might have led to syncope), and the blood pressure had to be monitored throughout the procedure. The patient felt flushed and for approximately 30 seconds also experienced "heart pounding," a normal side effect of the drug. Such manipulations are potentially dangerous and belong to the pre-echocardiography era.

Mitral Valve Prolapse

86. What is mitral valve prolapse?

This entity has had many names; currently the most common is **prolapsed mitral syndrome**. It is called syndrome because it is also associated with a complex clinical presentation characterized by arrhythmias, atypical chest pain, and abnormal EKG. The valvular abnormality is typically a ballooning and prolapsing of the mitral valve into the left atrium during systole. This finding is due to a redundancy of either one or both mitral valve leaflets and leads to mitral regurgitation. The ballooning also may cause a sharp systolic extra sound (click), which may occur in either mid or late systole and may be followed by a regurgitant murmur. The murmur usually extends into the second sound (A2).

The most commonly involved mitral leaflet is the posterior leaflet, which often has myxomatous degeneration. Myxomatous degeneration is commonly seen in patients with Marfan syndrome, who often have mitral valve prolapse. However, many patients with mitral valve prolapse have no features of Marfan syndrome, although 20–30% of such patients have minor characteristics, such as tall stature, straight back, pectus excavatum, and other skeletal or joint abnormalities. Often the degeneration of the mitral valve is accompanied by a similar degeneration of the tricuspid valve.

87. What is the differential diagnosis of mitral valve prolapse?

Papillary muscle dysfunction due to myocardial infarction, which may lead to a similar phenomenon of prolapse. Because of the unequal length of the chordae tendineae, HOCM also may lead to prolapse of the mitral valve.

88. What is the cause of the click heard in a patient with mitral valve prolapse?

The click appears to be caused by a sudden stretch of the chordae tendineae as they try to hold back the ballooning of the leaflet into the left atrium. This sound has been appropriately defined as a **chordal snap**. Other authors argue that the contraction of the papillary muscles may prevent the chordae from snapping during systole. They believe that the ballooning of the valve leaflet itself causes the snap, much like the sound produced by a sail suddenly filled with wind.

89. Can the regurgitation of mitral valve prolapse be hemodynamically severe?

Usually the regurgitation is mild to moderate and starts toward mid systole. With time, however, the degree of regurgitation may worsen gradually from mild to moderate to severe. Severe regurgitation may be caused by the rupture of abnormal and malformed chordae or, even more frequently, the development of infective endocarditis on the abnormal valve. In fact, infective endocarditis may be the presenting manifestation of a mitral valve prolapse that previously remained clinically silent.

90. What does a murmur of mitral valve prolapse sound like?

The murmur tends to be loudest at the apex and usually has a crescendo shape, starting in mid systole immediately after the click and peaking toward the end of the second sound. It tends not to be loud in intensity (usually no greater than 3/6). It may have, however, some systolic musical features, usually described as honks or whoops. Honks refer to the honking of a goose. Such murmurs almost always reflect mitral valve prolapse. They tend to change (and may even totally disappear) with different positions and different phases of respiration. Either the click or the murmur may be missing. Often bedside maneuvers, such as simple exercise, may bring them back, either together or separately.

91. What maneuvers lead to a change in the auscultatory characteristics of the click and murmur of mitral valve prolapse?
The most important variable affecting the regurgitation of a prolapsing mitral valve is the size of the left ventricular chamber. A larger left ventricle pulls down (through the chordae) the ballooning leaflet and therefore leads to less prolapse and regurgitation. Conversely, a smaller left ventricle facilitates the ballooning into the left atrium and therefore leads to more regurgitation. Maneuvers that lead to a decrease in left ventricular size are squatting and then standing, inspiration, and the straining phase of the Valsalva maneuver. Both the click and the murmur become louder and start earlier. For example, in many patients only squatting/standing or a Valsalva maneuver can unmask the murmur or click. These maneuvers are also useful to differentiate the murmur of mitral valve prolapse from the murmur of papillary muscle dysfunction (which does not become louder or longer during sitting or standing or the Valsalva maneuver). Drugs that decrease the left ventricular size and peripheral vascular resistances (such as amyl nitrite) may lead to an earlier location of the click during systole, although the click may become softer and even disappear (because of the low systolic blood pressure). Similarly, an increase in peripheral vascular resistance, such as that produced by vasopressors, leads to a decrease in the loudness of the murmur and the severity of regurgitation. Finally, drugs that slow the heart rate and therefore increase left ventricular size cause the click and the murmur to diminish in intensity or disappear altogether.

Tricuspid Regurgitant Murmurs

92. Where are tricuspid regurgitant murmurs best heard?
Tricuspid regurgitant murmurs are best heard in the left lower sternal border or in the epigastric area. When the right ventricle is large enough to displace the left ventricle laterally and posteriorly, tricuspid regurgitant murmurs at times may be best heard over the right sternal border or apex. In patients with severe chronic obstructive pulmonary disease and air trapping, the murmur of tricuspid regurgitation usually can be heard only over the free edge of the liver.

93. What are the classic diagnostic characteristics of a murmur of tricuspid regurgitation?
The murmur spans throughout systole, is best heard over the epigastrium, and becomes louder with inspiration (see above). The murmur of tricuspid regurgitation remains louder as long as inspiration is held (inspiratory apnea) because throughout inspiration venous return and blood flow to the right ventricle are increased. The murmur of tricuspid regurgitation becomes louder in response to other situations that increase venous return to the right side, such as exercise, passive elevation of the legs, or bending the knees toward the chest. Finally, the presence of a whooping or honking pattern in tricuspid regurgitation usually indicates the presence of pulmonary hypertension with an increase in regurgitant flow.

94. What are the characteristics of a murmur of acute tricuspid regurgitation?
Whenever regurgitation is sudden, the murmur of tricuspid regurgitation may have low intensity and even a decrescendo pattern. This pattern may occur, for example, during rupture of the chordae tendinae, causing such acute and severe regurgitation that the right atrium does not have enough time to enlarge. As a result, atrial pressure increases rapidly to the point of stopping regurgitation at mid systole. If regurgitation becomes so severe that the atrium and ventricle become almost a single chamber, there may be no systolic murmur.

95. How can one distinguish tricuspid from mitral regurgitation?
It is often difficult to separate the two entities. For example, the area of maximal intensity of the murmur of mitral regurgitation may become the left sternal border instead of the apex because

of the rotation of the heart. Similarly, an enlarged right ventricle may expand from the right sternal border toward the apex. The easiest way to distinguish the two murmurs is to use the inspiratory maneuver (which makes tricuspid regurgitation louder than mitral regurgitation) and to note a change in the intensity of the murmur after the release from the Valsalva strain. The murmur of tricuspid regurgitation becomes louder within about 1 second into the release phase, whereas it takes longer for the murmur of mitral regurgitation to reach its peak intensity (usually 3 seconds).

96. What are the most common causes of tricuspid regurgitation?

Primary tricuspid regurgitation is usually due to a primary abnormality of the valve without evidence of pulmonary hypertension. This abnormality may be due to trauma, endocarditis, or congenital abnormalities such as Epstein's disease. Infective endocarditis in such patients is almost always due to intravenous drug abuse.

Secondary tricuspid regurgitation usually requires both pulmonary hypertension (with a thick, hypertrophic left ventricle) and large right ventricular volume (as may be seen in patients with atrial septal defects). The presence of both pressure and volume load leads to tricuspid regurgitation. This condition may be seen in patients with mitral stenosis and pulmonary hypertension, in patients with atrial septal defect and pulmonary hypertension, in patients with primary pulmonary hypertension and right ventricular failure, and in patients with left ventricular failure so severe that it leads to pulmonary hypertension and right ventricular dilatation.

97. What other findings are present in patients with tricuspid regurgitation?

Giant V waves associated with deep Y descents (Lancisi's sign), bobbing motion of the earlobes (80% sensitivity), positive abdominojugular reflux test with an increase in the intensity of the murmur (Vitum's sign; 56% sensitive and 100% specific), and a pulsatile liver (sensitivity of 17%).

Miscellaneous Ejection Murmurs

Ventricular Septal Defect Murmur

98. What are the characteristics of the murmur of ventricular septal defect (VSD)?

The murmur of VSD is similar to both regurgitant and ejection murmurs. Indeed, a VSD murmur may cover the entire systole with a plateau, crescendo/decrescendo, decrescendo, or crescendo pattern. The decrescendo shape of a VSD murmur usually occurs when there is a defect in the muscular part of the septum. The contraction of this portion closes the defect toward the end of systole and therefore causes a decrescendo murmur. If, on the other hand, the hole is located in the membranous septum, no such reduction in flow occurs during systole and the murmur remains constant and holosystolic.

99. Is there any relationship between the intensity of the murmur and the size of the defect?

No. Murmurs of varying intensity may be heard with either small or large defects. Yet when the defect is large, the intensity of the murmur usually is loud. A soft murmur, however, may be due to a large defect if the patient has severe pulmonary hypertension. In this case the murmur is usually preceded by an ejection sound (the hallmark of high pulmonary pressures) and ends with a loud single second sound, followed by an early diastolic murmur of pulmonary regurgitation (Graham Steell murmur).

100. Where is the murmur of VSD best heard?

Along the left lower sternal border.

101. How can one differentiate a murmur of mitral regurgitation from a VSD murmur?

A mitral regurgitation murmur may be delayed in onset and exhibit a crescendo pattern toward the second sound. This pattern is never heard with a ventricular septal defect: although some VSD murmurs may exhibit a crescendo pattern, they always start immediately after S1. The early crescendo/decrescendo shape is not typical of MR but usually is seen in very small congenital muscular VSDs.

Pearl. *The key to recognition of a VSD murmur is that, in contrast to mitral regurgitation murmurs, it always starts immediately after the mitral component of the first sound.*

Continuous Murmurs

102. What are continuous murmurs?

Continuous murmurs are murmurs that never end. They are present throughout systole and diastole with no evidence of a silent pause. On the other hand, a murmur that increases in intensity, peaks on S2, and decreases in intensity immediately after, ending before the next S1, is not a continuous murmur, even though it envelopes the second sound and extends slightly beyond it. Murmurs that cover systole and diastole but are not continuous are called to-and-fro murmurs. Examples include the murmurs of aortic stenosis and regurgitation. They are called to-and-fro because the flow goes in opposite directions with systole and diastole. Although the most important continuous murmur is the murmur of patent ductus arteriosus (PDA), other forms of abnormal connection between the aorta and the pulmonary artery can create a continuous murmur. The murmur of PDA (often called a machine-like murmur or train-in-tunnel murmur) is continuous because the constant pressure gradient throughout systole and diastole causes the blood to flow from the aorta into the pulmonary artery. Over time the development of pulmonary hypertension gradually decreases the gradient between the aorta and pulmonary artery and eventually leads to the gradual disappearance of the diastolic component and, finally, to reversal of the shunt with total disappearance of the murmur. Such patients become cyanotic, have no murmur and have instead severe pulmonary hypertension (Eisenmenger's syndrome). They often have clubbing and cyanosis, and the clubbing may be more pronounced in the feet than in the hands because the reversed shunt involves the dependent portion of the aorta instead of the upper portion.

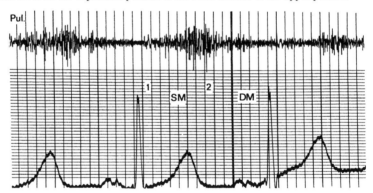

Continuous murmur of patent ductus arteriosus. (From Fyler DC: Nadas' Pediatric Cardiology. Philadelphia, Hanley & Belfus, 1992, with permission.)

DIASTOLIC MURMURS

Diastolic Atrioventricular Valve Murmurs

Mitral Stenosis

103. What are the common causes of mitral stenosis?

Mitral stenosis is usually due to rheumatic fever, which leads to chronic inflammation with fibrosis and fusion of the valve leaflets, often with superimposed calcification. This inflammatory process also involves the chordae tendinae, which become shorter and thickened. Less common causes of mitral stenosis are congenital conditions in which one papillary muscle has chordae attached to both leaflets (parachute mitral valve) and less frequently, myxomas of the left atrium or calcified bacterial vegetation that may obstruct the mitral valve. Mitral stenosis may be mimicked by the early diastolic murmur that occurs in settings of large flow across the mitral valve, such as in patients with severe mitral regurgitation or ventricular septal defect. Such murmurs are *not* murmurs of mitral stenosis; they are not even Austin Flint murmurs.

104. What is an Austin Flint murmur?

It is a diastolic rumble that truly resembles a murmur of mitral stenosis except that it is due to functional closure of the anterior leaflet of the mitral valve, caused by an aortic regurgitation stream pushing back the leaflet itself. Thus, the Austin Flint murmur is usually heard in diastole, at the apex, and in patients with severe aortic regurgitation.

105. How can one differentiate the Austin Flint murmur from the murmur of mitral stenosis?

Some auscultatory features may help to differentiate the two murmurs. For example, the presence of an opening snap tends to favor the presence of mitral stenosis. The opening snap, however, may be absent in the presence of thickened and calcific mitral valve (which was actively sought by fluoroscopy in pre-echocardiography years). Thus, the absence of an opening snap in a noncalcific valve favors the diagnosis of an Austin Flint murmur. The presence of a third sound is also more likely to favor an Austin Flint murmur; an S3 is extremely rare in mitral stenosis. Of course, an echocardiogram of the mitral valve is the definitive way to differentiate the two processes.

106. Is the presence of an Austin Flint murmur an indication of severe aortic regurgitation?

Not necessarily. Although an Austin Flint murmur usually requires an aortic regurgitant flow volume of at least 50 ml, it has been heard in patients with moderate aortic regurgitation. However, the presence of an Austin Flint murmur does indicate the presence of a high left atrial mean pressure and high left ventricular end-diastolic pressure.

107. Who was Austin Flint?

Austin Flint (1812–1886) was an American physician who studied at Harvard, where he was greatly influenced by one of the first American followers of Laennec. A superb teacher, he taught in Buffalo (where he helped to found the local medical college), Chicago, New Orleans, and New York.

108. What is the timing of the diastolic murmur of mitral stenosis? What is its relationship to the second sound?

The murmur of mitral stenosis is called a mid-to-late diastolic murmur because it does not start immediately after the second sound. It starts instead after the opening snap, which may or may not be audible. Therefore, there is usually a slight pause between the second sound (A2 component) and the diastolic rumble of mitral stenosis. (See figure on following page.)

109. Is there a slight pause between the opening snap and the diastolic murmur of mitral stenosis?

Yes. There is a slight pause between the opening snap and the diastolic murmur.

110. What is the shape of the diastolic rumble of mitral stenosis?

An initial crescendo pattern usually results from the fact that the most rapid phase of ventricular filling occurs during the early part of diastole. The initial crescendo is followed by a decrescendo phase with a late diastolic crescendo (also called the presystolic accentuation of the diastolic rumble). This accentuation is due to contraction of the left atrium and is therefore absent when no valid atrial contraction occurs (as in atrial fibrillation). The pattern of early crescendo, mid-diastolic rumble, and presystolic accentuation, therefore, results from the pressure gradient changes between left atrium and left ventricle.

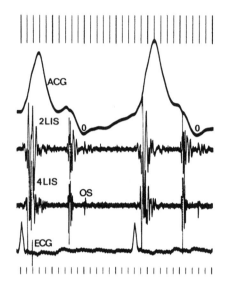

Opening snap (OS) in a child with mitral stenosis. (From Fyler DC: Nadas' Pediatric Cardiology. Philadelphia, Hanley & Belfus, 1992, with permission.)

111. What is the pitch of the mitral stenosis rumble?

The murmur of mitral stenosis is so low-pitched that it is audible only with the bell of the stethoscope. The murmur is produced more by the flow than by the pressure gradient between atrium and ventricle. Even in severe stenosis, the maximal pressure gradient is only 30 mmHg at the beginning of diastole and 10 mmHg at the end of diastole. These values are definitely much lower than the peak gradient encountered with significant systolic obstruction, such as aortic stenosis, where the pressure gradient may reach 50 mmHg. Because flow, more than pressure gradient, is usually responsible for the production of low-frequency murmurs, the murmur of MS is low-pitched. The typical low-pitch characteristic is further defined by adjectives that have been attached to the murmur of mitral stenosis throughout its history, such as rumbling or laboring (as in the terminology initially used by Austin Flint in 1884).

In certain situations, however, high-frequency components are also present in a mitral diastolic murmur, usually due to high forces across the orifice. High forces may be seen in patients with good circulatory time or strong atrial contraction or with the presence of mitral regurgitation in the previous systole that increase the volume crossing the valve in the following diastole.

112. Does an intense murmur reflect severe stenosis?

It depends. If the patient does not have concomitant mitral regurgitation, a strong, loud IV/VI murmur, usually accompanied by a thrill, reflects severe stenosis. On the other hand, the presence of a loud murmur almost always signifies the absence of significant pulmonary hypertension. In fact, by decreasing the flow of blood from the right into the left chambers, pulmonary hypertension normally decreases the intensity of the mitral stenosis murmur.

113. Which maneuvers can be used to increase the flow across the mitral valve?

Exercise followed immediately by auscultation with the patient in left lateral decubitus definitely helps. Listening while the patient is squatting during a hand-grip maneuver also helps because of the increase in cardiac output produced by hand grip and squatting. Finally, listening to the patient while the legs are raised also may help. If straightening the legs is too difficult, one may ask the patient to raise the legs with the knees bent toward the chest. Finally, listening after the patient has coughed a few times or completed a Valsalva straining maneuver (during the release phase) also may help.

All of these maneuvers increase flow across the stenotic valve. In the olden days, amyl nitrite was used to make the murmur of mitral stenosis louder. This drug decreased peripheral resistance but also increased cardiac output and flow/gradient across the stenotic valve, thereby increasing the loudness of the murmur.

114. Which bedside maneuvers can be performed to make the murmur of mitral stenosis louder?

1. Maneuvers that bring the left ventricle closer to the stethoscope. The most common is a left lateral decubitus position.

2. Maneuvers that increase the flow across the stenotic valve also help to increase the loudness of the murmur. Ask the patient to engage in brief exercise immediately before auscultation.

3. Exhalation also may be used to increase murmur intensity. During exhalation the stethoscope is closer to the heart (because of diminished lung aeration) and blood is squeezed from the lungs into the left atrium, then into the left ventricle, thereby increasing flow across the stenotic valve.

All left-sided findings tend to increase in expiration, whereas all right-sided findings tend to increase in inspiration. The reasons are physiologically different but grounded on the same principle: increased venous return.

4. The concomitant presence of mitral regurgitation also increases the loudness of a mitral stenosis murmur independently of the pressure gradient. Mitral regurgitation increases not only left ventricular size (thereby bringing the left ventricle closer to the stethoscope) but also left atrial volume (because of regurgitation during systole). This, in turn, increases diastolic flow through the mitral valve and therefore the loudness of the MS murmur.

In general, the best bedside maneuver to increase the loudness of the mitral stenosis murmur is to place the patient in a left lateral decubitus position (which moves the left ventricle closer to the chest wall) and to listen at the end of exhalation, over the apex, and after short exercise (which increases flow across the stenotic valve). Finally, applying the bell with a light pressure also helps (a strong pressure may completely eliminate the low-frequency murmur of mitral stenosis).

115. Which conditions are associated with a softer murmur of mitral stenosis?

The most common is emphysema. A thick emphysematous chest is typically associated with muffling of the murmur, which becomes soft even in the presence of severe mitral stenosis. Similarly, low flow across the valve typically manifests with a soft murmur. Severe stenosis causes a low flow, but severe pulmonary hypertension and cardiomyopathy due to rheumatic valve disease may have the same effect. Tricuspid stenosis may be present in 5% of patients with mitral stenosis and also cause low flow across the stenotic mitral valve. Finally, a large right ventricle, which may result from pulmonary hypertension late in the course of mitral stenosis, pushes the left ventricle posteriorly away from the anterior wall and the stethoscope. Thus the murmur becomes softer. Atrial fibrillation also often softens the murmur because of its associated tachycardia and the absence of valid atrial contraction (which may increase cardiac output by about 25% in patients with significant mitral stenosis). It is also important to make sure that one is listening at the proper apical location. In mitral stenosis this site may be quite displaced; therefore, it is important to palpate the apex beat with the patient in the left lateral decubitus position before placing the stethoscope bell.

Mitral Diastolic Flow Murmur

116. What are mitral diastolic flow murmurs?

They are murmurs produced by excessive flow through a mitral valve. Thus, they are literally "flow murmurs." They may be encountered in mitral regurgitation of moderate-to-severe degree; a high alpha state, such as thyrotoxicosis; or even when the patient has a left-to-right shunt flow either at the ventricular or arterial level (VSD or PDA). The large amount of blood flowing through the pulmonary artery and reaching the left atrium creates a characteristic early diastolic flow murmur, which may resemble mitral stenosis. Such murmurs also may be heard in patients who simply have a slow heart rate, which creates a large rush of blood during diastole.

They are similar to mitral stenosis: low-pitched, rumbling in quality, and following the second sound after a slight delay. They also are heard at the apex, in the left lateral decubitus position and by using the bell. In contrast to mitral stenosis, however, such murmurs tend to occur at the same time as the S3, remaining primarily early diastolic, whereas a murmur of mitral stenosis tends to rumble through diastole and has a presystolic accentuation. Sometimes a mitral diastolic murmur can be heard in patients with acute rheumatic fever, mitral regurgitation, and cardiomegaly. It is preceded by an S3 and called a Carey Coombs murmur (from the English physician who described it in 1924). This early-to-mid diastolic murmur can be mimicked by the presence of a summation gallop, when an S3 and an S4 are so close together that they become fused and resemble a mid-diastolic sound.

Tricuspid Diastolic Murmurs

117. What is the mechanism for a tricuspid diastolic murmur?
It is the same mechanism as for the mitral valve. The tricuspid valve may be the site of stenosis and stenosis-related diastolic murmur. It also may be the site of a diastolic flow murmur in the absence of mitral stenosis.

118. Where are tricuspid diastolic murmurs mostly located?
They are usually located over the right ventricular area (epigastrium) and right and left parasternal areas. When the right ventricle is highly dilated, it may displace the left ventricle and therefore place itself over the true apex.

119. What are the most common causes of a tricuspid diastolic flow murmur?
Increased flow through the tricuspid valve may occur in atrial septal defects and thereby produce a diastolic flow murmur. In addition, a tricuspid diastolic flow murmur also may be heard in tricuspid regurgitation, again caused by increased flow. All such murmurs can be increased by exercise, such as holding up or bending the legs or taking deep inspirations (panting). The most common differential diagnosis of this diastolic flow murmur is the murmur of tricuspid stenosis. The hallmark of tricuspid stenosis is an accentuated presystolic component, which is typical of tricuspid stenosis and absent in tricuspid diastolic flow murmur. Tricuspid stenosis also tends to occur without S3, whereas the tricuspid diastolic flow murmur tends to occur with an S3.

120. How frequently does tricuspid stenosis occur?
Tricuspid stenosis may be heard in as many as 5% of patients with mitral stenosis. It is usually recorded over the same area where tricuspid diastolic flow murmurs are recorded.

121. How can one differentiate a murmur of tricuspid stenosis from a murmur of mitral stenosis?
Besides having a different location, the murmur of tricuspid stenosis tends to increase with inspiration, whereas the murmur of mitral stenosis tends to soften with inspiration. In addition, the murmur of tricuspid stenosis is louder in the right lateral decubitus position, whereas the murmur of mitral stenosis is louder in the left lateral decubitus. Finally, the murmur of mitral stenosis tends to have a low-pitched quality, whereas the murmur of tricuspid stenosis tends to have a scratchy quality. The murmur of tricuspid stenosis has no presystolic accentuation, whereas it is present in almost all murmurs of mitral stenosis.

122. Why is the murmur of tricuspid stenosis accentuated during inspiration?
This feature is common to all right-sided findings. The murmur of tricuspid stenosis increases during both held and moving inspiration. Inspiration reduces intrathoracic pressure, which has a sucking effect on venous return, thereby increasing the flow of blood across the tricuspid valve. This, in turn, leads to an increase in the intensity of the murmur.

Diastolic Semilunar Valve Murmurs

Aortic Regurgitation

123. What is the primary characteristic of a murmur of aortic regurgitation?

It tends to occur immediately after the aortic component of the second sound and has a decrescendo, tapering quality.

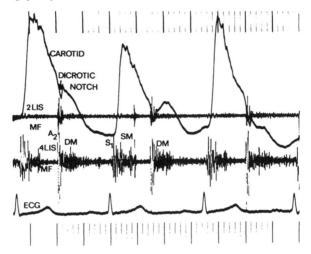

The murmur of aortic regurgitation. (From Fyler DC: Nadas' Pediatric Cardiology. Philadelphia, Hanley & Belfus, 1992, with permission.)

124. What is the typical pitch of the murmur of aortic regurgitation?

The pitch is variable, depending on the severity of regurgitation. The murmur of severe aortic regurgitation has quite a few medium- to high-pitched components. On the other hand in mild aortic regurgitation the murmur is purely high-pitched.

125. What maneuvers can be used to increase the loudness of a soft aortic regurgitation murmur?

Position. For example, ask the patient to sit up and lean forward; then press hard with the stethoscope diaphragm during held expiration. An increase in peripheral vascular resistance increases the loudness of the murmur. The same affect can be achieved by having the patient squat (which also increases peripheral vascular resistance) or by administering vasopressor agents.

126. When is the murmur best heard?

The murmur is best heard over the left sternum at what is called Erb's point (the third or fourth intercostal space). At times it can be heard in the second or third right interspace, when a tortuous and dilated aorta beyond the stenosis pushes the ascending aorta anteriorly and to the right.

127. How far into diastole does the murmur of aortic regurgitation extend?

It varies, depending on the severity of regurgitation. The murmur may extend throughout diastole or be present only in early-to-mid diastole. It starts immediately after the second sound, whereas the murmur of mitral stenosis starts after the second sound with a slight delay. Moreover, the murmur of mitral stenosis has a presystolic accentuation, whereas the murmur of aortic regurgitation does not.

128. What are the causes of aortic regurgitation?

The most common causes in adults are rheumatic heart disease, syphilis, and bicuspid aortic valve. Bicuspid valves occur in as many as 2% of men and 1% of women. Severe hypertension also may lead to aortic regurgitation of some degree (in as many as 60% of patients). In this setting, either a bicuspid aortic valve or dilation of the aortic ring is the most likely cause of the regurgitant murmur. Other causes include the aortic regurgitation associated with arthritis (such as Reiter's syndrome or ankylosing spondylitis), Marfan syndrome, and dissecting aneurysms of the ascending aorta. Infective endocarditis (often involving a bicuspid valve) also may cause acute and severe aortic regurgitation.

129. What are the auscultatory signs of sudden, severe aortic regurgitation?

As a result of sudden, severe aortic regurgitation, the left ventricle does not have enough time to expand as well as it does in chronic aortic regurgitation. Hence, the pressure in the left ventricle and diastole may rise so high and so fast that it quickly reaches the aortic diastolic pressure. Therefore, the murmur of acute aortic regurgitation is almost never holodiastolic but stops in mid diastole. Thus, the murmur is much more difficult to recognize. Usually the auscultatory sign of sudden aortic regurgitation is a softer or absent S1.

130. What is the significance of a systolic murmur associated with a murmur of aortic regurgitation?

It indicates either concomitant aortic stenosis or severe aortic regurgitation.

Pearl.   Whereas mitral regurgitation is diagnosed in systole, but its severity is assessed in diastole, aortic regurgitation is diagnosed in diastole, but its severity is best assessed in systole, looking for a companion flow murmur.

131. What is Landolfi's sign?

In aortic insufficiency, it is the systolic contraction and diastolic dilation of the pupil.

132. What is the Graham Steell murmur?

It is an early diastolic murmur of pulmonic regurgitation secondary to pulmonary hypertension. It is best heard in the second left interspace and may be indistinguishable from the murmur of aortic regurgitation. It occurs in 12% of patients with tricuspid regurgitation.

133. Who was Graham Steell?

A Scottish physician and author of a 1906 cardiology textbook that won the praise of Sir James MacKenzie. Graham Steell described the murmur that still carries his name in 1888 in the *Medical Chronicle*. Steell was an animal lover and one of the first promoters of physical exercise as the key to a long, productive life. This approach worked quite well, considering that he lived well into his nineties. He died in 1942.

PERICARDIAL FRICTION RUBS

134. What are the auscultatory characteristics of a pericardial friction rub?

A pericardial friction rub usually has three components that may resemble a murmur. One component is systolic (due to ventricular contraction) and two are diastolic (due to atrial contraction and ventricular filling). The two diastolic components occur early in diastole (at the time of the S3) and late in diastole (at the time of the S4). In other words, a rub has basically one atrial component (corresponding to atrial contraction) and two ventricular components.

The rub is usually described as a crunchy, squeaky, creaking, grading, scratching, scrapping noise. Given the presence of three components, a rub may resemble an S3 gallop. In general, the systolic component is almost always present, the atrial systolic component is often present, and the ventricular diastolic component is often absent. Rubs should be heard at the left sternal border in the third and fourth left interspace, with the patient sitting up, leaning forward, and holding the breath in inspiration to stretch the pericardium over the ventricular wall and thus increase the chance of producing the sound.

135. What are the most common causes of a pericardial friction rub?

Usually pericarditis, most commonly viral or due to lupus or uremia. The most common cause of localized pericarditis, however, is acute myocardial infarction. Neoplastic implants are another important cause of pericardial friction rubs.

BIBLIOGRAPHY

1. Abrams J: Essentials of Cardiac Physical Diagnosis. Philadelphia, Lea & Febiger, 1987.
2. Constant J: Bedside Cardiology. Boston, Little, Brown, 1976.
3. Danford D, Nasir A, Gumbiner C: Cost assessment for the evaluation of heart murmurs in children. Pediatrics 91:365–368, 1993.
4. Etchells E, Bell C, Robb K: Does this patient have an abnormal systolic murmur? JAMA 277:564–571, 1997.
5. Lembo N, Dell'Italia L, Crawford M, O'Rourke R: Bedside diagnosis of systolic murmurs. N Engl J Med 318:1572–1578, 1988.
6. Lombard JT, Selzer A: Valvular aortic stenosis. Ann Intern Med 106:292–298, 1987.
7. Perloff JK: Physical Examination of the Heart and Circulation, 2nd ed. Philadelphia, W.B. Saunders, 1990.
8. Rivera-Carvallo JM: Signo para el diagnostico de las insuficiencias tricuspideas. Arch Inst Cardiol Mex 16:531, 1946.
9. Rothman A, Goldberger AL: Aids to cardiac auscultation. Ann Intern Med 99:346–353, 1983.

13. CHEST INSPECTION, PALPATION, AND PERCUSSION

Salvatore Mangione, M.D.

According to a German physician, if the chest covered with a simple shirt is struck with the hand, it gives back a dull sound on the side where vomica is, as if one was striking a flesh piece, whereas if the chest opposite side is struck, it gives back a resonant sound, as if one was striking a drum. However, I still doubt that this information is generally correct.

Tissot SAAD, *Avis au peuple sur sa santé*. Paris, Didot le Jeune, 1782

A most violent and startling knocking was heard at the door . . . . The object that presented itself to the eyes of the astonished clerk was a boy—a wonderfully fat boy—standing upright at the mat, with his eyes closed as if in sleep. He had never seen such a fat boy, and this, coupled with the utter calmness and repose of his appearance, so very different from what was reasonably to have been expected of the inflictor of such knocks, smote him with wonder . . . . The extraordinary boy spoke not a word; but he nodded once and seemed to the clerk's imagination to snore feebly.

Charles Dickens, *Pickwick Papers*

Continued on following page

CONVENTIONAL TEACHING WATCH

Inspection, palpation, and percussion are the foundations of physical examination. Percussion is 15 years older than the United States, the brainchild of a German innkeeper's son who figured out that patients' chests behave like barrels of wine. Although ancient, these maneuvers retain considerable value. Careful use of inspection, palpation, and percussion in fact may provide valuable pieces of diagnostic information. Indeed, bedside diagnosis of lung diseases requires all of these maneuvers to yield useful information.

MANEUVERS		CONVENTIONAL TEACHING REVISITED
Modifications of respiration	⇑	Abnormal rales, depths, and rhythms of respiration provide important clues to functional status.
Use of accessory respiratory muscles	⇑	As above.
Abnormal respiratory postures	⇑	As above.
Modifications of chest morphology	⇔	Abnormalities in spinal column, ribs, and sternum are valuable clues. They often can be observed while patients are still dressed.
Abnormalities in chest surface	⇔	Look for collateral circulation and skin discolorations or hyperpigmentations.
Examination of the neck	⇑	Assessment of tracheal shift and mobility is part of chest exam.
Palpation	⇑	As above, plus assessment of hemithoracic expansion and tactile fremitus.
Percussion	⇑	A little older than the United States but still valuable.

1. What are the main components of the chest exam?

They are the same as for any other section of the physical exam: (1) inspection, (2) palpation, (3) percussion, (4) auscultation, and (5) contemplation. The last (but not least) component was added by William Osler and refers to the pondering of information gathered through the preceding four steps. Pondering was so important for Sir William that several portraits and pictures actually depict him at the bedside, deeply engrossed in his own contemplative thoughts. With the fading of bedside rounds, contemplation at the side of the patient seems to have particularly suffered, one of the latest casualties in the never-ending feud between science and art for the soul of medicine.

Pearl. *In pulmonary diseases, a bedside diagnosis usually is not achieved by auscultation alone (although it may provide important diagnostic information) but requires a comprehensive and competent performance of all parts of the chest exam. In cardiac diseases, on the other hand, diagnosis often can be achieved by auscultation only.*

INSPECTION

2. What information can be gathered through inspection?

1. Observation of the patient allows us to evaluate the vital signs of the respiratory pump, including the pattern of breathing and its three main components: (1) rate, (2) depth, and (3) rhythm.

Each of these may be abnormal, and each may be evaluated simply by observing the patient during the interview.

2. Observation of the patient before undressing also may allow identification of possible dysfunctions in lung mechanics, which usually consist of either abnormal thoracic cage morphologies or compensatory postures designed to improve the efficiency of the respiratory pump. Patients with chronic obstructive pulmonary disease (COPD), for example, tend to sit up and lean forward so that they can better tense their accessory respiratory muscles, thereby improving contractility. In these compensatory attempts patients with COPD lean forward so much that they have to prop themselves up by resting the elbows on the thighs. The protracted pressure applied by the elbows leads eventually to the formation of two patches of hyperpigmented calluses immediately above the knees (Dahl's sign).

3. Patients with COPD also may use accessory muscles of expiration (internal intercostals) and may have to breathe through pursed lips to maintain adequate intraairway pressure and prevent bronchioloalveolar collapse. Other valuable findings that can be gathered through astute observation include smoker's face (see chapter 1) and the presence of nicotine stains on the fingers, both of which are useful to spot the unrepentant smoker even before obtaining a history.

Abnormalities of Respiration

3. What are the main abnormalities in respiratory rate?

The major abnormalities are an increase and a decrease in rate. A normal respiratory rate in an adult should be 10–19 breaths per minute. **Tachypnea** indicates a faster rate, whereas **bradypnea** indicates a slower rate.

4. Can tachypnea be considered normal?

Yes and no. A respiratory rate equal to or greater than 20 breaths per minute at times is seen in elderly nursing home residents with chronic conditions but no active disease.

5. What is the clinical significance of tachypnea?

Tachypnea indicates moderate-to-severe disease of the cardiorespiratory system with a need for compensatory increase in the work of breathing. Clinically, tachypnea is usually more valuable if absent than present because it is so common in chest diseases that its presence adds relatively little information. Conversely, its absence significantly challenges a cardiac or respiratory diagnosis. For example, tachypnea is so common in pulmonary emboli (92% of patients) that its absence makes the diagnosis much less likely. In patients with an acute abdomen, on the other hand, the presence of tachypnea may direct the physician's attention to a supradiaphragmatic rather than a subdiaphragmatic process.

6. What is the clinical significance of bradypnea?

Bradypnea usually is seen in patients with hypothyroidism but also may be seen in patients with central nervous system diseases and patients taking narcotics or sedatives.

7. What is pursed-lip breathing?

It is a pattern of breathing often observed in patients with obstructive lung disease, primarily emphysema. Given their reduced lung elasticity and alveolar hyperinflation, patients with emphysema are at higher risk for airway closure and greater air trapping. As a result, they resort to pursed-lip respiration, which increases intraairway pressure by inducing auto-PEEP (positive end-expiratory pressure) and prevents expiratory airway closure. This pattern of breathing often is accompanied by audible expiratory sounds, such as wheezing or grunting (see figure at top of following page).

8. What is a rale de la mort?

The rale de la mort is a grunting and gurgling sound produced toward the end of life by patients who are unable to clear respiratory secretions. It literally means death rattle (*rale* = rattle in French). This distressing noise represents a clear sign of respiratory disease and a frequent harbinger of

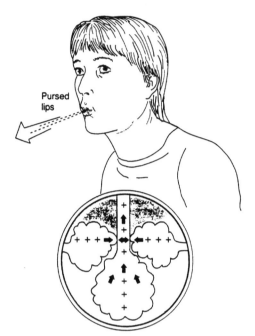

Pursed lips

Demonstration of pursed-lip breathing in patients with COPD and its effects. The weakened bronchial airways are kept open by the effects of positive pressure created by pursed lips during expiration. (From Hillegass EA, Sadowsky HS (eds): Essentials of Cardiopulmonary Physical Therapy. Philadelphia, W.B. Saunders, 1994, with permission.)

death. It is also the main culprit behind the botched respiratory sound nomenclature of Laennec (see chapter 14). In fact, he was so sensitive to the emotional overtones of the term *rale* that he eventually chose to use at the bedside the more politically correct Latin equivalent of *rhonchus*. This decision created tremendous, ongoing confusion in terminology.

9. What are the main abnormalities in depth of breathing?

1. **Hyperpnea** is characterized by an increase not only in respiratory rate but also in tidal volume. In other words, hyperpnea is rapid and deep respiration. The classic form was described by Kussmaul in patients with metabolic acidosis (primarily diabetic ketoacidosis), who attempt to compensate for pH by hyperventilating. Kussmaul's respiration is not only the hallmark of diabetic ketoacidosis but also may be observed in any of the other anion-gap metabolic acidoses, which can be recalled with the mnemonic **MAKE UP** a **L**ist: **m**ethanol poisoning, **a**spirin intoxication, **k**etoacidosis, **e**thylene glycol ingestion, **u**remia, **p**araldehyde administration, and **l**actic acidosis.

2. **Hypopnea** is characterized by shallow respirations. It is usually a hallmark of impending respiratory failure or of obesity-hypoventilation (pickwickian syndrome).

3. **Apnea** is the absence of respiration for at least 20 seconds while the patient is awake or 30 seconds while the patient is asleep. It often is seen in patients with either neuromuscular dysfunction (central apnea) or airway obstruction induced by rapid-eye-movement (REM) sleep (obstructive sleep apnea). Apnea remains the final event of all respiratory failure, whether due to pulmonary or neuromuscular disease.

10. Who was Kussmaul?

Adolf Kussmaul (1822–1902) was a graduate of Heidelberg and Würzburg (where he studied under Virchow) and a part-time army surgeon. Kussmaul was the first to describe periarteritis nodosa and progressive bulbar paralysis. He also was responsible for introducing pleural tapping and peritoneal lavage. His name is linked not only to Kussmaul's respiration but also to Kussmaul's sign, the inspiratory increase in jugular venous pressure in patients with tricuspid stenosis, constrictive pericarditis, or COPD. A meticulous and precise man, he was famous for complaining that none of his colleagues could write good German.

11. What are the main abnormalities in rhythm of respiration? What is their significance?
Abnormal rhythms of respiration usually result from lesions in the neurogenic control of the respiratory pump. They are valuable to recognize because they may help to localize the site of neurologic lesions. Moving downward in a rostrocaudal fashion from the uppermost to the lowermost neurologic center, abnormalities of respiratory rhythm are found in the following sequence:

1. Cheyne-Stokes respiration
2. Biot's respiration
3. Apneustic breathing
4. Central hyperventilation
5. Ataxic (agonal) respiration

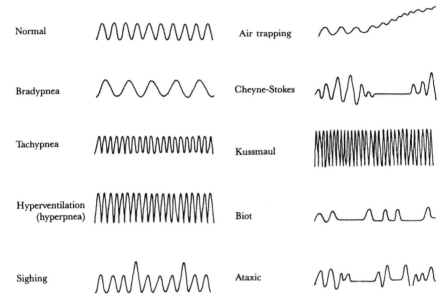

Patterns of respiration. The horizontal axis indicates the relative rates of these patterns. The vertical swings of the lines indicate the relative depth of respiration. (Adapted from Seidel HM, Ball JW, Bains JE, Benedict GW: Mosby's Guide to Physical Examination, 3rd ed. St. Louis, Mosby, 1995, with permission.)

12. What is orthopnea?
Orthopnea literally means upright respiration (from the Greek *orthos* = upright and *pneo* = breathing). Thus, orthopnea is characterized by discomfort in breathing that is brought on or aggravated by lying flat and relieved by sitting upright. It is seen most commonly in patients with congestive heart failure (primarily left-sided). Sitting upright pools blood in the dependent areas of the body, thereby decreasing venous return and reducing right- and left-ventricular preload. Orthopnea, therefore, is a quick and effective way to relieve pulmonary congestion, a poor man's phlebotomy. A patient with longstanding left-ventricular failure and history of orthopnea, however, may suddenly breathe better in the supine position if she or he has developed biventricular failure, because failure of the right ventricle provides a useful "unloading" to left-ventricular filling, thereby relieving pulmonary congestion.

13. Can orthopnea be due to lung disease?
Yes and no. Although usually the result of heart disease (as many as 95% of cases), orthopnea also may be encountered in patients with bilateral apical lung diseases, usually bullous. When such patients sit up, they increase perfusion to the lower lung fields (as a result of gravity). Because these fields are also the best ventilated (as a result of bilateral apical disease), a sitting-up position improves ventilation/perfusion matching and gas exchange. This improvement, in turn, makes the patient less dyspneic.

In patients with COPD (who often have apical bullae), sitting up improves not only gas exchange but also lung mechanics because of the increased tension applied to the accessory respiratory muscles. For this reason patients with COPD often breathe better while sitting upright and leaning forward. Patients unconsciously choose a position in which they can support their arms, fix their shoulder and neck muscles, and therefore help the respiratory muscles. They do so by sitting up and either clasping the side of the bed or pushing over their thighs (see Dahl's sign, question 2).

Orthopnea is also an important sign of asthma severity. In fact, when present at the time of initial emergency department evaluation, it is a good predictor of poor outcome. Patients who cannot lie flat have worse pulmonary function and a greater need for admission. The same is true for the presence of diaphoresis. Both findings were reported by Brenner in acute asthmatics and represent the scientific validation of the time-honored dictum that patients who "do not look good" (usually because they are sweaty and upright) tend to do poorly.

14. What is PND?

PND is paroxymsal nocturnal dyspnea, which consists of a spell (paroxysm) of acute dyspnea (air hunger) occurring at night, usually after an hour or two of sleep. The patient wakes up, sits upright, puts his or her legs down the side of the bed, often opens the window to catch some fresh air, and after a few minutes feels better and goes back to sleep.

The key, of course, is the upright posture, not the cold, fresh air (although cold air blowing in the face of the patient has been shown to give a refreshing feeling in cases of cardiac or pulmonary disease). Upright posture effectively decreases venous return, thereby reducing pulmonary capillary pressure and lung congestion. PND is, therefore, a sign of left-ventricular failure but, similar to orthopnea, also may be seen in pulmonary patients (usually with bullous bilateral apical disease). Basilar perfusion and lung mechanics are improved when patients sit upright and lean forward.

15. What is platypnea?

Platypnea, the opposite of orthopnea, literally means supine respiration (from the Greek *platy* = flat and *pneo* = respiration). Platypnea is difficulty with breathing in the erect position; it is relieved promptly by recumbency. Indeed, patients with platypnea feel much better when supine. Platypnea often is associated with orthodeoxia, which is a hemoglobin oxygen desaturation produced by upright posture.

16. What causes platypnea?

Unlike orthopnea, platypnea is not due to cardiac disease but to a bilateral pulmonary process. This process is a disease of the lower lobes rather than the upper lobes (as with orthopnea). An upright posture increases perfusion to the lower lobes and therefore worsens ventilation/perfusion (V/Q) matching. This, in turn, leads to orthodeoxia and dyspnea. Conversely, a supine posture improves V/Q matching and relieves dyspnea.

Platypnea has been described not only in patients with multiple recurrent pulmonary emboli (which, because of gravity, tend to involve primarily the lung bases) but also in patients with pleural effusion or bibasilar pneumonia (both of which tend to cause bibasilar atelectasis because of accumulation in the dependent portions of the chest). Platypnea also has been described in cirrhosis (as a result of bibasilar arteriovenous shunting) and atrial septal defect. The latter leads to platypnea only when associated with an increase in pulmonary vascular pressure, as may be caused by surgical resection (lobectomy, pneumonectomy) or pleural effusion. This increase in pulmonary pressure, in turn, increases the right-to-left shunt, thereby making the patient more dyspneic. An upright posture makes the shunt easier by anatomically redirecting the blood toward the atrial septum. A supine posture has the opposite effect.

17. What is trepopnea?

Trepopnea literally means twisted respiration (from the Greek *trepo* = twisted and *pneo* = breathing). It is characterized by the patient's inability to lie supine or prone and by preference for a lateral decubitus position.

18. What is the meaning of "down with the good lung"?

It is a less fancy term for trepopnea. "Down with the good lung" refers to patients who can breathe better in the lateral decubitus position with the good lung in a dependent position because gravity increases perfusion to the dependent lung. If the dependent lung is the good lung (in unilateral lung disease), the patient has better V/Q matching, better oxygenation, and more comfortable respiration.

19. In which conditions should the patient lie with the good lung in a dependent position?

All such conditions involve unilateral disease. The classic example is unilateral lung collapse due to either an endobronchial obstructing lesion or massive pleural effusion, which compresses the lung extrinsically. In both processes the patient feels better and has improved oxygenation with the good lung in the dependent position. Conversely, in unilateral lung diseases in which pus or blood may spill from the bad into the good lung (such as pneumonia or alveolar hemorrhages), lying with the good lung in a dependent position is highly detrimental. Patients with such diseases in fact should lie with the bad lung in a dependent position. Protection of the good lung against intrabronchial spillage is more important than improved oxygenation. Finally, lying with the good lung in a dependent position is *not* physiologically beneficial in small children with unilateral lung disease; in fact, it is detrimental.

20. What are respiratory alternans and abdominal paradox?

They are abnormalities in the function of the respiratory pump characterized by muscular weakness and fatigue, involving primarily the diaphragm but also the intercostal muscles. Paradoxical respiration (abdominal paradox) reflects the fact that both chest and abdomen usually rise in inspiration (as a result of lung expansion and contraction of the diaphragm, which pushes down the abdominal content). Conversely, in paradoxical respiration the abdomen does not rise in inspiration but instead collapses. Both signs can be detected by simple inspection. Even better, they can be detected by laying one hand over the chest of the patient and the other over the abdomen and observing their rocking motion.

21. Can inspection identify an asymmetry in thoracic expansion?

Yes, although not as effectively as palpation (see below). Asynchronies and asymmetries in expansion between the two hemithoraces occur in many lung conditions, such as atelectasis, severe pneumonia, and pleural effusion. Yet it is only in severe conditions (such as a large pneumothorax, complete lung collapse, or massive pleural effusion) that the degree of change in the volume of one hemithorax is large enough to be detectable by inspection alone. Protracted lung collapse may even lead to a deviation in spinal curvature, causing a concavity toward the side of disease.

Pearl.   The best way to detect asynchrony and asymmetry in expansion of the two hemithoraces by inspection alone is to ask the patient to inhale deeply while the examiner looks for local lagging in chest expansion. Such lags are undetectable during quiet respiration.

Abnormalities of the Chest Cage

22. What type of information about the chest cage should be gathered through inspection?

The morphology of the chest cage and its three main components: (1) spine, (2) ribs, and (3) sternum. Some of this information can be gathered from fully clothed patients during the interview.

23. What are the main chest cage abnormalities?

Chest cage abnormalities vary, depending on whether they affect the spine, sternum, or rib cage. Often more than one component of the chest cage is involved.

1. If the **spine** is affected, abnormalities may be on either the sagittal or frontal plane (see below).

2. If the **sternum** is affected, possible abnormalities include pigeon chest and barrel chest, both of which may alter lung mechanics severely enough to affect lung function adversely.

- **Pigeon chest**: a flattening on either side of the chest with forward projection of the sternum so that it resembles the keel of a ship (= *carina* in Latin; hence the term pectus carinatum). Although this abnormality occasionally is associated with specific diseases (such as rickets, acromegaly, or Marfan syndrome), it is more commonly familial or sporadic.
- **Funnel chest:** the opposite of pigeon chest. It is characterized by a backward displacement of the xiphoid cartilage with hollowing of the lower part of the chest (pectus excavatum, which is Latin for hollow chest). This abnormality also may be isolated or associated with other diseases (such as rickets, Marfan or Noonan syndrome). Because of the retraction of the distal portion of the sternum, a funnel chest may impinge mechanically on the heart, possibly leading to arrhythmias or even mitral valve prolapse.

3. If the **ribs** are affected, the most common abnormality is related to slope and shape (see below).

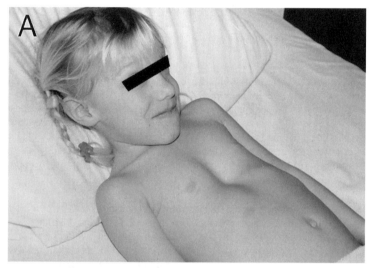

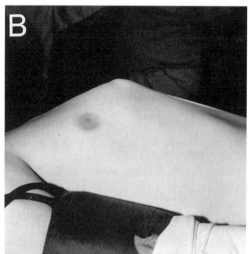

Pectus excavatum *(A)* and pectus carinatum *(B)*. (From James EC, Corry RJ, Perry JF: Principles of Basic Surgical Practice. Philadelphia, Hanley & Belfus, 1987, with permission.)

24. Which modifications of the spinal column can be detected by inspection?

1. **Abnormalities on the sagittal plane:** either increased convexity of the spin (lordosis) or increased concavity (kyphosis). Both may be present in the same patient.

2. **Abnormalities on the frontal plane:** mostly lateral curvatures of the spine, also called scoliosis (from the Greek word for crookedness). Depending on the etiology, scoliosis may be characterized by only one curvature or by a primary and a secondary curvature (the secondary curve has a compensatory function). Scoliosis may be fixed (as a result of muscle and/or bone deformity) or mobile (as a result of unequal muscle contraction).

Most patients actually have a combination of kyphosis, lordosis, and scoliosis.

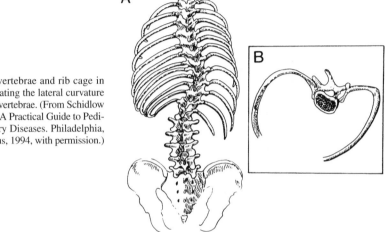

Deformity of vertebrae and rib cage in scoliosis illustrating the lateral curvature and rotation of vertebrae. (From Schidlow DV, Smith DS: A Practical Guide to Pediatric Respiratory Diseases. Philadelphia, Hanley & Belfus, 1994, with permission.)

25. What are the consequences of spinal column abnormalities?

The consequences may be quite dramatic. In fact, if severe enough, any of the above abnormalities can compromise respiratory mechanics sufficiently to cause profound derangement in ventilation. The resulting V/Q mismatch may lead to hypoxemia, pulmonary hypertension, and right-sided congestive heart failure. Kyphoscoliosis (scoliosis associated with kyphosis), for example, may be severe enough to lead to cor pulmonale.

26. How common is kyphoscoliosis?

Very common—and becoming more so as the population ages and osteoporosis becomes an increasing menace. The incidence of spinal deformities in the U.S. is 1 in 1000 for mild cases and 1 in 10,000 for severe cases. As a result, it is quite common to encounter on the medical wards delightful little old patients (usually women) with cor pulmonale due to severe spine deformity. In the compassionate jargon of busy house officers, such patients are often called "pretzel ladies."

27. What are the most common causes of kyphoscoliosis?

Idiopathic

Neuromuscular
　Muscular dystrophy
　Poliomyelitis
　Cerebral palsy
　Friedreich ataxia

Vertebral
　Osteoporosis
　Osteomalacia
　Vitamin D-resistant rickets

Vertebral *(continued)*
　Tuberculous spondylitis
　Neurofibromatosis

Disorders of connective tissue
　Marfan syndrome
　Ehlers-Danlos syndrome
　Morquio syndrome

Thoracic cage abnormality
　Thoracoplasty
　Empyema

28. What is a gibbus?

Gibbus is the Latin word for hump or hunch, the lay terms for a spinal deformity character-ized by a sharply angulated segment with the apex of the angle pointing posteriorly. In medical terminology, a hunchback or humpback is a patient with extreme kyphosis.

29. How clinically significant are chest cage abnormalities?

Quite significant. Indeed, anatomic abnormalities of one or more chest cage components may lead to hypoventilation of selected areas of the lung. This, in turn, may lead to localized pul-monary vasoconstriction. If severe enough, vasoconstriction eventually leads to pulmonary hy-pertension and cor pulmonale.

Pearl.   *Chest cage abnormalities are among the few conditions that may result in cor pulmo-nale in patients with entirely normal lungs. The others are obesity-hypoventilation and sleep apnea.*

30. What kind of rib abnormalities can be detected by inspection?

1. The **slope** of the ribs is normally oblique at a 45° angle. Patients with emphysema or status asthmaticus may horizontalize the slope. This deformity may be severe enough that the anteropos-terior (AP) diameter of the chest becomes almost equal to the transverse diameter. A chest so shaped is usually called a **barrel chest**. This sign has an interobserver reliability of about 70% and may be due to the fact that emphysematous patients tend to be so underweight that their flattened bellies and abnormally decreased AP diameter give the illusion of an increased transverse diameter. A horizontal slope of the ribs may compromise lung function by making ventilation less efficient.

2. The **shape** of the ribs may become quite deformed as a result of thickening of the osseous-cartilaginous junction. Rib deformities of this kind carry the name **rachitic rosary** because they are common in rickets and because the two lines of beading across the costochondral junction re-semble a rosary. Another rib abnormality typically encountered in rickets is a groove in the thorax extending laterally from the xiphoid process to the axillae. This deformity was first described in 1798 by the English physician Edwin Harrison and is still called Harrison's groove (see below).

31. Does chest examination allow adequate assessment of kyphoscoliosis?

No. It allows detection of the abnormality but is of little value in quantifying severity and degree. To do so, one must rely on chest radiography and determination of the Cobb angle of sco-liosis, which can be calculated by drawing two lines parallel to the upper border of the highest and the lower border of the lowest vertebral bodies of the primary curvature, as seen on an AP film of the spine. The angle is measured at the intersection points of lines drawn perpendicular to the original lines. A Cobb angle > 100° is considered a severe deformity and may be used to pre-dict the risk of developing pulmonary hypertension and respiratory failure.

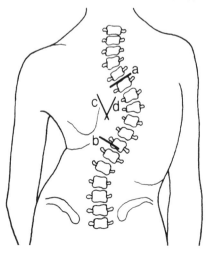

How to draw and measure the Cobb angle. (From Staheli LT: Pediatric Orthopaedic Secrets. Philadelphia, Hanley & Belfus, 1998, with permission.)

32. Why is it important to observe the characteristics of the chest surface?

To identify specific disorders. Both skin and chest surface can yield valuable clues:

1. The **color** of the skin helps to identify patients with ineffective oxygenation and/or ventilation. Cyanosis is a hallmark of hypoventilation or ineffective ventilation, whereas pallor, diaphoresis, and agitation are hallmarks of ineffective oxygenation. An increase in carbon dioxide acts as a depressor, whereas a decrease in oxygen acts as a stressor.

2. Patients with lung dysfunction who are hypercapnic also may exhibit **asterixis** (flapping tumor) and **clubbing**. Clubbing is a feature not only of lung diseases but also of several chronic inflammatory conditions not necessarily limited to the lungs (see chapter 23). In fact, clubbing has been described in patients with infective endocarditis, lung abscess, bronchiectasis, and even amyloidosis. It also has been described in chronic inflammatory conditions of the intestine, such as Crohn's disease and ulcerative colitis. Although it has been described in patients with hypercapnia (and therefore patients with chronic bronchitis), clubbing is *not* a feature of emphysema. Clubbing has been described in patients with hypoxemia due to shunts, whether cardiogenic or pulmonary in nature, and in patients with sex hormone imbalance, such as pregnant women and cirrhotics. Finally, clubbing has been described in patients with lung cancer.

3. Patients who are hyperpigmented over the chest with tightly drawn skin and multiple telangiectasias often have areas of **hyper- and hypopigmentation** and patches of vitiligo. Such patients are likely to have abnormal hands and fingers and a tight mouth opening. All of these features are typical of scleroderma and important to recognize because they are clues to severe underlying lung diseases, such as vasculitis with pulmonary hypertension and cor pulmonale.

33. How much information can be gathered through inspection of the neck?

Quite a bit. Inspection of the neck is, in fact, an integral part of the chest exam and should be included in the evaluation of all patients with pulmonary diseases.

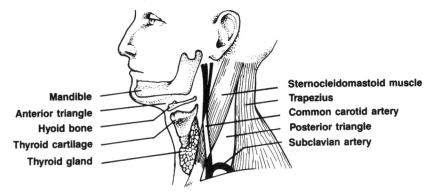

Mandible
Anterior triangle
Hyoid bone
Thyroid cartilage
Thyroid gland

Sternocleidomastoid muscle
Trapezius
Common carotid artery
Posterior triangle
Subclavian artery

Surface anatomy of the lateral neck region. (From James EC, Corry RJ, Perry JF: Principles of Basic Surgical Practice. Philadelphia, Hanley & Belfus, 1987, with permission.)

The first step is to assess whether the accessory muscles of respiration (such as the scalene, sternocleidomastoid, and trapezius) are being used and whether they appear hypertrophic. Hypertrophy is a valuable sign of increase in work of breathing, as may be seen in patients with chronic lung diseases. The scalene tends to be used before the sternocleidomastoid; both are used in patients exhibiting retractions.

Use of the sternocleidomastoid leads to an upward motion of the clavicle during inspiration. Upward motion in excess of 5 mm is a valuable sign of severe obstructive disease. In acute asthma an upward movement of the clavicles has been correlated with severity of airflow obstruction. In fact, it is clinically detectable when the forced expiratory volume in one second (FEV_1) falls below 1 liter. Inspiratory retractions of the suprasternal and supraclavicular fossa also may be seen in patients who have excessive swings in intrathoracic pressures, such as those with COPD. The mechanism is the same as for retraction of the intercostal spaces.

Finally, inspection of the neck should include evaluation of the neck veins. Distention of neck veins can be seen in patients with superior vena cava syndrome and often is associated with swelling of face, neck, shoulders, and even hands. Distention of the neck veins also may be seen in patients with right-sided heart failure or biventricular failure and can be elicited by applying pressure over the abdomen (hepatojugular reflux). An increase in venous filling during expiration is a sign of positive intrathoracic pressure and therefore is seen in patients with COPD. Conversely, an increase in venous filling during inspiration is a sign of obstruction to right-ventricular filling and therefore is seen in patients with obstruction of the superior vena cava, tricuspid stenosis, constrictive pericarditis, or pulmonary hypertension (Kussmaul sign).

34. What information can be gathered from the remainder of chest inspection?

1. Focal expiratory bulging of the intercostal spaces is seen in patients with pneumothorax. Diffuse expiratory bulging is seen in patients with obstructive disease. Focal inspiratory sinking (tirage) is seen in patients with focal airway obstruction. Diffuse tirage is seen in patients with upper airway obstruction.

2. Areas of collateral circulation may be seen over the chest wall of patients with obstructions in either the superior or inferior vena cava. Impeded venous return leads to cephalad or caudad formation of collateral vessels.

3. Dermatomic herpes zoster lesions.

4. Chest wall fistulas may be seen in patients with empyema necessitatis, a form of empyema in which pus burrows to the outside, producing a subcutaneous abscess that finally ruptures. The drainage may be beneficial, allowing relief of a closed-space infection and often spontaneous recovery.

5. The posture of the patient (such as an obligatory orthopnea; see above).

6. Nasal flaring (outward inspiratory motion of the nares) is a valuable sign of respiratory distress.

7. Pursed lip respiration (see above).

8. Finally, throughout inspection the physician should observe whether the patient coughs, sighs, or has any pain accompanying coughing, hiccuping, or sighing.

PALPATION

35. What are the main components of palpation of the chest?

1. Assessment of the trachea
2. Assessment of vocal tactile fremitus
3. Assessment of expansion of the hemithoraces, with attention to possible asymmetries and asynchronies.

36. What is the clinical value of palpation?

1. To supplement information gathered through inspection, either confirming or rejecting it, through palpation of the trachea and assessment of expansion of the hemithoraces. Both maneuvers provide valuable information about lung anatomy and chest mechanics.

2. To provide new information related to lung parenchyma and pleura, primarily through assessment of the vocal tactile fremitus.

37. How do you assess the trachea?

By assessing shifts and mobility.

38. How do you assess tracheal shifts?

By inserting your small finger into the pouch between the medial end of the sternocleidomastoid muscle and the lateral aspect of the trachea. By doing so, you find a little recess that can be easily probed by the tip of your finger. With the patient sitting up and leaning forward with head straight, the recesses should be symmetric. If not (i.e., the pouch is larger on one side than on the other), the patient has a tracheal shift. A smaller pouch on the left indicates shift of the trachea toward the left and vice versa.

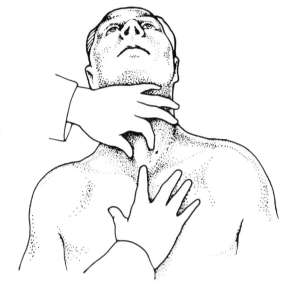

Palpation of the trachea (tracheal shift). (From James EC, Corry RJ, Perry JF: Principles of Basic Surgical Practice. Philadelphia, Hanley & Belfus, 1987, with permission.)

39. What are possible causes of a tracheal shift?

The two major causes are (1) an increase in the volume of the contralateral lung or (2) a decrease in the volume of the ipsilateral lung. A decrease in volume is usually due to atelectasis, whereas an increase in volume may be seen in patients with pneumothorax, large pleural effusions, or severe consolidation. Palpation of the trachea without the other steps of chest examination is usually unable to identify the reasons for a shift.

40. How do you assess mobility of the trachea?

1. **Spontaneous mobility** consists of a rostrocaudal tug of the trachea, which is synchronous with each heartbeat (Oliver's sign). It is usually a sign of a large and aneurysmatic aortic arch that overrides the left main bronchus and pulls down the tracheobronchial tree at each cardiac contraction.

2. **Induced mobility** consists of pushing the trachea sideward to see if indeed it is mobile. A rigid and fixed trachea indicates upper mediastinal fibrosis, which is often a sequela of mediastinitis but also may be seen in patients with carcinomatosis.

41. What is the significance of a tracheal descent with inspiration?

Tracheal descent with inspiration (Campbell's sign) usually suggests chronic airflow obstruction. It is best felt by placing the tip of the index finger on the thyroid cartilage during inspiration. Campbell's sign correlates well with severity of airflow obstruction and duration of symptoms but is not specific for COPD. It also may be seen in any patient with acute respiratory distress.

42. What is vocal tactile fremitus?

Vocal tactile fremitus (VCT) is the Latin for palpable thrill produced by the patient's voice. VCT can be detected by placing the hand sequentially over various areas of the chest and feeling the thrill transmitted through the chest whenever the patient voices sounds. Most commonly the patient is asked to say "E" or "1, 2, 3" or even "99." It really does not matter what you ask the patient to say, but it is important to understand the physiology behind the thrill. In VCT the larynx generates the sound. The acoustic signal is then transmitted downward along the tracheobronchial tree through the pleura, pleural cavity, and chest wall and eventually upward into the hand of the examiner. Any abnormality along this path may compromise transmission, thus creating a softer and less palpable thrill. For example, an obstruction in a distal bronchus (due to either tumor or mucus plug), a large collection of fluid or air in the pleural space, or even thick skin compromises transmission of the fremitus and makes it softer.

43. Can any disease process increase the VCT?

Yes—alveolar pneumonia (i.e., a rim of fluid-filled tissue surrounding a patent bronchial tree). Fluids or solids around a patent airway transmit sound better than air (in old western movies the arrival of the cavalry was heard first on the ground, then in the air). For this reason an area of alveolar consolidation (such as a patch of pneumonia) increases the VCT. However, if the pneumonia involves not only the alveoli but also the bronchi (bronchopneumonia), as is typically seen in pulmonary infections with *Hemophilus influenzae*, bronchial mucus plugs dampen the transmission of the tactile fremitus and make it softer.

The hallmark of a tactile fremitus is the difference between the two sides of the chest. Therefore, each side should be compared carefully, level by level. Detection of a localized area of abnormality (whether with an increased or decreased fremitus) is key to diagnosis.

Pearl. *Pneumonia increases VCT only if it is alveolar; it decreases VCT if it is broncho-alveolar.*

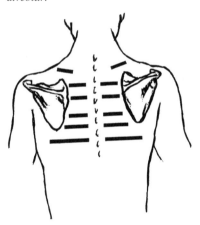

Locations on the the posterior aspect of the chest for evaluating tactile fremitus. (Adapted from Swartz MH: Textbook of Physical Diagnosis, 3rd ed. Philadelphia, W.B. Saunders, 1997.)

44. How good is agreement among physicians for evaluation of VCT?

Not too good. Two studies suggest that agreement among physicians about VCT is a little better than chance. Agreement among physicians for chest findings detected by inspection also has been shown to be poor. Both areas of physical examination have high inter- or intraobserver variability.

45. What information can be gathered through assessment of expansion of hemithoraces?

Palpation may allow the assessment of the synchrony and symmetry of expansion. A lag suspected on inspection is confirmed by palpation of both hemithoraces during respiration. Similarly, abnormalities in respiration (such as respiratory alternans or paradoxical respiration) can be confirmed with this maneuver. Therefore, palpation may confirm an abnormal respiratory dynamic that is suspected on inspection by observing the flaring of the nostrils, pursed-lip respiration, asynchrony in chest or abdominal movements, or use of accessory muscles.

46. Describe the technique for assessing expansion of hemithoraces.

Stand behind the patient, and grab both hemithoraces with your open and extended hands, laying your palms on the chest wall. Ask the patient to exhale while closing in with your hands and juxtaposed thumbs. On subsequent deep inspiration, your thumbs will move outward, acting as pointers to the degree of expansion, symmetry, and synchrony of the two hemithoraces.

47. What is Hoover's sign?

Hoover's sign often is seen in patients with COPD. The diaphragm is sufficiently flattened that both costal margins are drawn toward the medial line during inspiration. Because the contraction of the diaphragm pulls the ribs inward and medially during inspiration, the subcostal angle (i.e., the angle between the xiphoid process and right or left costal margins) becomes more acute. Hoover's sign also is called Hoover's groove (see above) because sometimes the examiner can observe a groove when the flattened diaphragm pulls inward. Hoover's groove typically is described in rachitic children as a constant groove occurring independently of respiration. Hoover's sign in COPD, on the other hand, occurs only during inspiration.

48. What are the other goals of palpation?

1. Palpation should identify areas of tenderness over the chest, ribs, or sternum. Tenderness may be seen in costochondritis (Tietze syndrome) and is an important sign in patients with atypical chest sign. Intercostal spaces and ribs also should be palpated to detect tumors.

2. Palpation should identify areas of crepitation (indicative of subcutaneous emphysema).

3. Palpation should identify areas of fluctuation or even fistulization (empyema necessitatis; see above).

4. Finally, palpation of the thorax is important to detect large lymph nodes and to assess systematically the supraclavicular and axillary fossae.

PERCUSSION

49. What is the value of percussion?

Although much less studied than auscultation, percussion remains a key component of the chest exam. Laennec suggested that percussion should complement auscultation in the differential diagnosis of emphysema, pneumothorax, and pleural effusion.

50. Who invented chest percussion?

An Austrian physician named Leopold Auenbrugger, a part-time musician who even wrote a libretto for Antonio Salieri (Mozart's rival). Auenbrugger was the son of an Austrian innkeeper and as a child used to help tap barrels of wine to see whether whether they were full or empty. Auenbrugger soon realized that patients' chests may well behave like barrels if appropriately percussed. In 1761 he published a small treatise of less than 100 pages, written in Latin, in which he suggested that by percussion alone a physician can obtain in the alive patient information about pathology that previously was confined to the autopsy table. As often happens with major revolutions in science, the book came out with a whimper, not a bang. Some authorities even ridiculed it. Percussion, however, was a major breakthrough and signaled the dawn of the golden age of physical diagnosis. In fact, until the invention of the stethoscope it was the only way for physicians to predict pathology in the alive patient.

Nonetheless, percussion remained silent for 50 years. It was rediscovered at the beginning of the nineteenth century by a charismatic and pompous Frenchman who also was Napoleon's personal physician. Baron Jean N. Corvisart became so enamored of this technique that he used it religiously during morning rounds to predict diseases that otherwise would have been found in afternoon autopsies. These predictions had remarkable accuracy and helped to establish percussion as the standard for bedside diagnosis. Incidentally, Corvisart taught percussion to Laennec, and Laennec, unsatisfied with the technique, developed a new diagnostic method: auscultation.

51. What is the physics behind percussion?

The physics is based on delivering a fixed amount of energy to the chest wall. The chest reflects this energy as a sound wave. The characteristics of this sound wave (amplitude and frequencies) are inversely related, and their product is constant. Both depend on the characteristics of the percussed tissues. In other words, the reflected sound has either high frequency and low amplitude or low frequency and high amplitude, depending on the characteristics of the underlying tissues:

1. *If the tissues are rich in air and poor in solid or fluid* (high air/fluid ratio), the percussion note is characterized by high amplitude and low frequency and is called a *resonant* percussion note. It is relatively loud and typical of the normal lung.

2. *If air is more abundant than normal,* the percussion note is called *hyperresonant or tympanic*. It has greater amplitude and lower frequency than a normal resonant percussion note. A hyperresonant note can be elicited by percussing the gastric bulla or a puffed cheek. It also can be heard in patients with pneumothorax, emphysema, or big blebs.

3. *If the tissue ratio between air and fluid/solid is low* (i.e., there is more fluid/solid than air), the percussion note is called *flat or dull*. It is characterized by high frequency and low amplitude and therefore is perceived as soft. This is the percussion note of consolidation, lung collapse, or pleural effusion.

Percussion can be accomplished by applying only the distal tip of the middle finger to the chest, lifting the other fingers (so that they will not dampen the vibrations), and gently percussing with the middle finger at a 90° angle the distal tip of the other middle finger, using the wrist as a fulcrum. Percussion provides valuable information that can be added to the data gathered through inspection and palpation.

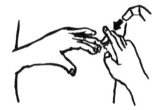

Method for percussion. (Adapted from DeGowin RL: DeGowin and DeGowin's Diagnostic Examination, 6th ed. New York, McGraw-Hill, 1994.)

Features of the Percussion Note

RELATIVE PITCH	RELATIVE INTENSITY	PERCUSSION NOTE
Low	Loud	Resonant
Lower	Very loud	Hyperresonant
Medium	Medium	Dull
High	Soft	Flat

52. What is direct percussion? Indirect percussion?

Direct percussion is Auenbrugger's original technique, which he developed while working in the Spanish Military Hospital of Vienna to guide thoracentesis. His technique consisted of striking a clothed chest with the tips of all fingers firmly held together. At times Auenbrugger even used a leather glove to strike the bare skin. Through this technique he came to observe that a healthy thorax is resonant, whereas an abnormal chest has either a higher- or lower-pitched sound. Percussion remained a medical curiosity without much support until it was made a standard part of bedside exam by Corvisart (who used the direct method of Auenbrugger).

The technique of **mediated or indirect percussion** was developed in 1828 by the French physician Piorry. It consisted of percussing the chest not directly but through a solid body applied to the chest wall. This solid body, called a plessimeter, was supposed to be made of ivory, 5 cm in diameter and 2.5 mm in thickness. Many plessimeters were literally screwed to the end of one of Laennec's stethoscopes to avoid their loss (which was common). William Stokes and James Hope, who had listened to Piorry's lessons, simplified this method by using their left middle finger as a plessimeter. Although disliked by Piorry, this variation eventually became the standard throughout Europe, thanks primarily to the influence of Skoda, who had become the chief advocate of mediated percussion. Skoda described the four major types of percussion note still taught today.

53. What is the current role of direct percussion?

It is still used at times as a quick screening exam. One form of direct percussion uses the clavicles as plessimeters to assess the lung apices.

54. Is there any difference between the percussion note of consolidation due to pneumonia and the percussion note of lung collapse secondary to pleural effusion?

Theoretically yes, practically no. Osler wrote that "the dullness of a pleural effusion has a peculiarly resistant, wooden quality, which is different from that of pneumonia and that can be readily recognized by skilled fingers." With all due respect for Sir William and his insistence on the role of the tactile sense in percussion, our ability to differentiate dull from flat is limited at best.

55. What is auscultatory percussion?

Auscultatory percussion is a modified variety of percussion developed by John Guarino. It consists of tapping lightly over the manubrium of the sternum with the distal tip of one finger while listening with the stethoscope over the chest wall posteriorly. A decrease in sound amplitude is considered a sign of lung abnormality. Guarino was able to detect lesions < 2 cm in diameter (which are almost impossible to detect with conventional bidigital percussion). Studies to confirm this technique, however, have produced conflicting results. Thus, no solid evidence suggests that auscultatory percussion should replace more traditional methods of percussion.

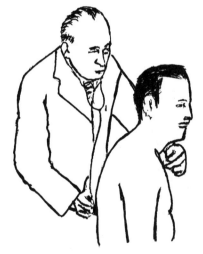

Method of auscultatory percussion. (Adapted from The Lancet, June 21, 1980, p. 1333.)

56. Summarize the role of the various techniques of chest examination in the diagnosis of disease.

Chest Examination Findings and Disease Processes

DISEASE	TRACHEA	FREMITUS	PERCUSSION NOTE	BREATH SOUNDS	ADVENT. BREATH SOUNDS	TRANSM. BREATH SOUNDS
Normal lung	Midline	Normal	Resonant	Vesicular	Late-inspiratory crackles at bases (resolve with deep breaths)	Absent

Table continued on following page

Chest Examination Findings and Disease Processes (Continued)

DISEASE	TRACHEA	FREMITUS	PERCUSSION NOTE	BREATH SOUNDS	ADVENT. BREATH SOUNDS	TRANSM. BREATH SOUNDS
Consolidation (pneumonia, hemorrhage)	Midline	Increased	Dull	Bronchial	Late-inspiratory crackles	All present
Pulmonary fibrosis	Midline	Normal/ increased	Resonant	Bronchovesciular	Late-inspiratory crackles	Absent
Bronchiectasis	Midline	Normal	Resonant	Vesicular	Mid-inspiratory crackles	Absent
Bronchitis	Midline	Normal	Normal to hyperresonant	Vesicular	Early-inspiratory crackles Possible rhonchi and wheezes	Absent
Emphysema	Midline	Decreased	Hyperresonant	Diminished vesicular	Usually-absent	Absent
Large pleural effusion	Shifted to opposite side	Absent	Flat	Bronchial immediately above effusion Absent over effusion	? Rub above effusion	May be present above effusion Absent over effusion
Pneumothorax	Shifted to opposite side	Absent	Tympanic	Absent	Absent	Absent
Atelectasis (patent bronchi)	Shifted to same side	Increased	Dull	Bronchial	Absent	All present
Atelectasis (plugged bronchi)	Shifted to same side	Absent	Dull	Absent	Absent	Absent
Status asthmaticus	Midline	Decreased	Hyperresonant	Vesicular	Inspiratory/ expiratory wheezes	Absent

BIBLIOGRAPHY

1. Maitre B, Similowski T, Derenne JP: Physical examination of the adult patient with respiratory diseases: Inspection and palpation. Eur Respir J 8:1756–1760, 1995.
2. McGee SR: Percussion and physical diagnosis: Separating myth from science. Dis Mon 41:641– 692, 1995.
3. Thompson DT: The art of percussion and auscultation of the chest reexamined. S Afr Med J 55:24–28, 1979.
4. Yernault JC, Bohadana AB: Chest percussion. Eur Respir J 8:1756–1760, 1995.

14. LUNG AUSCULTATION

Salvatore Mangione, M.D.

Those who advise that all stethoscopes should be "scrapped" may be influenced by the fact that they do not know how to use their own.

Sir James Kingston Fowler of the Brompton Hospital

Auscultation of breathing sounds with a cylinder (stethoscope) produces easily interpreted auditory signals capable of indicating the presence and extent of most disorders of organs in the thoracic cage.

Laennec RTH: Treatise on diseases of the chest in which they are described according to their anatomical characters and their diagnoses, established on a new principle by means of acoustic instruments. London, England, C. Underwood, 1821 [translated by Forbes JT, Underwood C].

TOPICS COVERED IN THIS CHAPTER

CONVENTIONAL TEACHING WATCH

Lung auscultation has suffered from a complex, confusing, and onomatopoeic terminology that goes back to Laennec. Recently, however, application of computer technology has rekindled this time-honored art. Even though we have granted most of these signs and findings a high pass, there is also little doubt that the clinical value of pulmonary auscultation is overall lower than that of cardiac auscultation. It is still quite valuable, however, even in our age of expensive and sophisticated diagnostic technology.

SOUNDS AND EXTRA SOUNDS		CONVENTIONAL TEACHING REVISITED
Vesicular breath sounds	⇔	Still informative and valuable, albeit not as much as the tubular sounds
Breath sound intensity (BSI)	⇑	Helpful in the assessment of airflow obstruction, whether monitored at the mouth or over the chest
Tubular breath sounds	⇑	Important clue to consolidation
Amphoric breath sounds	⇔	Rather specific but not sensitive indicator of cavitary disease
Bronchovesicular breath sounds	⇓	Do they really exist?
Crackles	⇑	The most valuable of all extra sounds. Remember to time and count them.
Crackles modifiers	⇓	A thing of the past, except for "fine" and "coarse"
Rales	⇓	As above
Posturally induced crackles	⇑	Important both diagnostically and prognostically
Wheezes	⇑	A little overrated, but still valuable
T_w/T_{tot}	⇑	The best way to assess severity of bronchospasm
Forced expiratory wheezes	⇓	Neither sensitive nor specific for the diagnosis of asthma

(Table continued on following page.)

SOUNDS AND EXTRA SOUNDS		CONVENTIONAL TEACHING REVISITED
Pleural rub	⇑	Important, although fleeting and at times difficult to recognize
Whispered pectoriloquy	⇑	Probably the most helpful (together with egophony) of all transmitted voice sounds
Egophony	⇑	As above
E-to-A changes	⇑	A variety of egophony
Bronchophony	⇔	Not as sensitive for consolidation as egophony or whispered pectoriloquy

1. Who invented lung auscultation?

Lung auscultation of the *direct* or immediate variety (that is, without the use of the stethoscope) has actually been known for a long time. References to breath sounds are in fact present in the Ebers papyrus (c. 1500 BC), the Hindu Vedas (c. 1400–1200 BC), and the Hippocratic writings.[1] Chest auscultation was taught and practiced by Hippocrates himself (fourth century BC), who used to advise physicians to apply their ear directly to the patient's chest to detect various diagnostic sounds. Since then, chest auscultation has been mentioned by Caelius Aeralianus, Leonardo Da Vinci, Ambroise Paré, William Harvey, Giovan Battista Morgagni, Gerhard Van Swieten, William Hunter and many others. The hypochondriacal Robert Hooke, an assistant to Robert Boyle and one of the first scientists to use the word *cell* (1664), even had a good insight in describing heart sounds. He wrote, "Who knows? It may be possible to discover the motions of internal parts . . . by the sound they make." This dream, however, had to wait for another century and a half before coming to realization.

In fact, during the late eighteenth and early nineteenth centuries direct auscultation fell rapidly out of favor, being replaced by a newer diagnostic technique: chest percussion. It took serendipity (and a lot of shyness) to rekindle the art of chest auscultation at the beginning of the nineteenth century. This time, however, the new modality of exam became *indirect* auscultation; that is, auscultation mediated by a newly invented cylindrical instrument, the *stethoscope*. The hero of this rediscovery was a shy, Catholic, introverted, asthmatic and tuberculotic French physician named René Theophile Iacynthe Laennec.

In 1816 (a year after the battle of Waterloo), Laennec had been summoned to the bedside of a young woman afflicted with a chest illness. Because chest percussion was technically difficult (given the large size of the woman's breasts) and because *direct* auscultation (i.e., placing the physician's naked ear over the patients' naked chest) was, in Laennec's own words, "inadmissible" because of the patient's young age and sex, Laennec figured out something totally new. He remembered that a few days before, while walking in the Tuileries garden in Paris, he had seen children scraping a stick of wood with a pin and listening to the other end. Imagining that something similar could easily be used with patients' chests, Laennec fetched a sheet of paper, rolled it into a cylinder, applied it to the young woman's chest, and to his amazement noticed that he could hear lung sounds without even touching her. Being quite handy (he used to make musical instruments, particularly flutes), Laennec quickly manufactured a flute-like wooden contraption, which he properly dubbed the *cylinder*. Being a cultured and sophisticated person who spoke Greek and Latin, Laennec subsequently gave his gadget a much more imposing name: the *stethoscope* (in Greek, inspector of the chest).

From September 1816 to August 1819 Laennec carried his new little tool all over Paris, detecting physical findings and establishing clinical-pathological correlations. Autopsy was indeed inevitable in times when tuberculosis killed as many as 30% of Parisians. Laennec was so taken by his little instrument and the information it provided that medical students used to call him the *cylindromaniac*. He was, in fact, cold and distant, not the epitome of charisma.

On August 15, 1819, the aloof cylindromaniac published a two-volume book chock full of clinicopathological observations titled *De l'Auscultation Mediate*. He gave a masterly description of several chest diseases, many of which had not been described before. Among them were bronchitis, bronchiectasis, pleurisy, lobar pneumonia, hydrothorax, emphysema, pneumothorax, pulmonary edema, pulmonary gangrene and infarction, mitral stenosis, esophagitis, peritonitis, cirrhosis (hence the eponym Laennec's cirrhosis), and, of course, tuberculosis.

The book also presented an entire new terminology, mostly originating from daily life examples and from Laennec's own knowledge of Greek and Latin. Among these neologisms were stethoscope, auscultation, rales, rhonchus, fremitus, crackled-pot sound, metallic tinkling, egophony, bronchophony, cavernous breathing, puerile breathing, veiled puff, and bruit.

The first edition of *De l'Auscultation* sold for thirteen francs. It came bundled with a wooden stethoscope for an additional cost of 3 francs. It sold badly. But by the time that the considerably rewritten second edition was in press (1826), the stethoscope had already become the standard method of chest examination. At the time of Laennec's premature death from tuberculosis (in 1826 at the age of 45), many young physicians were already carrying a stethoscope. Almost all of these stethoscopes were the product of Laennec's own hands.

In 1831 and 1837 the posthumous third and fourth editions came into print. Both sold quite well, establishing the stethoscope not only as a symbol of medicine as an art but also as the centerpiece of bedside diagnosis. To reach a diagnosis, Medicine could now rely on "objective" findings (instead of subjective symptoms reported by patients). A new era had begun.

2. How do modern stethoscopes differ from Laennec's original cylinder?

Not a lot. The binaural stethoscope (invented in 1954 by Camman of New York) clearly helped. Yet even today's fancy and expensive binaural stethoscopes remain primarily simple conduits for sound transmission between the patient's chest and the examiner's ears. Even as conduits, they are not that good. For example, instead of faithfully transmitting all sounds, most stethoscopes tend to selectively amplify or attenuate certain frequencies: they amplify sounds below 112 Hz (a welcome feature for cardiologists dealing with low-pitched S3s and S4s), but they also accentuate higher-pitched sounds (a not-so-welcome feature for pulmonologists dealing with higher-frequency respiratory sounds). For this reason the field of pulmonary auscultation has tremendously benefited from the recent application of objective computer technology to the analysis of sounds.

3. What are lung sounds?

Lung sounds (also called respiratory sounds) are sounds generated by the lungs, whereas transmitted voice sounds are generated by the larynx and then transmitted downward via the lungs. We shall discuss these two groups of sounds separately.

4. What is the interobserver variability in recognizing lung sounds?

Quite large. In a study by Shilling et al., two observers disagreed 24% of the time in reporting the abnormal lung sounds of 187 cotton workers.[2] A similar interobserver variability was reported by (1) Fletcher et al. in the specialists' recognition of emphysema[3]; (2) Smyllie et al. in the assessment by nine physicians of the rales and rhonchi of 20 patients[4]; (3) Schneider and Anderson for the presence of decreased breath sounds.[5]

Pearl. *Although this variability seems too high to be acceptable, it is actually not much higher than that found in data collection in general,[6] including interpretation of the chest radiograph.[7,8]*

5. How are lung sounds conventionally categorized?

They are subdivided into two major groups: (1) basic lung sounds (also called breath sounds) and (2) adventitious (i.e., extra) lung sounds. Each of these two subgroups contains in turn various other sounds (see table, top of next page).

6. How are lung sounds generated?

Lung sounds are generated by two major mechanisms:

1. Movement of air along the tracheobronchial tree, which is usually responsible for the production of basic lung sounds (or breath sounds).

2. Vibration of solid tissue, which is usually responsible for the production of adventitious (or extra) lung sounds.

*Categories of Respiratory Sounds**

RESPIRATORY SOUND	MECHANISMS	ORIGIN	ACOUSTICS	RELEVANCE
Basic sounds				
Normal lung sound	Turbulent flow vortices, unknown mechanisms	Central airways (expiration), lobar to segmental airway (inspiration)	Low-pass filtered noise (range < 100 to 1,000 Hz)	Regional ventilation, airway caliber
Normal tracheal sound	Turbulent flow, flow impinging on airway walls	Pharynx, larynx, trachea, large airways	Noise with resonances (range < 100 to > 3,000 Hz)	Upper airway configuration
Adventitious sounds				
Wheeze	Airway wall flutter, vortex shedding	Central and lower airways	Sinusoid (range ~ 100 to > 1,000 Hz; duration, typically > 80 ms)	Airway obstruction, flow limitation
Rhonchus	Rupture of fluid films, airway wall vibrations	Large airways	Series of rapidly dampened sinusoids (typically < 300 Hz and duration > 100 ms)	Secretions, abnormal airway collapsibility
Crackle	Airway wall stress-relaxation	Central and lower airways	Rapidly dampened wave deflection (duration typically < 20 ms)	Airway closure, secretions

• This table lists only the major categories of respiratory sounds and does not include other sounds such as squawks, friction rubs, grunting, snoring, or cough. Current concepts on sound mechanisms and origin are listed, but these concepts may be incomplete and unconfirmed.
From Pasterkamp H, Kraman SS, Wadricka GR: Respiratory sounds. Am J Respir Crit Care Med 156: 974–987, 1997, with permission.

BASIC SOUNDS: DEFINITION AND TERMINOLOGY

7. What are basic lung sounds?
   Basic lung sounds are the sounds heard over the chest of healthy (and diseased) people. They represent the underlying and background noise over which adventitious (or extra) sounds are occasionally superimposed.

8. What are the major types of basic lung sounds?
   1. Vesicular breath sounds   3. Bronchial breath sounds
   2. Bronchovesicular breath sounds   4. Amphoric (cavernous) breath sounds
      (see below)   5. Tracheal breath sounds)
This traditional classification, reported in most textbooks, is based on the sounds' site of production and physical characteristics. A more recent classification reports only two types of basic

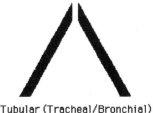

Tubular (Tracheal/Bronchial)

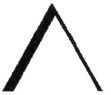

Bronchovesicular

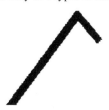

Vesicular

sounds[9]: (1) the normal lung sound (or vesicular breath sound) and (2) the normal tracheal sound (or tubular breath sound). The latter category consists of the subvarieties of tracheal, bronchial, and amphoric breath sounds.

9. What type of air movement is responsible for the production of basic lung sounds (breath sounds)?

It depends on the size of the airway. Overall, three types of air movement may take place along the tracheobronchial tree. Some are silent and some are noisy:

1. **Laminar airflow.** This very slow and organized air movement is characteristic of the small peripheral airways. It is so slow that flow in the alveoli almost comes to an end. This airflow is characteristically silent.

2. **Vorticose airflow.** This air movement is a bit faster than laminar airflow and is characteristic of branching airways. Branching separates the airflow in different layers with different velocities. Interaction of these layers then generates noisy eddies and vortices. This airflow is therefore noisy and is often called mixed (or transitional) because it resembles both laminar and turbulent airflow.

3. **Turbulent airflow.** This movement of air is very rapid and complex. It is characteristic of the large central airways (trachea and major bronchi). Air molecules randomly collide against each other and also impact on the airways' wall. This airflow is characteristically noisy.

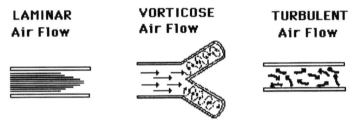

10. Why is a laminar flow called laminar?

Because it can be compared with a series of concentric and coaxial cylinders. Laminar flows are slow and silent. They are characterized by streamlines that run parallel to the walls of the airway, have the same axis, and slide over each other. Because the streamlines in the center move faster than those in the periphery, the profile of the flow is parabolic.

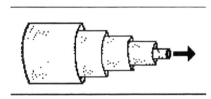

11. What are the characteristics of a vorticose (i.e., transitional or mixed) airflow?

As the name implies, the characteristics are mixed. They are in fact similar to both laminar and turbulent airflow. Indeed, a vorticose flow per se is relatively slow up to the point of the branching airways. The branching, however, modifies the flow, separating the main airstream in several layers, each moving at a different velocity. The impact against each other of these high-velocity and low-velocity streams creates, in turn, vortices and sounds.

Pearl. *In summary, laminar (and silent) airflow occurs in the very small peripheral airways. Turbulent (and noisy) airflow, on the other hand, occurs in the central airways, such as the trachea and major bronchi. Finally, transition (vorticose) airflow occurs in the remainder of the tracheobronchial tree.*

12. Why is airflow in the trachea and central bronchi turbulent and noisy, whereas airflow in the smaller and more peripheral airway is laminar and silent?

Because of the Reynolds number—a dimensionless number that determines whether the flow in a hollow tube is laminar and silent or turbulent and noisy. The Reynolds number is a ratio of several factors and is quite complicated. For simplification, however, it may be said that the Reynolds number is related *directly* to the rate of airflow (velocity of air) and *inversely* to the radius of the airway. Therefore, turbulence and noise are more likely to occur when the airflow is rapid and the airway is small.

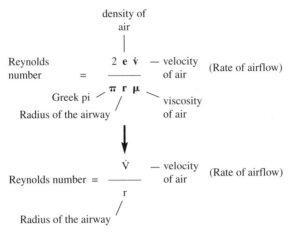

A Reynolds number greater than 2000 is usually characteristic of turbulence and noise.

13. Do the sounds produced by the lungs have the same acoustic characteristics as the sounds that we hear over the chest?

Not necessarily. The characteristics of the sounds we hear over the chest are due not only to their unique modality of production (see above) but also to their modality of transmission. The latter depends entirely on the different physical characteristics of the lung tissues that the sounds have to cross, particularly the air-to-liquid/solid ratio of the tissue.

14. Which breath sounds are louder: those heard over the chest or those heard over the neck and mouth?

Those heard over the neck and mouth. Although breath sounds are produced in the trachea and central bronchi, they still have to be transmitted. This transmission occurs both *downward* (therefore the sound is heard over the chest) and *upward* (therefore the sound is heard over the neck and mouth). Sounds heard over the neck and mouth are usually louder than those heard over the chest because they maintain all of their high frequencies. Sounds transmitted through the lungs and chest wall, on the other hand, lose components with the higher frequencies because of the presence of alveolar air, which acts as a high-frequency filter (a bit like the equalizer in home stereo equipment), eliminating all sounds with frequencies above 200 Hz. Because the remaining frequencies are in a very low range (e.g., ≤ 200 Hz), they are poorly perceived by the human ear. As a result, the breath sounds transmitted over the aerated chest are extremely soft. On the contrary, the breath sounds heard at the mouth maintain all of their components (equally distributed between 200 and 2000 Hz) and therefore are perceived as loud.

Pearl. *Thus, high-pitched breath sounds (such as those heard over the neck and mouth) are louder than low-pitched breath sounds (such as those heard over the chest) (see graph, top of next page).*

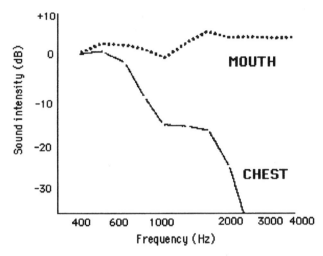

Adapted from Forgacs P: Lung Sounds. London, Baillière Tindall, 1978.

15. Is the ability of the lung to act as a high-frequency filter a constant phenomenon?

No. This filtering ability can be eliminated by the alveoli with a medium that transmits sound better than air, such as a liquid. Examples include pus (pneumonia), serum (pulmonary edema), or blood (alveolar hemorrhage). Alternatively, air can be simply "squeezed out" of the alveoli, as in the case of alveolar collapse. Both mechanisms are responsible for the formation of an airless lung (= con-*solid*-ation).

Pearl. *Replacement of alveolar air by liquid or solid allows the lung to transmit sounds better, including high-frequency components (normally filtered out) that are responsible for the perception of a sound as loud.*

16. How are the sounds transmitted by a consolidated lung?

They sound louder. Because solids and liquids transmit sounds better than gases, the consolidated lung no longer muffles the intensity of breath sounds. Breath sounds heard over a consolidated chest are therefore louder and similar in characteristics to the breath sounds heard over the mouth or the neck.

VESICULAR BREATH SOUNDS

17. What are vesicular breath sounds?

Vesicular breath sounds are basic lung sounds. More specifically, they are the breathing-associated sounds normally heard over the chest of healthy people.

18. Why are they called "vesicular"?

They were called vesicular by Laennec himself, who believed that the site of production was in the alveoli (= vesicles). Laennec described them as "a slight but extremely distinct murmur corresponding to the entrance of air into and out of the air cells of the lungs." This description, however, is wrong. Vesicular breath sounds are not produced by the alveoli. They are still generated in the airways. They are, however, filtered by the alveoli. Thus, the alveoli play an important role in these sounds but only in modifying their transmission: aerated alveoli eliminate most of the high-frequency components and allow the passage only of low-pitched and soft sounds.

19. Are vesicular breath sounds the same as normal breath sounds?

Yes. Because vesicular breath sounds represent the breathing-associated sounds of normal people, some authors have indeed suggested that they should be renamed normal breath sounds.[10]

20. What do vesicular breath sounds sound like?
They have three major characteristics:
1. They are soft and muffled (graphically represented by thin inspiratory and expiratory lines).
2. They have a short expiratory phase, with disappearance of the last two-thirds of exhalation (inspiratory-to-expiratory ratio approximately 3:1).
3. They have no silent pause between inspiration and expiration. Thus expiration immediately follows inspiration.

21. What are the physical characteristics behind these auscultatory features?
The major characteristic is the very low frequency of the vesicular breath sounds. The air-filled alveoli behave like a "low-pass" filter, thereby allowing transmission only of low-frequency sounds. Because of this filtering effect, vesicular breath sounds have frequencies that range between only 100 and 500 Hz, with a steep cut-off above 200 Hz and a maximal sound intensity below 100 Hz. The other striking characteristic of vesicular breath sounds, however, is the remarkable difference in the *component frequencies* of inspiration and expiration. Because the components with lowest pitch and lowest intensity are usually concentrated in expiration, the expiratory limb of vesicular breath sounds is very soft. Indeed, the last two-thirds of exhalation are usually entirely silent. As a result, expiration is much shorter than inspiration, and the inspiratory-to-expiratory ratio of these sounds is 3:1.

22. How are vesicular breath sounds produced?
They are produced by turbulent airflow in the large central airways (the inspiratory component is produced probably a little more peripherally than the expiratory component). The sounds so generated are then transmitted through the air-filled alveoli surrounding the bronchi. As mentioned before, the mantle of alveolar air acts as an equalizer, eliminating all frequencies greater than 600 Hz and allowing the transmission only of muffled and low-pitched sounds.

23. Are vesicular breath sounds heard throughout the chest?
No. Although vesicular sounds are heard over most of the lung fields of a normal patient, there are still two narrow areas (corresponding anteriorly and posteriorly to the trachea and central bronchi = parascapular areas, see figure) in which the vesicular sounds are replaced by bronchovesicular breath sounds. Outside these limited and narrow areas, the presence of vesicular breath sounds remains a sine qua non for a healthy lung.

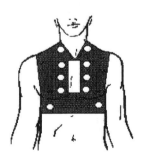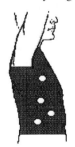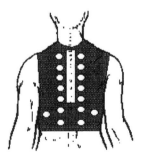

Adapted from Lehrer S: Understanding Lung Sounds. Philadelphia, W.B. Saunders, 1984.

24. How do vesicular breath sounds change with age?
They change primarily in regard to frequency. Vesicular breath sounds of children (up to the age of 9 years) are louder and higher-pitched than those of adults. Vesicular breath sounds of adults, on the other hand, are higher-pitched than vesicular breath sounds of the elderly.[11] Laennec first noticed this phenomenon, writing that the sound intensity of children was higher than that of adults (he dubbed this phenomenon "puerile respiration"). This acoustic difference is probably due to the different resonance behavior of small thoraces, leading to less power in the low

frequencies of children's breath sounds.[12] Alternatively, the smaller radius of children's airways may be responsible for the increased turbulence and loudness of their vesicular breath sounds.

25. What is the clinical significance of soft vesicular breath sounds?

Very important. In fact, assuming that the thickness of the chest wall is normal (i.e., no obesity), that the pleural space is also normal (i.e., no pleural collection of either air or fluid), and that the respiratory muscles are functioning normally, a reduced intensity of the vesicular breath sounds usually indicates reduced air flow. This finding is typical not only of patients whose right main bronchus has been selectively intubated by a misplaced endothracheal tube but also of patients with chronic obstructive pulmonary disease.

Pearl.   Thus, diminished breath sounds (often referred to as distant) are good indicators of obstructive lung disease. Conversely, vesicular breath sounds of normal intensity virtually exclude a severe reduction in FEV₁.

26. Is the intensity of breath sounds in airflow obstruction also diminished at the mouth?

No. The intensity of breath sounds heard at the mouth is actually increased in airflow obstruction (see below). Only over the chest is the intensity of breath sounds diminished.

27. How should the breath sound intensity (BSI) be assessed at bedside?

The patient should be seated and asked to take fast and deep inspirations from residual volume while breathing through the mouth. This maneuver generates as loud a breath sound as possible. Auscultation should then be carried out in the upper anterior zones, midaxillae, and posterior bases bilaterally. Sounds should then be classified as 0, absent; 1, barely audible; 2, faint but definitely audible; 3, normal; 4, louder than normal.[13] The sum of the sound intensities recorded in each area generates the BSI score. The BSI score, therefore, ranges from 0 to 24 (= 4 in each of the 6 auscultatory areas).

28. What is the interobserver reliability of this maneuver?

Quite good. A correlation coefficient of 0.966 was obtained in two observers examining 20 patients independently.[14]

29. Should the intensity of the extra sounds be considered in the calculation of the BSI?

No. In fact, to use this method effectively, one should disregard any superimposed adventitious lung sound (such as rhonchi, wheezes, or crackles) because these sounds often have a louder intensity than the underlying breath sound and thus obfuscate the BSI calculation.

30. How accurate is the BSI in predicting airflow obstruction?

Quite accurate. There is already a strong correlation between unscored lung sound intensity over the chest and percent predicted FEV_1 on spirometry.[15,16] The BSI score correlates even more strongly with FEV_1 and FEV_1/FVC.[17]

31. What is the physiology behind the BSI?

It is the strong correlation between the intensity of breath sounds heard over the chest and regional distribution of ventilation, as measured by radioactive gas.[18] For this reason the BSI is such an accurate finding. Indeed, in a group of 13 patients with obstructive disease examined by 9 physicians, the BSI was the best single index of "obstructive emphysema" compared with 14 other physical findings and signs[19] and when judged against the gold standard of airflow obstruction.[20]

Pearl.   Thus, BSI is an excellent bedside tool for the assessment of airflow obstruction when pulmonary function tests are either not available or cannot be performed.

32. Can a change in lung sounds' intensity be used to monitor the patient's response to airway challenge?

Yes. A progressive decrease in the intensity of breath sounds heard over the chest is a common feature of progressive airflow obstruction induced by respiratory challenge (such as inhalation of histamine or methacholine), even in the absence of wheezing.[21] Thus, a decrease in BSI is a good tool for monitoring airway challenge. Remember, however, that the pitch of the breath sounds may paradoxically increase with the development of airflow obstruction (see below).

33. What mechanism is responsible for the reduced BSI of patients with obstructive lung disease?

It is probably more a reduction in sound transmission (due to the parenchymal destruction and air-trapping so typical of COPD) than in sound production (due to diminished airflow). This explanation is intuitive, considering that the airflow limitation of patients with obstructive lung disease is usually more expiratory than inspiratory; thus, the diminished sound intensity of inspiration is probably due more to "muffling" than to diminished airflow.

Pearl. *The hyperinflated and hyperaerated lungs of patients with airflow obstruction filter the high-frequency components of breath sounds, causing a reduction in sound amplitude and a softening of sounds.*

34. Can airflow obstruction be quantitatively assessed by using lung auscultation?

Yes. In addition to the increased intensity of the breath sounds heard at the mouth and the diminished intensity of breath sounds heard over the chest, airflow obstruction can be accurately quantified by using a simple stopwatch and a stethoscope.[22] To do so, the patient should perform a forced-expiratory maneuver (take a deep breath and blast it out as quickly and forcefully as possible) while the bell of the stethoscope is over the patient's suprasternal notch. The duration of audible expiration (FETo) is then timed to the nearest half-second. An FETo greater than 6 seconds corresponds to an FEV_1/FVC less than 40%. Conversely, an FETo less than 5 seconds indicates an FEV_1/FVC greater than 60%. This simple test is a good equivalent of a poor man's spirometry and can help in the bedside assessment of airflow obstruction.

35. What is the clinical significance of breath sounds heard at the mouth?

Very important. The intensity of the breath sounds heard at the mouth by the unaided ear is in fact related directly to the spirometric degree of airway obstruction.[23] Intensity of breath sounds heard over the chest, by contrast, is related inversely to the spirometric degree of airway obstruction. This concept is not new at all. Laennec noticed the association between loud breath sounds at the mouth and dyspnea, reporting a patient whose breath sounds could be heard at a distance of 20 feet. He devoted a full page to this phenomenon in *De l'Auscultation Mediate*, explaining in detail that what he meant by "loud breath sounds at the mouth" was simply loud breathing and not the noise of rattling, whistling, or other adventitious lung sounds.

36. What is the mechanism of production of the breath sounds heard at the mouth?

It is probably turbulent airflow in the proximal bronchi and trachea.[24] In the normal person this turbulence is limited so that the noise generated at the mouth is barely audible. In patients with obstructive lung disease, on the other hand, the narrowing of the airways leads to much more turbulence and therefore to much noisier mouth breathing (even in the absence of crackles or wheezes). The intensity is so increased that the inspiratory breath sounds of patients with obstructive lung disease can easily be heard across the room, even when the patients are breathing at rest.

Pearl. *Thus, the intensity of breath sounds heard at the mouth by the unaided ear is an important physical finding in the evaluation of patients with suspected obstructive lung disease. The louder the sounds, the more severe the obstruction.*

37. What are the physical characteristics of the breath sounds heard at the mouth?

They have a spectrum of frequencies ranging between 200 and 2,000 Hz, very much resembling white noise.

38. Is the intensity of the breath sounds heard at the mouth increased in all patients with obstructive lung disease?

No. Only in patients with asthma or chronic bronchitis. In these two diseases the loudness of inspiratory sound correlates well with the severity of airflow obstruction as measured by airway resistance, forced expiratory volume in one second (FEV_1), or peak expiratory flow rate (PEFR).[25] In emphysema, on the other hand, the inspiratory breath sounds heard at the mouth are paradoxically quiet because patients have no direct narrowing of the bronchi, but only a dynamic expiratory airflow obstruction produced by loss of elastic recoil.

Pearl.   Thus, the difference in intensity of the breath sounds heard at the mouth is a useful method for differentiating emphysema from chronic bronchitis or asthma. Noisy mouth inspiration is even more reliable than chest wheezing in the diagnosis of chronic bronchitis and asthma, in which it reflects accurately the degree of airflow obstruction. Conversely, a soft or silent inspiration at the mouth in patients with airflow obstruction is a good clue that such obstruction is due to emphysema.

39. What are the auscultatory findings of patients with chronic bronchitis?

The first finding is the increased intensity of the breath sounds at the mouth. Paradoxically, patients with chronic bronchitis may have diminished breath sound intensity over the chest. More often, however, their chests are noisy, not because of the intensity of the breath sounds (which are, indeed, softer), but because of the many adventitious sounds that are commonly encountered. These extra sounds include early crackles and rhonchi (both of which may clear with coughing) and end-expiratory wheezes.

Changes in Lung Sounds with Pulmonary Disease

LUNG DISEASE	BREATH SOUNDS	ADVENTITIOUS LUNG SOUND
Pneumonia	Bronchial or absent	Inspiratory crackles
Atelectasis	Harsh/bronchial	Late inspiratory crackles
Pneumothorax	Absent	None
Emphysema	Diminished	Early inspiratory crackles
Chronic bronchitis	Normal	Wheezes and crackles
Pulmonary fibrosis	Harsh	Inspiratory crackles
Congestive heart failure	Diminished	Inspiratory crackles
Pleural effusion	Diminished	None
Asthma	Diminished	Wheezes

From Wilkins R: Lung Sounds. St. Louis, Mosby, 1996, with permission.

40. How accurate is auscultation in identifying patients with chronic bronchitis?

Quite accurate, particularly if computer-aided. Indeed, in one large study testing a total of 493 subjects,[26] computerized lung sound analysis added to a screening program based on symptom questionnaire, and spirometry increased the sensitivity for detection of respiratory diseases from 71% to 87%. One-half of the subjects with normal spirometry but symptoms of chronic bronchitis had abnormal lung sounds (primarily wheezing). Of interest, among the 24 subjects who only had abnormal lung sounds (but normal spirometry and not symptoms), three developed heart or lung disease at a 12–18-month follow-up.

41. If crackles and rhonchi of airflow obstruction clear with coughing, should all patients with these findings be asked to cough?

Yes. According to an old saying, you can tell a chest specialist from a generalist because the generalist never asks patients to cough during auscultation, whereas the specialist always does. Indeed, extra sounds originating from air-fluid interfaces of large-to-medium airways (such as early inspiratory crackles and some rhonchi) clear with coughing. Coughing, therefore, is a good clue to the site of origin of these sounds and should be routinely elicited.

42. What type of breath sounds are heard over a pleural effusion?
It depends on the location:

1. **Above the effusion** (where the alveoli are fully expanded and aerated) vesicular breath sounds are heard.

2. **At the upper margin of the effusion** (where there is only a thin layer of fluid, small enough to compress the alveoli but not large enough to collapse the bronchi) bronchial (or tubular) breath sounds are heard. The loss of alveolar filter favors the transmission of higher frequencies, giving the breath sound a typically tubular quality. The improved transmission is also responsible for the production of voice sounds of a nasal or bleating timbre, such as egophony.

3. **Over the rest of the effusion**, where the fluid is large enough to collapse both bronchi and alveoli, auscultatory silence is the norm.

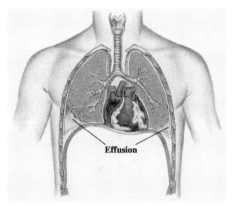

From Seidel HM, Ball JW, Dains JE, Benedict GW: Mosby's Guide to Physical Examination, 3rd ed. St. Louis, Mosby, 1995, with permission.

43. What type of breath sounds are heard in patients with a pneumothorax?
Very distant breath sounds. In fact, if the pneumothorax is large enough to compress the lung entirely, the hemithorax is completely silent. Of course, the percussion note in such patients is increased, whereas it is diminished in patients with pleural effusion. The diminished intensity of breath sounds in pneumothorax is the result not only of reduced generation of sound (due to the diminished airflow in the collapsed lung) but also of reduced transmission of sound (due to the cushion of air in the pleural space).

Pearl. *Thus, air (or fluid) in the pleural cavity forms an acoustic barrier to sound transmission and usually muffles the breath sounds. The only exception is a layer of fluid so thin that it compresses only the alveoli and not the bronchi (see above).*

TUBULAR BREATH SOUNDS

44. Why are these sounds called "tubular"?
Because they resemble the sounds that can be produced by blowing air through a hollow tube. The tubular sounds normally heard over the trachea are called tracheal (because they are produced in the trachea). Thus, tubular sounds heard over the chest in situations of consolidation are usually called bronchial (that is, they are produced in the bronchi and subsequently well transmitted by airless, consolidated lung).

45. What are tubular breath sounds?
They are basic breath sounds. Tubular breath sounds include various subtypes (see above). The most important of these subtypes are (1) tracheal breath sounds and (2) bronchial breath sounds. Tracheal breath sounds are physiologic, but bronchial breath sounds are always pathologic.

Tracheal Breath Sounds

46. What are tracheal breath sounds?

Tracheal breath sounds are produced by the flow of air in the upper airways (pharynx, glottis, and subglottic region). They are heard over the lateral neck and suprasternal notch of all normal people. They are loud and high-pitched.

47. What is the importance of tracheal breath sounds?

It is indirect and mostly linked to their resemblance to other, more clinically relevant tubular breath sounds: the bronchial breath sounds.

48. What are the acoustic characteristics of tracheal breath sounds?

1. Loudness (graphically represented by thick inspiratory and expiratory lines

2. A long expiratory phase, usually as long as inspiration (inspiratory-to-expiratory ratio approximately 1:1)

3. A silent pause between inspiration and expiration

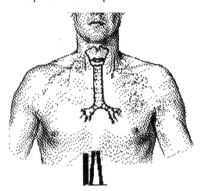

Adapted from Netter, the Ciba Collection.

49. What are the physical characteristics of tracheal breath sounds?

The most important is the higher frequency of tracheal breath sounds compared with vesicular breath sounds. Indeed, tracheal breath sounds consist of frequencies between less than 100 and more than 1,500 Hz (with a maximal intensity usually below 800 Hz). Although the component frequencies of inspiration and expiration are similar, exhalation tends to have a slightly higher intensity. Because of these high-frequency components, tracheal breath sounds are well perceived by the human ear and appear loud.

Pearl.   *Thus, a tracheal breath sound is normally heard over the neck, very high-pitched, and therefore much louder than the vesicular breath sound.*

50. How are tracheal breath sounds produced and transmitted?

Tracheal breath sounds are produced by turbulent airflow in the upper airways. Because they are generated close to the surface of the neck and upper retrosternal area, the absence of aerated lung tissue around the sound source prevents the filtering of the soundwave. As a result, tracheal sounds are transmitted with all of their components (including the high-frequency components). Thus, they remain unchanged, high-pitched, and loud.

Pearl.   *Tracheal sounds, therefore, are a more pure and less filtered type of breath sound than vesicular breath sounds.*

51. Does the monitoring of tracheal breath sounds have any clinical value?

Yes. It is, for example, routinely used as part of commercial apnea monitoring devices. It also may be used for the assessment of snorers with or without obstructive sleep-apnea.[27]

52. Do tracheal breath sounds change in relation to pathologic changes in the lungs?

No. Because tracheal breath sounds are produced in the trachea (i.e., outside the chest), they remain constant.

Bronchial Breath Sounds

53. What are bronchial breath sounds?

Bronchial breath sounds, like tracheal breath sounds, are basic lung sounds of the tubular variety. They are loud and high-pitched and are never heard in normal people. They are present over areas of airless lung and patent bronchi. Thus, they are a sign of consolidation (i.e., loss of aerated alveoli), indicating improved transmission of the high-frequency sounds generated in the airways.

Pearl. *When the lung surrounding the airways is either consolidated or fibrotic, the range of sound frequencies transmitted to the chest surface is increased to the point that the breath sounds start resembling the sounds heard over the trachea. As we will see later, this is also the acoustic basis for other clinical signs of consolidation, such as egophony, bronchophony and whispered pectoriloquy.*

54. How are bronchial breath sounds generated?

Like all breath sounds, bronchial breath sounds are generated by air rapidly flowing through the airways (in this case, the larger and more central airways). Thus bronchial breath sounds are generated centrally. Their peculiar quality and high intensity, however, are due to their abnormal transmission through the periphery of the lung. More specifically, their higher intensity is due to the preservation of their high-frequency components through airless lung, usually as a result of lung consolidation or fibrosis. To generate bronchial breath sounds, consolidation and/or fibrosis must extend all the way from the chest surface to 4–5 cm toward the hilum (where the central airways are located).

55. How do bronchial breath sounds differ from vesicular breath sounds?

They are louder and higher-pitched because consolidated lungs conduct high-frequency sound better than aerated lungs.

56. What do bronchial breath sounds sound like?

They have a peculiar hollow or tubular quality. They are louder than vesicular breath sounds (thus the respiratory cycle is diagrammatically represented by thick lines) and have a silent pause between inspiration and expiration and a longer expiratory phase. Because of the length of the expiratory phase, the inspiratory-to-expiratory ratio of bronchial breath sounds is usually 1:1 (instead of the 3:1 or 4:1 ratio of vesicular breath sounds).

57. Which pathologic processes are associated with a bronchial breath sound?

Bronchial breath sounds are usually heard in situations of consolidation. Con-*solid*-ation indicates the loss of alveolar air and its replacement by a mantle of solidified lung, which better transmits the high-frequency sounds. Consolidation occurs whenever there is alveolar collapse or alveolar fluid-filling.

- **Alveolar collapse** (with patent airways) occurs usually in situations of pleural effusion, when the amount of fluid is enough to compress the alveoli but not enough to compress the airways.
- **Alveolar fluid-filling**, on the other hand, occurs in situations such as pneumonia (= alveolar pus), alveolar hemorrhage (= alveolar blood), or pulmonary edema (= alveolar serum).

Finally, bronchial breath sounds also may be heard in the setting of pulmonary fibrosis. This phenomenon, however, requires severe fibrosis and tends to be more rare than consolidation.

58. What does the chest radiograph look like in patients with bronchial breath sounds?

It may show several disease processes, although all are characterized by patches of airless lung. Often, chest radiographs and chest CTs may show air bronchograms (air-filled bronchi, silhouetted out against airless consolidated parenchyma).

59. Can bronchial breath sounds produced by alveolar fluid-filling be differentiated from bronchial breath sounds produced by alveolar collapse?

Bronchial breath sounds produced by alveolar collapse tend to occur by themselves, whereas bronchial breath sounds produced by alveolar fluid-filling tend to be associated with crackles. In turn, crackles produced by interstitial fluid also tend to be associated with bronchial breath sounds, whereas crackles produced by interstitial scarring (= fibrosis), tend to occur with vesicular breath sounds.

60. What are the physical characteristics of bronchial breath sounds?

The most striking characteristic is their high frequency. Consolidation is associated with an overall increase in the density of the lung, which prevents the lung from functioning as a low-pass filter (i.e., an equalizer that eliminates sound frequencies > 200 Hz). Because airless lung allows high-frequency sounds to pass unaltered, bronchial breath sounds are perceived as quite loud. Both inspiration and expiration have similar component frequencies, ranging between 100 and 1200 Hz, with maximal intensity below 900 Hz. These frequencies are much higher than those found in vesicular breath sounds and, in fact, are similar to those found in other tubular breath sounds, such as tracheal breath sounds.

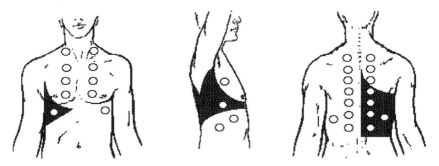

Location of bronchial breath sounds in a case of right lower lobe pneumonia with consolidation. (Adapted from Lehrer S: Understanding Lung Sounds. Philadelphia, W.B. Saunders, 1984.)

Amphoric Breath Sounds

61. What are amphoric breath sounds?

Amphoric breath sounds are a variety of tubular breath sounds. They are very high-pitched, loud, and quite resonant. They are typically generated by air flowing into pulmonary cavities, cysts, or blebs of large size.

BRONCHOVESICULAR BREATH SOUNDS

62. What are bronchovesicular breath sounds?

Bronchovesicular sounds are "transitional" sounds that possess characteristics typical of both vesicular and tubular breath sounds. Many authors even dispute their existence. Although we shall discuss them in some detail, we agree that this finer gradation of breath sounds probably should be abandoned.

Pearl.   Thus, basic lung sounds include only the vesicular breath sound (or normal lung sound) and the tubular breath sound (with its subvarieties of tracheal, bronchial, and amphoric breath sounds).

63. What do bronchovesicular breath sounds sound like?

Like tubular breath sounds, they have a long and well-preserved expiratory phase (inspiratory:expiratory ratio of 1:1); like vesicular breath sounds, they lack a silent pause between inspiration and expiration. They are softer and lower-ptiched than tubular breath sounds but harsher and higher-pitched than vesicular breath sounds.

64. What is the reason behind these "half-way" characteristics?

The half-way characteristics are due to the peculiar way of transmission of bronchovesicular sounds. After being produced by turbulent airflow in the large and central airways (distal trachea and main bronchi), bronchovesicular breath sounds have to cross a thin mantle of alveolar air before reaching the stethoscope. Thus, in contrast to tracheal breath sounds, which are heard immediately over the neck, bronchovesicular breath sounds still have to undergo *some* physical changes (mostly filtering of high frequencies) before they can reach the surface of the chest wall. Yet this filtering is not of the degree undergone by vesicular breath sounds.

Pearl. *Because the mantle of alveolar air that they have to cross is not as thick as that faced by vesicular breath sounds, bronchovesicular breath sounds are therefore louder and higher-pitched than vesicular breath sounds but still softer and lower-pitched than tubular breath sounds.*

65. Where are bronchovesicular breath sounds heard?

Many authors do not even believe that these semitransitional breath sounds truly exist. Yet, if sought carefully, they may be heard over the anterior and posterior parasternal areas of normal people (from the third to the sixth intercostal space).

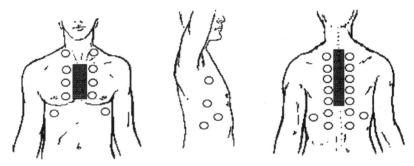

Adapted from Lehrer S: Understanding Lung Sounds. Philadelphia, W.B. Saunders, 1984.

66. What is the clinical significance of bronchovesicular breath sounds?

Their significance depends on the location. As indicated above they are normally heard only over the parasternal areas and parascapular areas of healthy people, both anteriorly and posteriorly. If detected in other areas, however, they indicate an underlying pathology, usually early consolidation (= enhanced transmission of high frequencies).

67. What are the pathologic and radiologic equivalents of bronchovesicular breath sounds?

If heard in locations other than the parasternal and parascapular areas, bronchovesicular breath sounds usually indicate a lung partially collapsed by a pleural effusion or showing early signs of consolidation.

ADVENTITIOUS LUNG SOUNDS

68. What are adventitious lung sounds?

They are extra (that is, adventitious) sounds that are normally absent in a respiratory cycle but that may become superimposed on the underlying breath sound in the presence of disease.

69. How were adventitious lung sounds initially classified?

They were first classified by Laennec himself, who called them "bruits étrangers" (foreign sounds). Laennec considered them to be extra sounds, superimposed on the regular underlying

Outline of Classification of Lung Sounds

ACOUSTIC CHARACTERISTICS	WAVEFORM	RECOMMENDED ATS* NOMENCLATURE	TERMS IN SOME TEXTBOOKS	A BRITISH USAGE	LAENNEC'S ORIGINAL TERM	LAENNEC'S MODEL
Discontinuous, interrupted explosive sounds Loud, low in pitch	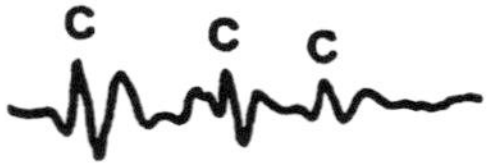	Coarse crackle	Coarse rale	Crackle	Rale muquex ou gargouillement	Escape of water from a bottle held with mouth directly downward
Discontinuous, interrupted explosive sounds Less loud than above and of shorter duration; higher in pitch than coarse rales or crackles	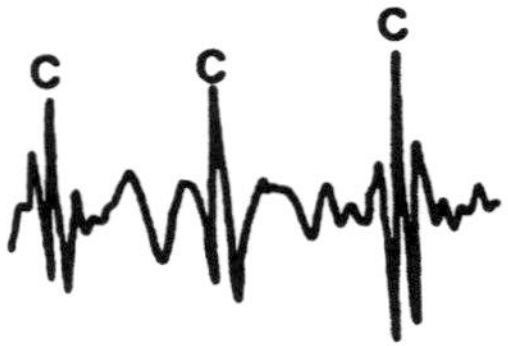	Fine crackle	Fine rale crepitation	Crackle	Rale humide ou crepitation	Crepitation of salts in a heated dish. Noise emitted by healthy lung when compressed in the hand
Continuous sounds Longer than 250 ms, high pitched; dominant frequency of 400 Hz or more, a hissing sound	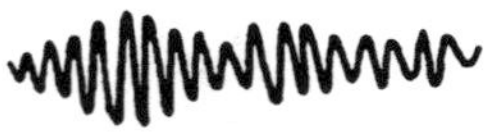	Wheeze	Sibilant rhonchus	High-pitched wheeze	Rale sibilant sec ou sifflement	Prolonged whisper of various intonations; chirping of birds; sound emitted by suddenly separating 2 portions of smooth oiled stone. The motion of a small valve
Continuous sounds Longer than 250 ms low pitched; dominant frequency about 200 Hz or less; a snoring sound	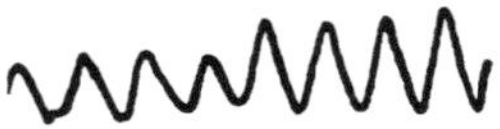	Rhonchus	Sonorous rhonchus	Low-pitched wheeze	Rale sec senore ou ronflement	Snoring; bass note of a musical instrument; cooing of a wood pigeon

* American Thoracic Society

Although the terms used to name the categories of lung sounds vary widely, the categorization scheme itself has changed little since Laennec. The most recent names recommended for adoption by the American Thoracic Society and terms used by others are shown here, accompanied by acoustic descriptions and examples of typical sound waveforms for each category.

vesicular or bronchial breath sound. Using painstaking clinical observations and accurate pathologic correlation, Laennec identified many of these bruits etrangers. Because many of his patients
had tuberculosis, rattling noises were the sounds that he most frequently heard. Laennec often referred to these bruits etrangers as "rales" (French for rattles).

When his treatise *De l'Auscultation Mediate* was first published in 1819, however, Laennec
became acutely aware that rales were much easier to recognize than to describe. Lacking, of
course, any recording equipment, he tried to help his readers by providing many examples from
daily life. They were quite odd, however. For instance, he compared coarse crackles to the gurgling of water from an upside down bottle. He added that these "mucous rales" were commonly
heard in patients with abundant secretions in the central airways. He then compared fine crackles
to the crackling of salt on a heated dish (!?!). He noted that these "humid rales" (or crepitations)
were commonly heard in patients with pneumonia, pulmonary edema, or hemoptysis. Finally, he
compared wheezes to the chirping of little birds and rhonchi to the cooing of a wood pigeon (?!?).

The problems with terminology and Laennec's odd examples were further compounded by
the fact that Laennec could not use the term rale at bedside. His patients, in fact, became very
scared whenever they heard it because it reminded them of the French expression "le rale de la
mort" (the death rattle), the snoring sound of dying patients who are unable to clear their respiratory secretions. Thus, to avoid any miscommunication (and possible legal repercussions),
Laennec elected to use at bedside the term rhonchus (rattle in Latin). Rales and rhonchi, however,
meant the same sound to him. But when Forbes translated Laennec's work into English, he decided that rhonchus should describe only *long* sounds, whereas rale should describe *short* sounds.
Not all translators, however, followed this example. This was the beginning of the end for
Laennec's classification. The confusion became so bad that in 1970 Fraser and Pare reported that
"every physician seems to have his own classification."[28]

70. When were adventitious lung sounds reclassified?

More than a century and a half after the initial classification by Laennec. The new classification was the brainchild of an international commission of experts that published its recommendation in 1977. The most striking feature of the new classification was the abandonment of Laennec's
beloved term "rale" in favor of a nomenclature based more on the acoustic characteristics of the
various adventitious sounds.[29,30] Priority was given to the duration of the sounds. As a result,
adventitious lung sounds are now divided into discontinuous (if they last less than 250 msec) and
continuous (if they last longer than 250 msec). In this classification crackles have replaced the
old French term rales and the old British term crepitations. Fine crackles are higher-pitched than
coarse crackles. Similarly, wheezes are higher-pitched than rhonchi.

ACOUSTIC CHARACTERISTICS	AMERICAN THORACIC SOCIETY NOMENCLATURE	COMMONLY USED SYNONYMS (OLD TERMINOLOGY)	LAENNEC EXAMPLE
1. Discontinuous (< 250 msec)	Coarse crackle	Coarse rale	Water gurgling from a bottle
	Fine crackle	Fine rale crepitation	Crackling of salt on a heated dish
2. Continuous (> 250 msec)	Wheeze	Sibilant rhonchus	The chirping of little birds
	Rhonchus	Sonorous rhonchus	The cooing of a wood pigeon

71. How accepted is this new terminology?

Not much. Although in common practice the terms crackles, wheezes, and rhonchi are used
to indicate the three major types of adventitious lung sounds, outdated terms such as rales or

crepitations are also used, confirmed by several surveys conducted among physicians, respiratory therapists, and even medical journals (review of case reports).

72. How are adventitious lung sounds produced?

They are produced by the vibration of respiratory structures, such as bronchi and pleura. These vibrations may occur in four major ways:

1. **Rupture of fluid films or bubbles** occurs whenever there is rapid air flow through secretions thinly coating the large central airways. This air-fluid interface causes the rupture of fluid films and bubbles and the generation of a popping sound. This mechanism is responsible for the generation of coarse crackles (discontinuous adventitious lung sounds), which are characteristic of acute and chronic bronchitis.

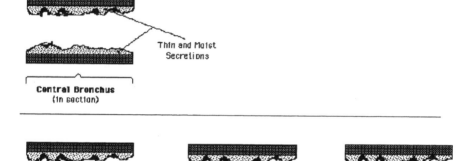

2. **Sudden equalization of intraairway pressure** occurs whenever partially collapsed small airways suddenly reopen in inspiration. This reopening causes a "pop" through a rapid equalization of intraairway pressures. This mechanism usually takes place whenever small airways are compressed by high interstitial pressure due to either scarring of the interstitium (pulmonary fibrosis) or fluid in the interstitium (pus, blood, or serum). This mechanism is responsible for the production of fine crackles (discontinuous adventitious lung sounds), which are characteristic of pneumonia, pulmonary hemorrhage, pulmonary edema, and pulmonary fibrosis.

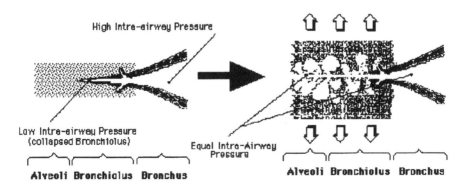

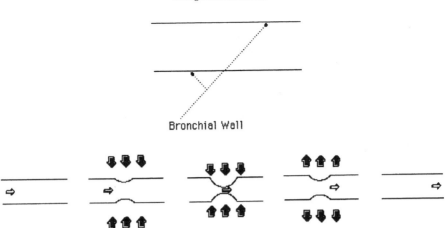

Bronchial Wall

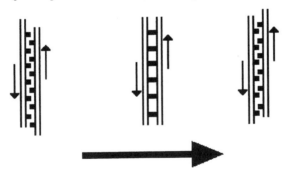

3. **Fluttering of the airway wall** is the mechanism responsible for production of wheezes and rhonchi. It occurs whenever air flows rapidly through a narrow airway (bronchospasm, thick secretions, edema), causing fluttering of the airway wall at one or more sites. The physical principle behind this mechanism is the Bernoulli principle, which also governs the water vacuum pump used in many biochemical labs. In the case of the pump, the rapidly flowing water through a narrow tube produces a sucking effect, which in turn sucks in air through a hole in the tube. In the case of wheezes, however, there is no hole in the airway wall. Thus, air flowing rapidly through the narrow bronchus simply sucks in the airway wall itself, thereby producing a wheeze. The recurrent closing and opening of the airway wall resemble very much the vibration of the reed of a toy trumpet and produce wheezes and rhonchi (continuous adventitious lung sounds).

4. **Rubbing of inflamed pleural surfaces.** In this case, the two pleural layers are roughened by an inflammatory process and covered with fibrinous layers. Whenever they slide against each other during respiration, they rub, producing a creaky leathery sound. Thus, the hallmark of a pleural friction rub is its presence during both inspiration and expiration.

DISCONTINUOUS ADVENTITIOUS LUNG SOUNDS

73. What are discontinuous adventitious lung sounds?
They are short (< 250 msec) and explosive extra sounds that are heard in certain disease processes. They are primarily inspiratory, even though they also may occur in expiration.

74. Why are they called discontinuous?
Because they last less than 250 msec. Given this short duration, the human ear cannot identify any musical attribute. Thus, discontinuous adventitious lung sounds are perceived simply as noises.

75. What are discontinuous adventitious lung sounds commonly called?

They are commonly referred to as crackles (see above for recent terminology changes and the demise of the term rales).

76. What do crackles sound like?

Forgacs vividly compared them to "miniature explosions."[31] In 1818 Laennec used various strange comparisons, such as the "gurgling sound of water leaving an upside-down bottle," or the sound of "salt crackling on a heated dish." In 1828 Williams compared them to the sound of "rubbing a lock of one's hair between the finger and thumb close-to-the-ear," and in 1876 Latham spoke of "dry and moist rales." The term crackle was actually first introduced by Robertson and Coope in 1957.[32] Currently we refer to crackles as either fine or coarse. Fine crackles have been compared to the crushing of fine leaves. A more recent comparison for fine crackles—and the one I particularly like—is the rubbing of Velcro or the crinkling of cellophane (examples that Laennec could not have anticipated, even in his wildest dreams).

77. Are crackles superimposed on a breath sound?

Yes. Like all adventitious lung sounds, crackles are superimposed on underlying breath sounds: (1) vesicular (for early and mid inspiratory crackles) and (2) either vesicular or bronchial for late inspiratory crackles (see below).

78. How are crackles graphically represented?

By a cluster of dots overriding the inspiratory or expiratory limb of the respiratory cycle (most commonly the inspiratory limb, considering that crackles are primarily inspiratory). Depending on their number, crackles may be scanty or profuse. Depending on their predominant frequency, they may be high- or low-pitched. Depending on the amplitude of their oscillations, they may be faint or loud. Finally, depending on their timing during inspiration, crackles may be described as early, mid, or late inspiratory (and are so represented graphically).

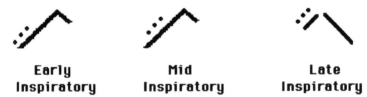

Early   **Mid**   **Late**
Inspiratory   **Inspiratory**   **Inspiratory**

79. How are crackles produced?

It depends on their location in the respiratory cycle[33]:

1. **Early and mid inspiratory crackles** are produced by the bubbling of air through thin secretions, coating, respectively, large and medium-sized airways (as in, respectively, bronchitis and bronchiectasis). These crackles are superimposed on the underlying vesicular breath sound and are heard mainly in the central portion of the chest, both posteriorly and anteriorly. Thus, early and mid inspiratory crackles are coarse, low-pitched, scanty, gravity-independent, well transmitted to the mouth (because they originate from more proximal airways), and strongly associated with obstructive physiology. They may vary in number (and even resolve) with coughing but cannot be extinguished with a change in posture.

2. **Late inspiratory crackles**, on the other hand, occur during the reopening of distal airways that became partially occluded by high interstitial pressure. Because the two ends of partially collapsed bronchioli have different intraairway pressures (a high central and a low distal pressure), the sudden inspiratory reopening of these bronchioli causes a rapid equalization of the intraairway pressure and, as a result, a pop.[34] The high interstitial pressure behind these crackles is usually due to either fluid in the interstitium (such as pus, blood, or serum) or scarring.

Pearl. *Thus, late inspiratory crackles are usually diagnostic of either interstitial fibrosis or interstitial edema (due to pneumonia, pulmonary hemorrhage, or congestive heart failure).*

Because gravity plays an important role in the airway collapse that is behind these sounds, late inspiratory crackles tend to occur in regions of high gravity: the lung bases and, mostly, the posterior regions. Thus, late inspiratory crackles are fine, high-pitched, profuse, gravity-dependent, poorly transmitted to the mouth (because they originate from more peripheral airways), and strongly associated with restrictive physiology. They can be extinguished with a change in posture but not by coughing. Otherwise they have a rather constant pattern.

Crackles

EARLY AND MID INSPIRATORY	LATE INSPIRATORY
Coarse	Fine
Low-pitched	High-pitched
Scanty	Profuse
Gravity-independent	Gravity-dependent
Do not change with posture	Change with posture
Clear with coughing	Do not clear with coughing
Well transmitted to the mouth	Poorly transmitted to the mouth
Associated with obstruction	Associated with restriction

80. Why is it important to separate early from late inspiratory crackles?

Because of their different clinical significance and association with different disease processes.

Early crackles tend to originate in the large central airways and therefore appear as low-pitched, coarse noises. Late crackles, on the other hand, originate in peripheral airways, which snap open during inspiration. Because these crackles originate more distally than early crackles, they are higher-pitched and fine. Finally, mid inspiratory crackles tend to originate in medium-sized airways and are usually pathognomonic of bronchiectasis. Thus, different timing means different disease processes. Given this correlation, early and late sounds are useful clinically. You should train your ear until you are able to time them accurately.

The ability to distinguish early vs. late crackles (and fine vs. coarse crackles) may even be enhanced by computer-assisted analysis of the waveforms.

81. What is the interobserver agreement in differentiating coarse from fine crackles?

Not too good. In a study by Piirila et al., observer agreement was only 60%.[35] In the same study an error in classification was even higher for patients with fibrosing alveolitis and bronchiectasis. This study suggests the importance of issues of nomenclature in determining interobserver agreement.

82. Can interobserver agreement be improved?

Yes. Murphy et al., for example, have shown that reasonable agreement can be obtained on the presence and quality of crackles if the observers are trained.[36]

Pearl.   Besides issues of terminology, interobserver agreement is usually quite good whenever the question concerns only the presence or absence of abnormal lung sounds. It is quite poor whenever the question concerns the grading or timing of these sounds. Interobserver agreement can indeed be improved with training.[37]

83. Can crackles occur in exhalation?

Yes. Although crackles tend to occur primarily in inspiration, expiratory crackles have been documented in patients with either obstructive or restrictive disease.[38] In patients with **obstructive disease**, such as chronic bronchitis or bronchiectasis, expiratory crackles tend to be coarse, to occur early in expiration, and to be gravity-independent and profuse.[39] They decrease in number after coughing. In patients with **restrictive disease**, such as fibrosing alveolitis or connective tissue disease, expiratory crackles tend to be fine, to occur in mid or late expiration, and to be gravity-dependent and scanty. They do not decrease in number with coughing.

84. What is the mechanism of production of late expiratory crackles?

There are two schools of thought:

1. Late expiratory crackles are produced by the closure (not by the reopening) of stiff and fibrotic small airways.

2. Late expiratory crackles are produced very much like late inspiratory crackles: by the reopening of small airways. Using the Forgacs model, the mechanism is as follows:
   • High interstitial pressure (from interstitial fibrosis, for example) collapses the lumen of a small airway.
   • The traction applied during inspiration snaps the airway open again. This "pop" coincides with a late inspiratory crackle.
   • The airway recoil in early exhalation then closes the airway lumen again. This, in turn, sets the airways up for a new reopening. This time, however, the reopening occurs in late exhalation and generates a late expiratory crackle.
   • This expiratory reopening occurs whenever the pressure of the air trapped within the airway exceeds the pressure in the adjacent airways.

Pearl. *Thus late inspiratory crackles are sounds generated by the reopening of small airways in inspiration. Late expiratory crackles, on the other hand, are sounds generated by either the reopening of small airways in exhalation or by their closure.*

85. Are crackles of bronchiectasis generated only by the bubbling of air through thin secretions?

No. Although in chronic bronchitis crackles are almost always produced by airway secretions and air-fluid interface, in bronchiectasis the mechanism may be different. The airways are abnormally dilated as a result of the destruction of the elastic and muscular components of the wall. Lacking its normal support, the bronchial wall therefore tends to collapse in expiration and then to reopen suddenly in inspiration. This mechanism plays an important role in the genesis of the inspiratory crackles and is responsible for crackles that do not clear with coughing (suggesting that secretions are not the causative mechanism).

86. Do the crackles of pulmonary fibrosis always occur late in inspiration?

No. Although they typically occur late in inspiration, crackles of pulmonary fibrosis may start in mid or even early inspiration. In fact, they may be *pan*inspiratory. Their hallmark, however, remains that they last until the end of inspiration. Similarly, crackles of bronchiectasis are typically mid inspiratory but also may start in early inspiration. Once again their hallmark is that they predominate in mid inspiration.

87. What are moist, dry, wet, sticky, atelectatic, close-to-the-ear, metallic, superficial, or consonating crackles?

Old and outdated modifiers. They are no longer recommended in the United States. Currently the only acceptable modifiers for crackles are fine and coarse (in addition, of course, to indicators of respiratory timing, such as early, mid, or late).

88. What about fine crepitations?

Same as above: an outdated term, except that this one used to be primarily a British favorite (and still is[40]). In fact, it used to be the English equivalent for the American and French rale and for the Italian rantoli. Still, it is a term to abandon.

89. How useful are crackles?

Very useful. Of all adventitious lung sounds they are probably the most clinically useful because of the strong correlation between inspiratory timing and site of production of the sounds (see above).

90. Which breath sounds are most commonly associated with crackles?

It depends. Early or mid inspiratory crackles are usually associated with vesicular breath sounds. Late inspiratory crackles, on the other hand, may be associated with either vesicular or bronchial breath sounds. This distinction may actually help in the differential diagnosis of the underlying disease process. For example, a fluid-filling process of the interstitial *and* alveolar compartments (such as pneumonia, pulmonary edema, or pulmonary hemorrhage) is much more likely to present with (1) late inspiratory crackles (due to interstitial fluid) and (2) bronchial breath sounds (due to alveolar fluid). To the contrary, a scarring process of the interstitium (pulmonary fibrosis) is much more likely to present with (1) late inspiratory crackles and (2) vesicular breath sounds.

Although a bit of an oversimplification, the algorithm below may help in the differential diagnosis of crackles.

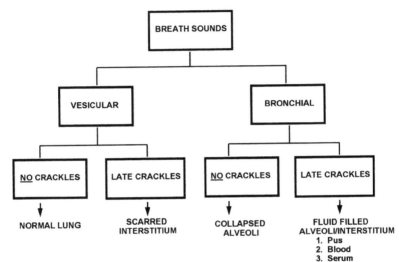

91. Can crackles be heard in healthy people?

Yes. Although usually a sign of disease, late inspiratory crackles also may occur in healthy people.[41] They may be found, for example, in dependent lung regions after prolonged periods of recumbence. They also have been detected in as many as 63% of 56 young nursing students using careful stethoscopic auscultation. This percentage increased to 92% when an electronic stethoscope with high-pass filtration was used.[42] In all these cases crackles were fleeting and heard only at the height of the first deep inspirations.

92. What is the mechanism of production of crackles in healthy people?

It is the reinflation of atelectatic lung units: the greater number of collapsed units, the greater the number of crackles generated. These crackles are generally limited to the posterior lung bases and occur quite frequently in people who have been breathing close to their functional residual capacity and then are suddenly asked to take a deep breath. Because a mild degree of basilar collapse is in fact common in any healthy person breathing shallowly below closing capacity, many basilar airways are collapsed. This collapse leads to the reabsorption of oxygen and further atelectasis. The sudden reopening of these airways in inspiration, in turn, generates the crackles.

Pearl. *"Normal" crackles are usually end-inspiratory and high-pitched and resemble the late inspiratory crackles of interstitial fibrosis. They usually resolve after a few deep inspirations.*

93. Are late inspiratory crackles common in all interstitial lung disease?

No. Although crackles have been reported in 65–91% of patients with chronic interstitial pulmonary disease,[43,44] late inspiratory and fine crackles are actually quite rare in sarcoidosis. In a survey of patients with various interstitial lung diseases, Epler et al. noted that bilateral fine crackles were present in approximately 60% of patients with either asbestosis or idiopathic pulmonary fibrosis but only in 18% of patients with sarcoidosis.[45] Fine crackles were also rare in other granulomatous disorders, such as miliary tuberculosis, eosinophilic granuloma, or allergic alveolitis, and in intra-alveolar processes, such as pulmonary alveolar proteinosis (20% of cases). When present, crackles of sarcoidosis still predominate at the bases, are fine in quality, and occur late in inspiration.

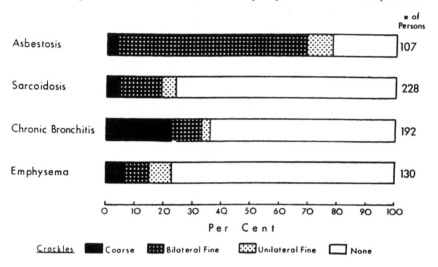

Incidence and types of crackles according to clinical diagnoses in 657 patients. (From Epler GR, Carrington CB, Gaensler EA: Crackles (rales) in the interstitial pulmonary diseases. Chest 73:333, 1978, with permission.)

94. Why are crackles so rare in sarcoidosis but so common in other fibrotic lung diseases?

Because the parenchymal fibrosis of the two types of diseases has a very different distribution, as seen clearly on high-resolution CT scans.[46] Idiopathic pulmonary fibrosis, for example, tends to be associated with lower lobar and subpleural fibrosis. Sarcoidosis, on the other hand, tends to be associated more with upper lobar and peribronchial fibrosis.

95. How common are late inspiratory crackles in patients with asbestosis?

Very common. In large population studies fine crackles are present in about 15% of asbestos workers compared with 3% of normal people.[47] Crackles are an early sign of the disease,[48] increasing in frequency and number with increased duration of exposure.[49] By the time asbestosis is clinically evident, late inspiratory, fine, high-pitched crackles are present in more than half of patients.[50] Crackles are a good marker of disease severity. In fact, they tend to be related to the duration of asbestos exposure more than the vital capacity itself. Thus, crackles can be a valuable tool in monitoring exposed workers.

96. Where are the crackles of asbestosis mostly localized?

They are first localized at the bases in the midaxillary lines and subsequently spread to the posterior bases.

97. Is the number of inspiratory crackles an indicator of disease severity?

Yes. As we have said in regard to asbestosis, the number of inspiratory crackles correlates with the severity of the underlying disease. This rule applies also to other interstitial diseases. Automatic crackle detection and counting methods have already been developed to help in the objective assessment of patients, for both diagnosis and follow-up.

98. Can late inspiratory crackles then be used for the assessment of severity of all interstitial lung disease?

Yes. In addition to the lower number of crackles, milder forms of the disease also tend to have crackles that are confined only to late inspiration and gravity-dependent areas of the lungs (such as the lung bases in upright patients). As the disease progresses, crackles may become paninspiratory (even though they still accentuate in end-inspiration), may persist despite changes in position, and may extend to involve higher levels above the bases. They also may become associated with late inspiratory squeaks.

99. What about expiratory crackles?

They are also valuable. Even if not as well documented as late inspiratory crackles, expiratory crackles may be present in many patients with interstitial lung disease. They tend to occur in mid or late inspiration. Their presence is very useful clinically. For example, Walshaw et al. have shown that the number of expiratory crackles is directly related to a reduction in diffusing capacity[51] of patients with fibrosing alveolitis. Thus, expiratory crackles (and their number) may be an important indicator of disease severity in patients with interstitial lung disease.

Pearl. As a matter of fact, because they are fewer in number than inspiratory crackles (and therefore easier to count), expiratory crackles may be an even more valuable sign than inspiratory crackles in assessing the severity of interstitial lung disease.

100. What are the characteristics of crackles in heart failure?

Very similar to those of crackles of pulmonary fibrosis (fibrosing alveolitis). Both tend to be profuse, fine, high-pitched, and late inspiratory. Both are predominantly located at the lung bases, are gravity- and posture-related and are difficult to separate clinically. Although a differentiation can usually be made on clinical grounds (and even better by using computerized sound analysis[52]), the examiner should still be aware of the similarity of these sounds when considering diuretics in patients with bibasilar crackles.

Pearl. As a rule of thumb, bibasilar fine crackles should be considered a sign of heart failure only in patients with no other clinical suggestion of pulmonary disease.

101. What are posturally induced crackles (PICs)?

A very useful finding. As indicated above, crackles are quite common in congestive heart failure. Recent evidence, however, indicates that crackles that occur only as a result of a recumbent posture have an even better diagnostic and predictive value.

102. How should PICs be elicited?

The standard procedure consists of the following:

1. Have the patient sit in bed upright for three minutes.
2. Place your stethoscope over the eighth, ninth, and tenth intercostal spaces along the posterior axillary line while the patient takes several deep breaths without forcing exhalation. The presence or absence of crackles should be noted during at least five consecutive breaths. For each breath special attention should be paid to the late inspiratory phase. Each inspiration should start from residual volume and end in total lung capacity.
3. Have the patient assume a supine position, maintaining it for three minutes.
4. Listen again to the patient's lungs using the same method outlined in 2.
5. Have the patient elevate both legs passively at an angle of 30° for three minutes.
6. Listen again to the patient's lungs using the same method outlined in 2.

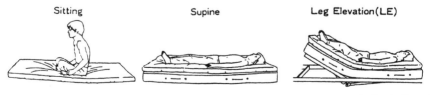

Standard procedure used to examine patients for PIC. (From Deguchi F, Hirakawa S, Gotoh K, et al: Prognostic significance of posturally-induced crackles. Long-term follow-up of patients after recovery from acute myocardial infarction Chest 103:1457–1462, 1993.)

103. How should the results of the PIC maneuver be interpreted?

Follow the schema illustrated in the table below:

1. If late inspiratory crackles are absent in the supine, sitting, and leg-elevated positions, the test is considered negative and the patient is given a score of 0.

2. If late inspiratory crackles are absent in the sitting position but become audible when the patient is either supine or has both legs elevated, the test is considered positive for PICs, and the patient is given a score of 1.

If late inspiratory crackles are already present in the sitting and the two supine positions, they are considered persistent, and the patient is given a score of 2.

Posturally Induced Crackles

	SITTING	SUPINE	LEG ELEVATION	SCORE
PIC-negative	–	–	–	0
PIC-positive (1)	–	–	+	1
PIC-positive (2)	–	+	+	1
Persistent crackles	+	+	+	2

(–) = late inspiratory and fine crackles are not audible. (+) = late inspiratory and fine crackles are audible. From Deguchi F, Hirakawa S, Gotoh K, et al: Prognostic significance of posturally-induced crackles. Long-term follow-up of patients after recovery from acute myocardial infarction Chest 103:1457–1462, 1993.

104. What is the clinical significance of PICs?

Very high, not only diagnostically but also prognostically. For example, Yagi et al. showed that PIC-positive patients have a significantly higher pulmonary capillary wedge pressure and a significantly lower pulmonary venous compliance than PIC-negative patients.[53] In a follow-up to this study, Deguchi et al. monitored 262 patients recovering from acute myocardial infarction. Over a period of 6 years, they found that PIC-negative patients had a significantly better long-term prognosis than PIC-positive patients. Only 3/78 (3.8%) of PIC-negative patients died of cardiac causes compared with 28/143 (19.6%) of PIC-positive patients. Cardiac death was, of course, even higher among patients with persistent crackles: 15/41 (36.6%).

Pearl. PIC is a noninvasive, simple, and valuable bedside test. After the number of diseased coronary vessels and the patient's pulmonary capillary wedge pressure (PCWP), PIC ranks third as the most important prognosticator for recovery after an acute myocardial infarction.[54]

Moreover, PIC is an independent variable. For example, PIC per se is not necessarily indicative of the number of diseased coronary vessels. In fact, when the number of disease vessels is constant, the presence of PIC consistently predicts a much lower survival rate. Similarly, in patients who had a higher PCWP ($\geq$ 13 mmHg), the presence of PIC consistently predicts a much lower survival rate.

Pearl. Thus, the lower survival rate of PIC-positive patients does not simply reflect an increased number of diseased vessels or a greater PCWP.

105. What are the characteristics of crackles in pneumonia?

Although Laennec considered the crackles of pneumonia very similar to the crackles of hemoptysis or pulmonary edema, their characteristics depend very much on the stage of pneumonia, as demonstrated by computerized sound analysis. In acute pneumonia crackles are predominantly coarse and mid inspiratory, resembling the crackles of bronchiectasis. During recovery, however, crackles tend to be shorter, more end-inspiratory, and more similar to the crackles of pulmonary fibrosis.[55]

106. What are the physical characteristics of crackles?

Crackles are high-pitched, short sounds of relatively high intensity. They usually last less than 20 msec in duration (hence the term discontinuous). Graphically they appear as sharp explosive spikes superimposed on the inspiratory limb (see figure on p. 321). Early inspiratory crackles tend to be louder, coarser, and of lower frequency than late inspiratory crackles.

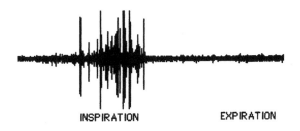

INSPIRATION   EXPIRATION

107. What are the radiographic findings in patients with crackles?

They depend on the etiology of the crackles. Considering that crackles may be heard in healthy people at end of a deep inspiration, chest radiographs may even be entirely normal. More commonly, however, crackles reflect either an air-fluid interface in the central airways (as in acute and chronic bronchitis or bronchiectasis) or a high interstitial pressure around the distal airways (as with interstitial scarring or edema). The radiographs of such patients therefore show the prominent and coarse interstitial markings of pulmonary fibrosis, the thickened airway walls and "tram-track lines" of bronchitis/bronchiectasis, or the fluffy consolidation of pneumonia, pulmonary hemorrhage, or pulmonary edema. In the last case, late inspiratory crackles (often associated with bronchial breath sounds and abnormally transmitted voice sounds) tend to be linked to the radiologic presence of air bronchograms (air-filled airways silhouetted out against consolidated and airless lung).

108. What is the lung pathology of patients with crackles?

It varies depending on the type of crackles and their mechanism of production. If the mechanism is air-fluid interface with rupture of thin films of secretions coating the large central airways, the pathology mostly shows bronchitis (acute or chronic) or bronchiectasis. This mechanism probably also plays a role in the crackles that Laennec referred to as "rales gargouillement," including the death rattle. If, on the other hand, the mechanism of production is the sudden equalization of intraairway pressure (as in the case of late inspiratory crackles), the pathology is pneumonia, pulmonary hemorrhage, pulmonary edema, or pulmonary fibrosis. This mechanism also plays a role in production of crackles in healthy people at the end of a deep inspiration; in this case, of course, the lung is entirely normal.

CONTINUOUS ADVENTITIOUS LUNG SOUNDS

109. What are continuous adventitious lung sounds?

Continuous adventitious lung sounds (CALs) are musical extra sounds superimposed on underlying breath sounds. They are usually expiratory but also may occur in inspiration or even cover the entire respiratory cycle. High-pitched CALs are called wheezes (dominant frequency of 400 Hz or more), whereas low-pitched CALs are called rhonchi (dominant frequency of 200 Hz or less[56]).

110. Why are these sounds called "continuous"?

They are called continuous not because they cover the entire respiratory cycle but simply because they are long. To be more precise, they are longer than the discontinuous adventitious lung sounds (i.e., crackles).

111. How long should the extra sounds last to qualify as CALs?

They should last more than 250 ms,[58] at least, according to the *American Thoracic Society Guidelines*. In reality, CALs are rarely that long; they usually last around 80–100 ms. This length, however, is just enough to give them a musical quality, which crackles lack.

112. What are the physical characteristics of CALs?

In addition to their long duration, CALs have a high frequency range (between less than 100 Hz to more than 1,000 Hz). An even higher frequency may be measured when CALs are recorded directly within the airways.

113. What are polyphonic and monophonic CALs?

Monophonic CALs are single musical tones, whereas polyphonic CALs are multiple distinct musical tones. This difference can be compared with the difference in the music generated by a solo singer and a polyphonic chorus. **Monophonic wheezes** consist of either a single note or of several notes starting and ending at different times. A good example of a monophonic wheeze is the rhonchus produced by a tumor that almost completely occludes a bronchus (see below). **Polyphonic wheezes** contain several notes, of which all start and end simultaneously, like a chord. Polyphonic wheezes may be heard in healthy people at the end of a forceful exhalation, but they usually are the hallmark of asthma. The narrowing of multiple airways is often responsible for the production of a real polyphonic chorus: the so-called concertus asthmaticus. Because in asthma the fluttering of large airway walls is a widespread phenomenon, CALs often may be heard throughout the lung fields.

114. How does one determine the pitch of a polyphonic wheeze?

By its fundamental frequency. In fact, a wheeze may contain several harmonically related frequencies, but the pitch of the wheeze is always set by its lowest (or fundamental) frequency.

115. How are CALs classified?

Based on their physical characteristics, they are classified into four categories: (1) sequential inspiratory CALs (or late inspiratory squeaks), (2) polyphonic expiratory CALs (or wheezes), (3) random monophonic CALs (or wheezes), and (4) fixed monophonic CALs (or rhonchi).

Sequential inspiratory CALs are simple (monophonic) or multiple (polyphonic) musical tones of various frequencies and different duration that occur toward the end of inspiration. They are produced by the airway as it reopens in partially collapsed lung areas, such as the bases in interstitial lung disease. Hence, they are often heard in association with the late inspiratory crackles so typical of interstitial fibrosis. These short, high-pitched, late inspiratory wheezes are usually localized at the more dependent lung fields (both laterally and posteriorly), have a high-pitched quality, and are often referred to as late inspiratory squeaks (or squawks in Britain, a term first coined by Earis et al.[59]).

Polyphonic expiratory CALs are multiple musical tones, each with a constant frequency and a similar duration. They occur only in expiration, have a high-pitched hissing quality, and are commonly referred to as wheezes. Because each tone has its own frequency (as indicated by the different height in the underlying schema), the communicative sound generated is called polyphonic (like the sound of a polyvocal chorus). Expiratory polyphonic wheezes are typically heard in mild asthma, but they may be heard even in healthy people at the end of a forced exhalation. Because they reflect alteration of airway mechanics throughout the lung, they can be heard equally over all lung fields.

| INSPIRATION | EXPIRATION |

Random monophonic CALs are single or multiple musical tones of various frequencies and different duration that occur randomly throughout the respiratory cycle. They have a high-pitched hissing quality and are often referred to as multiple monophonic wheezes. They are classically heard in severe asthma and are equally present throughout the chest. They can be heard during expiration, although more typically they cover the entire respiratory cycle. They are never present only in inspiration, which is the hallmark of either stridor or late inspiratory squeaks (see above). They are produced by the fluttering of central airways, narrowed by bronchospasm or inflammation.

INSPIRATION   EXPIRATION

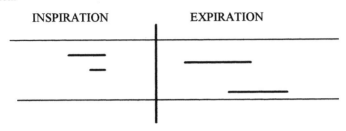

Fixed monophonic CALs are single musical tones of constant frequency and long duration. They are usually generated by the vibration of a large, partially obstructed bronchus. The obstruction may be due to tumor, inflammation, secretions, or a foreign body. These CALs have a low-pitched snoring quality and are often referred to as rhonchi. Their auscultatory site reflects the location of the underlying pathologic process. They may soften or disappear when the patient changes position.

Pearl. *A localized, persistent rhonchus may be the only abnormal physical finding in a patient with lung cancer.*

116. How are CALs produced?

CALs are *not* produced like the tone of an organ pipe. In an organ pipe, the sound is produced by the vibration of the air in the pipe, whereas the pitch of the tone is determined by the length and diameter of the pipe (the larger and longer the pipe, the lower-pitched the tone). If the same mechanism produced CALs:

- Our airways would have to be as long as 4–8 feet to produce some of the lowest-pitched wheezes heard in asthma. In reality, the longest axial pathway of the bronchial tree is less than 1 foot.
- The frequency of a wheeze generated by a particular airway would remain constant throughout respiration. In reality, it may differ by as much as an octave between inspiration and expiration.
- The pitch of a wheeze would change when the patient inspires a mixture of helium and oxygen (just as the pitch of an organ pipe rises when blown with helium). In reality, the pitch of a wheeze remains constant.

Therefore, the model for generation of CALs is not the organ pipe but the reed of a toy trumpet— or, even better, the reeds of an harmonica. In this model the flow of air sets the reed into oscillation between opening and closure, generating a note of constant frequency. Air moving at high velocity through a narrow bronchus also has a sucking effect on the airway wall, which is pulled inward and begins to flutter (i.e., wheeze). This fluttering delivers a note of constant frequency that depends on the mass and elasticity of the bronchial walls, the tightness of the narrowing, and the rate of gas flow through it.

117. What is the physical principle behind this mechanism?

Bernoulli's principle, which centers on the local drop in intraairway pressure that occurs whenever air flows at high velocity through a narrowed bronchus. The faster the flow at the point of constriction, the lower the pressure locally. Eventually, this drop in pressure becomes severe enough to cause a collapse of the airway wall. Because the collapse also reduces flow, the airway then reopens and the fluttering cycle starts again, repeating itself indefinitely.

Pearl. *Thus, wheezes are not produced by vibration of the air (as in organ pipes or wood-wind instruments), but by vibration (fluttering) of airway walls. This vibration is facilitated by fast jets of air, forced by high expiratory pressures through tightly compressed airways.*

Postulated wheeze mechanism. The stability of the airway wall depends on a balance between internal air pressure and external forces, and on the mechanical characteristics of the airway itself. When a narrowing of the lumen occurs, the air velocity must increase through the constricted region to maintain a constant mass flow rate. According to the Benoulli principle, the increased air velocity leads to a decrease in air pressure, thus allowing external forces to further collapse the airway. When the lumen has been reduced so much that the flow decreases, the process begins to reverse itself as the pressure inside the airway begins to increase and reopen the lumen. When conditions are right, the airway wall flutters between nearly occluded and occluded positions and produces wheezing. Short open arrows indicate slower flow; long open arrows indicate faster flow. Large closed arrows indicate higher pressure; small closed arrows indicate lower pressure. Modified from Murphy and Holford (32); reproduced with permission.

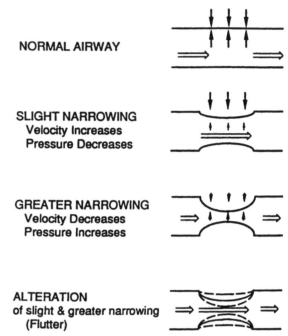

NORMAL AIRWAY

SLIGHT NARROWING
Velocity Increases
Pressure Decreases

GREATER NARROWING
Velocity Decreases
Pressure Increases

ALTERATION
of slight & greater narrowing
(Flutter)

118. What is a late inspiratory squeak?

It is a single, short, high-pitched wheeze heard at the very end of inspiration. Laennec described it as "le cri d'un petit oiseau" (the chirp of a little bird). Late inspiratory squeaks at times may be multiple and of different pitch. In this case they follow each other, sequentially and throughout inspiration. Squeaks often occur in association with late inspiratory crackles and usually follow them at the end of inspiration.

119. What are the causes of a late inspiratory squeak?

Not many. A squeak usually indicates either pulmonary fibrosis, allergic alveolitis, or bronchiolitis obliterans. The association between squeaks and late inspiratory crackles suggests that squeaks are produced much like late inspiratory crackles: by the reopening of a partially collapsed distal airway. It is likely that air passing through a newly reopened but still narrowed airway will cause a crackle (as the airway opens abruptly) and a wheeze (as the air rushes through an airway that is still narrowed).

120. How can CALs be graphically represented?

They can be represented by bars in a way similar to the representation of musical notes.

1. The **pitch** of the CALs is graphically indicated by the height of the bar (that is, the vertical location of the bar above the respiratory cycle; the higher the pitch, the higher the bar and vice versa).

2. The **loudness** is represented by the thickness of the bar (the thicker the bar, the louder the sound and vice versa).

3. The **duration** is represented by the length of the bar (the longer the bar, the longer the sound and vice versa).

4. Finally, the **timing** of the CALs is represented by their location within the respiratory cycle. CALs may be early expiratory, late expiratory, or even panrespiratory when they cover the entire length of the respiratory cycle.

121. Is the pitch of a wheeze related to its site of production?

No. This widely held belief is based on an erroneous analogy with orchestral wind instruments: wheezes are not produced like the sounds of wind instruments (see above). Thus, the pitch of a wheeze does not depend on anatomic location but on the degree of obstruction of the bronchus in which the wheeze is generated. Wheezes, therefore, are produced whenever the bronchial diameter is narrowed to the point of dynamic compression by bronchospasm, peribronchial edema (due to left ventricular failure), accumulation of secretions, or closure of the airway lumen by a partially obstructing tumor.

Pearl.   Therefore, in contrast to crackles, high-pitched wheezes do not originate in small peripheral airways, and low-pitched wheezes are not produced by large central bronchi.

122. Is the pitch of a wheeze related to the degree of anatomic narrowing of an airway (that is, the higher the pitch, the worse the narrowing)?

Yes and no. As we said before the pitch of a wheeze reflects the degree of dynamic narrowing of the airway and the rate of flow through that airway, in accordance with Bernoulli's effect. For example, forced expiratory flow through a normal airway may produce a wheeze even in a healthy person, and diminished flow in a narrowed airway may remain totally silent (hence the conventional teaching, "Beware of the asthmatic who stops wheezing while turning blue").

Nonetheless, the pitch of a wheeze *does* correlate with the degree of airflow obstruction. Shim and Williams, for example, showed that more severe asthmatics tend to have higher-pitched wheezes.[60] Similarly, a decrease in the frequency content of wheezes has been shown to result from bronchodilator therapy. Thus, the pitch of a wheeze is an indicator of the severity of asthma. The length of wheezes, on the other hand, is even a better indicator (see below).

123. Describe the breath sounds of asthmatic patients.

They vary, depending on the degree of bronchospasm. For example, a decrease in frequency as a result of bronchodilator therapy is typical not only of wheezes, but also of their underlying breath sounds. Conversely, an increase in the frequency of the vesicular breath sound is one of the first signs of bronchospasm, even before the onset of audible wheezing.

Pearl.   Thus, the breath sounds of patients with asthma are diminished in intensity but often have a higher frequency than regular vesicular breath sounds.

124. Describe the breath sounds of patients undergoing bronchoprovocation.

A positive bronchial provocation usually produces a decrease in the intensity of inspiratory breath sounds, unaccompanied by wheezing. This decrease is as common in positive responders as the appearance of a wheeze.[61] An overall increase in frequency is also characteristic of the breath sounds of patients undergoing an asthmatic attack.[62]

Pearl.   Thus, the breath sounds of patients developing bronchospasm tend to be softer (because of diminished regional air flow) but higher-pitched (because of the effect of stiffer airway walls on sound transmission at low frequencies).

125. How can one assess the severity of asthma based on wheezing?

This question was answered by Baughman and Loudon,[63] who studied patients admitted to the emergency department for acute asthma, recorded their lung sounds at four standard chest sites, and correlated the auscultatory findings with spirometric data (FEV_1 and FVC) before and after treatment. They found that the intensity of wheezing and the simultaneous presence of wheezes of different pitch (polyphonic wheezing) were *not* correlated with the severity of the obstruction.

Pearl.   Only two variables correlated consistently with the degree of airflow obstruction: (1) the proportion of the respiratory cycle occupied by the wheeze and (2) the frequency content of the highest-pitched wheeze. Thus, only the pitch and length of wheezes are clinically useful parameters to assess the degree of airflow obstruction: higher-pitched and longer wheezes reflect a more severe obstruction.

126. How can one best express the length of a wheeze?

By the proportion of the respiratory cycle occupied by the wheeze (T_w/T_{tot}). In adults with moderate-to-severe obstruction T_w/T_{tot} is inversely related to the FEV_1.[64]

Pearl. *Thus, wheezing that occurs only in exhalation is not as severe as wheezing that occurs both in exhalation and inspiration; similarly, longer expiratory wheezes reflect worse obstruction than shorter expiratory wheezes.*

127. What are the features of a resolving asthmatic attack?

A decrease in the frequency of the highest-pitched wheeze[65] and a decrease in T_w/T_{tot}.

128. In summary, what are the auscultatory findings in patients with asthma?

They depend primarily on the degree of asthma severity. Overall, the most prominent finding is a high-pitched continuous sound (wheeze), first heard in exhalation and then, as the disease worsens, in both inspiration and exhalation. Wheezes tend to be monophonic initially and polyphonic as the disease progresses. More specifically:

1. In **mild asthma** the site of dynamic obstruction is in the central airways. The fluttering of bronchi generates random monophonic wheezes that are loud and well transmitted both upward (to the mouth) and downward (to the chest wall).

2. In **more severe asthma**, on the other hand, the site of dynamic obstruction is in the more peripheral airways. Because the airflow rate in these structures is too low to cause a major fluttering, the sounds generated are random monophonic wheezes that are too weak to be transmitted to the mouth and barely audible at the chest well.

3. The airflow obstruction of **status asthmaticus** is due to a combination of bronchial edema, bronchospasm, and mucus plugging. These changes usually start in the central airways and cause at first only expiratory, random, monophonic CALs (wheezes). Subsequently, however, the site of airway fluttering moves gradually toward the periphery of the tracheobronchial tree. Because the airflow rate of small and peripheral airways is too low to generate adequate fluttering, the chest of a patient with advanced status asthmaticus may become paradoxically silent.

129. How sensitive and specific are wheezes in the diagnosis of airflow obstruction?

Neither sensitive nor specific. Forced exhalation, for example, can produce wheezing in healthy people (see below), whereas patients with severe airflow obstruction may not wheeze at all. Indeed, Godfrey et al. found wheezing in only 70% of patients with a forced expiratory volume in one second (FEV_1) < 1 L.[66] Wheezes are more frequent in patients with asthma than patients with chronic obstructive pulmonary disease.[67] Yet wheezing may resolve while airflow obstruction remains quite severe. In a study by McFadden et al., wheezing disappeared with emergency care when the FEV_1 was still only 63% of predicted value.[68] In another study of emergency care, wheezing among asthmatics was one of the least discriminating factors in predicting either hospital admission or relapse.[69] Absence of wheezing in status asthmaticus, on the other hand, may have an ominous meaning. For example, it may indicate that flow rates are so low that wheezing cannot be generated (hence the aforementioned dictum, "Beware of the asthmatic who stops wheezing while turning blue.").

Pearl. *Thus wheezes, although useful, are not perfect diagnostic findings. From the clinical standpoint, they are less valuable than crackles.*

130. What is the differential diagnosis of wheezing?

Rather broad. The famous dictum, "Not all that wheezes is asthma," is an important reminder that we should always exclude other causes of wheezing before concluding that the patient has asthma (see table below). In an epidemiologic study, for example, wheezes were present in 25% of the population, whereas the prevalence of asthma was only 7%.[70] Among the extrathoracic causes of wheezing, it is important to keep in mind vocal cord dysfunction and, of course, stridor.

Considering that wheezes originating extrathoracically tend to be louder over the neck than over the chest, auscultation over the trachea should help. Vocal cord dysfunction may be associated with either inspiratory or expiratory wheezes. Stridor, of course, is primarily inspiratory.

Clinical Conditions Associated with Wheezing

• Infections (croup, whooping cough, laryngitis, tracheobronchitis)	• Chronic obstructive pulmonary disease
• Laryngo-, tracheo-, or bronchomalacia	• Bronchorrheal states (such as chronic bronchitis, cystic fibrosis, bronchiectasis)
• Laryngeal or tracheal tumors	• Bronchiolitis obliterans*
• Tracheal stenosis	• Interstitial fibrosis*
• Vocal cord dysfunction	• Hypersensitivity pneumonitis*
• Foreign body aspiration	• Pulmonary edema
• Large airway compression or stenosis	• Forced expiration in normal subjects
• Asthma	

* All of these conditions tend to be associated with a late inspiratory squeak (or squawk); see below.
From Meslier N, Charbonneau G, Racineaux JL: Wheezes. Eur Respir J 8:1942–1948, 1995, with permission.

131. How helpful are forced expiratory wheezes?

Not much. Forced expiratory wheezes originate in the large central airways[71] and totally lack specificity for asthma. In fact, forced expiratory wheezes can be generated in entirely healthy people by asking them to take a deep breath and "blast out really fast."

Pearl.   *Wheezing on maximal forced exhalation has a sensitivity of only 57% and a specificity of only 37%.[72] Thus, a forced expiratory maneuver aimed at "unmasking silent bronchospasm" should not be relied on for the clinical diagnosis of airflow obstruction.[73]*

132. What is cardiac asthma?

It is the wheezing heard in patients experiencing left ventricular failure. Based on conventional teaching, it is not a sign of pulmonary disease (i.e., asthma) but of cardiac disease. The mechanism is narrowing of the airways as a result of edema of the bronchial wall and interstitium. In reality, various studies have indicated that cardiac asthma is really asthma—that is, airflow obstruction produced by reactive airways disease in patients experiencing edema of the airway wall. For this reason, the majority of patients with left-ventricular failure develop crackles, whereas only a minority develop wheezing.

133. What is the significance of wheezes heard only in inspiration?

They are not wheezes; they are **stridor**. In fact, with the sole exception of the sequential inspiratory wheeze (the so-called late inspiratory squeak of interstitial fibrosis or allergic alveolitis), wheezes heard only in inspiration represent stridor.

134. What are the acoustic differences between stridor and wheezes?

Baughman and Loudon analyzed the physical characteristics of wheezes and stridor.[74] They found that the best discriminators were timing and location. Stridor is more prominent over the neck and exclusively inspiratory. Wheezes, on the other hand, are either expiratory or inspiratory *and* expiratory; they are never inspiratory only.

135. Is the stridor a higher-pitched sound than a wheeze?

No. Baughman and Loudon found no differences in the frequency characteristics of stridor compared with wheezes. There were only two distinct separations between the two sounds: timing and location.

136. What are the radiographic characteristics of a patient with CALs?

They depend on the physical characteristics of the CALs. For example, **sequential inspiratory CALs** (or squeaks) are usually encountered in patients with interstitial fibrosis or bronchiolitis obliterans. The chest radiograph may show prominent interstitial markings, usually at both lung bases. **Polyphonic expiratory CALs** are usually encountered in patients with mild asthma, although at times they can be heard in healthy people at the end of forced exhalation. The chest radiograph of most asthmatics is usually normal. **Random monophonic CALs** are usually encountered in patients presenting with severe asthma (status asthmaticus). The chest radiograph is usually normal, although hyperinflation tends to be a more common finding. **Fixed monophonic CALs** (rhonchi) are usually encountered in patients with chronic bronchitis or even asthma. They also may be encountered in patients with a normal chest radiograph and an unsuspected endobronchial lesion, which is responsible for the production of the localized expiratory rhonchus. Localized rhonchi, therefore, are important findings. At times they may be the only clinical evidence for an early bronchogenic carcinoma.

PLEURAL RUB

137. What is a pleural rub?
A pleural rub is a special type of adventitious lung sound. It is loud and creaky and is generated by two inflamed pleural surfaces rubbing against each other.

138. How does a rub sound?
It has been compared to a violin bow striking a string in a to-and-fro mode.[75] According to this model, the chest wall, because of its large mass and springiness, behaves like the body of a string instrument. As a result, it continues to vibrate for a short time after each impulse transmitted by the pleural friction. As a result, the various components of the rub lengthen and even merge into a continuous and often musical sound, similar to a rhonchus or a wheeze.

139. Is a pleural rub inspiratory, expiratory, or both?
The pleural rub is usually both inspiratory and expiratory because it is generated by the sliding and rubbing against each other of the two pleural layers. However, because of the faster sliding and rubbing of the pleural surfaces during inspiration, the inspiratory component tends to be louder than the expiratory component. At times it may even be the only audible component.

140. How can a rub be graphically represented?
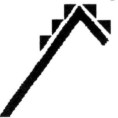
It is usually represented by small triangles superimposed on the underlying respiratory cycle.

141. How can one distinguish a pleural rub from a crackle?
With great difficulty. Pleural rubs, in fact, are often misdiagnosed as crackles because the two share many similar physical characteristics. To help differentiate them, one needs to remember that a rub (1) occurs in both inspiration and expiration; (2) does not change with coughing; is usually (3) longer, (4) louder, and (5) lower-pitched; (6) is often palpable; and (7) is usually highly localized and present in only a small area of the chest wall.

142. How can one distinguish a pleural rub from a wheeze?
This distinction is a little easier. Rubs can indeed be confused with a polyphonic medium- or low-pitched wheeze. Differentiation, however, may be facilitated by remembering that rubs never occur only in expiration, whereas most wheezes do. Indeed, rubs are usually present during both inspiration and expiration. They may occur during inspiration only, but they never occur only in expiration.

Pearl.   *Therefore, an adventitious sound that is audible (or louder) only in inspiration is more likely to be a rub. Conversely, an adventitious sound that is audible only in exhalation is more likely to be a wheeze (or rhonchus).*

143. How can one distinguish a pleural rub from a pericardial rub?

By asking the patient to hold his or her breath. If the rub persists, it is much more likely to be pericardial.

144. Are rubs transient or long-lasting findings?

Rubs are transient. They usually disappear when enough pleural fluid accumulates to separate the two pleural layers, preventing them from rubbing against each other. Thus, if not carefully and frequently sought after, a fleeting rub may be easily missed.

145. What is the pleural histology in patients with a rub?

The visceral pleura and the parietal pleura are normally lined with a single layer of flat mesothelial cells. These layers are smooth and lubricated by a thin film of fluid, which allows them to slide easily and silently on each other during respiration. The smoothness of the pleural surface, however, is lost with inflammation, when fibrin deposits of either neoplastic or inflammatory cells cover the two pleural layers. The friction produced by the roughened pleural surfaces sliding and rubbing against each other is responsible for the generation of the pleural rub. Whenever fluid accumulates in the pleural cavity, the two pleural layers become widely separated and the rub disappears. Pleural rubs, therefore, are pathognomonic of pleural inflammation. Thus, noninflammatory effusions, such as those associated with congestive heart failure, nephrotic syndrome, or cirrhosis, are never associated with a rub.

146. What are the disease processes most commonly associated with a pleural rub?

Common diseases that may be associated with a pleural rub include cancer, pneumonia, pleuritis, and pulmonary embolism. Serositis, such as that seen in collagen vascular diseases, may produce a rub even when the chest radiograph is entirely normal. Rubs are common in lupus pleuritis but rare in rheumatoid pleural effusion. They are common in thromboembolic disease and parapneumonic pleuritis but relatively rare in tuberculous pleurisy. Similarly, the frequency of rubs in neoplastic pleural involvement is variable. Neoplastic involvement of the pleura may produce a rub either directly (as a direct invasion of pleural layers) or indirectly (as an inflammatory process of the pleura overlying a lung cancer). Finally, pleural rubs often occur in lobar pneumonia, such as pneumococcal, staphylococcal, or gram-negative pneumonias. Because rubs are fleeting and highly localized findings, a thorough search may be necessary to detect them.

147. What are the physical characteristics of a pleural friction rub?

The most important characteristic is the presence of several extra sounds of short duration and relatively high frequency, all superimposed on the underlying breath sound. From this standpoint, the sound wave of a rub is quite similar to the sound wave of a crackle (although the rub tends to span inspiration and expiration, whereas crackles predominate in inspiration).

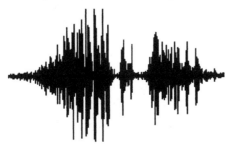

INSPIRATION   EXPIRATION

Frequencies represented in the pleural rub tend to vary in range. Although most are medium- to high-pitched, they are not as high as the frequencies of crackles. Because of their relatively high frequency, rubs are well perceived by the human ear and appear loud. The inspiratory components of the rub usually have higher intensity and sometimes may be the only audible sounds. The rub is also characterized by what Forgacs defines as the "mirror image effect," which refers to the apparent reverse sequence of the expiratory component of the rub compared with the inspiratory component.

Pearl. *Thus, a pleural rub is composed of a series of short, loud, and creaky sounds that often have been compared to the sound of leather. They can be visualized in a sound wave as tall "spikes" superimposed on both inspiration and expiration.*

TRANSMITTED VOICE SOUNDS

148. What are transmitted voice sounds?

Transmitted voice sounds are sounds that, unlike other respiratory sounds (whether they be breath sounds or adventitious lung sounds), are not produced by the patient's lungs; instead, they are produced by the patient's larynx. These voice-generated sounds may become abnormally transmitted in certain disease processes, thus providing an important clue to the underlying diagnosis.

149. List the abnormally transmitted voice sounds.

1. **Bronchophony** (Greek for the sound of the bronchi) indicates a clear voice sound—at least as clear as it can be when heard over the bronchi or larynx. In bronchophony, however, the voice sounds are heard over the chest and in areas remote from either bronchi or larynx. The words spoken by the patient remain unintelligible; only the sound becomes loud and clear.

2. **Pectoriloquy** (Latin for the voice of the chest) indicates the clear and intelligible words heard over the chest when a patient is either whispering (whispered pectoriloquy) or speaking (spoken pectoriloquy).

3. **Egophony** (Greek for the voice of the goat) is the bleating and goatlike sound produced by the patient's voice when heard over the chest.

4. **E-to-A changes** are a more recent variant of egophony.

150. Is there any magic word that one should ask patients to say to elicit these sounds?

Not really. In the U.S. we usually ask patients to say "ninety-nine" (which is the same number used to elicit tactile fremitus). In Italy (a smaller country) "thirty-three" is the number of choice. As Sapira points out, the custom of having patients say "ninety-nine" comes from the English translation of the German "neun und neunzig."[76] This translation actually changed the physical characteristics of the sound, making it possibly less fit for the task. Another alternative is to ask the patient to say "one, two, three." For eliciting abnormally transmitted voice sounds, any sound will do (unless, of course, you are trying to elicit the E-to-A change; see question 157).

151. What is the significance of abnormally transmitted voice sounds?

All of them reflect an abnormal transmission of spoken or whispered words or vowels through the lungs. More specifically, they indicate that the lung parenchyma has become airless and consolidated.

152. Are the bronchi of patients with abnormally transmitted voice sounds closed or open?

Open. If the bronchi were closed, there would be no transmission of sounds to the chest surface. Hence, there would be no egophony, bronchophony, or pectoriloquy.

153. When should one elicit transmitted voice sounds?

Only when one suspects abnormal sound transmission along the tracheal bronchial tree and across the lungs—in general, when one suspects consolidation.

154. What are the production and transmission characteristics of voice sounds?

Normal voice sounds are generated by vibration of the vocal cords, which is produced by the flow of exhaled air. Although normal voice sounds are mostly transmitted upward to the mouth, they are also simultaneously transmitted downward to the chest. In the chest the air-filled lungs act as a low-pass filter, eliminating high-frequency components and allowing only the low-frequency sounds to reach the chest wall surface. This low-pass filtering, therefore, eliminates the high-pitched components of the vowels, the so-called formants. Because the recognition of vowels is essential to the comprehension of words (vowels have been called the spice of a language), the elimination of formants transforms voice sounds into a muffled and low-pitched mumble. Although detectable through the stethoscope, this mumble is soft and unintelligible.

Solids and fluids, on the other hand, can transmit high frequencies better than air. Thus, consolidation of the lung parenchyma improves transmission of the higher-pitched components of vowels, making the vowels and the voice sounds louder, clearer, and even intelligible.

Pearl. Voice sounds change physical characteristics depending on whether they are transmitted through aerated or consolidated (airless) lung. Thus, they provide a useful sign for the bedside recognition of consolidation.

155. What is egophony?

Egophony is Greek for the voice of a goat. No, this is not a Freudian slip—egophony has nothing to do with the voice of the ego. It refers instead to Αιξ (aix), which is Greek for goat. Thus, egophony indicates the bleating and goatlike sound produced by the human voice when it is heard over consolidated lungs. Laennec was the first to describe this phenomenon (and, of course, to give it its complicated Greek name): "Egophony . . . possesses, moreover, one constant characteristic from which it has seemed to me suitable to name the phenomenon; it is quavering and jerky like the bleating of a goat."

156. What are the E-to-A changes?

They are a variant of egophony and another type of abnormally transmitted voice sound.

157. Who first described the E-to-A changes?

A British missionary named Shibley was working as a physician in China in the 1920s. He auscultated his patients' chests while asking them to say "one, two, three." Since his patients were obligingly Chinese, "one, two, three" was said in Chinese: "i, er, san." There is, however, another important clue in this story: the Chinese word for "one" ("i") was pronounced "E" in the province of China where Shibley was working. Soon Shibley noticed that whenever his patients had either pneumonia or pleural effusion, they developed a localized area of the chest in which the sound "E" changed surprisingly and consistently into an "A." In fact, he noticed that *all* five vowel sounds (A, E, I, O, U) became "A" in cases of consolidation or pleural effusion. He reported these findings in the *Chinese Medical Journal* (1922),[77] and we now refer to them as the E-to-A change.[78]

In the same year (1922), Froschels and Stockert reported a similar finding in Vienna. Of course, they wrote it in German, not in English, but they observed that in cases of consolidation one vowel sound seems to be transformed into another without any particular predictability.[79]

158. What is the mechanism behind the E-to-A changes?

It is, of course, consolidation—more precisely, consolidation that extends from the auscultated chest wall to the tracheobronchial tree.[80] Less extensive consolidation (as, for example, the consolidation of a pulmonary nodule) does not create a bridge long enough to cause either E-to-A changes or egophony.

159. What are the most common causes of extensive consolidation?

Either filling of the alveoli by a medium that transmits sound better than air (such as pus, blood, or serum) or collapse of the alveoli. The layer of pleural fluid is thick enough to compress the alveoli and to make them airless but thin enough to leave the airways patent.

160. How does consolidation change an E into an A?

Consolidation creates a change in the filtering properties of the lung, allowing it to transmit sounds of higher frequency. The fact that an E may sound like A when auscultated over an area of consolidation remains, nonetheless, almost an acoustic paradox. In fact, when heard at the mouth, E is higher-pitched than A. Thus, it appears contradictory that a consolidated lung, which is capable of transmitting high frequencies better than a normal lung, should change a high-pitched sound like an E into a low-pitched sound like an A.

The explanation for this apparent paradox is that the sound E is a mixture of both high- and low-frequency components. The high-frequency components are in the 2,000–3,500 Hz range, whereas the low-frequency components are in the 100–400 Hz range. The sound A also has both low- and high-frequency components; the only difference is that the low-frequency components of A have a range that is a bit higher than the low-frequency components of E (in A they reach 600 Hz).

When E or A is heard over the chest, none of their high-frequency components are audible, regardless of whether the underlying lung is consolidated. Thus, even though a consolidated lung can transmit higher frequencies better than a normal lung (close to 1,000 Hz instead of 400), it still cannot transmit the highest frequencies (such as the 2,000–3,500 frequencies) that are so typical of E.[81]

Pearl. Thus, consolidated lung better transmits the low frequencies that are very important features of A (the ones up to 600 Hz), but does not transmit well the higher frequencies that are unique to E. As a result, an E can now become an A, as do all other vowels when similarly analyzed. All vowels, in fact, sound like an A when heard over a consolidated lung.

161. What is the mechanism of whispered pectoriloquy?

Still consolidation. Remember that whispered sounds consist almost entirely of high-frequency components. Therefore, they are not transmitted by the aerated lung; they become audible only when the loss of alveolar air from consolidation allows their transmission.

162. What kind of breath sounds accompany abnormally transmitted voice sounds?

Tubular (bronchial) breath sounds—because egophony, bronchophony, and pectoriloquy require consolidated lungs. Consolidated lungs, in fact, transmit breath sounds differently, giving more prominence and better transmission to the higher-frequency components. This is also the mechanism behind the generation of tubular (or bronchial) breath sounds. These tubular sounds are associated with late inspiratory crackles in patients who are consolidated because of alveolar fluid-filling, whereas they are isolated in patients who are consolidated because of alveolar collapse.

163. Is there any radiographic equivalent for abnormally transmitted voice sounds?

Yes. Abnormally transmitted voice sounds are typically associated with air bronchograms, which are air-filled and patent bronchi silhouetted against the white background of airless and consolidated alveoli. This radiographic finding is nonspecific and may be seen with atelectasis, lung hemorrhage, pneumonia, or pulmonary edema.

164. Which is the most useful of all these transmitted voice sounds?

Probably egophony, closely followed by whispered pectoriloquy. In some patients whispered pectoriloquy may be the first finding to appear in case of consolidation.

REFERENCES

1. Bishop PJ: Evolution of the stethoscope. J R Soc Med 73:448–456, 1980.
2. Schilling RSF, Highes JPW, Dingwall-DeFordyce I: Disagreement between observers in an epidemiologic study of respiratory disease. BMJ 1:65, 1995.
3. Fletcher CM: The clinical diagnosis of pulmonary emphysema. A experimental study. Proc R Soc Med 45:577, 1952.

4. Smyllie HC, Blendis LM, Armitage P: Observer disagreement in physical signs of the respiratory system. Lancet 2:412, 1965.
5. Schneider IC, Anderson AE: Correlation of clinical signs with ventilatory function in obstructive lung disease. Ann Intern Med 62:477, 1965.
6. Koran LM: The reliability of clinical methods, data, and judgment. N Engl J Med 293:642–701, 1975.
7. Cochrane AL: Observer error in the interpretation of chest films. Lancet 2:505–509, 1952.
8. Felson B, Morgan WKC, Bristol LJ, et al: Observations on the results of multiple readings of chest films in coal miners pneumoconiosis. Lintonow's Reger RB Radiol 109:19–23, 1973.
9. Pasterkamp H, Kraman SS, Wodicka GR: Respiratory sounds. Am J Respir Crit Care Med 156:974–987, 1997.
10. Forgacs P: The functional basis of pulmonary sounds. Chest 3:399–405, 1978.
11. Hidalgo HA, Wegmann MJ, Waring WW: Frequency spectra of normal breath sounds in childhood. Chest 100:992–1002, 1991.
12. Pasterkamp H, Powell RE, Sanchez I: Characteristics of lung sounds at standardized air flow in normal infants, children and adults. Am J Respir Crit Care Med 154:424–430, 1995.
13. Pardee NE, Martin CJ, Morgan EH: A test of the practical value of estimating breath sound intensity. Breath sounds related to measured ventilatory function. Chest 70:341–344, 1976.
14. Bohadana AB, Pesliln R, Uffholtz H: Breath sounds in the clinical assessment of airflow obstruction. Thorax 33:345, 1978.
15. Pardee NE, Martin CJ, Morgan EH: A test of the practical value of estimating breath sound intensity. Breath sounds related to measured ventilatory function. Chest 70:341–344, 1976.
16. Purhoit A, Bohadana AB, Kopferschmitt-Kubler MC, et al: Lung auscultation in airway challenge testing. Respir Med 91:151–157, 1997.
17. Bohadana AB, Pesliln R, Uffholtz H: Breath sounds in the clinical assessment of airflow obstruction. Thorax 33:345, 1978.
18. LeBlanc P, Macklem PT, Ross WRD: Breath sounds and distribution of pulmonary ventilation. Am Rev Respir Dis 102:10–16, 1970.
19. Scheider IC, Anderson AE: Correlation of clinical signs with ventilatory function in obstructive lung disease. Ann Intern Med 62:477–485, 1965.
20. Scheider IC, Anderson AE: Correlation of clinical signs with ventilatory function in obstructive lung disease. Ann Intern Med 62:477–485, 1965.
21. Bohadana AB, Peslin R, Uffholtz H, Pauli G: Breath sound intensity in patients with airway provocation challenge test positive by spirometry but negative for wheezing : A preliminary report. Respiration 61:274–279, 1994.
22. Lai S, Ferguson AD, Campbell EJM: Forced-expiratory time: A simple test for airway obstruction. BMJ 1:814, 1964.
23. Forgacs P, Nathoo AR, Richardson HD: Breath sounds. Thorax 26:288–295, 1971.
24. Forgacs P: The functional basis of pulmonary sounds. Chest 3:399–405, 1978.
25. Forgacs P: Lung Sounds. London, Bailliere Tindall, 1978, p 34.
26. Gavriely N, Nassan M, Cugell W, Rubin AH: Respiratory health screening using pulmonary function tests and lung sound analysis. Eur Respir J 7:35–42, 1994.
27. Pasterkamp H, Schafer J, Wodicka GR: Posture-dependent change of tracheal sounds as standardized flows in patients with obstructive sleep apnea. Chest 110:1493–1498, 1996.
28. Fraser RG, Pare JAP: Diagnosis of Diseases of the Chest. Philadelphia, W.B. Saunders, 1970.
29. American Thoracic Society Ad Hoc Committee on Pulmonary Nomenclature: Updated nomenclature for membership reaction. ATS News 3:5–6, 1977.
30. Cugell DW: Lung sounds: Classification and controversies. Semin Respir Med 6:210–219, 1985.
31. Forgacs P: Crackles and Wheezes. Lancet 2:203–205, 1967.
32. Robertson AJ, Coope R: Rales, rhonchi, and Laennec. Lancet 2:417–423, 1957.
33. Nath AR, Capel LH: Inspiratory crackles: Early and late. Thorax 29:223–227, 1974.
34. Nath AR, Capel LH: Inspiratory crackles and mechanical events of breathing. Thorax 29:695–698, 1974.
35. Piirila P, Kallio K, Katila T, et al: Crackle sound intensity in the auscultation of crackling sounds in fibrosing alveolitis and heart failure. In Proceedings of the 17th International Conference on Lung Sounds. Helsinki, Finland, 1992, p 26.
36. Murphy RLH, Gaensler EA, Holford SK, et al: Crackles in the early detection of asbestosis. Am Rev Respir Dis 129:375–379, 1984.
37. Shirai F, Kudoh S, Shibuya A, et al: Crackles in asbestos workers: Auscultation and lung sound analysis. Br J Dis Chest 75:383–396, 1981.
38. Walshaw MJ, Nisar M, Pearson MG, et al: Expiratory lung crackles in patients with fibrosing alveolitis. Chest 97:407–409, 1990.
39. Nath AR, Capel LH: Lung crackles in bronchiectasis. Thorax 35:694–699, 1980.
40. Bunin JN, Loudon RG: Lung sound terminology in case reports. Chest 76:690–692, 1979.

41. Thatcher RE, Kraman SS: The prevalence of auscultatory crackles in subjects without lung disease. Chest 81:672–674, 1982.
42. Workum P, Holford SK, DelBono EA, Murphy RLH: The prevalence and character of crackles (rales) in young women without significant lung disease. Am Rev Respir Dis 126:413–415, 1982.
43. DeRemee RA, Harrison EG, Andersen HA: The concept of classic intestinal pneumonitis-fibrosis as a clinicopathological syndrome. Chest 61:213–220, 1972.
44. Crystal RG, Fulmer JD, Roberts WC, et al: Idiopathic pulmonary fibrosis. Ann Intern Med 85:769–788, 1976.
45. Epler GR, Gaensler EA, Carrington CB: Crackles (rales) in the interstitial pulmonary disease. Chest 73:333–339, 1978.
46. Baughman RP, Shipley RT, Loudon RG, Lower EE: Crackles in interstitial lung disease: Comparison of sarcoidosis and fibrosing alveolitis. Chest 100:96–101, 1991.
47. Huuskonin MS: Clinical features, mortality and survival of patients with asbestosis. Scand J Work Environ Health 4:265, 1978.
48. Leathart GL: Pulmonary function tests in asbestos workers. Trans Soc Occup Med 18:49–53, 1968.
49. Epler GR, Gaensler EA, Carrington CB: Crackles (rales) in the interstitial pulmonary disease. Chest 73:333, 1978.
50. Epler GR, Gaensler EA, Carrington CB: Crackles (rales) in the interstitial pulmonary disease. Chest 73:333–339, 1978.
51. Walshaw MJ, Nisar M, Pearson MG, et al: Expiratory lung crackles in patients with fibrosing alveolitis. Chest 97:407–409, 1990.
52. Piirila P, Sovijarvi ARA, Kaisla T, et al: Crackles in patients with fibrosing alveolitis, bronchiectasis, COPD and heart failure. Chest 99:1076–1083, 1991.
53. Yagi Y, Ohshima S, Osamura M, et al: Incidence of occurrence of posturally-induced crackles (PIC) in various diseases, with particular reference to the ischemic heart disease. In Proceedings of the Tenth International Conference on Lung Sounds, 1985, p 35.
54. Deguchi F, Hirakawa S, Gotoh K, et al: Prognostic significance of posturally-induced crackles. Long-term follow-up of patients after recovery from acute myocardial infarction Chest 103:1457–1462, 1993.
55. Piirila P: Acoustic properties of cough and crackling lung sounds in patients with pulmonary disease [doctoral thesis]. Helsinki University, Helsinki, 1992.
56. Meslier N, Charbonneau G, Racineux JL: Wheezes. Eur Respir J 8:1942–1948, 1995.
57. American Thoracic Society Ad Hoc Committee on Pulmonary Nomenclature: Updated nomenclature for membership reaction. ATS News 3:5–6, 1977.
58. American Thoracic Society Ad Hoc Committee on Pulmonary Nomenclature: Updated nomenclature for membership reaction. ATS News 3:5–6, 1977.
59. Earis JE, March K, Pearson MG, Ogilvie CM: The inspiratory "squawk" in extrinsic allergic alveolitis and other pulmonary fibroses. Thorax 37:923–926, 1982.
60. Shim CS, Williams MH: Relationship of wheezing to the severity of obstruction in asthma. Arch Intern Med 143:890–892, 1983.
61. Purhoit A, Bohadana AB, Kopferschmitt-Kubler MC, et al: Lung auscultation in airway challenge testing. Respir Med 91:151–157, 1997.
62. Pasterkamp H, Consuniji-Araneta R, Oh Y, Holbrow J: Chest surface mapping of lung sounds during methacholine challenge. Pediatr Pulmonol 2:21–30, 1997.
63. Baughman RP, Loudon RG: Quantitation of wheezing in acute asthma. Chest 86:718–722, 1984.
64. Baughman RP, Loudon RG: Lung sound analysis for continuous evaluation of airflow obstruction in asthma. Chest 88:364–368, 1985.
65. Marini JJ, Pierson DJ, Hudson LD, Lakshminarayan S: The significance of wheezing in chronic airflow obstruction. Am Rev Respir Dis 120:1069–1072, 1979.
66. Godfrey S, Edwards RHT, Campbell EJM, et al: Repeatability of physical signs in airways obstruction. Thorax 24:4–9, 1969.
67. Marini JJ, Pierson DJ, Hudson LD, Lakshminarayan S: The significance of wheezing in chronic airflow obstruction. Am Rev Respir Dis 120:1069–1072, 1979.
68. McFadden ER, Kiser R, DeGroot WJ: Acute bronchial asthma: Relations between clinical and physiologic manifestations. N Engl J Med 388:221–224, 1973.
69. Fischl MA, Pitchemik A, Gardner LB: An index predicting relapse and need for hospitalization in patients with acute bronchial asthma. N Engl J Med 305:783–789, 1981.
70. Dodge RR, Burrows B: The prevalence and incidence of asthma and asthma-like symptoms in a general population sample. Am Rev Respir Dis 122:567–575, 1980.
71. Kraman SS: The forced-expiratory wheeze: Its site of origin and possible association with lung compliance. Respiration 44:189–196, 1983.
72. King DK, Thompson BT, Johnson DC: Wheezing on maximal forced exhalation in the diagnosis of atypical asthma. Ann Intern Med 110:451–455, 1989.

73. King DK, Thompson BT, Johnson DC: Wheezing on maximal forced exhalation in the diagnosis of atypical asthma: Lack of sensitivity and specificity. Ann Intern Med 110:451–455, 1989.
74. Baughman RP, Loudon RG: Stridor: Differentiation from asthma or upper airway noise. Am Rev Respir
Dis 139:1407–1409, 1989.
75. Forgacs P: Crackles and wheezes. Lancet 2:203–205, 1967.
76. Sapira JD: The Art and Science of Bedside Diagnosis. Baltimore, Urban & Schwarzenberg, 1990.
77. Shibley GS: New auscultatory sign found in consolidation, or collection of fluid in pulmonary disease.
Chin Med J 35:500, 1922.
78. McKusick VA, Jenkins JT, Webb GN: The acoustic basis of the chest examination: Studies by means of
sound spectrography. Am Rev Tuberc 72:12–34, 1955.
79. Froschels E, Stockert FG: Ueber ein neues Symptom bei Lungen- und Pleuraerkrankungen. Wien Klin
Wochenschr 35:500, 1922.
80. Sapira JD: About egophony. Chest 108:865–867, 1995.
81. Baughman RP, Loudon RG: Sound spectral analysis of voice-transmitted sound. Am Rev Respir Dis
134:167–169, 1986.

15. THE ABDOMEN

Salvatore Mangione, M.D.

> *It's this damned belly that gives a man his worst troubles.*
> Homer, *Odyssey*, XV.344

TOPICS COVERED IN THIS CHAPTER

Abdominal Wall
Abdominal contour and umbilicus
Sister Joseph's nodule
Abdominal paradox and respiratory
  alternans
Abdominal wall ecchymoses
Abdominal wall striae
Collateral venous circulation
Caput medusae
Light and deep palpation techniques
Abdominal auscultation
  Bowel sounds
  Systolic murmur (bruit)
  Continuous murmur
  Friction rub
  Succussion splash
Liver
Assessment of liver size
The "scratch" test
Auscultation
  Hepatic friction rub
  Hepatic bruit
  Hepatic venous hum
Gallbladder
Murphy's sign(s)
Courvoisier's law
Spleen
Assessment of splenomegaly
  Palpation
  Percussion
Auscultation
Kehr's sign

Stomach
Clapotage
Succussion splash
Pancreas
Grey Turner's sign
Cullen's sign
Kidneys
Costophrenic tenderness
Arterial bruits
Urinary Bladder
Assessment of enlargement by palpation
Assessment of enlargement by percussion
Assessment of enlargement by auscultatory
  percussion
Acute Abdomen (Peritoneal Signs)
Guarding (local and induced)
Modified induced guarding (Carnett's sign)
Rebound tenderness (Blumberg's sign)
Referred rebound tenderness
Jar tenderness (Markle's sign)
Boas sign
Obturator test
Reverse psoas maneuver
Assessment of Ascites
Fluid wave
Shifting dullness
Bulging flanks
Auscultatory percussion
Puddle sign
Ballottement

CONVENTIONAL TEACHING WATCH

Conventional teaching has long recognized the abdomen as "the grave of the internist." Indeed, much more than the chest, this cavity has been impenetrable and unyielding to bedside physical examination. All maneuvers devised by generations of physicians in an attempt to prod, explore, and unlock the secrets of its many and important organs have been for the most part wanting. Only a limited number of bedside techniques and findings, therefore, have passed our conventional teaching test.

ORGANS/TISSUES/ BODY FLUIDS		CONVENTIONAL TEACHING REVISITED
Abdominal wall	⇔	Inspection is worth the time.
Liver	⇓	Definitely a down-the-hill revisitation. Should we still bother?
Gallbladder	⇔	Murphy's sign is cool, but Courvoisier's law may not apply to obese patients.
Spleen	⇔	More science (and less folklore) than for the liver.
Stomach	⇓	Not much here (and never was).
Pancreas	⇓	It was traditionally a secret for physical diagnosis, and it still is.
Kidneys	⇓	Forget it!
Urinary bladder	⇑	Not too bad. Physical exam is informative and useful.
Peritoneum	⇑	All pertinent maneuvers are informative and important. Be good at them!
Ascites	⇑	A wealth of helpful techniques, but only in skillful hands.

ABDOMINAL WALL

Here too their sisters dwell.
And they are three, the Gorgons, winged
With hair of snakes, hateful to mortals.
Whom no man shall behold and draw again
The breath of life.

Aeschylus, *Prometheus Bound* (refers to question 19)

CONVENTIONAL TEACHING WATCH

Inspection, palpation, and auscultation of the abdominal wall still allows the detection of useful findings. Other findings, however, belong more to the art (and folklore) than to the science of medicine. Percussion of the abdomen is not included in this section, because it is pertinent to the examination of other abdominal organs (mainly liver, spleen, kidneys, and bladder).

MANEUVER/FINDING		CONVENTIONAL TEACHING REVISITED
Cullen's sign	⇓	Low sensitivity and low specificity for acute hemorrhagic pancreatitis
Grey Turner's sign	⇓	Same as above
Sister Joseph's nodule	⇓	More part of the medical folklore, but useful if present
Abdominal paradox	⇑	Sensitive and specific indicator of impending respiratory failure
Respiratory alternans	⇑	Same as above
Collateral venous circulation	⇑	An important sign. Remember to identify direction of blood flow
Caput medusae	⇔	Part of the folklore of medicine: how can we abandon it?
Increased bowel sounds in intestinal obstruction	⇓	Neither sensitive nor entirely specific. Probably not worth your time
Search for bruit/murmurs/rubs	⇔	Its value depends on the location and characteristics of these auscultatory findings

Inspection

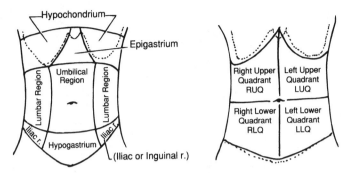

Topographic divisions of the abdomen. On the left are the regions of the abdomen as defined in the BNA terminology. Most of the nine regions are too small so that enlarged viscera and other structures occupy more than one. On the right is a simpler plan with four regions; it is preferred by most clinicians and is employed in this book. Many occasions arise when the quadrant plans need supplementing by reference to the epigastrium, the flanks, or the suprapubic region. (From De Gowin RL: De Gowin and De Gowin's Diagnostic Examination, 6th ed. New York, McGraw-Hill, 1994, with permission.)

Wall Contour and Umbilicus

1. What information can be gathered from the lateral inspection of the abdominal contour?

- A typical Cupid's bow profile has been described in patients with acute pancreatitis. In this condition the point connecting the two branches of the bow coincides with the umbilicus of the patient and produces a central dimple in the abdominal contour.

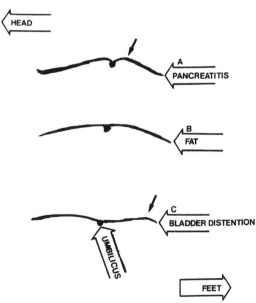

- A localized bulge in the epigastric area is sometimes described in patients with a large pericardial effusion (a condition that carries the eponym of Auenbrugger's abdomen). This sign should not be confused with a fat abdomen, which presents on the lateral view as a uniform arching of the abdominal contour peaking at the level of the umbilical scar.
- Distention of the bladder usually produces a flat abdominal contour with a localized bulge at the level of the hypogastric area.
- Finally, small bowel obstruction produces a "ladder" pattern of abdominal distention, whereas large bowel obstruction produces an inverted-U pattern of abdominal distention.

Lateral abdominal contours. *A,* Cupid's bow of pancreatitis; *B,* fat; *C,* bladder distention. (Adapted from Sapira J: The Art and Science of Physical Diagnosis. Baltimore, Williams & Wilkins, 1990.)

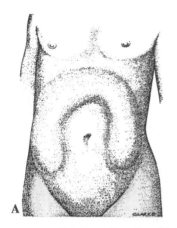 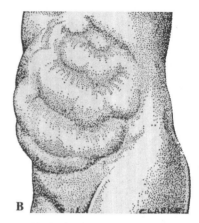

A, The appearance of moderate distension of the large gut. *B,* The ladder pattern of abdominal distension (indicating obstruction of the lower ileum). (From Silen W: Cope's Early Diagnosis of the Acute Abdomen, 19th ed. New York, Oxford University Press, 1996, with permission.)

2. What are the major abnormalities of the umbilicus?

(1) A protuberance of the umbilicus; (2) a purplish discoloration of the umbilicus; and (3) a shift of the umbilicus along the vertical line.

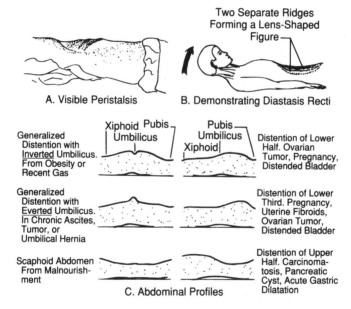

A, Visible peristalsis. Peristaltic waves in the stomach or small bowel sometimes can be seen in the upper abdomen. They usually appear as oblique ridges in the wall that begin near the left upper quadrant and gradually move downward and rightward. Occasionally parallel ridges form a "ladder" pattern. Visibility may be caused by normal waves showing through a thin abdominal wall or by abnormally powerful waves beneath a normal wall. The latter indicates obstruction of a tubular viscus. *B,* Diastasis recti. This is abnormal separation of the abdominal rectus muscles. It is frequently not detected when the patient is supine unless the patient's head is raised from the pillow so the abdominal muscles are tensed. *C,* Abdominal profiles. Careful inspection from the side may give the first clue to abnormality, directing attention to a specific region and prompting search for more signs. (From De Gowin RL: De Gowin and De Gowin's Diagnostic Examination, 6th ed. New York, McGraw-Hill, 1994, with permission.)

3. What is Sister Joseph's nodule?

It is a metastatic nodule of the umbilicus, named after Sister Joseph of the St. Mary's Hospital (and therefore often referred to erroneously as the "Sister Mary Joseph's nodule"). It was Sister Joseph who, in the early days of the Mayo Clinic, first drew the attention of William Mayo to this physical diagnostic abnormality when she could predict the outcome of a celiotomy based on the presence or absence of the nodule. Because of its relations and its generous vascular and embryologic connections, the umbilicus is a highly susceptible site of metastases from intraabdominal malignant disease. These lesions appear as irregularly nodular or exfoliative, often completely replacing the umbilicus. Often a paraumbilical node is palpable through the navel. In decreasing order of frequency, the primary sites of umbilical metastases are stomach, ovary, colon, rectum, and pancreas.[1]

4. What type of protuberances may be present in an umbilicus?

The most common protuberance is the eversion of the umbilical scar, usually seen in conditions of increased intraabdominal pressure (because of either fluid or masses). The most common cause is ascites. Eversion of the umbilical scar may be seen even in patients who have neither ascites nor intraabdominal masses; usually such patients are very obese and have a lax abdominal wall.

5. What is the significance of a purplish discoloration of the umbilicus?

It represents a sign of retroperitoneal bleeding, usually the result of acute hemorrhagic pancreatitis. A periumbilical ecchymosis is usually referred to as Cullen's sign. It is often encountered in association with the Grey Turner's sign (bilateral flank reddish/purplish discoloration).

Pearl. *Discolorations are poorly sensitive and poorly specific markers of hemorrhagic pancreatitis.*

6. What type of shifts along the vertical line may be present in an umbilicus?

The most common is a downward displacement, usually seen in patients with ascites or hepatomegaly, particularly if the condition is long-standing. The abdominal scar is not localized midway between the xyphoid and the pubic symphysis, as it normally should be, but it is pushed downward toward the symphysis pubis. The umbilicus may instead be displaced upward, particularly in pregnant women; this also may occur in patients with pelvic tumors.

7. What other information can be gathered from inspection of the abdomen?

The abdominal surface should be sequentially checked for (1) abdominal respiratory motion; (2) abnormal markings, such as ecchymoses, striae, and surgical scars; and (3) abnormal venous patterns.

8. How should the abdominal wall behave during normal respiration?

The abdominal wall should be synchronized with the chest wall, expanding in inspiration and contracting in exhalation. In some conditions, however, abdomen and chest walls may not be synchronized. Thus, the abdomen expands while the chest is pulled inward and vice versa. This "rocking motion" of chest and abdomen, which has been labeled abdominal paradox, paradoxical respiratory breathing, or respiratory paradox, indicates paralysis or weakening of the diaphragm. As a result, the diaphragm behaves as a passive membrane, sucked upward into the chest during inspiration and pushed downward into the abdomen during exhalation.

9. How sensitive is abdominal paradox in predicting respiratory failure?

Highly sensitive. It usually precedes deterioration of arterial blood gases in patients with impending respiratory failure.

10. What is respiratory alternans?

It is another sign of respiratory muscle weakness and impending respiratory failure. It may be present in place of or in combination with the abdominal paradox. Patients with respiratory alternans exhibit alternate use of either the diaphragm or the intercostal respiratory muscles. Occasionally they may actually cycle from respiratory alternans to abdominal paradox and vice versa.

11. What respiratory movements can be noticed in the abdominal wall of patients with peritonitis?

In patients with peritonitis the abdominal wall may remain immobile during respiration. These movement limitations are diffuse in patients with generalized peritonitis and localized in patients with focal peritonitis. For example, in a patient with diverticulitis the motionless area is the left lower quadrant, whereas in a patient with appendicitis it is the right lower quadrant.

12. What abnormal skin markings can be seen on the abdominal wall?

The most common are *ecchymoses* and *striae*. An abnormal venous pattern is a different type of abnormal marking of the abdominal wall and should be discussed separately.

13. What are ecchymoses?

They are soft tissue bruises, commonly seen with retroperitoneal or intraperitoneal subcutaneous blood leaks. They have been described more frequently in the periumbilical and flank areas, and carry the names of the two physicians who first described them (Cullen and Grey Turner, respectively).

Pearl. *These bruises may occur in as many as 3% of patients with acute pancreatitis,[3] usually within a few days after onset of the condition. They also may occur in ruptured ectopic pregnancies, with a sensitivity of less than 1%.[4] Overall their specificity is low, because they are seen in many other intraabdominal and intrapelvic catastrophes, such as strangulation of the ileum, strangulation of an umbilical hernia, hemorrhagic ascites, and bilateral salpingitis.*

14. What are striae?

Striae are stretch marks usually located either on the flanks or lateral aspects of the abdomen. They may be multiple, 1–6 cm long, and are often encountered in other regions of chronic stretching (such as shoulders, thighs, and breasts). Although they are usually due to rapid weight gain (or loss), they may represent simply a sequela of pregnancy. They also may be seen, however, in Cushing's syndrome, including its iatrogenic variety. Because patients with Cushing's syndrome have erythrocytosis, the striae of this condition tend to be purplish, a hue usually lacking in other disease processes.

15. What about surgical scars?

Every surgical scar should be investigated and inquired about. They also should be reported in the patient's record, using a sketch to delineate the four abdominal quadrants.

Surgical incisions

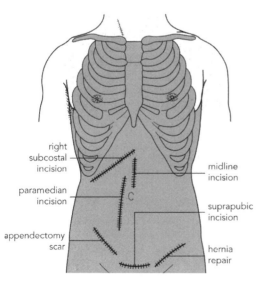

Surgical scars seen commonly on the abdomen. (From Epstein O, Perkin GD, de Bono DP, Cookson J: Clinical Examination, 2nd ed. St. Louis, Mosby, 1998, with permission).

Collateral Venous Circulation

16. What collateral venous circulations may be seen on the abdominal wall?

There are three important networks of collateral venous circulation. They are due to obstruction of (1) the superior vena cava, (2) the inferior vena cava, or (3) the portal venous system.

17. How can you distinguish the three venous networks?

By identifying their location and the direction of their blood flow (see figure):

1. **Obstruction of the superior vena cava** is characterized by the presence of engorged veins on the upper abdominal wall, with flow directed downward.

2. **Obstruction of the inferior vena cava** is characterized by the presence of engorged veins on the lateral abdominal wall (flanks), all draining upward.

3. **Obstruction of the portal system** is characterized by the presence of a network of periumbilical veins, with the upper abdominal veins draining upward and the lower abdominal veins draining downward.

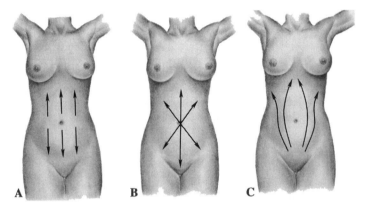

Abdominal venous patterns. *A,* Expected. *B,* Portal hypertension. *C,* Inferior vena cava obstruction. (From Seidel HM, Ball JW, Dains JE, Benedict GW: Mosby's Guide to Physical Examination, 3rd ed. St. Louis, Mosby, 1995, with permission.)

18. How can one demonstrate direction of flow in an engorged collateral vein?

The examiner first should place his or her two index fingers over the engorged vein and collapse it, then slide the fingers apart, producing a 1-inch stretch of empty vein. By releasing first the pressure on the caudal end and then on the rostral end of the vein, the examiner can see the direction of refilling (upward or downward, respectively).

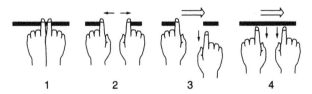

Testing direction of blood flow in superficial veins. The examiner presses the blood from the veins with his index fingers in apposition (1). The index fingers are slid apart, milking the blood from the intervening segment of vein (2). The pressure upon one end of the segment is then released (3) to observe the time of refilling from that direction. The procedure is repeated and the other end released first (4). The flow of blood is in the direction of the faster flow. (Adapted from De Gowin RL: De Gowin and De Gowin's Diagnostic Examination, 6th ed. New York, McGraw-Hill, 1994.)

19. What is caput medusae?

This is the name given to one of the abnormal venous networks seen on the abdominal wall of patients with portal hypertension. It is most commonly encountered in patients with cirrhosis of the liver who have reopened their old umbilical veins. Caput medusae presents as a tuft of engorged abdominal veins radiating from the umbilicus and resembling a nest of snakes. Some of these veins drain in a cephalad fashion into the internal mammary vein, whereas others drain caudally into the inferior mammary vein.

The expression caput medusae refers to Medusa and her peculiar head ("caput" in Latin). Medusa was one of the three Gorgon sisters and a rather wicked figure in Greek mythology. She had snakes in place of hair and such a horrible face that whoever gazed upon it was turned into stone. Perseus eventually slew her by looking at her image across a polished shield he had received from Athena, goddess of wisdom (a metaphor for the value of rationality as a shield against the wickedness of life). After slaying her, Perseus pinned Medusa's head on his shield and used it as a sort of biologic weapon, turning enemies into stone. His example was followed by many Greek foot soldiers, who traditionally painted the Gorgon's head on their hoplite shield.

Palpation

20. How should the abdomen be palpated?

The abdomen should be palpated in a clockwise sequence, starting from the right upper quadrant, moving to the left upper quadrant, down to the left and right lower quadrants, and ending with the periumbilical region, where special attention should be given to palpation of the aorta. The examiner should first use a lighter technique and then a deeper technique of palpation. Areas of abdominal tenderness should be examined last. Tension in the abdominal wall musculature may be minimized by having the patient bend both knees.

21. What are light and deep palpation techniques?

- In a **light palpation technique** the palm of the hand rests gently on the abdomen, while the fingers are pressed into the abdomen at a depth of 1 cm.
- A **deep palpation technique** is the same as light palpation, except that the examiner presses his fingers more deeply than 1 cm. This technique is usually carried out by reinforced palpation, i.e., by pushing on the fingers of the palpating hand with the fingers of the other hand.

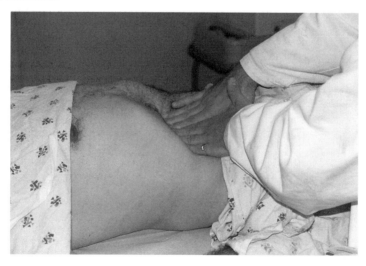

Technique for deep palpation

22. How can one distinguish between an intraabdominal and an intramural mass?
This distinction can be made by palpating the mass while the patient raises his or her head from the pillow. The raising of the head tenses the muscles of the abdominal wall and pushes away an intraabdominal mass but not an intramural mass (i.e., a mass localized in the abdominal wall).

Auscultation

23. Should abdominal bowel sounds be searched for before or after palpating the abdomen?
Definitely before palpating or even percussing the abdomen. Both maneuvers, in fact, may silence the abdomen.

24. What is the significance of increased bowel sounds?
Contrary to conventional teaching, the typical high-pitched, loud, bowel sounds of small intestinal obstruction (usually described as high-pitched rushes interspersed with periods of silence) are a relatively specific but not highly sensitive finding. Indeed, the examiner would have to listen to the abdominal wall for a very long time before being able to detect such sounds.[5] Moreover, bowel sounds of increased (or diminished) intensity can be heard in many other medical conditions.
Pearl. *Thus bowel sounds lack both sensitivity and specificity; they are not a very useful finding.*

25. What is the significance of hearing an abdominal systolic murmur?
It depends on the location and timing of the murmur. Abdominal murmurs may be systolic or continuous and may occur in the left upper quadrant, right upper quadrant, or epigastric area.

26. How frequently are such murmurs encountered?
Overall, about 1–2% of unselected patients on a medical ward may have an abdominal murmur or bruit of some sort.[6]

27. What is the significance of a systolic murmur over the epigastric area?
A systolic murmur in the epigastric area is not uncommon and in selected cases may be encountered in as many as 16% of patients. Usually this murmur indicates an aneurysmatic lesion of either the upper aorta, celiac axis, or mesenteric artery, although it also may be encountered in pregnancy and in as many as one-fifth of normal, thin women. Such murmurs are quite rare in men.

28. What is the significance of a systolic murmur over the right upper or left upper quadrant?
A systolic murmur heard over the right upper quadrant usually reflects the presence of hepatic tumors, such as hepatomas. It also may indicate an arteriovenous malformation or, occasionally, the presence of tricuspid regurgitation. Similarly, a left upper quadrant systolic murmur may indicate an anomaly of the spleen, usually a vascular anomaly. Renal vascular diseases of the right or left kidney also may produce systolic murmurs in these two areas.

29. What is the significance of a continuous murmur?
A continuous murmur (particularly if heard over the epigastric area) is usually encountered in patients with portal hypertension. It is called the Cruveilhier-Baumgarten murmur. This murmur becomes louder during the forced expiratory phase of a Valsalva maneuver and indicates reopening of the umbilical veins. A humming systolic noise, on the other hand, can be heard over the umbilical region in patients with congenital patency of the umbilical vein, even in the absence of portal hypertension or other liver disease (Cruveilhier-Baumgarten disease).

30. What is the significance of a friction rub?
Rubs usually indicate infarcts or tumors of the liver and spleen. They are heard over the right upper and left upper quadrant, respectively.

31. What is a succussion splash?
It is the sound produced by a large collection of air and fluid, often detected by the unaided ear during the exam of a normal patient. If very loud, a succussion splash indicates intestinal obstruction or gastric dilatation.

LIVER AND GALLBLADDER

Zeus' winged hound, an eagle red with blood,
Shall come a guest unbidden to your banquet.
All day long he will tear to rags your body,
great rents within the flesh,
feasting in a fury on the blackened liver.
Look for no end to this agony,
Until a God will freely suffer for you,
will take on Him your pain, and in your stead
Descend to where the sun is turned to darkness,
the black depths of death.

Aeschylus, *Prometheus Bound*

CONVENTIONAL TEACHING WATCH

Based on recent evidence, the role of physical diagnosis in the examination of the liver has become more and more questionable. Assessment of hepatomegaly, for example, seems to be highly unreliable, and some authors have even wondered whether it should not be abandoned altogether. Exam of the gallbladder, on the other hand, has not been under much indictment and still occupies an important role in the abdominal exam.

MANEUVER/FINDING		CONVENTIONAL TEACHING REVISITED
Palpate the enlarged bottom of the gallbladder (Courvoisier's law)	⇑	Valuable sign of olden days (but may not apply to obese patients)
Elicit and recognize Murphy's sign	⇑	Specific for cholecystitis, but not highly sensitive
Palpate lower edge of the liver at rest and deep inspiration	⇔	Only helpful to assess the surface characteristics of the liver edge; not useful to assess hepatomegaly
Palpation of the liver edge for consistence and surface characteristics	⇓	Huge interobserver reliability
Locate the dome of the liver by percussion	⇔	The only game in town for locating the upper liver edge
Measure the width of hepatic dullness by percussion	⇔	Probably unreliable in different hands (huge interobserver variability)
Pulsatile liver and hepatojugular reflux	⇑	Helpful maneuvers
Scratch test	⇑	Needs more validation, but overall an accurate maneuver to locate the lower liver edge
Auscultation for bruits and rubs	⇔	Rare sign, although quite specific for tumors

Liver

Palpation

32. What is the best way to palpate the lower edge of the liver?
The patient lies supine, ideally with flexed knees and hips (to relax the abdominal wall musculature). The examiner places a hand on the abdomen, keeping it parallel to the rectus muscle, with fingers pointing toward the head. The hand then should be moved in a cephalad direction,

while the patient is instructed to take a deep breath. The respiratory excursion of the diaphragm displaces the liver edge downward, allowing it to encounter the examiner's fingertips. If the edge is not felt, the exam of the liver should end there. If the edge is felt, the examiner should determine its consistency and contour; look for nodules, tenderness, pulsations, or thrills, and then listen for the presence of rubs or bruits. Alternatively, the examiner may point his or her fingers toward the patient's feet, while trying to hook the liver gently.

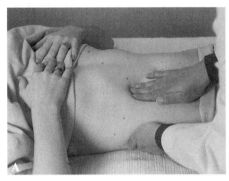
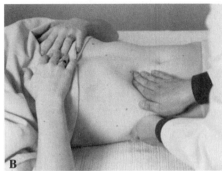
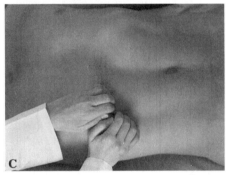

A, Palpating the liver. Fingers are extended, with tips on right midclavicular line below the level of liver tenderness and pointing toward the head. B, Alternate method for liver palpation with fingers parallel to the costal margin. C, Palpating the liver with fingers hooked over the costal margin. (From Seidel HM, Ball JW, Dains JE, Benedict GW: Mosby's Guide to Physical Examination, 3rd ed. St. Louis, Mosby, 1995, with permission.)

33. What can be learned from palpation of the liver?

Palpation of the liver allows assessment of characteristics of the lower liver edge, such as (1) consistency and contour, (2) abnormalities of its surface (e.g., presence of nodules), (3) tenderness, (4) presence of systolic pulsations, and (5) presence of frictions and thrills.

34. How reliable is palpation of the liver edge as a measure of hepatic consistency?

Not very. Interobserver reliability varies widely. In two studies of alcoholic and jaundiced patients, multiple experts had an 11% chance-corrected agreement for abnormal consistency of a palpable liver edge and a 26–29% agreement for the presence of nodules. Only agreement on tenderness reached a more acceptable 49%.[8,9]

35. What is the significance of liver tenderness?

It usually indicates distention of the hepatic capsule, such as may be encountered in patients with passive liver congestion. It is, however, a nonspecific finding that also may be caused by inflammation or even tension of the abdominal wall muscles.[10]

36. What is the significance of a firm and hard liver edge?

A very hard edge suggests tumor, whereas a sharp edge suggests cirrhosis. A firm liver, neither sharp-edged nor stone-hard, is usually passively congested. Nodules indicate cirrhosis, but they also may be related to cancer. The size of the nodules usually distinguishes the two conditions (the larger nodules are more likely neoplastic).

37. What is the meaning of a pulsatile liver edge?

It usually indicates the presence of one of two conditions: (1) tricuspid regurgitation or (2) constrictive pericarditis.

38. How can one distinguish the two conditions?

An inspiratory increase in the magnitude of the pulsations may help to distinguish patients who have true tricuspid regurgitation from patients with constrictive pericarditis. Pulsatility in the setting of hepatomegaly, on the other hand, is a good indicator of constrictive pericarditis. In a total of 55 patients with constrictive pericarditis, 35 (64%) had pulsatile hepatomegaly.[11,12] Pulsations are best appreciated in a held mid-inspiratory or end-inspiratory phase. They are usually felt as a double pulsation of the liver edge, usually in synchrony with the jugular venous pulse, with a strong diastolic dip immediately following the carotid pulse.

Pearl.   Because this finding is highly sensitive, its absence makes a diagnosis of constrictive pericarditis very unlikely. It is not, however, highly specific and in fact may represent aortic pulsations transmitted through an enlarged liver.

39. What is hepatojugular reflux?

It is a bedside maneuver commonly used to diagnose congestive heart failure. While the patient lies supine and breathes quietly, the examiner's hand exerts firm and sustained pressure over the lower liver edge. This pressure should be applied immediately below the right costal margin, both inward and cephalad. A positive hepatojugular reflux is signaled by filling of the neck veins.

Pearl.   This maneuver is also used either to augment or to unmask a murmur of tricuspid regurgitation. It has a specificity of 100% and a sensitivity of 66%, whereas the Rivero-Carvallo maneuver (inspiratory increase in intensity of the tricuspid regurgitation murmur) has a specificity of 100% and a sensitivity of 80%. When combined, the two maneuvers have a sensitivity of 93%[13] and a specificity of 100%.

Assessment of Size

40. Is assessment of liver size another goal of palpation of the liver?

No. Determination of liver size is not accomplished by palpation alone but by a combination of percussion and palpation (with the possible addition of the scratch test).

41. How reliable is palpation of the liver edge as a measure of hepatic enlargement?

It is totally inaccurate. Although many physicians screen for hepatic enlargement by just feeling whether the liver is palpable at peak inspiration (and, if so, by measuring the number or centimeters or finger breadths below the costal margin), palpability of the liver edge is a highly inaccurate marker for hepatomegaly. A normal liver, for example, may become palpable just because it is pushed downward by an emphysematous lung. Palmer[14] in 1958 found a palpable liver in 57% of military personnel with normal liver tests and no history of liver disease. In 28% the liver edge was palpable ≥ 2 cm below the right costal margin. Similarly, Riemenschneider et al.[15] found hepatomegaly at autopsy in less than one-half of all patients who had a palpable liver on physical exam. Finally, Naftalis et al.[16] demonstrated no correlation between palpability of the liver and liver scan or autopsy data.

Pearl.   Thus, palpability of the lower hepatic margin is a common and nonspecific finding. Although palpable livers are more likely to be enlarged (whereas nonpalpable livers are more likely to be normal), palpability of the lower liver edge does not necessarily indicate hepatomegaly. Its primary value consists in localizing the lower hepatic border. This finding can be interpreted only if linked to percussion of the superior liver border and to determination of the longitudinal liver span.

42. Should the lower liver edge be assessed by percussion alone?

This technique has been suggested by a few authors. It is counterintuitive, considering that percussion is notoriously inaccurate even in locating the upper liver border, particularly when used with light intensity. Indeed, most errors in assessing liver span are made when the lower liver edge is not palpable and the examiner has to rely on percussion alone to locate both upper and lower edge.[17]

43. What is the best way to determine liver size on physical exam?

It is definitely not palpation alone, because one-half of all palpable livers are not enlarged. Liver size should be determined by measuring the longitudinal (or vertical) liver span, i.e., the distance in centimeters between the lower and upper liver borders along the midclavicular line (MCL).

- The **lower liver border** is located by palpation, percussion, or the scratch test. The last two maneuvers are usually conducted along the MCL. This reference to the MCL has to be precise, because inaccuracies may lead to an interobserver variability as high as 10 cm.
- The **upper liver border** is located only by percussion.

44. How can one determine hepatic size by percussion?

There are two techniques: direct and indirect percussion. Both can be performed during quiet breathing. The **direct technique** refers to a light percussion of the abdominal wall by the index finger alone. **Indirect percussion**, on the other hand, refers to the more traditional combination of a plexor and pleximeter as the striking and stricken fingers, respectively. The pleximeter finger is applied to the abdominal wall only by its distal interphalangeal joint to avoid dampening of vibrations. The middle finger of the other hand is then used to tap firmly (not lightly) the pleximeter finger, usually along the right MCL. The hepatic area is identified by a change in percussion note from resonant (pulmonary parenchyma) to dull (liver) to resonant again (air-filled bowel loops). The distance between the two points along the MCL, either during quiet breathing or at the same phase of respiration, represents the vertical liver span.

Although direct percussion performed by attending gastroenterologists has been found to be more accurate than indirect percussion in measuring liver span,[18] a normal range of liver span for direct percussion has not been determined. Thus, until we know more about this technique, indirect percussion should be the maneuver of choice.

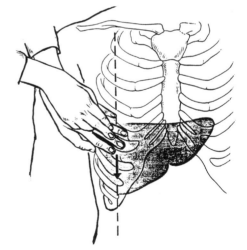

Technique for liver percussion. (Adapted from Swartz MH: Textbook of Physical Diagnosis, 3rd ed. Philadelphia, W.B. Saunders, 1997.)

45. What is a normal liver span?

Liver size depends on body size and shape. As a rule of thumb, a normal liver span is < 12–13 cm on the MCL, as assessed by light percussion or a combination of percussion and palpation.

46. What is the scratch test?

It is a combined auscultatory/percussive maneuver that can be used to localize the inferior hepatic border. The stethoscope is placed either beneath the xiphoid or over the liver just above the costal margin in the MCL. "Scratches" are then administered in a cephalad fashion by moving the finger from the right lower quadrant toward the costal margin along the MCL.[19] The point at which the scratching sound intensifies indicates a change in the underlying tissue and therefore the presence of the lower liver edge (see figure). A variation of the scratch test is auscultatory percussion, in which the examining finger does not scratch but gently percusses (or flickers) the abdominal wall.

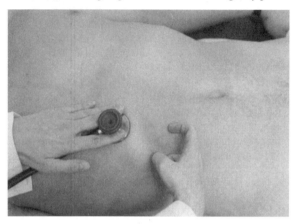

Scratch technique for auscultating the liver. With stethoscope over the liver, lightly scratch the abdominal surface, moving toward the liver. The sound will be intensified over the liver. (From Seidel HM, Ball JW, Dains JE, Benedict GW: Mosby's Guide to Physical Examination, 3rd ed. St. Louis, Mosby, 1995, with permission.)

47. How reliable is the scratch test in localizing the lower liver edge?

The scratch test has been found to be as accurate (or possibly even more accurate) than percussion or palpation in localizing the lower liver edge.[20] Most studies of liver span, however, have used only percussion. Thus, more validation is needed before the scratch test may become more than an adjunct to either palpation or percussion.

48. How accurate are these bedside techniques in diagnosing hepatomegaly?

Palpation of the lower liver edge has an interobserver variability of 6 cm and an intraobserver variability of 1–2 cm. Similarly, determination of liver span by percussion alone has an interobserver variability of 2.5–8 cm and an intraobserver variability of 1–2 cm.[21] Variability in measurement by percussion is usually due to variations in the intensity of percussion, which may yield differences in liver span as high as 3 cm,[22] primarily because of the difficulty in localizing the upper liver edge through interposed lung tissue.

Direct percussion was shown by Skrainka et al. to be as accurate as ultrasound in estimating liver span, but this study relied only on skilled gastroenterology consultants. Other studies conducted among less skilled practitioners suggest more disappointing results. Overall, indirect percussion underestimates liver size (the lighter the percussion, the greater the underestimation). This limitation may be overcome by using a firm technique and by comparing the measured span to the span predicted by nomograms, which take into account patients' weight and height. A span greater than the 95% confidence intervals predicted by these tables most likely represents hepatomegaly. Nomograms are also available for a light percussive maneuver.[23]

Pearl.   Because each clinician's technique may be so different (and interobserver variability as high as 30–50%), some authors have suggested that measurement of liver span by physical diagnosis should be abandoned altogether.[24]

49. What is the recommendation about assessment of liver size by physical diagnosis?

Light percussion underestimates liver size compared with firm percussion; measurements by direct and indirect percussion vary significantly; palpability of the lower liver edge is a totally inaccurate marker of hepatomegaly; the scratch test needs further validation; liver span measured by physical exam does not correlate with the actual size of the liver. Hence, the bedside examination of the liver provides highly inaccurate information about size. Based on this disappointing evidence one may make the following recommendations:

1. A physician may use serial examinations of the liver to detect changes over time because the low intraobserver variability permits accurate follow-ups.

2. A physician cannot, however, use physical examination to assess liver size accurately and objectively. The interobserver variability is so high that a diagnosis of hepatomegaly by physical exam lies more in the eyes (and fingers) of the beholder. The gold standard, therefore, should remain ultrasound, which not only allows quantitative and reproducible estimate of liver span but also permits a calculation of total liver volume by means of reconstruction techniques.[25,26]

3. The primary role f physical examination of the liver should be to determine by palpation the characteristics and consistency of the lower edge.

Auscultation

50. What is the role of auscultation of the liver?
Its role is limited to the detection of friction rubs, venous hums, and arterial bruits.

51. What is the significance of a hepatic friction rub?
Friction rubs can be heard in hepatomas but also in as many as 10% of metastatic tumors.[27] They are less commonly associated with localized or disseminated inflammatory processes, such as liver abscesses and hepatitis. Overall, rubs are rare and nonspecific findings.

52. What is the significance of a hepatic bruit?
Arterial bruits over the liver and epigastrium have been described in patients with neoplasms (primary and metastatic) and in patients with hepatitis. Their prevalence in the general population is low (less than 3%)[28] but may be as high as 10–56% in patients with liver cancer.[29,30] Therefore, auscultation should be carried out only in patients with high pretest probability of disease, based on history and other physical findings.

53. What is the significance of a hepatic bruit associated with a rub?
A bruit associated with a rub is almost always a sign of neoplasia.[31]

54. What is the significance of a hepatic venous hum?
It indicates the presence of portal venous hypertension.

55. How can one differentiate a venous hum from an arterial bruit?
The differential diagnosis is based on the presence or absence of a diastolic component. While arterial bruits are primarily systolic, venous hums are both systolic and diastolic. They originate in a communication between the umbilical veins and the abdominal wall veins. True continuous murmurs (and not hums) are due to either an arteriovenous fistula or a hepatic hemangioma.

Gallbladder

56. What is Murphy's sign?
It is a painful arrest in inspiration, triggered by palpation of the edge of an inflamed gallbladder. To elicit this sign, the patient lies supine and takes a deep breath, while the examiner touches the right lower costal margin along the midclavicular line (point of location of the gallbladder). The encounter between the examiner's fingertips and the inflamed edge of the gallbladder causes pain and a reflex arrest in inspiration.

57. What are Murphy's signs?
In addition to Murphy's sign there are other maneuvers that carry Dr. Murphy's name. Two of these are still being used. Dr. Murphy considered these various techniques "the most valuable contributions I have made to medicine and surgery in the way of aids to diagnosis." One of these

methods (percussion of the costovertebral angle to determine the presence of kidney pathology) has long lost its linkage with Murphy's name, even though it is still routinely performed in bedside diagnosis. The other two maneuvers are deep-grip palpation of the gallbladder (the real Murphy's sign) and hammer stroke percussion of the gallbladder. He used this last maneuver on more obese patients and considered it indisputably "the best test of all." In this technique

> . . . the examiner sitting at the right side of the recumbent patient presses the tip of the second finger of the left hand, flexed at a right angle, firmly up under the costal arch at the tip of the ninth cartilage . . . The patient is instructed to take a deep breath, and at the height of the inspiration, when the gall bladder is forced below the costal guard, the flexed finger is struck forcibly with the ulnar side of the open right hand of the examiner, and if there be an inflammation or a retention in the biliary tract, the patient will announce that the blow caused him severe pain. One is again striking an overdistended or inflamed viscus that contains extremely sensitive nerve filaments.[32]

Dr. Murphy used deep-grip palpation routinely in the examination for suspected biliary disease, even though he did not consider it to be "as good a test as the perpendicular finger percussion test, i.e., the hammer stroke percussion." Dr. Murphy described the deep-grip palpation technique in 1903:

> Hypersensitiveness of the gallbladder is present in all varieties of *infection* and *calculous* obstruction, but not in the neoplastic, torsion, flexion, cicatricial, or valvular obstructions. The hypersensitiveness is elicited by deep palpation just below the right ninth costal cartilage, or in a line from that point to the middle of Poupart's ligament, as this is the common track of gallbladder enlargement. Deep percussion along the same line, with the patient in forced inspiration, gives pronounced pain. The most characteristic and constant sign of gallbladder hypersensitiveness is the inability of the patient to take a full, deep inspiration, when the physician's fingers are hooked up beneath the right costal arch below the hepatic margin. The diaphragm forces the liver down until the sensitive gallbladder reaches the examining fingers, when the inspiration suddenly ceases as though it had been shut off. I have never found this sign absent in a calculous or infectious cause of gall bladder or duct disease.[33]

58. Who was Murphy?

John B. Murphy of Chicago (1857–1916) was an acclaimed leader in American surgery. He was regarded by many as the greatest clinical teacher of surgery of his day. Murphy linked his name to several diagnostic maneuvers for the evaluation of the acute abdomen.[34]

59. How accurate is Murphy's sign in predicting cholecystitis?

It is a specific but not too sensitive sign, being positive in only 27% of all patients with cholecystitis.[35]

60. What is the recommendation for evaluation of acute cholecystitis?

Murphy's sign is definitely cool but a bit passé in the era of sophisticated ultrasonography. In a 1914 article Murphy boasted that "you can make the differential diagnosis at the bedside. You do not have to go home for your instruments; you do not have to have a blood count made. You just have to use your brain and your fingers." Yet ultrasound has become the current gold standard for evaluation of the patient with right upper quadrant abdominal pain, having a 95–99% accuracy in the detection of cholelithiasis.[36]

61. What is the sonographic Murphy's sign?

Because discovering stones by ultrasound does not in itself establish that an episode of acute abdominal pain is due to acute cholecystitis, a sonographic Murphy's sign has been proposed to confirm the diagnosis. Under ultrasonic guidance, the examiner locates the gallbladder and then ascertains whether this site corresponds to the point of maximal tenderness by pressing the ultrasound transducer directly over the gallbladder.

Pearl. *A positive sonographic Murphy's sign is thought to be 87% accurate in diagnosing acute cholecystitis.*[37]

62. Do patients with cholecystitis exhibit other findings?

They also may have an area of hypersensitivity over the right costophrenic angle (Boas' sign; see section on acute abdomen) and, at times, an audible rub over the edge of the gallbladder.

63. What is Courvoisier's law?

Courvoisier's law (or, better, Courvoisier's gallbladder) states that an enlarged and palpable gallbladder in a setting of painless jaundice is not due to cholelithiasis but to cancer of the biliary tract or head of the pancreas.

64. Why should the gallbladder of patients with cholelithiasis remain small?

There are two possible explanations. The first mechanism was proposed by Courvoisier himself and is probably not as accurate as the second mechanism.

1. Recurrent biliary colics caused by stone migration tend to lead to chronic cholecystitis and stiffening of the gallbladder wall. This stiffening, in turn, prevents the gallbladder from enlarging when a new biliary duct obstruction is caused by the passage of a stone. To the contrary, the slow growth of a biliary duct cancer (or of a head of the pancreas cancer) and the pliability of the gallbladder lead to painless jaundice *and* a palpable, enlarged gallbladder.

2. Biliary colics caused by stones are less likely to produce a complete ductal obstruction. They are also more likely to be symptomatic and acted upon quickly, whereas malignant obstructions are severe and lead to higher intraductal pressures over longer periods.[38]

65. How accurate is Courvoisier's law?

It may not be as sensitive or specific as originally claimed. In the original series by Courvoisier (187 cases of jaundice due to common duct obstruction, 87 due to stone, and 100 to other causes), the gallbladder was enlarged in as many as 92% of common duct obstructions not due to stones, but also in 20% of cases due to cholelithiasis. To the contrary, the gallbladder was not enlarged in 80% of common duct obstructions due to cholelithiasis and 8% of cases not due to stones.[39]

More recent series suggest a lower specificity and sensitivity than Courvoisier's original data. For example, only 50% of patients with jaundice caused by pancreatic carcinoma had a clinically palpable gallbladder (this incidence increased to 80% if operative or autopsy enlargement was taken into consideration[40]). Similarly, 42% of patients with common duct stones and jaundice had an enlarged gallbladder at surgery, opposed to 80% of patients with a pancreatic tumor and jaundice.[41]

66. Who was Courvoisier?

Contrary to his French-sounding name, Ludwig G. Courvoisier was born in Basel, Switzerland, in 1843. Not only was he not French; he actually fought against France in the Franco-Prussian war of 1870. After the war he became professor of surgery at the University of Basel, where he published extensively in the field of biliary tract surgery. Courvoisier's law had its origin in a monograph entitled "The Pathology and Surgery of The Biliary Tract," in which he reviewed 109 cases of gallbladder dilatation.

SPLEEN

The neighbouring organ [the spleen] is situated on the left-hand side, and is constructed with a view of keeping the liver bright and pure, like a napkin always ready prepared and at hand to clean the mirror.

Plato, *Timaeus*, 72C

CONVENTIONAL TEACHING WATCH

Physical diagnosis does not fare much better in the assessment of splenomegaly than in the assessment of hepatomegaly. Palpation or percussion may have good sensitivity in detecting splenomegaly, but the sensitivity varies enormously, depending directly on the size of the spleen. These techniques are also among the most difficult to master in the entire physical diagnosis armamentarium, and examiners' skills play an important role.

MANEUVER/FINDING		CONVENTIONAL TEACHING REVISITED
Palpation for splenomegaly	⇔	More specific than percussion, but less sensitive
Percussion for splenomegaly	⇔	More sensitive than palpation, but less specific
Auscultation for bruits and rubs	⇓	Not too common; usually indicative of infarcts but also present in simple splenomegaly

67. Is there any contraindication to palpation of the spleen?
A relative contraindication is infectious mononucleosis, which involves a small risk of splenic rupture as a result of energetic and vigorous palpation.

68. What can be learned from palpation of the spleen?
The major goal, of course, is to ascertain whether the tip of the spleen is palpable. If the tip is palpable, the examiner should then determine the characteristics of the tip, such as consistency. A firmer spleen indicates a more protracted and possibly fibrotic splenomegaly as may be encountered in patients with cirrhosis of the liver.

69. What is the best way to palpate the spleen?
There are four methods: (1) bimanual palpation, (2) ballottement, (3) palpation from above, and (4) one-hand hook technique.

1. **Bimanual palpation.** The patient should lie supine. The examiner, standing at the right of the patient, applies gentle pressure with the right hand to the left upper abdominal quadrant (the examiner's hand is parallel to the rectus muscle with fingers pointing toward the patient's head). The examiner's left hand is placed on the lower left rib cage. The patient breathes in slowly, and at peak inspiration the spleen edge will touch the examiner's fingertips. If the edge is not felt, examination of the spleen should end here. If the edge is felt, the examiner should determine its consistency and contour. Ideally he or she should then listen for the presence of rubs and bruits.

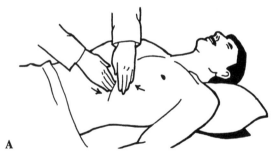

A, The spleen is palpated bimanually with the patient in a supine position and the examiner at the patient's right side. The examiner's left hand is placed on the lower left rib cage, and the right hand explores for the spleen. (From Yang JC, Rickman LS, Bosser SK: The clinical diagnosis of splenomegaly. West J Med 155:47–52, 1991, with permission.)

A

2. **Ballottement.** The patient should lie supine. The examiner's left hand reaches over and around the patient's left hemithorax, lifting it up. At the same time the examiner's right hand is used to receive any impulse transmitted by an enlarged spleen (see figure *B*, top of next page).

3. **Palpation from above.** The examiner keeps all fingers pointing toward the patient's feet, trying to hook the spleen gently with both hands while the patient takes a deep breath. The examiner should be standing at the patient's left, and the patient ideally should be in right lateral decubitus. It also can be done with the patient in a supine position (see figure *C*, top of next page).

4. **One-hand hook technique.** This method, although not validated, should allow detection of an enlarged spleen weeks before it becomes palpable by the other, more conventional methods. In the words of Dr. Hedge, who first described this technique[43]:

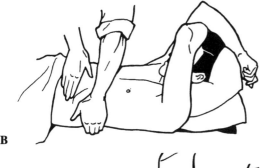

B, The drawing shows the positioning of the examiner's hands during ballottement of the spleen. (From Yang JC, Rickman LS, Bosser SK: The clinical diagnosis of splenomegaly. West J Med 155:47–52, 1991, with permission.)

B

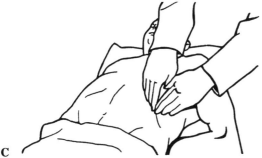

C, The spleen is palpated from above. (From Yang JC, Rickman LS, Bosser SK: The clinical diagnosis of splenomegaly. West J Med 155:47–52, 1991, with permission.)

C

The examiner stands on the left side of the bed, facing the patient's head at the level of the patient's chest. The patient should be in right lateral decubitus. The examiner's left hand is placed on the patient's left costal border. The fingers should be flexed around the left subcostal margin of the patient with the middle finger around the top of the 11th rib. The patient is asked to breathe slowly and deeply, and early splenic enlargement may be noted when the soft splenic edge hits the tip of one of the flexed fingers of the examiner's left hand.

In any technique, it may be helpful to have the patient flex knees and hips to relax the abdominal wall musculature.

70. If the tip of the spleen is palpable, how can one estimate the extent of splenomegaly?

Hacket has proposed a semiquantitative assessment of spleen size, using as a reference point three lines passing through the left costal margin, umbilicus, and symphysis pubis.[44] The size of the spleen is progressively numbered from 0–5. A spleen may not be palpable (0) or may be palpable only after deep inspiration (1). It may reach between the left costal margin and a line halfway to the umbilical line (2); to the umbilical line (3); halfway between the umbilical line and symphysis (4); or beyond the umbilical line (5). This system may help standardization of chart documentation and sharing of information among physicians.

71. How accurate are these bedside techniques in diagnosing splenomegaly?

Not very. Splenomegaly detected by physical diagnosis raises two main questions: (1) is the splenomegaly real? and (2) is the splenomegaly pathologic or simply an incidental finding? Many palpable spleens are not really enlarged, and many enlarged spleens are not really pathologic. For example, splenomegaly may be found in as many as 3% of college students,[45] 12% of postpartum women,[46] 10.4% of hospitalized patients undergoing liver scans,[47] and 2.3–3.8% of patients in an office practice.[48] Similarly, many palpable spleens turn out to be nothing more than a conglomerate of colonic feces, miraculously disappearing after an enema.

Pearl. *Overall, bedside palpation of the spleen has a wide range of sensitivity for detection of splenomegaly (as low as 28%[49] and as high as 100%[50]). Sensitivity is directly proportional to enlargement of the spleen, increasing from 50% (for spleens of 600–750 gm to almost 100% (for spleens > 2350 gm[51,52]). Interobserver variability is low. In a study of 32 patients, four observers* *agreed 88% of the time on the presence or absence of splenomegaly.*[53] *False-positive results may occur in patients with chronic obstructive lung disease and spleens pushed downward into the abdomen. False-negative results, on the other hand, may occur in patients with obesity, ascites, or narrow costal angles.*

72. What is the best way to percuss the spleen?

There are three methods: (1) Nixon's technique, (2) Castell's technique, and (3) percussion of Traube's semilunar space.

1. **Nixon's technique** consists of percussing the entire spleen outline while the patient is in right lateral decubitus. The decubitus position allows the spleen to lie above the stomach and colon, permitting determination of both upper and lower margins. Nixon described this technique in 1954[54]:

> Percussion is initiated at the lower level of pulmonary resonance in approximately the posterior axillary line and carried down obliquely on a general perpendicular line toward the lowest mid-anterior costal margin. Normally the upper border of dullness is measured 6 to 8 centimeters above the costal margin. Dullness increased over 8 cm is indicative of splenic enlargement in the adult.

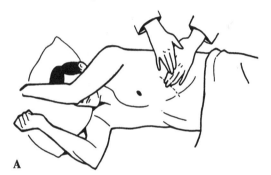

A, The drawing depicts Nixon's method of percussing the spleen. (From Yang JC, Rickman LS, Bosser SK: The clinical diagnosis of splenomegaly. West J Med 55:47–52, 1991, with permission.)

A

2. **Castell's technique** consists of percussing the lowest left intercostal space (eighth or ninth) along the anterior axillary line. The patient is instructed to breathe in deeply and then to exhale. Percussion is carried out during both inspiration and exhalation. Spleens that are either undetectable or just barely palpable yield a dull percussion note. This sign is present only on deep inspiration. Castell described this technique in 1967[55]:

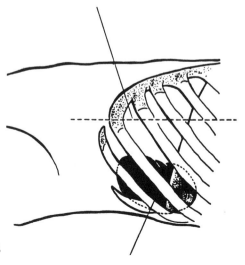

B, In Castell's method of percussing the spleen, the examiner percusses at the intersection of the left anterior axillary line and 9th intercostal space (marked). The lower diagonal line points to normal spleen. (From Yang JC, Rickman LS, Bosser SK: The clinical diagnosis of splenomegaly. West J Med 55:47–52, 1991, with permission.)

B

With the patient in the supine position, percussion in the lowest intercostal space (eighth or ninth) in the left anterior axillary line usually produces a resonant note if the spleen is normal in size. Furthermore, the resonance persists with full inspiration. As the spleen enlarges the lower pole is displaced inferiorly and medially. This may produce a change in the percussion note in the lowest left interspace in the anterior axillary line from resonance to dullness with full inspiration. The percussion sign is considered positive, therefore, when such a change is noted between full expiration and full inspiration.

3. **Percussion of Traube's semilunar space** was described by Barkun et al. in 1989.[56] Traube's space is defined as an area bordered by the left sixth rib superiorly, the left midaxillary line laterally, and the left costal margin inferiorly.

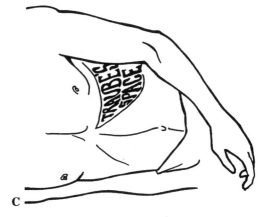

C, Traube's space is shown, as defined by Barkun et al. (From Yang JC, Rickman LS, Bosser SK: The clinical diagnosis of splenomegaly. West J Med 155:47–52, 1991, with permission.)

Pearl. *Barkun compared percussion of Traube's space with ultrasonography and found it 62% sensitive and 72% specific for the detection of splenomegaly.*

73. Who was Traube?

Ludwig Traube (1818–1876) belongs to the school of great German clinicians of the nineteenth century who were, above all, excellent pathologists and often outstanding bacteriologists as well. Trained at the Berlin clinic, Traube's interest was the pathology of fever and the connections between diseases of the heart and kidneys. He introduced the use of the thermometer into the clinic and described the dullness over the gastric air bubble area (usually tympanitic) that still carries his name. Traube described this finding as a sign of left pleural thickening (usually due to tuberculous empyema in his day). He did not name the area after himself, however, nor did he associate dullness of the left upper quadrant with splenomegaly.

74. How accurate is percussion of the spleen in diagnosing splenomegaly?

In a study of 65 patients undergoing liver scan, Sullivan and Williams compared the accuracy of palpation versus percussion (by Nixon's and Castell's methods).[57] Castell's method was found to be more sensitive than palpation (82% vs. 71% false-negative rate) but less specific (16% vs. 10% false-positive rate). Nixon's technique was less sensitive than palpation (59% vs. 71%) but more specific (6% vs. 16%).[57] Castell's technique appeared, therefore, to be more sensitive than Nixon's method (82% vs. 59%, respectively). Overall Castell's and Nixon's methods had a combined false-positive rate of 16.6%. In another study, Halpern et al. found a sensitivity of only 28% and a specificity of 1.4% for physical examination in detecting splenomegaly (compared with nuclear scintigraphy). This study, however, was flawed by the lack of a standardized method for physical examination. So far, the best comparison of palpation, percussion, and technology-based assessment remains the study by Sullivan and Williams.

Although still widely cited, Castell's technique was validated in only 10 male patients who had a positive percussion sign and an otherwise nonpalpable spleen. In this study, the gold standard was nuclear scan, and the controls were male patients with disease in which hepatosplenomegaly was not "expected." It is also not certain whether the technique of percussion (light vs. heavy) interferes with the sensitivity of this maneuver. Castell himself wrote a paper demonstrating that this variable is important in determining liver size by percussion.

75. What are the recommendations for assessment of spleen size by physical diagnosis?

Both percussion and palpation have good sensitivity but a high false-positive rate. Percussion with Castell's technique may be more sensitive than palpation and may help to unmask patients with barely palpable spleens. Percussion thus should serve as an adjunct to palpation. The two techniques are indeed complementary; each may fail to detect splenomegaly and therefore may be rescued by the other.

Technologic alternatives. Plain films of the abdomen are unreliable and poorly sensitive methods to assess splenomegaly; they are helpful only in cases of gross splenomegaly. Ultrasonography, on the other hand, is probably the gold standard: quick, reliable, cheap, noninvasive, safe, and highly sensitive and specific. In a study of more than 3,000 patients, Leopold and Asher found ultrasonic assessment to be a reliable index of splenomegaly in more than 90% of patients.[58] Nuclear scintigraphy is also highly accurate in predicting and assessing splenic size, although it is limited by long acquisition time, need for immobility, vascular integrity and function of the spleen, and cost. CT scan is a highly accurate (albeit expensive) method to assess splenomegaly, producing a mean error of 3.59% (using 1-cm cuts) or 3.65% (using 2-cm cuts).[59] Its major limitation is cost and exposure of the patient to radiation. Magnetic resonance imaging seems to offer no clear advantage over CT scanning.[60]

Bedside and Technology-based Methods to Assess Splenomegaly

EXAMINATION	REFERENCE	SENSITIVITY (%)	SPECIFICITY (%)
Palpation	Holzbach et al. (1962)	—	62
	Halpern et al. (1974)	28	99
	Sullivan and Williams (1976)	71	90
Percussion			
Nixon's method	Sullivan and Williams (1976)	59	94
Castell's method	Sullivan and Williams (1976)	82	83
Traube's method	Barkun et al. (1989)	62	72
Plain film	Whitley et al. (1966)	—	—
Ultrasonography	Leopold and Asher (1975)	—	> 90
Nuclear scans	Rollo and DeLand (1970)	93	—
Computed tomography	Heymsfield et al. (1979)	> 95	—
	Breiman et al. (1982)	96.4	—

76. What is the role of auscultation of the spleen?

It should be limited to the detection of rubs (usually indicative of splenic infarcts) or murmurs. Murmurs can be encountered in patients with massive splenomegaly, or, more commonly, in patients with carcinoma of the pancreas compressing the splenic artery (sensitivity 39%).[61]

77. What is Kehr's sign?

It is referred pain or hyperesthesia to the left shoulder. It is a sign of irritation of the left hemidiaphragm, usually the result of splenic rupture with free blood in the peritoneal cavity. The shoulder pain and hyperesthesia are not elicited by pressure or movement of the joint. Instead they are triggered by allowing the intraperitoneal blood to reach the diaphragm (such as having the patient lie supine for 10–15 minutes in reverse Trendelenburg position).

STOMACH

The stomach is the distinguishing part between an animal and a vegetable; for we do not know any vegetable that has a stomach, nor any animal without one.

J. Hunter (1728–1793),
Principles of Surgery, Chapter V

CONVENTIONAL TEACHING WATCH

The stomach has been traditionally off limits to physical diagnosis. It still is. The only value of physical examination may be in auscultation, which is useful to confirm the position of endotracheal nasogastric tubes.

MANEUVER/FINDING		CONVENTIONAL TEACHING REVISITED
Clapotage	⇓	Helpful (but not much) in detecting gastric stasis or retention
Succussion splash	⇓	As above
Auscultation	⇑	Useful for ascertaining position of endotracheal and nasogastric tubes

78. What is the role of physical diagnosis in the assessment of the stomach?
Very small. It is usually limited to the detection of gastric stasis or retention.

79. What maneuvers can be used to test for gastric retention?
Clapotage and succussion splash.

80. What is a clapotage?
Clapotage ("splashing sound") due to fluid in the stomach is produced by tapping the relaxed epigastric area with fingertips held together. The tapping should begin in the lower abdomen (slightly to the left of the midline) and then move upward gradually until approaching the ensiform cartilage. The splash should be detected as soon as the first few blows are struck, because afterward voluntary muscle guarding interferes with the test.

81. What is a succussion splash?
A succussion splash is elicited by placing a stethoscope over the stomach and then moving the patient quickly from side to side. This splash is absent in the empty stomach. If present 5 hours after a full meal or 2 hours after a glass of water, it indicates a delay in gastric emptying. It is not a highly sensitive test, however, nor is it specific (as opposed to the chest, the abdomen contains many viscera that may be responsible for a succussion splash). Overall a flat and upright film of the abdomen (which will show air-fluid levels in patients with gastric stasis) is a much more valuable tool. Yet the succussion splash should remain in our bag of tricks as a simple and economic way of screening for gastric stasis.

82. Is there any role for auscultation of the stomach?
Only to determine whether a nasogastric tube has been successfully placed in the stomach. If the tube is placed correctly, air injected through the tube produces a gurgling sound over the stomach.
Similarly, auscultation over the stomach (and lungs) should be performed after placement of an endotracheal tube to make sure of its correct position.

PANCREAS

Many a diabetic has stayed alive by stealing the bread denied him by his doctor.

M. H. Fischer (1879–1962),
Principles of Surgery, Chapter V

CONVENTIONAL TEACHING WATCH

The pancreas has been traditionally off limits to physical diagnosis. It still is. The only value of physical examination is detection of pancreatic enlargements, such as pseudocysts and possibly cancer. The retroperitoneal subcutaneous hemorrhages that may accompany acute hemorrhagic pancreatitis have a sensitivity that is too low to be valuable.

MANEUVER/FINDING		CONVENTIONAL TEACHING REVISITED
Grey Turner's sign	⇓	Low specificity and disappointing sensitivity (3% for acute pancreatitis)
Cullen's sign	⇓	As above
Detection of pseudocysts	⇔	Palpable in as many as one-half of the patients

83. What is the role of physical diagnosis in the assessment of the pancreas?
Very small. It is usually limited to pathologic processes because the normal pancreas cannot be examined. Acute pancreatitis may lead to any of the following:

- Retroperitoneal hemorrhage, which is visible on the abdominal wall as Cullen's and Grey Turner's signs. These signs have low sensitivity (3%) and low specificity. They also are encountered in a host of obstetric-gynecologic conditions, such as ruptured ectopic pregnancies, ovarian cyst hemorrhage, and bilateral acute salpingitis.
- Arching of the abdominal wall, also referred to as the Cupid's bow profile (see above under abdominal wall inspection).
- Tenderness to percussion of the thoracolumbar spine or to palpation of the left upper quadrant. The latter is encountered in patients lying in the right lateral decubitus position with knees flexed to the chest (Mallet-Guy's sign).
- Sequelae. The most common sequela is a pseudocyst, which may manifest as a deformation of the abdominal wall. At times a pseudocyst may even become palpable (in as many as 50% of patients).[62]

KIDNEYS

Bones can break, muscle can atrophy, glands can loaf, even the brain can go to sleep, without immediately endangering our survival; but should the kidneys fail . . . neither bone, muscle, gland, nor brain could carry on.

Homer Smith, *From Fish to Philosopher,* Chapter 1

CONVENTIONAL TEACHING WATCH

Kidneys are hidden within the retroperitoneal fat, far from the reach of the physician's fingers (especially in typical, overweight patients). Physical diagnosis should concede to ultrasonography the role of assessing renal size, and keep for itself the detection of costophrenic tenderness in patients with acute renal inflammation and identification of arterial bruits in patients with renal vascular disease.

MANEUVER/FINDING		CONVENTIONAL TEACHING REVISITED
Palpation for kidney enlargement	⇓	Sensitivity is too low. Ultrasound is in, palpation is out!
Costophrenic tenderness	⇑	Still a valuable sign of pyelonephritis
Arterial bruits	⇑	Sensitive and overall specific; still a good maneuver to keep as part of our armamentarium

84. What is the role of physical diagnosis in the assessment of the kidneys?

Palpation, percussion, and auscultation of the kidneys have lost ground since the introduction of ultrasonography.

85. What is the best way to assess renal size?

The best way to assess renal size is to get an ultrasound. (It is our bias that palpation of the kidneys should step down and concede to ultrasonography.) In the absence of ultrasonic equipment, various techniques of kidney palpation may be tried. Although they may detect polycystic kidney disease (bilateral renal enlargement) or hydronephrosis and carcinoma of the kidney (unilateral renal enlargement), these techniques are difficult to perform and have a low yield in any patient who is not very skinny.

86. What is the value of testing for costophrenic tenderness?

Percussion of the costophrenic (or costovertebral) angles is still a valuable maneuver for identifying patients with presumed pyelonephritis or other conditions associated with distention of the renal capsule or pelvis (such as perinephric abscess, renal calculus, and renal infarction). In J. B. Murphy's original description (see section on gallbladder), this technique served well in differentiating renal from biliary, appendiceal, and pancreatic pathology.

87. How is percussion of the costophrenic angle carried out?

The examiner uses the ulnar aspect of the hand to strike the patient's flanks (between lumbar column and costal margin). Alternatively, in Murphy's original method, the examiner uses both hands:

> placing the left hand flat upon the back of the patient over the kidney region, care being taken to have the hand pressed firmly upon the back. The clenched right hand of the examiner is then brought down with considerable force upon the dorsum of the fixed hand, and if an acute congestion, or urethral obstruction exists in that kidney, the patient will cry out with the pain of the blow.[63]

88. What is the thumb pressure test?

Application of pressure with the thumb to the costophrenic angles. This maneuver is an alternative to testing for costophrenic tenderness and may allow distinction between tenderness due to inflammation of the kidneys and tenderness due to inflammation of the abdominal wall.

89. What is the role of auscultation of the kidneys?

It has an important role in the detection of patients with renal vascular disease. Approximately one-half of such patients have a systolic bruit, which is heard anteriorly along a horizontal band crossing the umbilicus. Although these anterior systolic bruits have high sensitivity for renal vascular disease, they also have a disappointing specificity (with a false-positive rate that may be as high as 30%, particularly in hypertensive patients).

Posterior systolic bruits (localized to the areas between the lumbar column and the costal margin) tend to be valuable only if present. Indeed, their specificity for renal vascular disease approaches 100%, but their sensitivity is only 10%.[64]

90. What is the significance of anterior continuous bruits?

Anterior continuous bruits have a sensitivity of approximately 50% for renal vascular disease, but this rate may reach 80–90% in hypertensive patients with fibromuscular hyperplasia of the renal artery.[65] The continuous bruit is also much more specific than the systolic bruit, with a false-positive rate less than 7%.[66]

URINARY BLADDER

You notice that the tabetic has the power of holding water for an indefinite period. He is also impotent—in fact two excellent properties to possess for a quiet day on the river.

Dr. Dunlop, Teaching at Charing Cross Hospital, London

CONVENTIONAL TEACHING WATCH

Physical diagnosis still plays an important role in assessment of the urinary bladder. Percussion, aided or unaided by auscultation, allows accurate assessment of bladder enlargement.

MANEUVER/FINDING		CONVENTIONAL TEACHING REVISITED
Percussion for enlargement	⇓	Still a good maneuver
Subjective palpation for enlargement	⇑	A recent, and useful, addition
Auscultatory percussion for enlargement	⇑	A recent addition; more sensitive than percussion alone

91. Is the urinary bladder palpable?

Only when distended and only in patients who are very thin (or whose bladder is fibrotic as a result of radiation therapy).

92. What is the gold standard for detecting a full bladder?

Percussion alone or auscultatory percussion.

93. What is subjective palpation of the urinary bladder?

It is a useful technique to identify a full bladder. The examiner gently pushes one finger perpendicularly into the lower abdomen, starting from above and going downward in a stepwise fashion toward the pubis. If this maneuver causes an urge to urinate at any point, the fundus is probably distended at that level.

94. How accurate is subjective palpation of the bladder?

The technique was evaluated in 50 consecutive patients undergoing cystoscopy. All 20 patients in whom suprapubic palpation evoked an urge to urinate had at least 100 ml of urine in the bladder. Only two of the bladders were objectively palpable and percussable. None of the 25 patients with negative findings had more than 200 ml of urine. Thus, when suprapubic pressure evokes a call to micturition, the bladder probably contains more than 100 ml of urine, whereas when suprapubic pressure does not evoke a call to micturition, the bladder probably contains less than 200 ml of urine.[67]

95. What is auscultatory percussion?

It is a combined auscultatory percussive maneuver used to locate the upper border of the bladder. The diaphragm of the stethoscope is placed just above the symphysis pubis in the midline. "Scratches" are then administered in a rostrocaudal fashion by moving the finger along the vertical midline from the umbilicus downward, 1 cm at a time. The point at which the scratching sound intensifies indicates a change in the underlying tissue and thus locates the upper edge of the bladder.

96. How accurate is auscultatory percussion in diagnosing a full bladder?

The likelihood of identifying a full bladder (defined as ≥ 250 ml of urine on catheterization) directly correlates with the distance above the symphysis pubis at which the percussion note changes. Thus, a distance ≤ 6.5 cm has a 0% likelihood, a distance of 6.5–7.5 cm has a 43% likelihood, and a distance > 7.5 cm has a 91% likelihood.[68]

ACUTE ABDOMEN (PERITONEUM)

The abdomen is like a stage
enclosed within a fleshy cage,
The symptoms are the actors who
Although they are a motley crew
Act often with consummate art
The major or the minor part;
Nor do they usually say
Who is the author of the play.

That is for you to try and guess
A problem which, I must confess
Is made less easy for the fact
You seldom see the opening act,
And by the time that you arrive
The victim may be just alive.

Sir Zachary Cope, *The Acute Abdomen in Rhyme*, 5th ed. London, H.K. Lewis, 1972

CONVENTIONAL TEACHING WATCH

The important maneuvers below help physicians to identify patients with an acute peritoneal process. They are an essential part of the laying on of the hands and remain valuable even in the era of MRIs and CT scan. Once more, individual skills and technique play an important role.

MANEUVER/FINDING		CONVENTIONAL TEACHING REVISITED
Guarding (local and induced)	⇑	Essential maneuver for the assessment of peritonitis
Modified induced guarding (abdominal wall tenderness or Carnett's sign)	⇑	As above
Blumberg's sign (rebound tenderness)	⇑	As above
Referred rebound tenderness	⇑	A more humane variety of the Blumberg's sign
Stethoscope sign	⇑	A nice little trick to recognize nonspecific abdominal pain (but do not rely on it too heavily)
Closed-eyes sign	⇑	It refers to the patient, of course (you should keep your eyes wide open)
Jar tenderness (Markle's sign)	⇔	Specific for peritonitis (only for ambulatory patients)
Obturator test	⇓	A nonspecific sign of appendicitis
Reverse psoas maneuver	⇓	Another nonspecific sign of appendicitis

97. What are the two most commonly used maneuvers for examining patients with suspected peritonitis?

Guarding (local and induced) and rebound tenderness.

98. What is guarding?

The guarding reflex is stiffness of the abdominal wall, which may be present at rest or, more commonly, after a deep gentle pressure is applied by fingertips. It is usually localized to areas of the abdominal wall that overlay an inflamed viscus.

99. What is the significance of localized guarding?

Localized guarding (or localized rigidity) of the abdominal wall (for example, absence of respiratory motion in those areas of abdominal wall overlying the inflamed viscus) is a good indicator of a focal area of peritonitis.

100. What is induced guarding?

Induced guarding is triggered by having the patient raise the head from the pillow until he or she can touch the chest with the chin. This maneuver tenses the abdominal musculature (voluntary or induced guarding) and thus forms a sort of cuirass that protects any inflamed intraabdominal organ against the examiner's hand or other offending palpation.

101. What is Carnett's sign?

Carnett's sign (from the author who first described it in 1926[69]) uses induced guarding to differentiate abdominal tenderness due to an inflamed intraabdominal viscus from abdominal tenderness due to an inflamed abdominal wall. The examiner localizes by palpation the area of abdominal tenderness and then asks the patient to contract the abdominal muscles by raising the head from the couch. During this maneuver, the pressure on the examining fingers is maintained and the patient is asked whether there is any change in tenderness. Pain originating from the abdominal wall increases (positive Carnett's sign), whereas pain originating from an intraabdominal viscus decreases (negative Carnett's sign).

102. What is abdominal wall tenderness?

It is a variation of Carnett's sign. The examiner first identifies the site of maximal abdominal tenderness while the patient is lying flat and relaxed. At that point, with the examining hand remaining in place, the patient is asked to cross arms and sit forward. With the patient midway between a sitting and recumbent position (and while the anterior abdominal wall muscles are tensed), the examiner renews pressure on the previously tender spot. If the tenderness is increased, the test is recorded as positive (positive abdominal wall tenderness); if it is made better, the test is recorded as negative (negative abdominal wall tenderness).

103. What is the significance of a positive abdominal wall tenderness?

Pain on abdominal palpation may arise from the abdominal wall, parietal peritoneum, and underlying viscus. Tensing of the abdominal muscles allows the physician to differentiate the first from the second two. If tenderness on palpation is increased by the tension of the abdominal muscles, the pain originates from the abdominal wall itself (positive abdominal wall tenderness) because the tension of the abdominal muscles protects parietal peritoneum and intraabdominal viscera against the pressure of the examiner's hand.

104. What are the causes of an abdominal wall tenderness (AWT)?

Often the cause remains a mystery. Possible culprits include muscular strain, viral myositis, fibrositis, nerve entrapment, and trauma. The most important aspect of a positive AWT, however, is that it usually indicates absence of intraabdominal pathology.

105. Does AWT have limitations?

1. It should not be used in children or elderly patients (because of the risk of misinterpretation).
2. It is useless and inhumane in patients with diffuse abdominal pain and rigidity.
3. It is possibly dangerous in patients with an intraabdominal abscess (straining and increased intraabdominal pressure may cause the abscess to burst).

106. What are the indications for AWT?

It should be used whenever laparotomy is considered in a patient with acute abdominal pain and always in the context of the clinical picture and in the setting of periodic reexaminations.

107. How accurate is AWT in differentiating peritonitis or intraabdominal pathology from inflammation of the abdominal wall?

The modified induced guarding technique (AWT sign) has been studied by several authors and found to be quite helpful clinically. Thomson and Francis used it in 120 patients admitted as surgical emergencies for acute localized abdominal pain.[70] Only 1 of the 24 patients with positive AWT had an intraabdominal inflammatory process (acute appendicitis). All 96 patients with a negative test, however, had intraabdominal pathology. Gray et al. studied 158 patients admitted to the hospital for acute abdominal pain.[71] They found AWT to be less accurate; it was present in only 28% of patients without intraabdominal pathology (true positive) and 5% of patients with intraabdominal pathology (false positive). The authors found a predominance of young females among patients with no intraabdominal pathology and a positive AWT. Finally, Thomson et al. revisited this sign for the evaluation of patients with chronic abdominal pain.[72] Over time patients with positive AWT underwent a great deal of studies (including surgical procedures) but only a small minority had serious pathology.

Pearl.   *Thus, the AWT sign is quite useful in assessing patients with either acute or chronic abdominal pain.*

108. What is rebound tenderness?

It is tenderness of the abdominal wall elicited indirectly by the sudden release of hand pressure. This test (also called Blumberg's sign) consists of gently palpating an area of abdominal tenderness as deeply as allowed and then suddenly releasing the pressure. The elastic abdominal wall suddenly springs back into its baseline position, eliciting an exquisite localized pain in patients who have a localized inflammation of the abdominal wall. The pain is due to the sudden tension of the inflamed peritoneum. This test is painful and not necessary in patients who already have a localized guarding.[73] A less painful alternative to the rebound tenderness maneuver may be light indirect percussion over the area of pain.

109. What is the referred rebound tenderness test?

It is a more humane variation of Blumberg's sign. The examiner compresses and then releases the abdominal wall of the quadrant contralateral to the quadrant where the patient complains of pain. This maneuver is positive only when it elicits pain in the site where the patient originally felt it. Pain at the site of palpation represents a negative test. A negative test, however, should not exclude a diagnosis of localized peritonitis. Thus, it must be followed up by a test of rebound tenderness.

110. What is the stethoscope sign?

It consists of palpating the abdomen twice, first with the hands and then with the stethoscope. In the second case, the patient should be informed in advance that the examiner is only trying to listen to the abdomen. This seems to distract the patient, often allowing the examiner to compress the anterior abdominal wall against the posterior abdominal wall in patients whose pain is either not real or exaggerated. In these same patients, even the light touch of the examiner's fingers had previously elicited a much more dramatic response characterized by flinching, grimacing, complaining, and quick tensing of the abdominal muscles.[74,75]

111. How reliable is the stethoscope sign?

It has not been studied prospectively. There is, however, a case report of a false-positive stethoscope sign in a patient with acute appendicitis.[76] As always, this sign should be evaluated in the context of the clinical picture and within the realm of periodic observation of the patient.

112. While performing these maneuvers, should the examiner look at the patient's face or at the patient's abdomen?

At the patient's face. It is essential that the physician observe the patient's expression while testing for guarding reflex or rebound tenderness. Any grimacing or reaction to even a gentle and light touch is sometimes the only clue to an acute abdomen.

113. What is the closed-eyes sign?

It refers to the particular face of patients with nonspecific abdominal pain (i.e., pain without a clear-cut intraabdominal pathology). Such patients often keep their eyes closed during abdominal palpation, and their face has an embalmed, beatific smile. This behavior is quite different from that of patients with true intraabdominal pathology, who keep their eyes wide open and monitor carefully what the examiner's hand is doing.[77]

114. What is the use and the cause of a closed-eyes sign?

It is an accurate test in diagnosing nonspecific abdominal pain. It is not clear why patients without intraabdominal pathology should keep their eyes closed. The authors who described this sign speculated that, unlike patients with true pathology, they may not need to monitor the physician's hand to avoid unnecessary pain. Similarly, it is possible that patients may be aware (either consciously or unconsciously) that palpation will not produce severe pain, implying that the pain has a psychological etiology. In either case, a positive closed-eye sign usually indicates absence of true intraabdominal pathology.

115. How accurate is the closed-eye sign in diagnosing nonspecific abdominal pain?

Gray et al. studied this sign in 158 consecutive patients admitted for acute abdominal pain. The eyes were closed in 6 of 91 patients with true pathology (6.5%), and 22 of the 67 patients with no pathology (33%). Twenty-two of 28 patients with a positive closed-eyes sign were females ($p < 0.01$), usually young. In summary, the predictive power of a positive closed-eyes test is 79% and that of a negative closed-eyes test is 65%.[78]

116. What is abdominal hyperesthesia?

It is hypersensitivity (hyperesthesia) to light touch in areas of the abdomen that overly an inflamed viscus.

117. How can one test for abdominal hypersensitivity?

Areas of hyperalgesia (increased pain) can be easily identified by lightly drawing across the abdominal wall a cotton wisp, a pin, or even a fingernail. Head was the first to describe these areas of hypersensitivity. Since his time these areas have been usually referred to as Head's zones. (See figures below and at top of next page.)

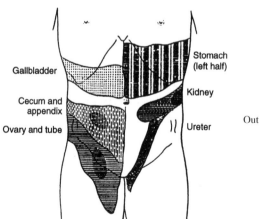

Outline of the zones of hyperalgesia.

118. Is abdominal hyperesthesia specific to localized peritonitis?

No. It may also be seen in herpes zoster infection (in which it usually precedes the cutaneous rash by several days) and at times in patients with peptic ulcer disease (usually as an area of circumscribed tenderness over the midepigastrium).

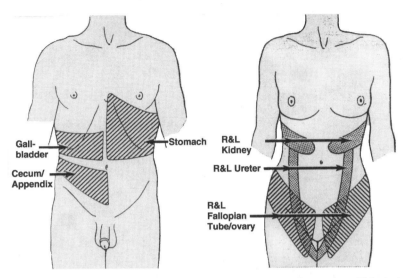

Sensitive areas for male (left) and female (right) organs. Men can have renal-ureteral sensitivity in the same distribution as women, involving the penis and scrotum. (From Willms JL, Schneiderman H, Algranati PS: Physical Diagnosis: Bedside Evaluation of Diagnosis and Function. Baltimore, Williams & Wilkins, 1994, p 368, with permission).

Pearl.   In an endoscopic study of 88 patients with peptic ulcer disease, the closed-eyes sign was found to be an insensitive indicator; it is also present in many normal people or in patients with functional disorders.

119. What is Boas' sign?

It is abdominal hyperesthesia as applied to the gallbladder. In Boas' sign, patients with acute cholecystitis experience referred pain and hyperesthesia of the right costophrenic angle (which is indeed the site of referred pain for the gallbladder). Even a light touch in this area elicits exquisite tenderness in patients with an inflamed gallbladder. The value of this sign, unfortunately, is limited by its low sensitivity of only 7%.[79]

120. What is jar tenderness?

It is another maneuver aimed at detecting and localizing peritoneal irritation. It is carried out in the ambulatory setting by asking the patient first to stand on outstretched toes and then to let body weight fall on the heels. This maneuver sets the abdominal wall into motion and allows the patient to localize any area of pain. This finding is specific for peritoneal irritation[80] and may represent a less painful and more humane alternative to a rebound tenderness maneuver.

121. What is the value of a Valsalva maneuver in a patient with an acute abdomen?

The Valsalva maneuver may allow a patient with an acute abdomen to identify a particular area of tenderness. For example, after a 20-second Valsalva maneuver a patient with acute appendicitis may be able to pinpoint with one finger the area of abdominal pain. This maneuver may be used as a screening method to guide (and possibly avoid) more painful maneuvers, such as rebound tenderness and guarding.

122. What is the obturator test?

This test consists in having a patient flex the thigh and rotate it fully inward while supine. Usually the examiner pulls the patient's ankle toward him- or herself while pushing the knee away. It should be carried out on both thighs, and it should be painless. Pain (usually referred to the suprapubic region) indicates inflammation in one of the organs surrounding the obturator muscle, usually retrocaecal appendicitis. Beside appendicitis, the obturator test may be positive in many obstetric-gynecologic conditions characterized by the presence of pus in the pelvis. In such cases the test is usually positive in both legs, whereas in appendicitis is positive only on the right leg.

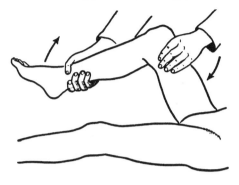

Method of performing the obturator test. (From Silen W: Cope's Early Diagnosis of the Acute Abdomen, 19th ed. New York, Oxford University Press, 1996, with permission.)

123. What is the reverse psoas maneuver?

This is another maneuver that can be used to detect irritation of the iliopsoas muscle due either to retrocaecal appendicitis or to some other localized collections of pus and blood. It is performed by having the patient roll toward the left side and hyperextend the right hip. The test is positive when it elicits pain.

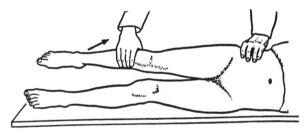

Method of performing the iliopsoas test. (From Silen W: Cope's Early Diagnosis of the Acute Abdomen, 19th ed. New York, Oxford University Press, 1996, with permission.)

ASCITES (DROPSY)[81,82]

I walk as I were girdled with my spleen
And look as if my belly carried twins
Wretch that I am! I fear me I shall burst.

Plautus, *Curculio*, Act II, Scene I

CONVENTIONAL TEACHING WATCH

These are important maneuvers that can help physicians to identify patients with ascites. Particularly if combined, these time-honored techniques are still valuable.

MANEUVER/FINDING		CONVENTIONAL TEACHING REVISITED
Fluid wave	⇑	Highly specific but poorly sensitive
Shifting dullness	⇓	Highly sensitive but poorly specific
Bulging flanks	⇔	No, we are not talking about Mae West
Auscultatory percussion	⇔	A recent addition to our armamentarium
Puddle sign	⇓	A not too sensitive and quite cumbersome maneuver
Ballottement (or dipping)	⇓	Folklore more than science

124. What is ascites?

It is the presence of free fluid in the abdominal cavity. It is an important clinical finding, usually suggestive of heart failure, liver disease, nephrotic syndrome, or malignancy.

125. What are the best clues to a diagnosis of ascites?

A focused history may provide important information to diagnose ascites, even before resorting to physical examination. The physician should inquire about any history of liver disease, which greatly increases the pretest probability of ascites. In addition, the physician should inquire about recent weight gain and especially about recent ankle edema or change in abdominal girth. If absent, the last two symptoms greatly decrease the likelihood of ascites, particularly in patients who already have a low pretest probability of disease. For example, in patients with less than a 20% chance of having ascites (because of the absence of liver disease by history), the absence of recent ankle swelling decreases the likelihood of ascites to less than 2.5%.

Pearl. *Thus, a diagnosis of ascites is unlikely in the absence of recent increase in abdominal girth and very unlikely in the absence of recent ankle edema (particularly in male patients).*

126. What is the role of physical diagnosis in the detection of ascites?

It represents a quick, convenient, and inexpensive way to diagnose ascites. Unfortunately, physical diagnosis is valuable only for relatively large volumes of fluid. For smaller amounts the diagnostic gold standard remains ultrasonography, which can detect as little as 100 ml of fluid at a cheaper cost than computed tomography.

127. What bedside maneuvers may be used to detect ascites?

Four classic maneuvers can be used to detect ascites: (1) inspection for bulging flanks, (2) percussion for flank dullness, (3) the shifting-dullness maneuver, and (4) the fluid-wave maneuver. In addition, two other maneuvers have been reported as useful for the detection of ascites: the puddle sign and auscultatory percussion.

128. What are bulging flanks?

This expression does not refer to Mae West's silhouette but rather to the peculiar abdominal shape of patients with ascites. Because of the weight of intraabdominal fluid, the flanks are pushed outward, almost looking like the belly of a frog. This same shape, however, may be seen in patients who are simply obese. To separate the two conditions, one needs to resort to the flank-dullness test, which is performed by percussing the abdomen in a radiating pattern from the umbilicus toward the flanks and symphysis. Because gas-filled intestinal loops (resonant) float on top of ascites (dull), the maneuver reveals a rounded area of tympany around the umbilicus, flanked by two areas of dullness on the flanks.

Pearl. *Bulging flanks and flank dullness are both very sensitive (≥ 72% and ≥ 80%, respectively) but poorly specific tests for ascites.*

129. How is the shifting-dullness maneuver performed?

The patient lies supine while the examiner percusses the abdomen from the umbilicus downward along one flank (see figure, top of next page). The examiner marks the level at which the percussion note turns from resonant to dull and then asks the patient to roll over on one side. At this point the percussion sequence is reinitiated, with the patient in right lateral decubitus and supported by a 45°-angle pillow. A gravity-dependent shift in dullness of at least 1 cm indicates that the dullness is due to fluid, whereas the absence of a shift indicates that the dullness is caused by a solid organ.

130. How accurate is this test?

This test has high sensitivity (≥ 83% in two separate studies) but low specificity (on average 50%, although one study showed a specificity of 90%).

Pearl. *Thus, a negative shifting dullness is a useful finding for ruling out ascites.*

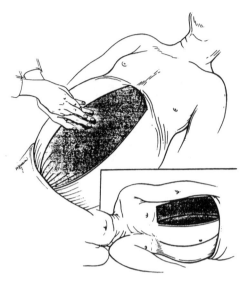

Technique for testing for shifting dullness. The colored areas represent the areas of tympany. (From Swartz MH: Pocket Companion to Textbook of Physical Diagnosis. Philadelphia, W.B. Saunders, 1995, with permission.)

131. How is the fluid-wave maneuver performed?

It requires two examiners or, more simply, one examiner assisted by the patient. While the patient lies supine, one examiner places one hand on one flank and taps gently on the opposite flank. In the mean time, the other examiner (if available) places the ulnar surface of both hands over the patient's umbilicus and along the abdominal vertical midline (from the xyphoid process to the symphysis pubis). This is done to prevent a false-positive fluid wave, which may occur when the thumping of the abdominal wall creates ripples of mesenteric fat (not of ascites) toward the contralateral side. If an assistant is not available, the patient may place the ulnar surface of one hand vertically over the umbilicus. The test is positive when the examiner feels a fluid wave emanating into the contralateral side. The wave must be of moderate-to-strong intensity (slight fluid waves have a high interobserver variability and should not be relied on for diagnosing ascites).

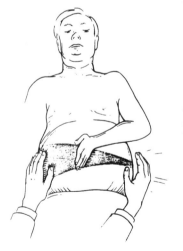

Technique for testing for a fluid wave. (From Swartz MH: Pocket Companion to Textbook of Physical Diagnosis. Philadelphia, W.B. Saunders, 1995, with permission.)

132. How accurate is this test?

The fluid-wave maneuver is 80–90% specific for ascites. In fact, it is probably the only truly specific bedside test for the diagnosis of ascites. Thus, a positive fluid wave is a useful finding for ruling in ascites. If the test is negative, on the other hand, the diagnosis of ascites should not be ruled out because of the low sensitivity of this maneuver (around 50%).

    Pearl.   *Thus, the fluid-wave maneuver detects only large amounts of ascitic fluid.*

133. What is the ballottement sign?

The ballottement or dipping maneuver is another method to determine the presence of ascites (and not a particularly sensitive one). The patient's body is tilted toward the side of the organ to be palpated (usually the liver or spleen). Then the examiner applies with his or her fingers a quick pushing motion to the chosen organ. A positive sign is characterized by a feeling of displaced fluid before the examiner's fingers can touch the organ in question.

134. How is the puddle sign elicited?

The patient lies on the belly for 5 minutes and eventually raises him- or herself by supporting body weight on the knees and stretched forearms. The middle portion of the abdomen, therefore, is dependent and pendulous. At this point the examiner places his or her diaphragm over the most dependent part of the abdomen and starts flicking a finger over a localized flank area. Then the examiner gradually moves the stethoscope over the opposite flank. A positive sign is a sudden increase in intensity and clarity of the sound just as the stethoscope moves beyond the edge of the peritoneal fluid.

    Pearl.   *This test was initially reported as having high sensitivity (capable of detecting as little as 140 ml of fluid). In reality, its sensitivity is much lower (40–50%), particularly for small amounts of ascites. Moreover, the test is cumbersome and difficult to perform. Therefore, it cannot be recommended in the routine evaluation of patients with ascites.*

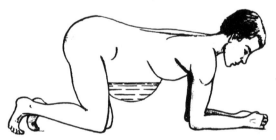

Patient positioning for eliciting the puddle sign. (From Dioguardi N, Sanna GP: Moderni Aspetti di Semeiotica Medica. Milan, Societa Editrice Universo, 1975, with permission.)

135. What is the auscultatory percussion maneuver?

This test has been reported too recently for adequate validation. It consists of having the patient sit or stand for 3 minutes after voiding. This maneuver allows free abdominal fluid to gravitate into the pelvis. The examiner then places the stethoscope in the abdominal midline, immediately above the pubic crest, while at the same time percussing the abdomen (by a finger-flicking technique) from the costal margin downward and perpendicularly toward the pelvis. The level at which the percussion note turns from dull to loud usually indicates the pelvic border. In patients with free fluid this level clearly is raised above the pelvic baseline.

136. What is the overall accuracy of these signs for ascites?

No single sign is both sensitive *and* specific. Many, however, are quite sensitive *or* quite specific. Moreover, there seems to be little interobserver variability in detection of these signs, suggesting that physicians tend to agree on their presence or absence. Overall, the most useful tools to *rule in* diagnosis of ascites are (1) the fluid wave maneuver, (2) the shifting dullness maneuver, and (3) the history of ankle edema. The least useful signs to *rule in* a diagnosis of ascites are (1) the puddle sign and (2) auscultatory percussion. The most useful signs to *rule out* a diagnosis of ascites are those with high sensitivity. Thus, absence of a history of ankle swelling or increased abdominal girth and absence of bulging flanks, flank dullness, or shifting dullness make the diagnosis of ascites very unlikely.

137. How can one improve the diagnostic accuracy of these maneuvers?

By combining them. For example, the fluid-wave maneuver has a low sensitivity (50%) but a high specificity (80–90%), whereas the shifting-dullness maneuver has a high sensitivity (≥ 83%) but a low specificity (55%).

Pearl.   *Thus, their combination provides a skillful physician with an excellent bedside tool for the diagnosis of ascites. Overall, the accuracy of both tests is around 80%.*

138. What is the role of the Bayes' theorem in the bedside diagnosis of ascites?

Very important. Interpreting each of these tests in light of the pretest probability of disease is the best way to improve accuracy. Because the predictive value of any test (including physical diagnostic tests) depends on the prevalence of the disorder in patients undergoing the test, a positive test in patients with low prevalence of the disease is more likely to represent a false positive than a true positive. This application of Bayes' theorem can be extended to the positive predictive values of shifting dullness and fluid wave for the diagnosis of ascites. As a result, the predictive value of these tests is enhanced when they are interpreted in combination with the patient's prothrombin time (PT). For example, a prominent fluid wave has a high positive predictive value for ascites (96%) in patients with a prolonged PT. This rate will be much lower (48%) in patients with normal PT. On the other hand, patients with normal PT and no shifting dullness rarely have ascites (2%).

Thus, a focused physical examination based on the shifting-dullness and fluid-wave maneuvers and interpreted in light of the patient's pretest probability of disease (as determined by PT) allows physicians to use ultrasonography more judiciously and cost-effectively.

Pearl.   *In summary, patients with a history of liver disease, prolonged PT, and positive fluid wave are likely to have ascites and do not need an ultrasound for confirmation. On the other hand, patients with normal PT and no shifting dullness are unlikely to have ascites even if they have a history of liver disease; therefore, they do not need an ultrasound.*

MANEUVER	SENSITIVITY (%)	SPECIFICITY (%)
History		
Increased abdominal girth	90	60
Recent weight gain	60	70
Ankle swelling	100	60
Physical examination		
Bulging flanks	70	60
Flank dullness	80	60
Shifting dullness	90	60
Fluid wave	60	90
Puddle sign	50	70

REFERENCES

1. Flynn VT, Spurrett BR: Sister Joseph's nodule. Med J Aust 1:728–730, 1969.
2. Macklem PT: The diaphragm in health and disease. J Lab Clin Med 99:601–610, 1982.
3. Dickson AP, Imrie CW: The incidence and prognosis of body wall ecchymosis in acute pancreatitis. Surg Gynecol Obstet 159:343–347, 1984.
4. Smith I, Wirght FJ: Cullen's Sign in ruptured ectopic gestation. Lancet 1:930–932, 1935.
5. Delp MH, Manning RT: Major's Physical Diagnosis. Philadelphia, W.B. Saunders, 1975.
6. Sherman HI, Hardison JE: The importance of a coexistent hepatic rub and bruit. JAMA 241:1495, 1979.
7. Naylor CD: Physical examination of the liver. JAMA 271:1859–1865, 1994.
8. Theodossi A, Knill-Jones RP, Skene A, et al: Interobserver variation of symptoms and signs in jaundice. Liver 1:21–32, 1981.

9. Espinoza P, Ducot B, Pellettier G: Interobserver agreement in the physical diagnosis of alcoholic liver disease. Dig Dis Sci 32:244–247, 1987.

10. Thomson H, Francis DMA: Abdominal wall tenderness: A useful sign in the acute abdomen. Lancet 2:1053–1054, 1977.

11. Bhatia ML, Tewari HL: Hepatic pulsations in constrictive pericarditis. Indian Heart J 26:165–170, 1974.

12. Manga P, Vythilingum S, Mitha AS: Pulsatile hepatomegaly in constrictive pericarditis. Br Heart J 52:465–467, 1984.

13. Maisel AS, Atwood JE, Goldberger AL: Hepatojugular reflux: Useful in the bedside diagnosis of tricuspid regurgitation. Ann Intern Med 101:781–782, 1984.

14. Palmer EC: Palpability of the liver edge in healthy adults. US Armed Forces Med J 12:1685–1690, 1958.

15. Riemenschneider PA, Whalen JP: The relative accuracy of estimation of enlargement of the liver and spleen by radiologic and clinical methods. Am J Roentgenol 94:462–468, 1965.

16. Naftalis J, Leevy CM: Clinical estimation of liver size. Am J Dig Dis New Series 8:236–243, 1963.

17. Peternel WW, Schaefer JW, Schiff L: Clinical evaluation of size and hepatic scintiscan. Am J Dig Dis 11:346–350, 1966.

18. Skraika B, Stahlhut J, Fulbeck CL, et al: Measuring liver span: Bedside examination versus ultrasound and scintiscan. J Clin Gastroenterol 8:267–270, 1986.

19. Sullivan S, Krasner N, Williams R: Clinical estimation of liver size. Am J Dig Dis New Series 8:236–243, 1963.

20. Fuller GN, Hargreaves M, King DM: Scratch test in clinical examination of the liver. Lancet i:181, 1988.

21. Malchow-Moller A, Rasmussen SN, Jensen AM, et al: Clinical estimation of liver size by percussion in normal individuals. Ann Intern Med 70:1183–1189, 1969.

22. Castell DO, O'Brien KD, Muench H, Chalmers TC: Estimation of liver size by percussion in normal individuals. Ann Intern Med 70:1183–1189, 1969.

23. Sapira JD, Williamson DL: How big is the normal liver? Arch Intern Med 139:971–973, 1979.

24. Zoli M, Magalotti D, Grimaldi M, et al: Physical examination of the liver: Is it still worth it? Am J Gastroenterol 90:1428–1432, 1995.

25. Gosink BB, Leymaster CE: Ultrasonic determination of hepatomegaly. J Clin Ultrasound 9:37–41, 1981.

26. Zoli M, Pisi P, et al: A rapid method for the in vivo measurement of liver volume. Liver 9:159–163, 1989.

27. Fenster LF, Klatskin G: Manifestation of metastatic tumors of the liver. Am J Med 31:238–248, 1971.

28. Zoneraich S, Zoneraich O: Diagnostic significance of abdominal arterial murmurs in liver and pancreatic disease: A photoarteriographic study. Angiology 22:197–205, 1971.

29. Motoki T, Hayashi T, Katoh Y, et al: Hepatic bruitis in liver tumours. Lancet ii:259, 1978.

30. Motoki T, Hayashi T, Katoh Y, et al: Hepatic bruits in malignant liver tumors. Am J Gastroenterol 71:582–686, 1979.

31. Sherman HI, Hardison JE: The importance of a coexistent hepatic rub and bruit: A clue to the diagnosis of cancer in the liver. JAMA 241:1495, 1979.

32. Dowdall GG: Five diagnostic methods of John B. Murphy of Chicago. Arch Diag 3:18–21, 1910.

33. Murphy JB: The diagnosis of gall stones. Med News 82:825–833, 1903.

34. Aldea PA, Meehan JP, Sternbach G: The acute abdomen and Murphy's signs. J Emerg Med 4:57–63, 1986.

35. Gunn A, Keddie N: Some clinical observations on patients with gallstones. Lancet ii:230–241, 1972.

36. Laing FC: Diagnostic evaluation of patients with suspected acute cholecystitis. Radiol Clin North Am 21:477–493, 1983.

37. Ralls PW, Halls J, Laplin SA, et al: Prospective evaluation of the sonographic Murphy's sign in suspected cholecystitis. Radiol Clin North Am 21:477–493, 1983.

38. Chung RS: Pathogenesis of the Courvoisier's gallbladder. Dig Dis Sci 28:33–38, 1983.

39. Courvoisier LG: Kasuistisch-statistiche Beitraege zur Pathologie and Chirurgie der Gallenwege. Leipzig, Vogel, 1980, pp 57–59.

40. Mikal S, Campbell AJA: Cancer of the pancreas: Diagnostic and operative criteria based on 100 consecutive autopsies. Surgery 18:963–967, 1950.

41. Viteri AL: Courvoisier's law and evaluation of the jaundiced patient. Tex Med 76:60–61, 1980.

42. Yang JC, Rickman LS, Bosser SK: The clinical diagnosis of splenomegaly. West J Med 155:47–52, 1991.

43. Hedge BM: How to detect early splenic enlargement. Practitioner 229:857, 1985.

44. Hackett LW: Spleen measurement in malaria: The importance of the spleen survey. J Nat Malaria Soc 3:121–133, 1944.

45. McIntyre RO, Ebaugh FG: Palpable spleens in college freshmen. Ann Intern Med 66:301–306, 1967.

46. Berris B: The incidence of palpable liver and spleen in the post-partum period. Can Med Assoc J 95:1319–1319, 1966.

47. Sullivan S, Krasner Williams R: The clinical estimation of liver size: A comparison of techniques and an analysis of the source of error. BMJ 2:1043–1044, 1976.

48. Lipp WF, Eckstein EH, Aaron AH: The clinical significance of the palpable spleen. Gastroenterology 3:297–291, 1944.

49. Halpern S, Coel M, Ashburn W, et al: Correlation of liver and spleen size: Determination by nuclear medicine studies and physical examination. Arch Intern Med 134:123–124, 1974.
50. Aito H: The estimation of the size of the spleen by radiologic methods. Ann Clin Res 15(Suppl 6):5–54, 1974.
51. Fisher J: Hypersplenism. Internist 12:176–186, 1971.
52. Fisher J, Wolf R: Die Milzszintigraphie. Deutsche Artzeblatt 7:401–408, 1973.
53. Blendis LM, McNeilly WJ, Sheppard L, et al: Observer variations in the clinical and radiological assessment of hepato-splenomegaly. BMJ 1:727–730, 1970.
54. Nixon: The detection of splenomegaly by percussion. N Engl J Med 250:166–167, 1954.
55. Castell DO: The spleen percussion sign. Ann Intern Med 67:1265–1267, 1967.
56. Barkun AN, Camus M, Meagher T, et al: Splenic enlargement and Traube's space. How useful is percussion? Am J Med 87:562–566, 1989.
57. Sullivan S, Williams R: Reliability of clinical techniques for detecting splenic enlargement. BMJ 2:1043–1044, 1976.
58. Leopold GR, Asher WM: Fundamentals of Abdominal and Pelvic Ultrasound. Philadelphia, W.B. Saunders, 1975.
59. Breiman RS, Beck JW, Korobkin M, et al: Volume determination using computer tomography. Am J Roentgenol 138:329–333, 1982.
60. Stark DD, Bradley WG: Magnetic Resonance Imaging. St. Louis, Mosby, 1988.
61. Bauerlein TC, De la Vega F: A diagnostic sign of carcinoma of the body and tail of the pancreas. Gastroenterology 44:816, 1963.
62. Shatney CH, Lillehei RC: Surgical treatment of pancreatic pseudocysts: Analysis of 119 cases. Ann Surg 189:386–394, 1979.
63. Dowdall GG: Five diagnostic methods of John B. Murphy of Chicago. Arch Diag 3:18–21, 1910.
64. Shapiro AP, Perez-Stable E, Scheib ET, et al: Renal artery stenosis and hypertension. Am J Med 47:175–193, 1969.
65. Hunt JC, Harrison EG, Kincaid OW, et al: Idiopathic fibrous and fibromuscular stenoses of the renal arteries associated with hypertension. Am J Cardiol 23:434–445, 1969.
66. Grim CE, Luft FC, Weinberger MH, Grim CM: Sensitivity and specificity of screening tests for renal vascular hypertension. Ann Intern Med 91:617–622, 1979.
67. Ashby EC: Detecting bladder fullness by subjective palpation. Lancet 2:936–937, 1977.
68. Guarino JR: Auscultatory percussion of the bladder to detect urinary retention. Arch Intern Med 145:1823–1825, 1985.
69. Carnett JB: Intercostal neuralgia as a cause of abdominal pain and tenderness. Surg Gynecol Obstet 42:625–632, 1926.
70. Thompson H, Francis DMA: Abdominal wall tenderness: A useful sign in the acute abdomen. Lancet ii:1053–1054, 1977.
71. Gray DWR, Dixon M, Seabrook G, Collin J: Is abdominal wall tenderness a useful sign in the diagnosis of non-specific abdominal pain? Ann Coll Surg Engl 70:2333–2334, 1988.
72. Thomson WHF, Dawes RFH, Carter S: Abdominal wall tenderness: A useful sign in chronic abdominal pain. Br J Surg 78:223–225, 1991.
73. Clain A (ed): Hamilton Bailey's Demonstration of Physical Signs in Clinical Surgery, 15th ed. Baltimore, Williams & Wilkins, 1973.
74. Meyerowitz BR: Abdominal palpation by stethoscope. Arch Surg 111:831, 1976.
75. Mellinkoff SM: Stethoscope sign. N Engl J Med 271:630, 1964.
76. Oldstone MB: Stethoscopic treachery. N Engl J Med 272:107, 1965.
77. Colling J, Gray DWR: The eyes closed sign. BMJ 295:1656, 1987.
78. Gray DWR, Dixon MJ, Colling J: The closed eyes sign: An aid to diagnosing non-specific abdominal pain. BMJ 297:837, 1988.
79. Gunn A, Keddie N: Some clinical observations on patients with gallstones. Lancet ii:230–241, 1972.
80. Markle GB: A simple test for intraperitoneal inflammation. Am J Surg 125:721–722, 1973.
81. Williams JW, Simel DL: Does this patient have ascites? JAMA 267:2645–2648, 1992.
82. Cummings S, Papadakis M, Melnick J, et al: The predictive value of physical examination for ascites. West J Med 142:633–636, 1985.

16. MALE GENITALIA, HERNIAS, AND RECTAL EXAM

Salvatore Mangione, M.D.

God gave man the penis and the brain as His two greatest gifts. Unfortunately, He made it so that he could only use one at a time.

Robin Williams

TOPICS COVERED IN THIS CHAPTER

Penis
Anatomic landmarks
Techniques of examination
Priapism
Phimosis/paraphimosis
Peyronie's disease
Hypospadias/epispadias
Penile skin lesions
   Ulcerating
   Nonulcerating
Scrotum
Anatomic landmarks
Techniques of examination
Skin lesions
Fordyce lesions
Scrotal edema/masses
Varicocele
Hydrocele
Spermatocele
Cryptorchidism
Small testes
Epididymitis and orchitis

Groin Hernias
Anatomic landmarks
Techniques of examination
Femoral hernias
Inguinal hernias
   Direct
   Indirect
Zieman's tridigital examination
Rectal Examination
Anatomic landmarks
Techniques of examination
                  Prostatic findings

CONVENTIONAL TEACHING WATCH

Examination of the male genitalia and rectum is important but often forgotten. It usually is conducted as the final part of the physical examination. There is no gain in being prudish about it (or, even worse, in skipping it altogether, while documenting in the chart: *Patient refused*). A wealth of information can be gained from completing this part of the physical exam.

FINDING/MANEUVER		CONVENTIONAL TEACHING REVISITED
Priapism	⇔	Intriguing but usually quite obvious physical finding; hard to miss (no pun intended).
Phimosis/paraphimosis	⇔	Relatively common, important findings; should not be missed.
Hypospadias/epispadias	⇔	As above.
Penile/scrotal skin lesions	⇑	Important findings with wide differential diagnosis.

Continued on following page

FINDING/MANEUVER		CONVENTIONAL TEACHING REVISITED
Urethral discharge	⇑	Important to obtain and analyze.
Fordyce lesions	⇓	Benign, common lesions; recognition and reassurance suffice.
Scrotal swelling/mass	⇔	Important problem with wide differential diagnosis.
Transillumination	⇑	Key maneuver for interpretation of scrotal masses.
Cryptorchidism	⇑	Important to detect as early as possible.
Varicocele	⇑	Frequent cause of reversible infertility.
Small testes	⇑	Important sign of atrophy.
Groin hernias	⇑	Common, important problems. Pertinent maneuvers to identify various types of groin hernias should be part of every physician's toolbox.
Rectal exam	⇑	Mandatory.

MALE GENITALIA

1. What are the main components of the male genital system?

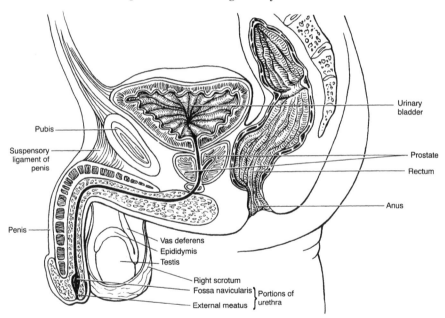

Male pelvic anatomy. (From Willms JL, Schneidermann H, Algranati PS: Physical Diagnosis. Baltimore, Williams & Wilkins, 1994, with permission.)

Penis

2. Describe the anatomy of the penis.

The penis consists of a **shaft** formed by three juxtaposed columns of spongy and vascular tissue, the **corpora cavernosa**. These structures can be temporarily filled with blood, thereby providing a unique erectile capacity. The distal tip of the penis consists of a cone-shaped structure called the **glans** (acorn in Latin), which contains the vertical slit-like opening of the urethra (**urethral meatus**). The glans is separated from the shaft by a circular sulcus called the **corona** (crown in Latin), which in uncircumcised men is covered in a hood-like fashion by the **foreskin** (**prepuce**). This fold of skin is surgically removed during circumcision.

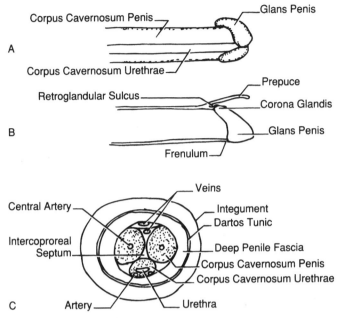

Structure of the penis. In *A* the shaft is diagrammed in its ventrolateral aspect, with integument removed. A sagittal section of the shaft is represented in *B* with integument included. *C* is a cross-section of the shaft. (From DeGowin RL: DeGowin and DeGowin's Diagnostic Examination, 6th ed. New York, McGraw-Hill, 1994, with permission.)

3. What steps should be taken to examine the penis properly?

The first step, of course, is precautionary: put on a pair of gloves. Some sexually transmitted diseases (including syphilis) can be acquired through simple skin abrasions. With gloves on, the physician examines the penis by first palpating the shaft, carefully looking for areas of induration or tenderness. The prepuce should be retracted to gain access to the glans and inspect its structure for possible abnormalities. Return the foreskin to its original position after completing the exam. Failure to do so may lead to severe edema in unconscious patients. Finally, the glans should be gently compressed between thumb and forefinger so that the urethral meatus can be visualized and secretions possibly expressed. Even in patients with a history of penile discharge, this maneuver may fail. In this case, milking of the shaft of the penis (from its base to the glans) may produce a few precious secretions for analysis.

4. What is priapism?

Priapism is a fancy term for a protracted erection, usually associated with pain. If we look at American history, we might conclude that priapism qualifies as an occupational hazard for a few American presidents were it not for the fact that priapism is not associated with sexual desire. The name priapism is rooted in Greek mythology, specifically in Priapus, one of the many illegitimate sons of Jupiter, King of Gods (which confirms our suspicion that power and sex may be linked, at least among American presidents and Greek gods). Juno (Jupiter's unhappy wife) found out about the illicit affair and promised to be present at the child's birth so that she could cast a mortal spell. When the child was finally born, however, he was so well endowed that Juno, taken by surprise, totally missed her chance. The baby's mother and her friends rushed the boy to safety, and a new medical term was born. Priapism eventually came to signify a condition charac-terized by chronic, protracted, and painful erections.

The Priapus story prompted a tremendous respect among ancient Romans for the penis, which became a symbol not only of fertility but also of luck. After all, his penis literally saved Priapus' life. As a result, Romans started wearing little gold phalluses around their neck as hope-ful lucky charms. They also carved phalluses on their buildings. For example, the great Roman wall erected (no pun intended) in northern England by Emperor Hadrian during the first century A.D. was riddled with with numerous carvings of penises. These penises (still visible today) were supposed to bring good luck to the wall's defenders. Unfortunately, they fell short of expec-tations: Hadrian's wall was pierced multiple times by Scots and Picts and eventually totally aban-doned. The reverence for the penis, however, continued unabated in many parts of the Mediterranean culture. Indeed, in some areas of southern Italy and Greece it is still not uncom-mon to see golden pricklets hanging from people's necks, a memento of the long-lasting value of Greek mythology.

5. What are the causes of priapism?

True priapism may reflect several abnormalities, either systemic or local. **Local abnormali-ties** may result from neoplastic or inflammatory diseases of the shaft. They also may reflect a thrombotic and/or hemorrhagic process involving the vasculature of the penis. **Systemic condi-tions,** on the other hand, may represent either neurologic lesions or various hematologic abnor-malities. Among these are several conditions favoring thrombosis, such as sickle cell anemia or leukemia.

6. What is phimosis?

Phimosis is a condition characterized by narrowness of the opening of the prepuce so that the foreskin cannot be retracted over the glans. The word derives from the Greek *phimos,* which means muzzle or snout. Phimosis is usually due to a congenital abnormality (such as the pres-ence of membranes binding the prepuce to the glans), but it also may due to acquired adhesions, often the sequelae of a previous infection (see figure on following page).

7. What is paraphimosis?

Paraphimosis is condition similar to phimosis: once the foreskin has been retracted, it cannot be brought forward again to cover the glans. Paraphimosis usually results from edema of the glans and often is an indication for circumcision to prevent possible infectious or vascular com-plications (see figure on following page).

8. What is Peyronie's disease?

It is a peculiar disease of unknown etiology, often referred to as penile fibromatosis or van Buren's disease. It may be associated with Dupuytren's contracture. Peyronie's disease is charac-terized by plaques or strands of dense fibrous tissue surrounding the corpora cavernosa of the penis. These may be detectable by palpation and often cause deformity of the penis with crooked and painful erections. The penis at rest is entirely normal; only when erect does it appear bent and deformed. The major significance of Peyronie's disease is usually psychological. In some cases, however, the deformity may be severe enough to interfere with erection, penetration, orgasm, and even fertility.

9. Who was Peyronie?

François de la Peyronie (1678–1747) was a well-respected French surgeon and the personal physician to the Sun King, Louis XIV. He astutely used his royal connection to have the king pass a law banning barbers and wigmakers from practicing medicine, thereby eliminating with the stroke of a pen the main competition to the surgical community. He subsequently founded the French Academy of Surgery and became one of the main forces in the establishment of Paris as a world center of surgery.

10. Define hypospadias and epispadias.

Hypospadias is a developmental anomaly characterized by a defect on the lower (ventral) surface of the penis. Consequently, the urethral meatus is located more proximally than normal, opening on the ventral aspect of the penis instead of the glans. **Epispadias** is characterized by a defect on the upper (dorsal) surface of the penis. Consequently, the urethral meatus opens dorsally. Both of these congenital malformations may lead to problems with fertility and represent a clue to the presence of other underlying abnormalities, such as an undescended testis (see cryptorchidism), Klinefelter's syndrome, or other chromosomal disorders. Hypospadias also may be induced by the mother's ingestion of estrogens or progesterone or congenital adrenal hyperplasia.

Structural abnormalities of the prepuce (foreskin). From DeGowin RL: DeGowin and DeGowin's Diagnostic Examination. New York, McGraw-Hill, 1994, with permission.)

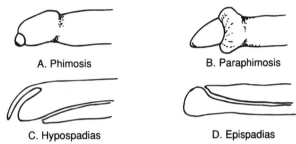

A. Phimosis   B. Paraphimosis

C. Hypospadias   D. Epispadias

11. What skin lesions can be visualized on the penis?

Nonulcerating lesions are typical of secondary syphilis. They present as as papulosquamous rash involving not only the penis but also the palms and soles. Psoriasis also commonly involves the penis; squamous lesions resemble those seen elsewhere on the body. Carcinoma of the penis presents as an indurated and nontender nodule, which at times may even be ulcerated. Scabies and lichen planus also may involve the penis with nonulcerating lesions. Finally, Reiter's syndrome may present with the penile skin lesion that carries the fancy name of circinate balanitis (*circinate* means round in Latin, and *balanitis* is the Greek term for inflammation of the glans). This painless inflammatory process involves not only the skin of the glans but also the sulcus and corona. It starts as tiny blebs, which eventually merge into a larger ring of inflammatory tissue that may completely circumscribe the glans. In addition to circinate balanitis, patients with Reiter's syndrome also may have mucocutaneous lesions (of palms, soles, and mouth), iridocyclitis, arthritis, and diarrhea. One or more of these conditions may recur at intervals of months or years, but the arthritis is usually persistent. Patients with Reiter's syndrome also may have urethritis with urethral discharge, which usually is scanty, thin, and whitish, thus quite different from the profuse, thicker, and more purulent discharge of gonorrhea. The discharge of Reiter's syndrome resembles the other nongonococcal urethritides, such as chlamydial infection.

Ulcerating lesions include (1) syphilis, which is characterized by a single nontender ulcer (chancre) with bilateral lymphadenopathy; (2) chancroid, which is characterized by multiple painful ulcers with lymphadenopathy; (3) granuloma inguinale, which is characterized by a single painless ulcer without lymphadenopathy; (4) lymphogranuloma venereum, which is characterized by a small nontender ulcer with unilateral tender lymphadenopathy; (5) herpes simplex, which is characterized by small multiple vesicular skin lesions that are painful and occur in clusters (these lesions are *not* associated with adenopathy); and (6) condylomata lata or acuminata, which are flat (lata) or arbor-like (acuminata) skin lesions produced by infection with human papilloma virus. Genital warts tend to be predominantly located in moist areas, such as the corona and sulcus.

12. Who was Reiter?

Hans C. Reiter (1881–1969) was a German physician, the son of a wealthy industrialist of Leipzig. He described his famous syndrome in 1916, while serving with First Hungarian Army in the Balkans during World War I. He encountered a young lieutenant affected by diarrhea, urethritis, arthritis, and conjunctivitis. Reiter first thought that the patient may have had syphilis but eventually changed his mind and recognized the new syndrome. The same syndrome was described by Sir Benjamin Brodie in 1818 in his textbook, *Diseases of the Bones and Joints*. Reiter is also famous for having identified the spirochete causing Weil's disease while stationed on the Western front. After the rise of Hitler to power, he became a member of the Nazi party and even signed an oath of allegiance to Adolf Hitler in 1932. In 1936 Reiter was appointed minister of health for the state of Mecklenburg.

Scrotum

13. Describe the anatomy of the scrotum.
The scrotum consists of a skin pouch, divided in the midline by a raphe extending from the ventral surface of the penis to the perineum. The scrotum is internally subdivided into right and left compartments, which house, respectively, the testicles and epididymis and the various structures of the spermatic cord (vas deferens with its vascular and nervous supply).

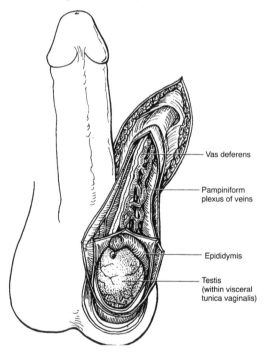

Vas deferens

Pampiniform
plexus of veins

Epididymis

Testis
(within visceral
tunica vaginalis)

Anatomy of the scrotum. (From Willms JL, Schneidermann H, Algranati PS: Physical Diagnosis. Baltimore, Williams & Wilkins, 1994, with permission.)

14. Which abnormalities can be visualized on the scrotum?
Mostly skin abnormalities, including lesions related to either sexually transmitted or fungal diseases. Tinea cruris, for example, is particularly common in the scrotum. It presents as a large erythematous area involving not only the scrotum but also the adjacent thighs. The lesions are usually a little scaly, with ragged margins. Candidal infection also may cause scrotal lesions, particularly in diabetics and patients who are grossly overweight. Finally, lice or sometimes even scabies can be visualized in the scrotal and pubic areas, often heralded by the presence of excoriations.

15. What are Fordyce lesions?
These tiny nodules, first described by the American dermatologist John Fordyce (1858–1925) are often referred to as Fordyce's angiokeratoma. Lesions are vascular papules of the scrotum, usually the size of the head of a pin. They are dark, totally asymptomatic, entirely benign, and quite common. In fact, they may be encountered in as many as 1 of 6 men over the age of 50.

Conversely, they are extremely rare below the age of 40. Because they are congenitally acquired, they usually occur in families. Yet they remain primarily a result of aging. Because of their vascular nature, Fordyce lesions should not be biopsied.

16. What are the causes of swelling of the scrotum?

Bilateral diffuse and painless swelling of the scrotum is usually a feature of systemic disease, most commonly anasarca. Ascites, pleural effusion, and edema of the scrotum are commonly seen in patients with severe congestive heart failure, nephrotic syndrome, or cirrhosis.

Unilateral edema of the scrotum is usually a sign of local pathology. The most common is a varicocele (from the Latin *varix* = dilated vein and Greek *kele* = tumor). This condition is caused by incompetent valves in the internal spermatic veins and therefore is characterized by venous engorgement along the spermatic cord. A varicocele resembles a nest of worms. It is present only when the patient is standing and resolves in a supine position with elevation of the scrotum. This condition is easily identifiable and clinically important because it is a common cause of reversible infertility. Varicoceles are much more common on the left than on the right because of the drainage characteristics of the testicular veins. Accordingly, a right varicocele should prompt investigation to rule out either anatomic abnormalities or an alternative diagnosis. Besides varicocele, localized scrotal swelling usually reflects pathology of either the testis or epididymis (see below). Painful and tender scrotal swelling usually indicates a much more acute process, such as torsion of the spermatic cord, strangulated inguinal hernia, acute orchitis, or acute epididymitis.

Pearl.   *The sudden appearance of varicocele in a patient with nephrotic syndrome should be considered due to renal vein thrombosis until proved otherwise.*

17. What is transillumination of a scrotal mass?

It is a good way to find out whether a localized swelling of the scrotum is caused by fluid or solid tissue (the maneuver, however, is not valid for examination of the testicles). The first step is to raise the penis so that the scrotum can be well visualized. Then the scrotal mass should be illuminated from behind with a penlight. Inability of the mass to transmit light suggests a solid lesion. Conversely, transmission of the light beam favors a fluid-filled mass, such as hydrocele or spermatocele. However, both hematocele (fluid-filled lesion caused by accumulation of blood) and varicocele (varicose veins of the spermatic cord) are transillumination-negative. Blood, in fact, does not transmit light.

18. What are the normal characteristics of the testes and epididymides?

The **testes** are paired organs, 2–3 cm in thickness and 5 cm in length (range: 3.5–5.5 cm). They have the shape of an egg; the vertical axis is the longest. All surfaces of both testes (with the exception of the posterior surfaces) are surrounded by a folded serous sheath with a potential cavity, the **tunica vaginalis**.

The **epididymides** (in Greek, the ones on top of the testicles) are two elongated structures attached to the posterior surface of the testes. In 7–10% of normal adult men, however, the epididymides are located anteriorly to the testicles. Each epididymis consists of a head (caput epididymidis), body (corpus epididymidis), and tail (cauda epididymidis). The tail turns sharply upon itself to become the **ductus** (or **vas**) **deferens**. Both the tail and the beginning of the ductus deferens represent a reservoir for spermatozoa. Secretions from the ductus deferens, seminal vesicles, and prostate combine to form the semen.

19. How should the testes and epididymides be examined?

Gently, of course, because these organs (especially the testes) are highly sensitive not only to touch but also to temperature. Thus, the best way to palpate them is by using the thumb and index finger. This technique also allows the examiner to gauge the length and thickness of each testicle, although a caliper is necessary for more accurate measurement. Finally, using great caution, the examiner should move cephalad and assess the upper and posterior pole of the testes and adjacent heads of the epididymides. Although the testicles can be examined in either a standing or supine position, a search for hernias for varicoceles requires the patient to stand.

20. What is a hydrocele?

A hydrocele (literally, a water tumor) is a collection of serous fluid in either the tunica vaginalis of the testis or in a separate pocket along the spermatic cord. It usually presents as a unilateral and painless scrotal swelling. It is easily recognized by transillumination.

21. What is a spermatocele?

A spermatocele (literally, a sperm tumor) is a spermatozoa-filled cyst of the epididymis. It presents as a unilateral, painless, and movable scrotal mass, located just above the testis and identifiable by transillumination. A true cyst of the epididymis is clinically similar but does not contain spermatozoa.

22. What is cryptorchidism?

It is a condition characterized by failure of one or both testes to descend (literally, the invisible testis in Greek). The undescended testicle may lie in either the inguinal canal or abdomen. Because of the high surrounding temperature, the undescended testis undergoes atrophy and even becomes susceptible to neoplastic degeneration. Because the other testis is fully functional, cryptorchidism usually does not affect fertility. It may, however, cause serious psychologic repercussions. For example, it has been suggested that Adolf Hitler's psychopathology may have resulted from cryptorchidism, a condition documented by a urologist that Hitler consulted before rising to power.

23. What is the most common cause of small testes?

The most common cause is atrophy. In fact, small testes (i.e., < 3.5 cm in length) tend to be atrophic. Atrophy may be due to either congenital diseases (such as Klinefelter's syndrome) or acquired conditions (such as alcoholic cirrhosis). Testicles in Klinefelter's syndrome tend to be small and firm, whereas in cirrhosis they are usually small and soft. Atrophy also may result from an inflammatory or infectious process (i.e., orchitis), which often is caused by viruses, such as mumps, but also by syphilis, filariasis, and even trauma.

24. What are the causes of an enlarged and solid testis?

Possibly cancer. Thus, an enlarged and firm testis should be transilluminated to exclude a fluid-filled mass, such as a hydrocele, spermatocele, or cyst of the epididymis. The presence of a confirmed solid lesion increases the likelihood of testicular cancer, which is the most common tumor in men between the ages of 20 and 35. Solid lesions of the testicles should be actively sought, not only by the physician but also by patients through self-examination.

25. What are the causes of a tender epididymis?

A tender epididymis usually reflects acute epididymitis, which may be associated with an enlargement of the epididymis to the point that separation from the testis is difficult to detect. Acute epididymitis often is associated with urinary tract infection, prostatitis, or urethritis. An enlarged, nodular, beaded, and nontender epididymis indicates tuberculous epididymitis, which often is encountered in patients with renal tuberculosis.

HERNIA EXAMINATION

26. Which are two possible sites of presentation of hernias in the groin?

1. **Femoral hernias** are less common, especially in males. Femoral hernias originate below the inguinal ligament and are located laterally to the site of inguinal hernias. They often are confused with femoral lymph nodes. They do not progress into the scrotum and on examination are associated with an empty inguinal canal.

2. **Inguinal hernias** are much more common. They may occur medially, in which case they are referred to as direct hernias. Direct hernias originate above the inguinal ligament, more

specifically in a congenital defect near the pubis tubercle and external inguinal ring. Such hernias usually affect men 40 years of age or older, rarely progress into the scrotum, and on examination bulge anteriorly, pushing the side of the finger forward. Inguinal hernias also may occur laterally, in which case they are referred to as indirect hernias. They are the most common of the groin hernias, affecting patients of all ages and both sexes. They are more common in children than adults. Indirect hernias originate above the inguinal ligament near its midpoint (the internal inguinal ring). They are due to a defect in the abdominal ring, through which the spermatic cord exits the scrotum and enters the pelvis.

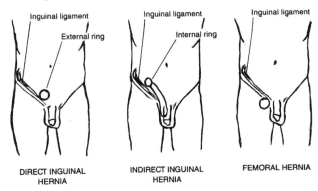

Sites of hernias in the groin. (Adapted from Swartz MH: Pocket Companion to Textbook of Physical Diagnosis. Philadelphia, W.B Saunders, 1995.)

27. What is the best way to detect a hernia?

The best way starts with inspection. The patient is asked to stand while the examiner sits comfortably in a chair and observes the external inguinal ring, looking for a localized bulge. The bulge can be elicited by asking the patient to cough or perform a Valsalva maneuver. Once inspection has been completed, palpation is carried out by using the small finger of the examiner's right hand for the patient's right side and the small finger of the examiner's left hand for the patient's left side. The finger is gently inserted through the invaginated scrotum and into the superficial inguinal ring, while the patient is asked to cough or strain. (See figure at top of next page.)

- A strong palpable impulse that pushes out the examiner's finger suggests the presence of a direct inguinal hernia.
- Conversely, a soft impulse without a bulge suggests an indirect inguinal hernia, gently descending the inguinal canal.
- Finally, an empty inguinal canal suggests the presence of a femoral hernia. This finding is substantiated by placing the index and middle fingers into the triangle lying medially to the femoral artery. A palpable bulge in this triangle, triggered by straining or coughing, confirms the presence of a femoral hernia.

28. What is Zieman's tridigital examination for hernia?

It is a procedure used to identify both femoral and inguinal hernias (direct and indirect). The examiner stands at the right side of the patient, who is also standing, and places the palm of the right hand over the patient's right lower abdomen. Consequently, the examiner's fingertips are near the right inguinal ligament. The tip of the long finger is in the external inguinal ring; the tip of the index finger is near the internal inguinal ring; and the tip of the ring finger is the femoral triangle. The patient is then asked to strain or perform a Valsalva maneuver. As a result of the increased intraabdominal pressure, a hernia in any of the three sites is perceived as either a gliding motion of the walls of the empty sac or as an impulse caused by the protrusion of the viscus into the sac. The maneuver should be repeated for the contralateral side.

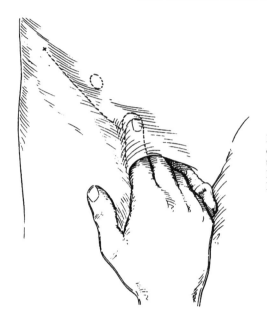

Examination of the inguinal floor by insertion of a finger through the invaginated upper scrotum. (From James EC, Corry RJ, Perry JF: Basic Surgical Practice. Philadelphia, Hanley & Belfus, 1987, with permission.)

RECTAL EXAMINATION

29. What findings can be detected by a rectal examination?

First of all, findings may be related to visible abnormalities in the rectal area, including skin lesions caused by sexually transmitted diseases, parasitic infestations (such as pinworms), or fungi (such as *Candida* sp.) Fissures or fistulas also may be detected by inspection (usually suggestive of Crohn's disease). Hemorrhoids also are detected by inspection, although they usually require palpation too. As for palpation, once the sphincter tone has been assessed (looking for localized tenderness and degree of resistance to the examiner's finger), one should examine the various internal structures, including not only the rectum per se but also the prostate and seminal vesicles. (See figure at top of facing page.)

Pearl.   *A rectal exam can be important in patients with appendicitis, particularly those with an inflamed and swollen retrocecal appendix. An appendix in this location is famous for not producing the classic findings on typical abdominal exam.*

30. Which prostatic characteristics should be assessed by rectal exam?

Mostly size, consistency, and surface characteristics. The size of the prostate is usually compared to that of a walnut, but in older men it may be larger simply because of benign prostatic hypertrophy. Thus, increase in size is not necessarily a sign of cancer. A prostatic nodule, on the other hand, should be considered suspicious until proved otherwise. The nodule may require evaluation by biopsy. In some series, only 50% of nodules turned out to be neoplastic; the remainder usually are due to benign prostatic hypertrophy. A localized area of induration is not necessarily typical of early cancer but more likely represents a late neoplastic phenomenon. Finally, although a rectal examination is valuable in detecting prostate cancers, it has a sensitivity of only 69%, a specificity of 89%, a positive predictive value of 67%, and negative predictive value of 91%.

31. Should rectal exam be deferred in patients with a myocardial infarction?

No. Although conventional teaching suggests that a rectal examination may worsen ischemia and even trigger arrhythmias in patients suffering an acute myocardial infarction, no scientific data support this assumption. A rectal exam may increase the acid prostatic phosphatase, but it

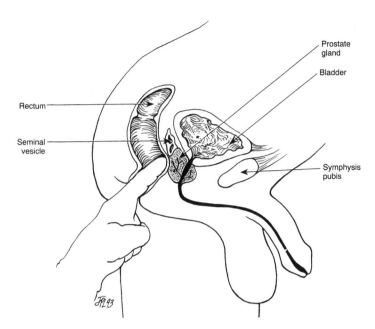

Prostatic palpation. Note the position of the examiner's finger relative to the median sulcus and lateral lobes of the gland. The depth of penetration of the examiner's index finger depends on the degree of flexion of the examiner's middle finger. (From Willms JL, Schneidermann H, Algranati PS: Physical Diagnosis. Baltimore, Williams & Wilkins, 1994, with permission.)

will do so only in patients with prostatic cancer, not in patients with benign prostatic hypertrophy. Thus, when screening for prostatic cancer, you should remember that the serum acid phosphatase should be obtained after a rectal exam, not before.

32. What causes prostatic nodules?

Prostatic nodules may be encountered in patients with benign hyperplasia of the prostate. They also may reflect various inflammatory processes and even infarct of the prostate. Of course, a prostatic nodule should raise concern about the presence of prostatic cancer. Because cancers often originate in the posterior lobe, they may present as palpable hard nodules.

33. What causes a tender prostate?

The most common causes are prostatitis and prostatic abscess. Patients with these conditions also may have palpable prostatic nodules.

BIBLIOGRAPHY

1. Bates B: A Guide to Physical Examination and History Taking, 6th ed. Philadelphia, J.B. Lippincott, 1995.
2. DeGowin, DeGowin: Bedside Diagnostic Examination, 6th ed. New York, McGraw-Hill, 1994.
3. Guinan P, Bush I, Ray V, et al: The accuracy of the rectal examination in the diagnosis of prostatic carcinoma. N Engl J Med 303:499–583, 1980.
4. Sapira JD: The Art and Science of Bedside Diagnosis. Baltimore, Urban & Schwarzenberg, 1990.
5. Willms JL, Schneidermann H, Algranati PS: Physical Diagnosis. Baltimore, Williams & Wilkins, 1994.

17. PELVIC EXAMINATION

Carol Fleischman, M.D.

A child of our grandmother Eve, a female; or, for thy more sweet understanding, a woman.

Shakespeare, *Love's Labour Lost*, Act I

TOPICS COVERED IN THIS CHAPTER

Vulva and Perineum
Anatomic landmarks
Techniques of examination
Female escutcheon·
Tanner's stages of sexual maturation
Enlarged inguinal nodes (differential diagnosis)
Normal appearance of the vulva
White lesions of the vulva
Premalignant white lesions
Other vulvar malignancies
Clitoral index
Bartholin glands and cysts
Skene's glands
Condyloma lata and acuminata
Genital warts
Genital herpes simplex
Vulvar ulcerations
Labial hernia
Vagina
Anatomic landmarks
Techniques of examination
Colpocele
Cystocele
Rectocele
Chadwick's sign
Gartner's duct cyst

Uterine Cervix
Anatomic landmarks
Techniques of examination
Duplication of the cervix
Endocervical polyps
Pap smear
Goodell's sign
Uterine Corpus
Anatomic landmarks
Techniques of examination
Retroversion and retroflexion
Hegar's sign
Uterine prolapse
Fundal height
Leopold maneuvers
Leiomyomata and fibroids
Adnexae
Anatomic landmarks
Techniques of examination
Adnexal mass
Cul-de-sac
Anatomic landmarks
Techniques of examination

CONVENTIONAL TEACHING WATCH

MANEUVER/FINDING		CONVENTIONAL TEACHING REVISITED
Pelvic examination	⇑	You will miss major diagnoses if you skip this part of the physical examination.

1. What is the value of pelvic examination?

The pelvic examination is an essential part of the physical examination of women. With good technique, an examiner can detect a wide variety of normal and pathologic conditions, including pregnancy, and screen for several kinds of cancer. All of this can be done on the basis of physical diagnosis with the aid of a few simple, low-tech laboratory techniques.

2. How can I make the pelvic examination painless and comfortable for my patient?

Pelvic examinations should be accomplished with a minimum of discomfort or embarrassment to the patient. The exam should not be painful except in the unavoidable circumstance in which a pathologic condition causes pain on palpation. Comfortable pelvic examinations are accomplished by the use of a few simple steps:

1. Instruct the patient to empty her bladder before the exam.
2. Position the patient comfortably in a way that maintains eye contact.
3. Use a drape sheet over the patient's abdomen and legs (unless she indicates that she does not prefer this).
4. Inform the patient of each step in the exam before proceeding.
5. Instruct the patient to breathe and relax perineal muscles before proceeding.

The importance of communicating with the patient continuously during the exam cannot be overstated. Some clinicians offer the patient a hand-held mirror so that she can observe the examination. Reassuring the patient that she may stop the exam if she feels uncomfortable gives her a sense of control and is also a useful technique.

3. When should a chaperone be present for pelvic examination?

In general, a chaperone should be present when the examiner is male, when the patient is a minor, when the patient requests a chaperone, or at the discretion of the examiner if the patient exhibits extreme apprehension.

4. What circumstances make pelvic examination difficult for women?

Women may be apprehensive about a pelvic exam for various reasons. A woman who is having her first pelvic exam may be nervous because the procedure is unfamiliar. A woman who has never had intercourse may have a small vaginal opening that makes speculum insertion difficult. Postmenopausal women, particularly if they are not sexually active, may have small, atrophic introita. Examiners also need to be mindful of the possibility that the patient may have experienced childhood or adult sexual abuse or rape. This information should be elicited in the course of the patient's history, preferably with the patient clothed and seated in a chair. It is not appropriate to attempt to obtain the history when the patient is on the exam table. A patient with a history of sexual abuse may exhibit signs of panic or dissociation during an exam. Women from a variety of cultures may have undergone some type of "circumcision" that alters their anatomy and makes examination difficult.

5. What techniques are helpful in the difficult pelvic examination?

Communication with the patient is essential. If the patient brings her knees together at the beginning of the exam, stop the exam and allow her to come to a sitting position with a drape sheet over her lap. Discuss what is making the exam difficult. If the exam is not urgently necessary, it can be rescheduled. The woman undergoing her first pelvic exam may be instructed to practice inserting tampons or a disposable speculum before the rescheduled exam. The postmenopausal woman with atrophy may be instructed to apply estrogen vaginal cream for a week before the rescheduled exam. The survivor of sexual abuse needs to be asked if she feels safe about having a pelvic exam and may want counseling before having one. The RAINBOW Foundation is a resource for clinicians and patients who have experienced "female circumcision," also known as female genital mutilation (FGM).

6. Who is qualified to perform a pelvic examination after sexual assault?

Examination of the victim of sexual assault should be undertaken only by professionals with training in forensic techniques. An incompletely documented exam can undermine the efforts of law enforcement authorities to arrest the perpetrator and prosecute the crime. Local authorities usually provide qualified examiners with evidence-collecting kits and the appropriate forms for documentation of the history and physical findings. Victims of sexual assault should be treated as supportively as possible. They should not change or bathe until a forensic examination can be done, because valuable evidence such as fibers, hairs, fingernail scrapings, blood, or body fluids may be lost.

7. What supplies are needed for an adequate pelvic examination?
- Padded exam table with heel rests
- Padded covers for heel rests (quilted oven mitts do nicely)
- Good light source (gooseneck or fiberoptic lamp)
- Examination gloves
- Plastic or metal speculums, including Pederson, Graves, and pediatric speculums
- Surgical lubricant

Although much information is gained from direct physical examination, physical diagnosis in the pelvic area is routinely supplemented by a few simple diagnostic procedures and the Papanicolaou smear, a cytologic examination for signs of inflammation, atypia, or dysplasia of the cervix. For this reason, the following supplies are needed:
- Glass slides for the Pap smear and wet mount
- Cytologic fixative
- Small test tube with a few drops of normal saline for the wet mount
- pH paper
- Cytobrush and wooden spatula for collecting the Pap smear
- Specimen collection tube for gonorrhea and chlamydial testing by DNA probe analysis
- Fecal occult blood test card

VULVA AND PERINEUM

The pelvic examination begins with inspection of external structures.

CONVENTIONAL TEACHING WATCH

MANEUVER/FINDING		CONVENTIONAL TEACHING REVISITED
Assessment of the shape of the escutcheon	⇓	Not a highly specific indicator of virilization and essentially a culturally biased definition of "normal."
Inspection of vulvar skin and mucosa for "white lesions" or moles	⇑	You may not make the diagnosis, but your referral for a biopsy may be critically important

8. What is the female escutcheon?
The female escutcheon is the characteristic triangular pattern of pubic hair growth in adult females. The escutcheon in males is rhomboidal and extends to the umbilicus. The presence of a male-type escutcheon in female patients may be a sign of virilization or a normal variant.

9. What are Tanner's stages for sexual maturation?
The Tanner stages are a method for assessing sexual maturation by observation of breast and pubic hair growth. This technique is useful mainly in pediatric and adolescent patients but also forms an important part of the evaluation of the patient with primary amenorrhea.

Tanner Stages of Sexual Maturation in Girls

STAGE	DESCRIPTION	MEAN AGE	AGE RANGE 5–95%
	Pubic Hair		
I	None	—	—
II	Countable; straight; increased pigmentation and length; primarily on medial border of labia	11.25	9–13.5
III	Darker; begins to curl; increased quantity on mons pubis	12	9.5–14.25
IV	Increased quantity; coarser texture; labia and mons well covered	12.5	10.5–15
V	Adult distribution with feminine triangle and spread to medial thighs	14	12–16.5

Table continued on following page

Tanner Stages of Sexual Maturation in Girls (Continued)

STAGE	DESCRIPTION	MEAN AGE	AGE RANGE 5–95%
	Breast Development		
I	None	—	—
II	Breast bud present; increased areolar size	11	9–13
III	Further enlargement of breast; no secondary contour	12	10–14
IV	Areolar area forms secondary mound on breast contour	13	10.5–15.5
V	Mature; areolar area is part of breast contour; nipple projects	15	13–18
Menarche		12.8	11–14.5

From Polin RA, Ditmar MF: Pediatric Secrets, 2nd ed. Philadelphia, Hanley & Belfus, 1997, with permission.

10. What is the differential diagnosis of enlarged inguinal lymph nodes?

Inguinal adenopathy may result from infection in the genital area, lower extremity, or the lymph node itself. It may indicate a primary neoplastic lesion (lymphoma) or metastatic invasion.

11. What is the normal appearance of the vulva?

The vulva includes several anatomic structures: mons pubis, major and minor labia, clitoris, vaginal vestibule, and vestibular (Bartholin's) glands.

12. What important physiologic information can be gained by inspection of the vulva?

The thickness and rugation of the mucosa of the vulva and vagina and the presence of mucus are indications of the degree of estrogenization of the urogenital tract.

13. What is the significance of white lesions of the vulva?

White lesions of the vulva may be benign, premalignant, or malignant. Benign and malignant white lesions frequently exist simultaneously. Therefore, it is important to evaluate vulvar white lesions carefully.

14. What are the benign white lesions of the vulva?

Benign causes of white lesions include vitiligo and inflammatory dermatitis such as psoriasis.

15. What are the premalignant white lesions?

The vulvar dystrophies are white lesions that may progress to malignancy. Atrophic dystrophy, or lichen sclerosus, may occur in all age groups but is more common in postmenopausal women. It consists of yellowish-blue papules or macules that eventually coalesce, forming areas of atrophic grayish mucosa that is smooth and thin. Extensive lesions may cause narrowing of the introitus. Hyperplastic dystrophy may appear as a similar gray-white plaque but is distinguished microscopically by epithelial hyperplasias or atypia. The vulvar dystrophies probably represent a continuum from benign to malignant, and benign and malignant white lesions frequently exist simultaneously. Therefore, it is important to biopsy dystrophic white lesions.

16. What are the malignant white lesions?

Vulvar intraepithelial neoplasia and Bowen's disease represent malignant white lesions.

17. What are the other vulvar malignancies?

Squamous cell carcinoma is the most common. Of importance, malignant melanoma is the second most common vulvar malignancy. Both patient and physician should be attentive to moles on the vulva, and this area should be included in the patient's regular self-examinations for moles. Other histologic types include adenocarcinoma (carcinoma of Bartholin's gland), basal cell carcinoma, and sarcoma.

18. What is the clitoral index?

The adult clitoral index is calculated by multiplying the vertical dimension of the clitoris by its horizontal dimension. The normal range is 9–35 mm. Enlargement of the clitoris is usually a sign of virilization. A clitoral index of 36–99 mm is considered borderline. An index > 100 mm is abnormal, and a source of androgenization should be sought.

19. What is the appearance of the vulva and clitoris in congenital adrenal hyperplasia?

Congenital adrenal hyperplasia is the generic term given to hereditary deficiency of any of a number of enzymes of glucocorticoid synthesis. Deficiencies of the 21-hydroxylase and 11-β-hydroxylase enzymes are most common. Decrease in hydrocortisone synthesis results in an increase in secretion of adrenocorticotropic hormone (ACTH), which causes an increase in adrenal steroids and a secondary increase in androgen. The final result is virilization of the female genitalia, which usually is apparent from birth. Signs include clitoral hypertrophy and fused labia. In untreated females, secondary sex characteristics fail to develop.

20. What is the normal location of Bartholin's glands?

Bartholin's glands are located deep in the lateral walls of the vulva, close to the posterior formix. They are normally not palpable. Formation of cysts and abscesses in Bartholin's glands is common and presents as a palpable, usually tender enlargement of one or both labia majora.

21. What is the technique for examining Bartholin's glands?

Place a gloved forefinger just inside the vaginal opening, with the thumb directly opposite on the outside. Palpate gently for any enlargement or tenderness.

22. What is the differential diagnosis of a mass or swelling of Bartholin's gland?

Bartholin's gland cyst, abscess, or adenocarcinoma.

23. Who was Bartholin?

Caspar Bartholin (1655–1738) was a Danish physician, the son of an anatomist famous for the first description of the intestinal lymphatics and their drainage into the thoracic duct. Bartholin is famous not only for the description of the homonymous glands (and their possible cystic degeneration), but also for the discovery of the sublingual glands and their ducts (that still carry his name). During the last part of his life he left medicine to dedicate himself to politics, becoming Procurator General and Deputy of Finance of Denmark.

24. What is the normal location of Skene's glands?

Skene's (paraurethral) glands are located on either side of the urethra.

25. Who was Skene?

Alexander J. Skene (1838–1900) was a native of Scotland. At the age of 18 he moved to Canada and subsequently to New York, where he obtained his M.D. degree in the middle of the American Civil War. He served in the army during that war (he even planned an army ambulance corps), and then he returned to the practice of gynecology, becoming one of the founders of the American Gynecological Society. His description of the homonymous gland in 1880 was, however, not entirely new. The glands had already been described by Reiner de Graf in 1672, but this description had been totally forgotten.

26. What are condyloma lata?

Condyloma lata, or flat warts, are lesions of secondary syphilis.

27. What are condyloma acuminata?

Condyloma acuminata, or genital warts, are caused by the human papillomaviruses (HPVs).

28. What is the significance of genital warts?

Genital warts, or condylomas, are flesh-colored papules with cauliflower-like papillations. They are caused by HPVs, which have been implicated in the pathogenesis of cervical cancer. There are over 70 serotypes of HPV. Serotypes 16, 18, 45, and 56 are thought to have the highest malignant potential.

29. What is the characteristic appearance of genital herpes simplex lesions?

Herpes lesions usually appear as clusters of small (1 mm or less) fluid-filled vessels on an erythematous base. The vesicles may appear ruptured or coalesced.

30. What is the differential diagnosis of ulceration of the vulva?

Painful ulceration may be due to ruptured, coalescent herpes simplex lesions or chancroid. A solitary painless ulcer is consistent with syphilis. A longstanding painless ulceration may be vulvar carcinoma.

31. What is a labial hernia?

The labial hernia is the uncommon occurrence of herniation of a bowel loop into the labium majus, analogous to an inguinal hernia in men.

VAGINA

CONVENTIONAL TEACHING WATCH

MANEUVER/FINDING		CONVENTIONAL TEACHING REVISITED
Maneuvers for detecting cystocele and rectocele	⇑	Sensitive and specific. Sensitivity can be enhanced by examining the patient when she is standing.

32. What is the technique for examining the vagina?

The vagina is visualized by inserting the speculum with gentle posterior pressure and opening the blades. Inspection of the vaginal vault is facilitated by the use of a clear plastic speculum. Assessment for cystocele or rectocele is accomplished by asking the patient to bear down and observing for bulging of the anterior or posterior vaginal wall.

33. What is the difference between a Pedersen speculum and a Graves speculum?

The Pedersen speculum is narrow with flat blades. It is a comfortable fit for most women and is more suitable for nulliparous women and menopausal women with a small, atrophic introitus. The Graves speculum has biconcave blades and is wider than the Pedersen speculum. It is most suitable for multiparous women or women in whom the Pedersen speculum is inadequate to retract the vaginal wall sufficiently to view the cervix. Pedersen and Graves speculums may be metal or plastic.

34. What about the hymen?

The hymen may or may not be apparent, even in women who have never had intercourse. Often hymeneal remnants may be visible as a posterior rim or a ring of small nubs of tissue around the vaginal opening.

35. What is an imperforate hymen?

The imperforate hymen is a congenital abnormality that often goes unrecognized until puberty, when the patient becomes symptomatic from retained menses. On exam, the hymen appears as an intact membrane bulging with retained fluid. If untreated, hematometrium and hematosalpinx may result.

36. What is a colpocele?

A colpocele is an outpouching of vaginal mucosa.

37. What is a cystocele?

A cystocele is a bulge in the anterior wall of the vagina that contains part of the bladder.

38. What is the technique for detecting a cystocele?

By observing and palpating the anterior vaginal wall as the patient coughs. A bulge in the anterior vagina with this maneuver is a sign of cystocele.

39. What is a rectocele?

A rectocele is a bulge in the posterior wall of the vagina that contains part of the rectum.

40. What are clues to the presence of a rectovaginal fistula?

The patient may relate a history of fecal contamination in the vagina. The fistula may be palpable as an area of induration in the posterior vaginal wall.

41. What is Chadwick's sign?

Chadwick's sign is a bluish-violet appearance of the vagina or cervix. It is a sign of pregnancy that may appear after the seventh week of gestation. It also may be seen in association with a pelvic tumor. It results from congestion of the mucosa and may be most notable in the anterior vaginal wall.

42. Who was Chadwick?

James R. Chadwick (1844–1905) was an American gynecologist. Born in Boston and schooled at Harvard, Chadwick traveled extensively in Europe after graduation, visiting the medical centers of Vienna, London, Paris, and Berlin. He eventually returned to Boston, where he became one of the founding fathers of the Boston Medical Library and the President of the American Gynecological Society.

43. What is the characteristic appearance of the vagina as a result of prenatal exposure to diethylstilbestrol (DES)?

Approximately 90% of women exposed to DES in utero have signs of vaginal adenomyosis, which is the presence of glandular columnar epithelium in the vagina. This condition is not premalignant but may be associated with the presence of clear cell adenocarcinoma of the vagina. Therefore, women with adenomyosis must be followed closely with clinical exams and colposcopy. DES was in use from 1938 to 1972.

44. What is a Gartner's duct cyst?

A Gartner's duct cyst is a benign tumor arising in the anterior or lateral vagina. It is a congenital lesion caused by retention of epithelial remnants of the Wolffian duct.

45. Who was Gartner?

Hermann T. Gartner (1785–1827) was a Danish surgeon. A native of St. Thomas, West Indies (when it was still a Danish possession), Gartner eventually returned to Denmark, graduated from Copenhagen Medical School, and worked as an army surgeon for most of his professional life.

46. What is normal vaginal pH?

Vaginal secretions are normally acidic with a pH of less than 4.5.

47. What is the significance of tenderness in the vaginal fornices?

Tenderness in either left or right vaginal fornix may indicate ipsilateral salpingitis. Tenderness of the right fornix may indicate appendicitis.

UTERINE CERVIX

CONVENTIONAL TEACHING WATCH

MANEUVER/FINDING		CONVENTIONAL TEACHING REVISITED
Papanicolaou smear	⇑	Although we are now defining instances in which the Pap smear can be skipped (e.g., after hysterectomy for benign disease), this test remains one of the major life-savers of women in this century. Efficacy and cost-effectiveness of "thin-prep" technology remains to be demonstrated.
Chadwick's sign	⇔	This sign is reliably present in early intrauterine pregnancy. However, readily available urine and serum human chorionic gonadotropin (hCG) assays have supplanted the art of physical diagnosis in this area.
Goodell's sign	⇓	Supplanted by hCG assays for the diagnosis of pregnancy.
Cervical motion tenderness	⇑	An important indicator of pelvic infection or inflammation. Should never be ignored.

48. What is the best method for locating and visualizing the cervix?

With the speculum pointing posteriorly, insert it with blades closed as far as it will go. Gently open the blades. In most cases the blades will frame the cervix. Occasionally the cervix is difficult to visualize because of a retroverted uterus or displacement of the cervix due to prolapse. If difficulty is encountered, perform the bimanual examination first with two gloved fingers lubricated with water only (other lubricants ruin the Pap smear). Once the cervix is located by palpation in this manner, the speculum can be aimed toward the correct location.

49. What is the normal appearance of the cervix?

The normal nonparous cervix is round and pink with a central os. The parous cervix has an os that is horizontal and may appear "fish-mouthed." The appearance of darker red columnar epithelium at the os is a variation of normal. Small yellowish Nabothian cysts also may be present.

50. What is the cause of duplication of the cervix?

Duplication of the cervix and uterus is caused by failure of müllerian duct fusion. It is commonly associated with a partially or fully septate vagina. On physical exam, the two cervices are often different sizes. They appear side by side in the coronal plane.

51. What is the squamocolumnar junction?

The squamocolumnar junction is the meeting of the external pink mucosa of the ectocervix with the columnar endothelium of the endocervical canal. The junction may or may not be visible on speculum examination. Cells of both types must be present on a Pap specimen for an adequate evaluation.

52. What is the significance of endocervical polyps?

Endocervical polyps are composed of columnar epithelium and appear as small, pedunculated masses protruding from the endocervical canal. Although they may be friable and cause bleeding, they are invariably benign.

53. What is the optimal technique for obtaining the Pap smear?

Endocervical canal cells are obtained using an endocervical brush inserted into the endocervical canal and rotated 360°. The brush is withdrawn and either brushed across a slide (standard method) or agitated in a tube of medium (thin-prep method). Squamous cells from the ectocervix are obtained by scraping the cervix circumferentially with the wooden spatula and also spread on a slide or in media. Pap smear slides must be fixed with cytology fixative as quickly as possible.

54. Which patients benefit from Pap smear screening?
Women who are sexually active should be screened with yearly or biennial Pap smears because they are at risk for HPV infection. Women who have had hysterectomies because of malignant disease should continue to be screened with vaginal Pap smears. Women who have had hysterectomies for benign indications (e.g., myomata) no longer need Pap smear screening.

55. Who was "Pap"?
George N. Papanicolaou (1883–1962) was an American pathologist. A native of Greece and a graduate of Athens University, Papanicolaou gained a medical degree only because of his father's wishes and only on the condition that he then would be free to pursue a career in history and philosophy. The Balkan War of 1912–1913 and the outbreak of World War I totally changed his plans. He decided to emigrate to the U.S., where he became Chair of Pathology at Cornell University.

56. What is the significance of purulent-appearing cervical discharge?
Purulent cervical discharge is the harbinger of purulent cervicitis, most often caused by gonorrhea or chlamydial infection. Left untreated, it may lead to pelvic inflammatory disease and serious sequelae.

57. What is the significance of cervical motion tenderness?
Cervical motion tenderness is an indicator of pelvic inflammatory disease. It is known informally as the "chandelier sign," indicating that the patient jumps for the chandelier when the cervix is palpated.

58. What additional laboratory tests should be obtained from the cervix?
In high-risk populations, some clinicians routinely culture the cervix for gonorrhea and chlamydial infection. Chlamydial infection, in particular, may be relatively asymptomatic; undiagnosed, it may lead to serious sequelae such as infertility. Therefore, a low threshold for screening is appropriate. A patient exhibiting any of the signs of purulent cervicitis outlined above should definitely be tested. The most convenient method for testing is the DNA probe (Genprobe).

59. What is Goodell's sign?
Goodell's sign is softening of the cervix associated with pregnancy. It usually occurs at about 8 weeks of gestation. It is said that whereas the cervix of a nonpregnant woman feels like the tip of the nose, the softer pregnant cervix has the same tactile quality as a lip.

60. Who was Goodell?
William Goodell (1829–1894) was an American gynecologist. Born in Malta (where his missionary father was temporarily stationed), he graduated from Jefferson Medical College in 1854. After practicing in Constantinople for 3 years (where he also married), he returned to the U.S. and became Chair of Gynecology at the University of Pennsylvania. A wealthy clinician and an insomniac, he suffered all of his life from gout.

UTERINE CORPUS

CONVENTIONAL TEACHING WATCH

MANEUVER/FINDING		CONVENTIONAL TEACHING REVISITED
Bimanual examination	⇑	Very informative, but may be limited in obese patients
Palpation for leiomyomata	⇑	Relatively sensitive and specific. However, any ambiguity in the adnexal area should be resolved with pelvic ultrasound.
Measurement of fundal height	⇔	Fairly accurate estimate of gestational age. When accuracy is critical, ultrasound should be used.

61. What is the normal shape and location of the uterus?

The uterus has the shape and size of a small pear. It is anteverted and anteflexed in approximately 80% of patients. Retroverted uterus, present in approximately 20% of patients, is a variant of normal and not pathologic.

62. What is the technique for examining the uterus?

The uterus is assessed during bimanual examination. With the examiner standing, the gloved index and middle fingers of one hand are inserted into the vagina with gentle posterior pressure into the posterior fornix. The examiner's other hand palpates the uterus through the abdominal wall.

63. What is the difference between uterine retroversion and retroflexion of the uterus?

Retroversion is a posterior angulation of the entire uterus, including the cervix. **Retroflexion** is posterior flexion of the uterine corpus with the cervix in its usual position. Both are normal variants, occurring in about 20% of women.

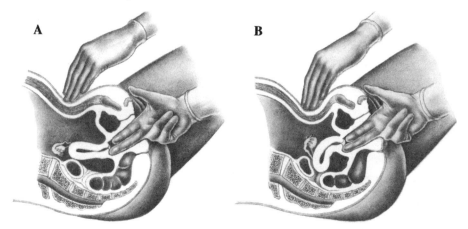

A, Retroversion of the uterus. *B,* Retroflexion of the uterus. (From Seidel HM, Ball JW, Dains JE, Benedict GW: Mosby's Guide to Physical Examination, 3rd ed. St. Louis, Mosby, 1995, with permission.)

64. What is Hegar's sign?

Hegar's sign is softening of the uterus at the junction between the cervix and the fundus. It occurs during the first trimester of pregnancy and may be elicited by placing two fingers in the posterior vaginal fornix, then compressing the uterus gently downward with the other hand.

65. What is uterine prolapse?

Uterine prolapse is a downward sagging of the uterus caused by gravity and weak pelvic floor musculature. In **first-degree prolapse**, the uterus has slipped downward but is still palpable relatively high in the vaginal vault. In **second-degree prolapse**, the uterus has descended the length of the vagina and the cervix presents at the introitus. **Third-degree prolapse**, also known as **procidentia uteri**, is descent of the uterus beyond the vaginal opening.

66. What is fundal height? How does it change with weeks of gestation?

Fundal height is the vertical dimension of the pregnant uterus. After 12 weeks of gestation, the uterine fundus is palpable above the pelvic brim. At 18 weeks it is palpable at the level of the umbilicus.

67. What are Leopold's maneuvers?

Leopold's maneuvers are four sequential palpations of the pregnant abdomen to determine the position of the fetus after the twenty-eighth week of gestation.

68. What are leiomyomata?

Leiomyomas, also known as uterine myomas or fibroids, are benign muscular tumors of the uterus. They range in size from impalpably small to very large. Size of leiomyomas is usually notated in weeks of gestation; for example, a myomatous uterus that is as enlarged as an 18-week pregnancy may be noted as an "18-week size fibroid." Leiomyomata on the lateral aspect of the uterus may be indistinguishable from adnexal masses. Large leiomyomas may be easily palpable in the lower abdomen.

69. Are fibroids ever malignant?

Rarely. Leiomyosarcomas account for less than 1% of uterine tumors.

ADNEXAE

CONVENTIONAL TEACHING WATCH

MANEUVER/FINDING		CONVENTIONAL TEACHING REVISITED
Palpation for ovarian malignancies	⇓	Sensitivity is low. Ovarian malignancies are difficult to detect in early stages. Value of other screening methods (ultrasound, CA-125 antigen testing) is unproved for routine use.

70. What are the adnexae?

The adnexae consist of the ovaries, oviducts (fallopian tubes), and supporting tissues.

71. What is the normal size of an ovary?

In young women, ovaries are usually 3.5–4 cm in their longest diameter. After menopause the ovaries shrink to about 2 cm and should not be palpable on examination.

72. What is the technique for examining the adnexae?

The adnexae are assessed during the bimanual examination after completion of the uterine exam. The examiner's vaginal fingers are shifted from the posterior fornix to each lateral fornix in turn, as the abdominal hand sweeps medially and inferiorly from the pelvic brim. This examination is markedly limited in obese patients.

73. What is the differential diagnosis of adnexal masses?

Adnexal masses may be physiologic cysts (follicular or corpus luteum cysts), polycystic ovaries, ectopic pregnancy, endometriomas, benign tumors (e.g., teratomas, serous or mucinous cystadenoma, Brenner tumor), malignant ovarian tumors, tuboovarian abscess, hydrosalpinx, or hematosalpinx. In some cases a mass palpated in the adnexa is actually not adnexal. Examples include uterine myomata that are lateral or pedunculated, appendiceal mass or abscess, pelvic kidney, or other abdominal tumor.

74. What is the differential diagnosis of adnexal tenderness?

Ectopic pregnancy and tuboovarian abscess must be excluded. Other causes include ovarian cysts, endometriomas, and other intraabdominal pathology such as appendicitis.

75. What are some characteristics of malignant ovarian tumors on exam?

Malignant tumors are more likely to be bilateral, larger, and less mobile and have a nodular, irregular quality on palpation. They may be associated with other physical findings such as abdominal distention and ascites.

CUL-DE-SAC

76. What is the cul-de-sac?

The cul-de-sac, also known as the pouch of Douglas, is the parietal peritoneum-lined space behind the uterus.

77. What information can be gained from rectovaginal examination?

Rectovaginal examination allows the examiner to palpate the posterior aspect of the uterus and the cul-de-sac for tenderness or presence of fluid.

BIBLIOGRAPHY

1. Bastian LA, Piscitelli JT: Is this patient pregnant? Can you reliably rule in or rule out pregnancy by clinical examination? JAMA 278:586–591, 1997.
2. Bates B: A Guide to Physical Examination and History Taking, 6th ed. Philadelphia, J.B. Lippincott, 1995.
3. Cotran RS, Kumar V, Robbins SL: Robbins Pathologic Basis of Disease, 5th ed. Philadelphia, W.B. Saunders, 1994.
4. DeGowin RL: DeGowin and DeGowin's Diagnostic Examination, 6th ed. New York, McGraw-HIll, 1994.
5. Fauci AS, Braunwald E, Isselbacher KJ, et al (eds): Harrison's Principles of Internal Medicine, 14th ed. New York, McGraw-Hill, 1998.
6. Frederickson HL, Wilkins-Haug L (eds): Ob/Gyn Secrets, 2nd ed. Philadelphia, Hanley & Belfus, 1997.
7. Mayeaux EJ, Spigener S: Epidemiology of human papillomavirus infections. Hosp Pract 15:39–41, 1997.
8. Moore KL, Persaud TVN: The Developing Human, 6th ed. Philadelphia, W.B. Saunders, 1998.
9. Pearce K, et al: Cytopathological findings on vaginal Papanicolaou smears after hysterectomy for benign gynecological disease. N Engl J Med 335:1559–1562, 1996.
10. Research Action and Information Network for Bodily Integrity of Women, 915 Broadway, Suite 1603, New York, NY 10010-7108.
11. Sapira J: The Art and Science of Bedside Diagnosis. Baltimore, Urban & Schwartzenburg, 1990.
12. Wallis L: Modern Breast and Pelvic Examinations. New York, National Council on Women's Health, 1996.

18. LYMPH NODES

Salvatore Mangione, M.D.

CONVENTIONAL TEACHING WATCH

The lymph nodes are an important area of physical examination. A methodical search for enlarged lymph nodes may yield invaluable information in patients with systemic disease or cancer. Some of these "sentinel" nodes have become part of the folklore of medicine, linked by eponym to the physicians who first described them.

ENLARGED LYMPH NODES		CONVENTIONAL TEACHING REVISITED
Head and neck lymph nodes	⇑	Of different clinical significance, depending on location.
Delphian nodes	⇔	Confusing term for small prelaryngeal nodes.
Axillary lymph nodes	⇑	If neoplastic, of breast or lung origin.
Supraclavicular lymph nodes	⇑	Very important; often known as Troisier's or Virchow's node.
Epitrochlear lymph node	⇔	Often tricky to find.
Inguinal and femoral lymph nodes	⇔	Of different clinical significance, depending on location.
Popliteal lymph nodes	⇓	Greatly overrated.
Sister Mary Joseph's nodule	⇑	Valuable sign of intraabdominal malignancy.

1. What important characteristics of a lymph node should be assessed by palpation?

1. **Size.** Size can be easily measured by using plastic calipers. Lymph nodes > 1 cm should be considered significant and possibly pathologic. There are, however, exceptions at both ends of this rule. For example, a node < 1 cm in the preauricular region is often pathologic; conversely, large and benign nodes are often encountered in intravenous drug users. Nodes > 5 cm are almost always neoplastic.

2. **Consistency.** Rock-hard nodes usually reflect neoplastic involvement, but there are exceptions. For example, the lymph nodes of Hodgkin's disease are typically rubbery in consistency. Fluctuant nodes, on the other hand, reflect necrosis and bacterial lymphadenitis. They may even fistulize through the skin, forming open sinuses (a common feature in tuberculosis). Nodes of this type are often referred to as *bubos*, particularly in inguinal locations. Nodes that feel like buckshot or tiny peas are often referred to as "shotty." Although the size of such nodes varies from patient to patient, they tend to be small and equal in size, firm but not stony-hard, mobile, nontender, and well demarcated.

3. **Matting.** Fusion and matting usually transform individual nodes into larger, masslike conglomerates. Matting is usually a feature of malignancy, but it also may occur in inflammatory processes, such as chronic infections or sarcoidosis. In addition to "fusion" of nodes into a scalloped mass, it is also important to identify whether the node is stuck to overlying skin, subjacent tissues, or both.

4. **Tenderness.** Tenderness is an important clinical feature, usually suggesting inflammation but at times even malignancy. Tuberculosis may vary in this regard.

Pearl. *Benign nodes tend to be small in size, soft, nontender, and well demarcated (discrete). Cancerous nodes, on the other hand, tend to be large, nontender, matted, and rock-hard. Inflammatory nodes tend to be tender, firm (but not rock-hard), occasionally fluctuant, and often matted.*

2. What other important features should be kept in mind in assessing the clinical relevance of lymph nodes?

The location of the node is, of course, important. As mentioned before, a node of any size felt in the preauricular area is usually significant compared with a node of similar size felt in other locations. Even more important is the distinction between generalized vs. localized lymphadenopathy, which usually reflects two separate processes, each carrying a unique differential diagnosis. **Generalized lymphadenopathy**, for example, usually indicates (1) disseminated malignancy, particularly hematologic (such as lymphomas and leukemias); (2) collagen vascular disease, including sarcoidosis; or (3) an infectious process (such as mononucleosis, syphilis, cytomegalovirus, toxoplasmosis, rheumatic fever, AIDS, tuberculosis, and, of course, the bubonic plague of olden days). Finally, other miscellaneous conditions, such as reaction to drugs (e.g., phenytoin) and use of intravenous drugs, also may cause generalized lymphadenopathy. **Regional (or localized) lymphadenopathy**, on the other hand, usually reflects conditions of local infection or neoplasm.

3. In what locations should the examiner look for lymph nodes?

Nodes should be looked for in (1) the axilla, (2) epitrochlear space, (3) cervical and neck areas, (4) supraclavicular fossa, and (5) inguinal and femoral regions. In addition lymph nodes of clinical significance also may be found in the popliteal fossa, paraumbilical area, and hilar regions.

4. What is the clinical significance of palpable nodes in the axilla?

Axillary nodes are usually not detectable, although at times small, mobile, soft, and nontender nodes can be felt in normal people. Larger, tender but still mobile axillary nodes usually reflect small wounds or infections of the arm (as simple as a cat scratch or skin infection). Harder, fixed, or matted axillary nodes, on the other hand, often indicate spread from malignancies, usually of pulmonary or breast origin.

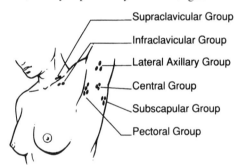

Supraclavicular Group

Infraclavicular Group

Lateral Axillary Group

Central Group

Subscapular Group

Pectoral Group

Lymph node groups in the axilla. (From De Gowin RL: De Gowin & De Gowin's Diagnostic Examination, 6th ed. New York, McGraw-Hill, 1994, with permission.)

5. What is the best way to search for axillary nodes?

Use the tip of your fingers to palpate deep into the axillary fossa and roof. Conduct this maneuver first with the patient's arm gently relaxed and passively abducted from the chest wall. Repeat the maneuver with the patient's arm gently and passively adducted.

6. What is the clinical significance of palpable nodes in the head and neck region?

The clinical significance depends on the location. For example:

- **Enlarged occipital lymph nodes**, located at the junction between head and neck, are usually common in childhood infections. They are, however, rare in adults unless there are clear signs of scalp infection. In the absence of infection, they usually reflect a generalized lymphadenopathy, such as may be encountered in HIV infection.
- **Posterior cervical lymphadenopathy** is usually seen as a result of dandruff.
- **Preauricular nodes**, on the other hand, can be encountered in lymphoma or on the same side as conjunctivitis (often referred to as Parinaud's syndrome, from Henry Parinaud, one of the founding fathers of French ophthalmology).

- **Nodes scattered around the two branches of the mandible** (submandibular and submental) tend to reflect localized pathology, usually dental (such as periodontitis or other teeth infection) rather than malignancies from outside the head and neck.

When the nodes are rock-hard:

- **High posterior cervical nodes** usually suggest a nasopharyngeal tumor.
- **Submental and submandibular nodes** reflect cancer of the nose, lip, anterior tongue, or anterior floor of the mouth.
- **Midjugular nodes** suggest cancer of the base of the tongue or larynx.
- **Lower jugular nodes** reflect a primary cancer of the thyroid or cervical esophagus.

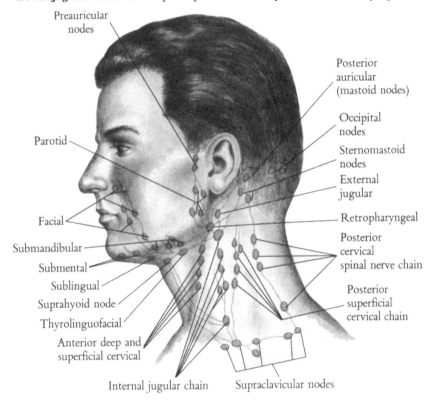

Lymph nodes and lymphatic drainage system of head and neck. (From Seidel HM, Ball JW, Dains JE, Benedict GW: Mosby's Guide to Physical Examination, 3rd ed. St. Louis, Mosby, 1995, with permission.)

7. What is scrofula?

Scrofula is an old term for cervical tuberculous lymphadenitis. The term refers to swollen cervical nodes that make the patient's neck appear as large as the neck of a piglet (*scrofa* = sow in Latin). Scrofula used to be common, particularly in children; it was spread by unpasteurized milk from infected cows. Scrofula often was treated by the king's touch: children were lined up in front of the king, who healed them by touching. This "cure," of course, reflected the overall benign nature of the disease rather than the healing powers of royalty.

8. What is the clinical significance of "shotty" nodes in the head and neck region?

Shotty nodes are small, pea-sized, nontender, mobile, and discrete lymph nodes. They are quite common, particularly in small children, and usually reflect a preexistent infection. They may even outlast the infection by several weeks. Their location usually reflects the site of infection:

• **Anterior cervical lymphadenopathy** reflects upper respiratory infections and inflammation of the anterior portions of the mouth.

• **Posterior cervical lymphadenopathy** reflects otitis media and infections of the scalp.

9. What are Delphian nodes?

Delphian nodes are a cluster of small, midline prelaryngeal lymph nodes, located on the thyrohyoid membrane. They are called Delphian presumably because of their prophetic tell-tale significance, similar to the oracle of Delphi in ancient Greece. When enlarged, they are indicative of thyroid disease, usually subacute thyroiditis, Hashimoto's disease, or thyroid carcinoma. They also may reflect tracheal carcinoma. Make sure, however, not to confuse Delphian nodes with a pyramidal lobe of the thyroid.

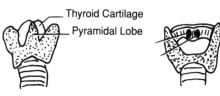

A. Pyramidal Lobe of Thyroid Gland   B. Delphian Nodes

Associated thyroid masses. *A,* Pyramidal lobe of thyroid gland, an upward projection of thyroid tissue, usually arising from isthmus or left lobe. It may follow the course of the thyroglossal duct as far as the hyoid bone. *B,* Delphian nodes are enlarged lymph nodes in the thyrohyoid membranes, usually involved only in thyroid carcinoma or subacute thyroiditis. (From De Gowin RL: De Gowin & De Gowin's Diagnostic Examination, 6th ed. New York, McGraw-Hill, 1994, with permission.)

10. What is the clinical significance of a palpable supraclavicular node?

A localized node in the supraclavicular fossa (either right or left) is an important finding. It usually indicates metastatic involvement from ipsilateral breast or lung cancers (a *right* supraclavicular node, however, also may indicate cancer of the *left* lower lobe of the lung because of bilateral crossed drainage). If located in the *left* supraclavicular fossa, a palpable lymph node also may represent spread from a large number of intraabdominal or intrapelvic tumors (see below). Thus, a large left supraclavicular node is often referred to as a *sentinel* node (signaling a deep-sited carcinoma) or Troisier's node.

11. What is Troisier's node?

Troisier's node (or sign) is a palpable single *left* supraclavicular node, frequently located behind the clavicular head of the sternocleidomastoid muscle. It may represent metastatic involvement from either an ipsilateral breast or lung carcinoma or from an esophageal tumor. Most commonly, however, it reflects spread from intraabdominal or intrapelvic malignancies, such as stomach, intestine, liver, kidneys, pancreas, and even testicles and endometrium. When it represents metastasis from a gastric carcinoma, it is often referred to as **Virchow's node**.

12. Who was Troisier?

Charles E. Troisier (1844–1919) was a graduate of the University of Paris and, subsequently, a professor at the same institution. A well-respected pathologist and an excellent clinician, Troisier's major contribution to medicine was in the study of lymphatic spread of cancer. He also wrote on other topics, including rheumatoid nodules, meningitis, deep vein thrombosis, and hemochromatosis. Indeed, bronzed diabetes (or hemochromatosis) is still often referred to as Troisier syndrome.

13. Who was Virchow?

Rudolf L. K. Virchow (1821–1902) was a graduate of the Friedrich-Wilhelm Institute for Army Doctors in Berlin, which he joined after realizing that his voice was not strong enough to support a career as a preacher. He was released from military service in 1847. After multiple rejections by various journal editors, Virchow founded a new medical journal, which eventually became known as *Virchow's Archiv*. His contributions to medicine were staggering, including hemostasis and pulmonary embolism (see Virchow's triad for venous thrombosis), leukemia, public health, and preventive medicine. At times a scientific reactionary, Virchow was politically an outspoken liberal with socialist sympathies. During the 1848 Berlin uprising, he even helped construct some of the barricades. He never missed a chance to castigate strongly the social injustice and poor hygienic conditions of his time, which he considered responsible for the frequent and recurrent epidemics. In a report to the government that became almost a political indictment against the industrial revolution, he asked, "Shall the triumph of human genius lead to nothing more than to make the human race miserable?" His interests included anthropology, archeology, and medical history. He died at the age of 81 from complications related to a hip fracture that he sustained by leaping from a moving tram.

14. What is the best way to palpate a supraclavicular node?

The best way is to have the patient sit up, with the head straight forward and the arms down (to minimize the risk of misidentifying a cervical vertebra or neck muscle for a node). Palpation from behind usually allows optimal adaptation of the examiner's hand to the patient's anatomy and is probably preferable. Palpation from the front, on the other hand, should be attempted in the supine patient (in this position, the change in gravity may mobilize the node, thus making it more accessible). Finally, asking the patient to perform a Valsalva maneuver or simply to cough may "pop out" a deeply seated node, bringing it within reach of the examiner's fingers.

15. What is the significance of an enlarged epitrochlear node?

An enlarged epitrochlear node usually reflects an inflammatory process of the hand or forearm. Epitrochlear nodes also may be enlarged in intravenous drug users or patients with sarcoidosis.

16. What is the best way to palpate an epitrochlear node?

The best way is to use your right hand to shake hands with the patient's right hand, while at the same time using your left hand fingertips to search for nodes in the epitrochlear region. You can repeat this maneuver on the other side by reversing hands.

17. What is the significance of enlarged inguinal and femoral nodes?

The significance depends on whether the affected nodes are inguinal or femoral. Inguinal nodes are located more laterally in the groin than femoral nodes (which are quite medial and close to the genital area). This distinction is not only anatomic but also clinical. In fact, femoral nodes are usually much less significant than inguinal nodes. Often enlargement of the femoral nodes reflects a simple dermatophytosis of the foot. Enlargement of the inguinal nodes, on the other hand, is usually much more relevant. The cause may even be malignant. Hence, biopsy of inguinal nodes often yields valuable diagnostic information, whereas biopsy of the femoral nodes usually yields simple reactive hyperplasia.

18. What is the clinical significance of popliteal nodes?

Very little. Some popliteal nodes are so deep that they may be impossible to palpate. Even if palpable, their clinical significance is highly questionable.

19. What is Sister Mary Joseph's nodule?

Sister Mary Joseph's nodule is a periumbilical nodule or hard mass, detectable by either inspection or palpation of the navel. It is clinically quite valuable. It represents metastatic involvement of the paraumbilical nodes from intrapelvic or intraabdominal malignancies, most commonly of the stomach or ovary. This finding was first reported in an article published in 1928 by W. J. Mayo. The article was based on an observation of Mayo's first surgical assistant, Sister Mary Joseph of St. Mary's Hospital.

20. Who was Sister Mary Joseph?

Sister Mary Joseph was born Julia Dempsey in Salamanca, New York in 1856. In 1878 she entered the congregation of Our Lady of Lourdes and was assigned to the St. Mary Hospital in Rochester, Minnesota. There she learned nursing, first working under the guidance of Edith Graham (who subsequently became the wife of Dr. C.H. Mayo) and eventually rising to the position of hospital superintendent, a title she kept until her death in 1939. From 1890 to 1915 she served as the first surgical assistant to Dr. W. J. Mayo. In this role she drew Dr. Mayo's attention to the sign that eventually carried her name.

BIBLIOGRAPHY

1. Ioachim HL: Lymph Node Biopsy, 2nd ed. Philadelphia, Lippincott-Williams & Wilkins, 1994.
2. Kuiper DH, Papp JP: Supraclavicular adenopathy demonstrated by the Valsalva maneuver. N Engl J Med 280:1007–1008, 1969.

19. NEUROLOGIC EXAMINATION

Loren A. Rolak, M.D., and Cameron Quanbeck, M.D.

Some seventy years ago a promising young neurologist made a discovery that necessitated the addition of a new word to the English vocabulary. He insisted that this should be knee-jerk, *and* knee-jerk *it has remained in spite of the efforts of patellar reflex to dislodge it. He was my father: Sir William Richard Gowers. So perhaps I have inherited a prejudice in favour of home-made words.*

Sir Ernest Gowers (1880–1966), *Plain Words*, Chapter 5

TOPICS COVERED IN THIS CHAPTER

Mental Status Examination
  Level of consciousness
  Memory
  Language and aphasias
Cranial Nerve Examination
  Bell's palsy
  Corneal reflex
Motor System Examination
  Muscle strength
  Muscle atrophy
  Fasciculations
  Deep tendon reflexes
  Babinski sign
  Muscle tone
  Abnormal involuntary muscle movements

Sensory System Examination
  Nociceptive sensations
  Proprioceptive sensations
  Assessment of pain/light touch/vibration
Cerebellum
  Assessment of cerebellar function in the
    upper extremities
  Assessment of cerebellar function in the
    lower extremities
  Cerebellar gait
Gait

CONVENTIONAL TEACHING WATCH

In times of MRI and CT it may seem almost anachronistic to rekindle the time-honored art of neurologic diagnosis. And yet this aspect of physical diagnosis (probably the most sophisticated of the entire bedside exam) is still able, if competently performed, to pinpoint the location of a lesion and deliver a diagnosis. Strong knowledge of neuroanatomy and neurophysiology is, of course, fundamental to the success of these maneuvers. Although our presentation for this book highlights the essentials, we have given high scores to all sections of the neurologic examination.

MANEUVERS/SIGNS		CONVENTIONAL TEACHING REVISITED
Mental status exam	⇑	Essential to detect and diagnose even very subtle changes.
Cranial nerves exam	⇑	Lots of eponyms and important reflexes in this section. Very valuable.
Motor system exam	⇑	Deep tendon reflexes are commonly used. Still very valuable.
Sensory system exam	⇑	A little less practiced than motor exam, but still essential.
Cerebellum	⇑	A plethora of signs in this section.
Gait	⇑	Allows diagnosis by just looking at patient.

1. What is the purpose of the neurologic examination?

The purpose of the neurologic examination is to localize lesions—that is, to identify the precise location in the nervous system where disease is present. The brain, spinal cord, and peripheral nerves possess a unique property termed *eloquence*. In other words, they "talk to us." Damage to a particular part of the nervous system produces a highly specific symptom. Similarly, because each section of the nervous system performs a discrete function, the loss of a particular function can be easily traced to the part of the nervous system responsible for it. Accordingly, signs noted on the neurologic examination often pinpoint precisely the site of neurologic damage.

2. What are the most important parts of the neurologic examination?

1. Mental status   4. Sensory system
2. Cranial nerves   5. Cerebellum
3. Motor system   6. Gait

MENTAL STATUS EXAMINATION

3. What are the most important parts of the mental status examination?

A complete and detailed examination of mental status can easily take several hours or even days. For clinical purposes, however, the most important aspects of the mental status exam include the following:

1. Level of consciousness   3. Memory
2. Orientation   4. Language

4. What are the most important levels of consciousness?

In patients suffering a progressive degree of deterioration, we encounter four levels of consciousness in the following sequence:

1. **Alertness** refers to an awake person with a normal level of consciousness (alert patient)

2. **Lethargy** indicates a patient who is sleepy and needs to be stimulated to remain awake (lethargic patient).

3. **Stupor** refers to a patient who cannot be aroused, although he or she may moan, withdraw, or roll around during examination (stuporous patient).

4. **Coma** refers to patients who offer no purposeful response to stimulations of any kind (comatose patient).

5. What is orientation? How is it assessed?

Orientation refers to the recognition of person, place, and time. It is assessed by asking patients to state their name and location and the day, date, month, and year during which the interview is conducted.

6. How is memory assessed?

Memory is assessed by asking the patient to remember three words, such as "apple, flag, ball." After 3–5 minutes of distraction, spent in other aspects of the examination, the patient is asked to repeat the same words. This is a reliable bedside test for recall. Most normal people can accurately remember three objects after a brief distraction.

7. What are the components of language? How are they assessed?

The ability to use language is one of the most complex functions of the human brain. It involves not just speech (verbal language) but also comprehension (understanding what is spoken to you), reading, and writing. A correct assessment of language must test all of these functions.

8. What is aphasia?

Aphasia (from the Greek *a* = lack of and *phasis* = speech) is an acquired disturbance of language. The expression was introduced by Armand Trousseau (1801–1867), one of the legendary figures of French medicine. It is used to indicate the many types of language disturbance encountered clinically.

Aphasia is different from **dysarthria** (from the Greek *dys* = difficulty and *arthros* = articulation), which is a disturbance of speech and language due to problems with the articulation of sound. Dysarthria may result from brain injury, paralysis, incoordination, spasticity of the muscles of phonation, or, more simply, emotional stress. **Cerebellar speech**, on the other hand, refers to sudden changes in tempo and volume in an otherwise slow and irregular speech. It is typical of patients with cerebellar disease. Finally, aphasia should not be confused with **mutism**, which is seen in patients without the ability to produce sounds. Both dysarthria and mutism preserve the capacity to read and write, whereas most types of aphasia do not.

9. What are the two most important types of aphasia?

Fluent aphasia and **nonfluent aphasia**. This classification, however, is a simplification. Neurologists in fact have identified many more disorders of language function.

10. What are the clinical differences between fluent and nonfluent aphasia?

Patients with **fluent aphasia** can talk readily and easily, but their words are often jumbled, nonsensical, and meaningless. In addition, they have difficulty in naming objects, repeating sentences, or comprehending. This type of aphasia is commonly referred to as Wernicke's aphasia or receptive, sensory, or posterior aphasia. The responsible lesion is in the temporal or parietal lobe.

Patients with **nonfluent aphasia**, on the other hand, struggle for words and have great difficulty with speaking. Their language is slow, often made up of monosyllabic sentences and characterized by latency. It has been compared with the labored use of English by not-too-fluent foreigners. Although patients with nonfluent aphasia have a hard time naming objects and repeating sentences, their comprehension of spoken and written material is often quite good. Nonfluent aphasia is commonly referred to as Broca's aphasia or expressive, motor, or anterior aphasia. The responsible lesion is in the frontal lobe.

Pearl.   Broca's aphasia is characterized by nonfluent speech, impaired repetition, and intact comprehension. Wernicke's aphasia is characterized by fluent speech with impaired comprehension and impaired repetition.

11. Who was Broca?

Pierre P. Broca (1824–1880) was a French surgeon with a prolific career in both medicine and neurology. He was a pioneer in many areas, even outside medicine. He described rickets as a nutritional disorder before Virchow; Duchenne's dystrophy before Duchenne; and the use of hypnotism as an adjuvant to surgery. He also was responsible for introducing the microscope to France for the diagnosis of cancer. An anthropologist with sympathy for Darwinian theories, Broca founded his own Anthropological Institute and the first Anthropological Society of France. He married the daughter of Dr. Lugol (of Lugol iodine fame) and died at 56 of a myocardial infarction.

12. Who was Wernicke?

Karl Wernicke (1848–1904) was a German physician born in what is now Poland. A graduate of the University of Breslau (now Wroclaw, Poland), Wernicke described his famous aphasia in a book that he wrote when he was only 26. His interest in localization of neurologic lesions was subsequently summarized in a three-volume textbook that he published in 1881. The book also contains the description of Wernicke's encephalopathy (confusion, ophthalmoplegia, nystagmus, ataxia, and peripheral neuritis due to alcoholic thiamine deficiency). A cold and aloof man, Wernicke died at age 56 as a result of a biking accident in the Thuringian forest.

13. How can the various aspects of mental status be examined efficiently?

Through a battery of carefully analyzed and validated questions, such as the Folstein Mini Mental Status Examination.

CRANIAL NERVE EXAMINATION

Conventional Wisdom.   All cranial nerves have specific functions that permit an accurate localization of lesions based only on neurologic exam. Detailed testing of all cranial nerves, however, is quite time-consuming. Therefore, unless a patient has symptoms pointing toward a specific cranial nerve, little information is obtained by a routine examination.

14. How is cranial nerve I (olfactory nerve) tested?

Ask the patient to close the eyes, occlude one nostril, and then smell a distinctive odor with the unoccluded nostril. Strong and typical scents, such as cinnamon, cloves, and peppermint, are commonly used. Yet the olfactory nerve is seldom tested in the routine exam because transient **anosmia** (from the Greek *a* = lack of and *osme* = sense of smell) is not uncommon in people who are otherwise normal. Transient anosmia usually results from intercurrent sinus problems or a simple head cold. Thus, an abnormal test result rarely indicates a true olfactory dysfunction. Conversely, a chronic (especially congenital) anosmia is quite important (see chapter 6).

15. How is cranial nerve II (optic nerve) tested?

By using two bedside maneuvers, each of which tests a separate functional aspect of the optic nerve:

1. **Visual acuity** is measured by asking the patient to read an eye chart from a set distance of 20 feet. Because we are testing the best corrected vision, glasses or contact lenses are allowed. A person capable of reading at a distance of 20 feet letters that others can read at a distance of 40 feet is said to have a visual acuity of 20/40. Conversely, a normal person, capable of reading at a distance of 20 feet letters that others can read at a distance of 20 feet, is said to have 20/20 vision.

2. **Visual fields** are an important test. In fact, damage anywhere from the retina to the occipital lobes may result in a loss of vision involving a discrete area (or field). The best way to detect such a cut in the visual field is by confrontation: place yourself head to head and eye to eye with the patient while both of you occlude the opposite eye. This maneuver is based on the principle that while looking into each other's eyes, both patient and examiner have the same peripheral vision. To determine whether the patient can see what the examiner sees, the examiner moves objects into his or her peripheral vision, starting from above, then below, then left and right. The patient should be able to see the objects at the same time as the examiner. Conversely, if the examiner can see objects at a point where the patient cannot, the patient probably has a visual field defect corresponding to the particular region of peripheral vision. (See figure at top of facing page.)

Pearl.   Various complex field defects can be produced by disease affecting various segments of the visual system, not just the optic nerve. Visual field testing is therefore useful for assessing many aspects of visual function.

16. How are cranial nerves III, IV, and VI tested?

The oculomotor (III), trochlear (IV), and abducens (VI) nerves are tested together because they work together to produce various eye movements. Ask the patient to hold the head stationary and at the same time to follow the examiner's finger as it moves through the main directions of gaze: left–up, left–middle, left–down and right–up, right–middle, and right–down. The eyes should move smoothly and symmetrically. Any restriction in eye movement or the development of double vision (due to the inability of the eyes to move in conjunction with each other) suggests damage to one of these three cranial nerves.

17. What abnormal eye movements are produced by damage to cranial nerves III, IV, or VI?

The abnormality depends on the involved nerve and its particular function:

1. The **oculomotor nerve** supplies the medial, superior, and inferior rectus; the inferior oblique; and the levator palpebrae (the muscle responsible for raising the eyelid). It also contains parasympathetic fibers that constrict the pupil. Thus, damage to cranial nerve III produces an eye that is partially abducted and difficult to adduct, elevate, or depress. The patient also has an eyelid droop (ptosis), and the pupil may be large (mydriatic) and difficult to constrict.

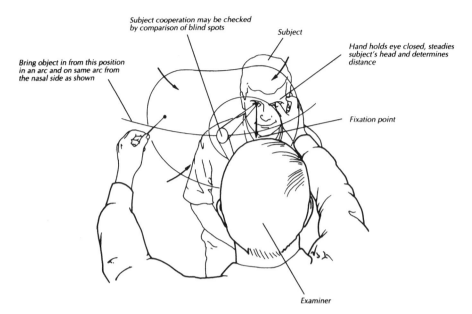

Visual field testing by confrontation. (From Patten J: Neurological Differential Diagnosis, 2nd ed. London, Springer, 1996, with permission.)

2. The **trochlear nerve** supplies the superior oblique muscle. Thus, damage to cranial nerve IV produces an eye that cannot be depressed when adducted. In other words, when the eye is adducted (moved inward toward the nose), the patient is not able to move it downward. This subtle abnormality often is difficult to detect.

3. The **abducens nerve** supplies the lateral rectus muscle. Thus, damage to cranial nerve VI causes an inability to abduct the eye.

18. What is nystagmus?

It is an involuntary oscillation of the eye (from the Greek *nystagmos* = nodding). It can be either vertical (like an up-and-down bouncing of the eye), horizontal (like a back-and-forth shaking), or rotatory (like a clockwise/counterclockwise twisting or rotating). Although usually detected in testing cranial nerves III, IV, and VI, nystagmus is *not* actually produced by damage to the cranial nerve directly responsible for eye movement, but rather by damage to the brain/brainstem mechanisms responsible for the coordination of the eye movements.

19. How is cranial nerve V (trigeminal nerve) tested?

By either pinprick or light touch over the three facial areas of distribution of the trigeminal branches: V1 (ophthalmic), V2 (maxillary), and V3 (mandibular).The trigeminal nerve is primarily sensory in function, providing sensation to the face. However, it also carries a small motor component, involved primarily in chewing. (See figure at top of following page.)

20. How is the motor function of cranial nerve V tested?

Ask the patient to clinch the teeth, and at the same time feel the patient's masseter muscles. The masseters should contract strongly and symmetrically.

21. How is cranial nerve VII (facial nerve) tested?

By assessing its unique territory of distribution: the muscles of facial expression. Accordingly, damage to cranial nerve VII causes an inability to wrinkle the forehead, close the eye tightly, or smile on the same side as the neurologic damage.

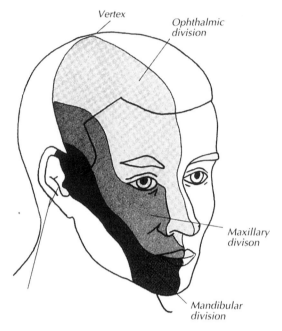

Vertex
Ophthalmic division
Maxillary divison
Mandibular division

The distribution of the ophthlamic, maxillary, and mandibular branches of the trigeminal nerve. Some cutaneous branches deep behind the ear are derived from cranial nerves IX and X. (From Patten J: Neurological Differential Diagnosis, 2nd ed. London, Springer, 1996, with permission.)

Because of the unusual representation of the facial muscles in the brain, central damage to cranial nerve VII (i.e., involving the cortical or upper motor neuron) results in weakness of the opposite facial muscles, but only in the lower half of the face. The lower motor neuron responsible for the innervation of the upper half of the face is supplied by both sides of the cortex. Thus, a patient with central damage to cranial nerve VII is unable to smile or open the mouth fully but can still use the muscles of the upper half of the face (such as wrinkling the forehead). Conversely, a patient with peripheral damage to cranial nerve VII that involves directly either the lower motor neuron (i.e., brainstem) or the nerve itself cannot smile, move the mouth well, or wrinkle the forehead.

Pearl. The distinction between facial weakness that is central in origin (i.e., due to central involvement of the nuclei of cranial nerve VII) and facial weakness that is peripheral in origin (i.e., involving the nerve itself) is clinically important.

22. What is Bell's palsy?

Bell's palsy is a common peripheral mononeuropathy of cranial nerve VII. Because it directly involves the nerve (peripheral damage), it causes paralysis of both lower and upper motor neurons. As a result, the patient cannot smile, move the mouth well, or wrinkle the forehead. Bell's palsy is usually idiopathic in origin, although it may be due to infectious mononucleosis, Guillain-Barré syndrome, diabetes, or, occasionally, a tumor of the cerebellopontine angle.

23. What is Bell's phenomenon?

Bell's phenomenon refers to the upward rotation of the eyeball triggered by contraction of the ipsilateral orbicularis muscle (with resulting closure of the eyelid). It is a normal phenomenon that occurs physiologically in everyone as a result of synkinesis (from the Greek *syn* = together and *kinesis* = movement). Synkinesis is an involuntary movement that accompanies a voluntary one, such as movement of a closed eye after movement of the open eye or movement of the arms with movement of the legs during walking. The only peculiar aspect of Bell's phenomenon is that in patients with paralysis of the lower cranial nerve VII, the eyelid on the affected side cannot be closed. As a result, the physiologic upward rotation of the eyeball becomes suddenly visible.

24. Who was Bell?

Sir Charles Bell (1774–1842) was a Scottish neurophysiologist and surgeon. He is *not* the same Dr. Bell who taught medicine in Edinburgh and impressed a young student named Arthur Conan Doyle, eventually becoming the model for Sherlock Holmes. The model for Holmes was Joseph Bell, a charismatic teacher who applied his analytical powers to the mystery of Jack the Ripper, the 1888 serial killer of London. Charles Bell was the son of an Episcopal minister; in 1801 he left Edinburgh for London after being denied a position at the local university. In London he made a name for himself through his artistic skills, particularly "Essays on the Anatomy of Painting." He attended the military hospital at Haslar, where he had plenty of opportunities to treat the many casualties of Wellington's peninsular campaign. This experience triggered a life-long fascination with war and what it can inflict on the human body. In 1815, while tirelessly operating on the many wounded soldiers returning from Waterloo, Bell made many sketches and drawings, some of which can still be viewed at the Royal College of Surgeons in Edinburgh. Bell eventually moved back to his native Scotland, but before leaving London he founded the Middlesex Hospital and Medical School. He is remembered not only for Bell's palsy and Bell's phenomenon but also for Bell's law, which states that the anterior spinal roots carry motor fibers, whereas the posterior roots carry sensory fibers.

25. What is the corneal reflex?

It is a useful bedside test of the integrity of cranial nerves V and VII. The test is carried out by asking the patient to look away from the examiner (so that the patient cannot see what the examiner is doing) while the examiner uses a wisp of cotton to touch the edge of the patient's cornea. The normal response is a protective reflex blinking, which requires integrity of both the fifth and seventh cranial nerves: the fifth must be intact to receive the sensation from the cornea, whereas the seventh must be intact to carry out the motor response (i.e., blinking of the eye).

26. How is cranial nerve VIII (acoustic/vestibularis nerve) tested?

In two different ways, depending on which function is to be tested. The eighth cranial nerve carries fibers mediating both vestibular and auditory function. **Vestibular dysfunction** produces symptoms of vertigo and dizziness that are usually quite obvious. Therefore, unless these symptoms are present, vestibular function should not be routinely tested as part of the neurologic examination. Auditory dysfunction, on the other hand, may be quite subtle. It is easily tested by simple bedside maneuvers, such as asking the patient if he or she can hear the soft noise of a ticking watch, fingers rubbing against each other near the ear, or whispered words.

Hearing loss can be recognized at the bedside as either sensorineural or conductive through the Rinne and Weber tests. In the Rinne test a vibrating tuning fork is pressed against the mastoid bone and then held next to the ipsilateral ear, testing respectively bone conduction (BC) and air conduction (AC). Normally AC lasts longer than BC because of the amplifying effects of the eardrum and middle ear. If BC is longer than AC, the patient is likely to have **conductive deafness** (such as hearing loss produced by impacted cerumen or middle-ear disease). Conversely, AC and BC are equally diminished in **sensorineural deafness**. For a more detailed description of these tests, refer to chapter 5.

27. How are cranial nerves IX (glossopharyngeal nerve) and X (vagus nerve) tested?

By asking the patient to say "ahhh" or "ehhh" (see chapter 6) while observing whether the palate rises symmetrically. Alternatively, one can touch the palate with a cotton swab, producing a gag reflex that also moves the palate and the pharynx. Axons from several brainstem nuclei mingle together to emerge from the brainstem through two separate nerves. Early neuroanatomists named them the glossopharyngeal (IX) and vagus (X) nerves. In reality, the origins of the two nerves is essentially identical. Their function is also similar: to control the palate and the pharynx.

28. How is the function of cranial nerve XI (spinal accessory nerve) assessed?

It depends on which muscle you are testing. Cranial nerve XI is composed of motor neurons from both the brainstem and the upper levels of the cervical spinal cord. The axons of the spinal neurons exit the cord and rise in the neck, where they join the axons of brainstem neurons to emerge through the foramen magnum as the spinal accessory nerve. This nerve supplies the trapezius and sternocleidomastoid muscles with motor function. To test the function of the **trapezius muscle**, ask the patient to shrug the shoulders. This maneuver rules in or out any weakness or atrophy. To test the function of the **sternocleidomastoid muscle**, ask the patient to turn the head to the side and then forcibly resist efforts to turn it back.

29. How is the function of cranial nerve XII (hypoglossal nerve) assessed?

By testing for movements of the tongue, which is innervated by cranial nerve XII. Thus, any weakness or atrophy can be easily determined by asking the patient to move the tongue from side to side or up and down or to press it into the cheek.

MOTOR SYSTEM EXAMINATION

30. How is muscle strength graded?

Muscle strength is graded on a 6-point scale:
1. 0/5 represents no muscle contraction and no joint movement.
2. 1/5 is visible contraction of a muscle without sufficient strength to move a joint.
3. 2/5 is strength sufficient to move a joint but not to overcome the resistance of gravity.
4. 3/5 is strength sufficient to move against gravity but not to withstand active resistance.
5. 4/5 is strength sufficient to move against gravity *and* to overcome some resistance offered by the examiner.
6. 5/5 is normal strength.

This system is well accepted and clinically useful but does have flaws.

31. What are the limitations of muscle grading?

The most important limitation involves the 3/5 rating, which is an uncommon event. Only a few patients can move against gravity yet be unable to offer any resistance to the examiner's action. The 4/5 rating is also flawed, because it is too broad for clinical application. Thus, it is generally subdivided into the following categories:
- 4–/5, which offers little resistance
- 4/5, which offers moderate resistance
- 4+/5, which offers strong resistance

32. What is muscle atrophy?

Atrophy (from the Greek *a* = lack of and *trophe* = nourishment) is the muscle wasting caused by damage of the muscle-supplying nerves. Because these nerves contain various trophic factors, damage causes degeneration and wasting of dependent muscle fibers. Disuse of the muscle or various muscle diseases also may cause atrophy. Yet the most common cause of muscle atrophy is damage to the supplying nerve.

33. What are fasciculations?

They are visible and irregular muscle flickerings caused by the spontaneous contraction of individual motor units. Like atrophy, fasciculations are a sign of denervation. In fact, interrruption of the nerve supply makes the muscle hyperexcitable, thereby favoring the spontaneous contractions of individual fibers.

34. How are muscle reflexes elicited?

By briskly tapping the muscle tendon with a reflex hammer. This maneuver produces a rapid stretch of the muscle itself, which is then sensed by the muscle spindles and relayed to the spinal cord. The cord, in turn, sends signals back to the muscle, making it contract reflexively.

35. How are reflexes graded?
Reflexes usually are graded on a 5-point scale:
1. 0/4 is absence of any reflex (areflexia).
2. 1/4 is a reduced or weak reflex.
3. 2/4 is a normal reflex.
4. 3/4 is a very brisk reflex (hyperreflexia)
5. 4/4 is extremely brisk hyperreflexia, usually accompanied by clonus (from the Greek *klonos* = tumult). A clonus is a rhythmic form of muscle movement, marked by contractions and relaxations that occur in rapid sequence and persist after the initial reflex.

36. What is the Babinski sign?
It is the dorsiflexion (or extension) of the great toe in response to stroking the lateral aspect of the sole of the foot. In other words, the great toes goes up. With the exception of infancy (in which it is a normal response), dorsiflexion of the great toe indicates an upper motor neuron lesion of the pyramidal (corticospinal) tract. The Babinski sign is an excellent physical examination maneuver: sensitive, specific, and capable of localizing the lesion precisely. In an effort to avoid eponyms, a Babinski sign (that is, a pathologic response) is often called an extensor plantar response. Conversely, a normal response (in which the great toe goes down) is often called a flexor plantar response.

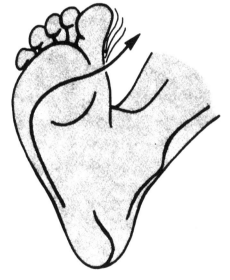

Eliciting the Babinski sign. (From Patten J: Neurological Differential Diagnosis, 2nd ed. London, Springer, 1996, with permission.)

37. Who was Babinski?
Joseph F. Babinski (1857–1932) was the son of Polish political refugees. He arrived in France at the age of nine, graduated from the University of Paris with a thesis on multiple sclerosis, and became one of the most famous neurologists of his time. He was a tall, handsome man and a true bon vivant who spent his evenings at the theater, opera, and ballet and even wrote a popular recipe book under the pseudonym Ali-Bab. He created the systematic approach to physical examination that has been part of the neurologic exam ever since. The last few years of his life were plagued by Parkinson's disease.

38. What is muscle tone? How can it be tested?
Muscle tone is the resistance to passive motion offered by all normal muscles. It can be tested by passively flexing or extending a joint, such as bending the arm at the elbow or the leg at the knee. By carrying out this maneuver (and by comparing sides), the examiner can easily estimate whether the resistance encountered is greater or less than normal.

39. What are the most common forms of altered tone?

1. **Rigidity** is an increase in muscle tone, diffusely present throughout the full range of motion of the joint. It is commonly seen in degenerative neurologic conditions, such as Parkinson's disease.

2. **Spasticity** is commonly seen in patients with damage to the pyramidal (corticospinal) tract. It is characterized by an increase in muscle tone, which becomes greater with progressive muscle stretch. Thus, initial resistance is low, but it increases gradually as the muscle is progressively stretched. Ultimately, when the muscle is under considerable tension, there may be a protective relaxation and giveaway phenomenon. This sudden "clasp-knife" loss of tone is highly characteristic of spasticity.

3. **Flaccidity** is a decrease in tone; muscles become unusually floppy. Flaccidity often results from damage to the peripheral nervous system and nerves supplying the muscles themselves.

40. What muscles should be tested during the neurologic examination?

For a screening neurologic examination, it is usually adequate to test one extensor and one flexor muscle, proximally and distally in each arm and leg, such as the biceps, triceps, wrist extensors, and grip in the arm and iliopsoas, hamstrings, anterior tibial, and gastrocnemius in the legs. Because it is impractical to test every muscle in the body, the examination should focus on the area where the patient reports symptoms.

41. What abnormal involuntary movements are most important to recognize?

1. **Tremor** is a rhythmic muscular oscillation around a joint in a to-and-fro or up-and-down fashion.

2. **Chorea** is an involuntary writhing and twisting motion.

3. **Myoclonus** is a sudden, shocklike, jerking or twitching motion of a joint.

4. **Dystonia** is a persistent, fixed contraction of a muscle, such as torticollis or wry neck.

These abnormal involuntary movements are usually quite characteristic of a selected group of neurologic diseases.

SENSORY SYSTEM EXAMINATION

42. How are nociceptive sensations carried in the nervous system?

They are carried by slow, unmyelinated fibers. Nociceptive fibers (which carry not only pain but also temperature sensations) synapse in the anterolateral columns of the spinal cord, then cross over to the opposite side of the cord, ascend and synapse in the thalamus, and finally reach the sensory cortex.

43. How are proprioceptive sensations carried in the nervous system?

They are carried by fast, myelinated fibers. Proprioceptive inputs (which carry vibration and joint-position sensations) travel in the posterior columns of the spinal cord, synapse in the gracile and cuneate nuclei of the upper cord, then cross over to the opposite side in the medial lemniscus, synapse in the thalamus, and finally end in the sensory cortex.

44. What are the dermatomes?

A dermatome (literally a *skin cutting* in Greek) is the area of the skin supplied by nerve fibers originating from a single dorsal nerve root. Thus, damage to a nerve root (radiculopathy) often causes sensory loss in a dermatomal distribution. For the neurologic examination it is useful to remember a few key dermatomes:

- C6 (thumb)
- T4 (nipple line)
- T10 (umbilicus)
- L5 (top of foot)
- S1 (bottom of foot)
- S2–S4 (perineum)

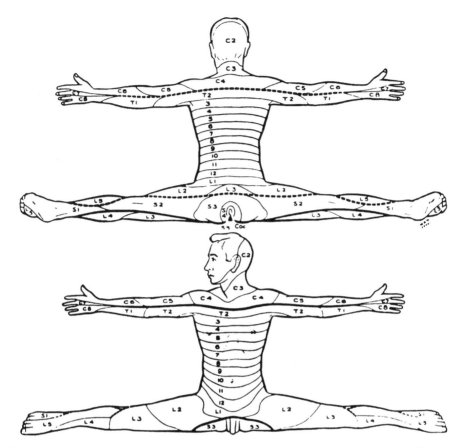

The sensory dermatomes. (From Garoutte B: Survey of Functional Neuroanatomy.Greenbrae, CA, Jones Medical Publishers, 1992, with permission.)

45. Which sensations should be tested during the neurologic examination?

A comprehensive neurologic examination should include testing of:
1. Pain (pinprick)
2. Touch
3. Vibration
4. Position

46. How is pain assessed?

By using a safety pin and testing the patient's ability to differentiate the sharp point from the blunt end. An abnormal pain response may include increased pain sensation (hyperesthesia); diminished pain sensation (hypesthesia); or numbness (anesthesia).

47. How is light touch assessed?

By using either the fingertips or a cotton swab to stroke the skin gently. Patients should perceive the touch as light and symmetric throughout.

48. How is vibration assessed?

By setting a 128-Hz tuning fork in motion, applying its end to a bony prominence of the hand or foot, and asking the patient whether he or she can feel the vibration.

CEREBELLUM

49. How is the sense of position best assessed?

By grasping the lateral aspect of the great toe or index finger between the examiner's thumb and forefinger while asking the patient to close his or her eyes. The digit is then moved slightly up or down while the patient guesses the direction of motion. If proprioception is intact, patients should be able to detect even slight movement in the joint.

50. What physical findings are produced by damage to the cerebellum?

Difficulty with smooth coordinated movements. As a result, patients have tremulous, jerky, and clumsy motions. Cerebellar damage can affect eye movements (nystagmus), speech, arms or legs, or walking.

51. How is cerebellar function tested in the upper extremities?

1. In the **finger-to-nose** test the examiner holds a finger in front of the patient and asks the patient to use the index finger to touch the tip of the patient's nose and the examiner's finger, back and forth, repeating the sequence several times. Each hand is tested separately, and the patient should extend the arm fully during the course of the test because tremors and incoordination may appear only with full extension.

2. **Rapid alternating movements** are particularly difficult to perform when the cerebellum has been damaged. This ability can be tested by instructing the patient to pat the knee alternately with the dorsum of the hand and the palm of the hand, pronating and supinating back and forth. Abnormalities in rate and rhythm are noted. Another technique is to have the patient touch the tip of the thumb to the tip of the each of the other fingers in sequence. Errors in speed and coordination should be noted.

52. How is cerebellar function tested in the lower extremities?

By the heel-to-shin test, which is performed by placing the heel of one foot on the opposite knee and then sliding the heel smoothly down the shin, over the dorsum of the foot, and then back up to the knee. This test can be performed several times, looking for wobbling or unsteadiness.

53. How is a cerebellar gait assessed?

Patients with cerebellar deficits are off balance and incoordinated; they walk with legs spread wide apart, suggesting a staggering "drunk" appearance. It is particularly difficult to perform tandem walking (walking with one foot directly in front of the other, as though on an imaginary tight rope).

GAIT

54. How is gait assessed?

Gait is tested by asking the patient to walk normally, then to walk on the heels and toes, and then to perform tandem walking. In this way it is possible to assess weakness, incoordination, dizziness, and many other deficits. Walking is a highly complex action that requires integration of motor, cerebellar, vestibular, sensory, visual, and other systems. Almost any abnormality in the nervous system thus appears in the patient's gait, and simply asking the patient to walk is an excellent way to assess all aspects of the neurologic exam. (See also chapter 1.)

APPLICATION OF THE NEUROLOGIC EXAMINATION

55. What is the best way to evaluate patients complaining of neurologic symptoms?

The first step is to localize the lesion, to determine specifically which part of the nervous system is affected. Only then should a cause be sought, since defining the anatomy usually implies certain causes.

56. How can neuroanatomy be applied clinically, given the great complexity of the nervous system?

For clinical purposes, the most important aspects of neuroanatomy consist of only a few large regions. Finer detail can be left to neurologic specialists. The regions in which lesions should be localized (proceeding from distal to proximal) include the following:

1. Muscle
2. Neuromuscular junction
3. Peripheral nerve
4. Root
5. Spinal cord
6. Brainstem
7. Cerebellum
8. Cerebral hemisphere

57. Which clinical features of muscle disease can be elicited by the history?

Muscle disease (myopathy) causes proximal symmetric weakness without sensory loss. Therefore, questions that elicit these symptoms should be asked:

1. Can the patient arise from a chair, get out of a car seat, get off the toilet, or go upstairs without using the hands? (This question checks proximal leg weakness.) Can the patient lift or carry objects, such as briefcases, school books, children, grocery bags, or garbage bags? (This question checks proximal arm weakness.)

2. Is the weakness relatively symmetric? (Minor differences are allowed because most generalized processes are slightly asymmetric, but weakness essentially confined to one limb or one side of the body is unlikely to be a myopathy.)

3. Is numbness or other sensory loss present? (Pain, cramping, and other sensations may occur with some myopathies, but there should be no sensory loss with disease confined to the muscle.)

58. After a history of muscle disease is elicited, what findings can be expected on physical examination?

The examination should show proximal symmetric weakness without sensory loss. Tone is usually normal or mildly decreased, reflexes are usually normal or mildly decreased, and atrophy is seldom significant unless the process is advanced.

59. Which clinical features of neuromuscular junction disease can be elicited by history?

Neuromuscular junction diseases closely resemble myopathies, causing proximal symmetric weakness without sensory loss. However, the hallmark of disease of the neuromuscular junction is fatigability; the weakness worsens with use and recovers with rest. Because strength improves with rest, fatigability does not usually present as a steady progressive decline throughout the day. Instead, it presents as variability or fluctuation in weakness as the muscle first fatigues, then recovers, then fatigues again. (Almost any medical symptom may be worse by the end of the day. Look for variability or fluctuation as the characteristic of neuromuscular junction fatigability).

In addition, symptoms of neuromuscular junction disease usually are extremely proximal. They often involve muscles of the face, resulting in drooping of the eyelids (ptosis), double vision, difficulty with chewing and swallowing, slurred speech, and facial weakness.

60. After a history of neuromuscular junction problems is elicited, what findings can be expected on physical examination?

The examination should show proximal symmetric weakness without sensory loss. With repetitive testing, muscles weaken, but after a minute or so of rest they regain strength. Similarly, sustained muscular activity (such as upward gaze) leads to fatigability and progressive weakness (such as ptosis). Tone, reflexes, and muscle bulk are normal.

61. Which clinical features of peripheral neuropathies can be elicited by history?

Peripheral neuropathies cause distal, often asymmetric weakness with sensory changes. Atrophy and fasciculations also may appear. Questions to elicit such symptoms include the following:

1. Does the patient wear out the toes of shoes or catch the toes and trip, as expected with a foot drop? (Checking distal weakness in the legs.) Does the patient have trouble with grip or frequently drop things? (Checking distal strength in the hands.)

2. Is the process asymmetric? Some neuropathies are distal, symmetric, stocking-and-glove neuropathies, but most are asymmetric.

3. Has the patient noticed a shrinkage or wasting of the muscle (atrophy) or quivering, twitching muscles (fasciculations)?

4. Does the patient experience numbness or tingling?

62. After a history of peripheral neuropathy is elicited, what findings can be expected on physical examination?

The examination should show distal, often asymmetric weakness with atrophy and fasciculations and sensory loss such as decreased pinprick, vibration, and occasionally position sense. Tone is normal or decreased, and reflexes are diminished. Some patients also have trophic changes, such as loss of hair and nails and smooth, shiny skin.

63. Which clinical features of root diseases (radiculopathies) can be elicited by history?

The hallmark of root disease is pain. In addition, radiculopathies usually have features similar to peripheral neuropathies: denervation (weakness, atrophy, and fasciculations) with sensory loss. The weakness may be proximal (the most common radiculopathies in the arms involve C5–C6 muscles, which are proximal) or distal (the most common radiculopathies in the legs involve L5–S1 muscles, which are distal). The history is therefore the same as for peripheral neuropathies but with the added element of pain. Pain is usually severe, often described as sharp, hot, or electric, and commonly radiates down an arm or leg.

64. After a history of radiculopathy is elicited, what findings can be expected on physical examination?

The neurologic examination shows weakness in one group of muscles, such as C5–C6 in the arm or L5–S1 in the legs, sometimes with atrophy and fasciculations. Tone is normal or decreased, and muscular reflex is diminished or absent. Sensory loss occurs in a dermatomal distribution. Sometimes maneuvers that stretch the root elicit the pain, such as straight leg-raising.

65. Which clinical features of spinal cord disease can be elicited by history?

Spinal cord lesions cause a triad of symptoms:

1. Sensory level, which may occur as a band of sensory change around the chest or abdomen or a sharp level below which sensation is lost, is the hallmark of spinal cord disease.

2. Distal, usually symmetric weakness

3. Bowel and bladder changes

Questions about spinal cord disease therefore should focus on eliciting these symptoms:

1. Does the patient drag the toe or trip because of distal leg weakness? Lesions in the pyramidal tract, also called the corticospinal tract or upper motor neuron, cause weakness that is usually greatest distally and thus may mimic a peripheral neuropathy.

2. Are the patient's legs stiff? Because pyramidal tract weakness causes spasticity, many patients report that their legs are stiff and that their knees will not bend when they walk.

3. Is a sensory level present? Some patients describe it as a belt or band or "tight swimming trunks" around their waist or chest.

4. Is either retention or incontinence of bowel and bladder present? The bladder is usually much more sensitive to spinal cord injury than the bowel.

66. After a history of spinal cord disease is elicited, what findings can be expected on physical examination?

The physical examination in a person with spinal cord disease shows distal weakness, usually worse in the legs than in the arms and usually worse in the extensors (dorsiflexors of the feet and extensors of the wrists and fingers) than in the flexors. Tone is increased, reflexes are brisk, and extensor plantar reflexes (positive Babinski signs) usually are present. A sensory level often can be found, below which all sensory modalities are diminished.

67. Which clinical features of brainstem disease can be elicited by history?

The brainstem is essentially a spinal cord with cranial nerves stuck in it. Cranial nerve abnormalities are the hallmark of brainstem disease. Symptoms of brainstem disease usually consist of a combination of long-tract findings (such as weakness from the pyramidal tract, numbness from the spinothalamic tract) plus cranial nerve findings. Because the long tracts have crossed (decussated), the weakness and numbness are not in the distribution of a level but rather present as hemiparesis or hemianesthesia. Because of the crossing of the long tracts, damage to one side of the brainstem, affecting the cranial nerves on that side, usually results in long-tract symptoms that affect the opposite side of the body. These crossed symptoms are another hallmark of brainstem disease—for example, weakness of one side of the face and the opposite side of the body. Cranial nerve lesions commonly cause the big Ds: diplopia (cranial nerve III, IV, or VI), decreased sensation in the face (cranial nerve V), decreased strength in the face (cranial nerve VII), dizziness and deafness (cranial nerve VIII), and dysarthria and dysphagia (cranial nerves IX, X, and XII). The history therefore should focus on eliciting such symptoms:

1. Does the patient report diplopia, facial weakness or numbness, dizziness, deafness, dysarthria, or dysphagia?

2. Are long-tract findings present, such as hemiparesis or hemisensory loss?

3. Are the findings crossed or bilateral?

68. After a history of brainstem disease is elicited, what findings can be expected on physical examination?

The physical examination shows a combination of cranial nerve and long-tract abnormalities. Checking the cranial nerves may reveal ptosis, abnormalities of extraocular movements, diplopia, nystagmus, decreased corneal reflexes, facial weakness or numbness, decreased hearing, dysarthria, paralysis of the palate, decreased gag reflex, or tongue deviation. Long-tract abnormalities usually result in hemiparesis, with a pyramidal pattern of distal weakness, increased reflexes, increased tone, and positive Babinski sign. Hemisensory loss may include decreased sensation to all modalities.

69. Which clinical features of cerebellar disease can be elicited by history?

Cerebellar disease causes clumsiness and lack of coordination. The cerebellum is responsible for smoothing voluntary movements, and impairments produce abnormalities in the rate and rhythm of movements. Questions, therefore, should focus on incoordination in the legs and arms:

1. Does the patient have a staggering, drunken walk? Most laymen understand what is meant by a "drunken" walk and use this term to describe cerebellar disease. Drinking alcohol, in fact, impairs the cerebellum, and the characteristic wide-based staggering gait of the person intoxicated by alcohol is caused by cerebellar dysfunction.

2. Does the patient have difficulty with putting a key in a lock, lighting a cigarette, or other target-directed movements? The cerebellar tremor is worse with voluntary, intentional movements, especially as the hand approaches the target object. Fine coordinated movements, such as extending a key and inserting it into the narrow slot of a lock, are perfect examples of difficult tasks for people with cerebellar lesions.

70. After a history of cerebellar disease is elicited, what findings can be expected on physical examination?

Patients with cerebellar disease have a staggering gait and difficulty with tandem walking. When they slide a heel down a shin, it wavers unsteadily. The arms may show a tremor and wavering when the patient touches the examiner's finger, his or her own nose, or other targets. Similarly, rapid alternating movements in the limbs are irregular in rate and rhythm.

71. Which clinical features of disease in the cerebral hemispheres can be elicited by history and neurologic examination?

Clinically, disease of the brain itself may cause a variety of symptoms:
1. Mental status changes and high-function disturbances such as aphasia
2. Hemiparesis
3. Hemianesthesia
4. Visual field defects
5. Involuntary movements
6. Seizures

Questions to elicit these features include the following:
1. Does the patient have aphasia or other altered mental status?
2. Do weakness and numbness affect the face, arm, and leg on the same side of the body?
3. Does the patient have a visual field defect? Visual fibers run subcortically (in the optic tract, lateral geniculate, and optic radiations) and terminate in the occipital cortex.
4. Does the patient have a movement disorder? A history of chorea, dystonia, or hemiballismus suggest a brain lesion.
5. Does the patient have seizures? Seizures arise from the paroxysmal discharge of neurons, almost exclusively in the cortex.

72. After a history of cerebral hemisphere disease is elicited, what findings can be expected on physical examination?

The examination may be expected to show aphasia or other mental status changes, hemiparesis, hemianesthesia, or visual field defects.

BIBLIOGRAPHY

1. Haerer AF: DeJong's The Neurologic Examination, 5th ed. Philadelphia, J.B. Lippincott, 1992.
2. Medical Research Council: Aids to the Examination of the Peripheral Nervous System. London, Her Majesty's Stationery Office, 1986.
3. Patten J: Neurological Differential Diagnosis, 2nd ed. London, Springer, 1996.
4. Strub RL, Black FW: The Mental Status Examination in Neurology. Philadelphia, F.A. Davis, 1977.

20. BEDSIDE DIAGNOSIS OF COMA

Salvatore Mangione, M.D.

> *Ignore death up to the last moment; then, when it can't be ignored any longer, have yourself squirted full of morphia and shuffle off in a coma.*
>
> Aldous Huxley, *Time Must Have a Stop*

TOPICS COVERED IN THIS CHAPTER

Assessment of the Upper Brainstem
Pattern of breathing
Response to painful stimuli
Posturing
Assessment of the Midbrain
Pupillary reflex
Anisocoria
Assessment of the Pons
Oculocephalic reflex (doll's eyes)
Corneal reflex

Assessment of the Medulla
Apnea testing
Toxic–Metabolic Comas
Patterns of Breathing and Coma
Rostral-caudal Herniation

CONVENTIONAL TEACHING WATCH

Diagnosis of coma is an important area of medicine. Bedside exam can localize the lesion and provide a diagnosis. Most maneuvers reported below are therefore important (almost essential) for the practicing physician.

MANEUVERS/SIGNS		CONVENTIONAL TEACHING REVISITED
Response to painful stimuli	⇑	Eliciting posturing is essential part of upper brainstem exam.
Response to light (pupillary reflex)	⇑	Key for assessment of midbrain.
Doll's eye maneuver	⇑	Poor term, but important reflex.
Corneal reflex	⇑	As above.
Apnea testing	⇑	Essential for assessment of medulla.
Patterns of respiration	⇔	Helpful, but may be a bit overrated.

1. What is coma?
Coma (from the Greek *koma* = deep sleep) is a disturbance of consciousness, characterized by the inability of the central nervous system to receive, integrate, and react to environmental signals.

2. Are the patient's eyes open or closed in coma?
The eyes are supposed to be closed because coma is a sleep-like state. On the other hand, in some forms of metabolic coma (such as hepatic or uremic) or in chronic post-traumatic encephalopathic states the patient's eyes are open and roving. In the later stage of hypoxic encephalopathy, for example, the patient's eyelids are open and the eyes rove around to the point of misleading friends and family into believing that the patient has finally emerged from coma when, in reality, the patient has entered **vigil coma (persistent vegetative state).**

421

3. What is the neurologic basis for coma?

By definition coma is a state of diffuse, bilateral cortical dysfunction. This dysfunction may be either primary or secondary to a disorder of the brainstem, particularly a disorder involving the reticularis activating system. This network of brainstem cells keeps the cortex active. By analogy with a computer, coma is a state in which either the chips (brain cortex) or the generating power (reticularis activating system) is not working. If the generating power (brainstem) is down, the computer will not work even if the chips (cortex) are intact.

4. Where is the reticularis activating system located?

It is located throughout the four layers of the brainstem.

5. Describe the neurologic exam of a comatose patient.

The neurologic exam of a comatose patient is quite simple. In fact, because the cortex of a comatose patient is, by definition, dysfunctional, the neurologic exam is tailored only to assess the function of the brainstem. This assessment is carried out in a rostral-caudal, level-by-level fashion. If all four layers of the brainstem are functionally and anatomically intact, the coma is a **cortical coma** (i.e., a coma in which the cortex is primarily dysfunctional). If, on the other hand, one or more layers of the brainstem are damaged, the coma is a **brainstem coma** (i.e., a coma in which the cortex is secondarily dysfunctional as a result of direct damage to the brainstem).

6. What is a level-by-level exam of the brainstem?

Each brainstem level is tested by using at least one neurologic reflex. If the reflex is abnormal, the corresponding layer of the brainstem is considered dysfunctional and damaged. Thus, the neurologic exam of coma relies on an armamentarium of four reflexes, each of which tests one of the four brainstem layers.

7. What is the first and uppermost level of the brainstem?

The uppermost level of the brainstem is the thalamus.

8. Which reflex tests thalamic function?

The response-to-pain reflex. The thalamus is an integrating center for all sensory inputs (with the exception of proprioceptive signals, which travel to the cerebellum). Thus, to test the function of the thalamus, administer a painful stimulus to the patient, such as compressing the ungual bed of one finger.

9. What are proper and improper responses of a comatose patient to a painful stimulus?

The proper response of a conscious, lethargic, or obtunded patient is to push away the offending source. Thus, in the case of a painful stimulus administered by compressing the ungual bed of one finger with a pencil, a proper response is to push away the hand of the examiner. An improper response, on the other hand, is to assume a particular posture, either decorticate or decerebrate.

A **decorticate** posture is a sign of mild thalamic dysfunction. It consists of flexion of the upper extremity and extension and internal rotation of the lower deformity. A **decerebrate** posture consists of extension and internal rotation of both the upper and the lower extremity. It is a sign of severe thalamic dysfunction. It is easy to separate decortication from decerebration by remembering that in de-*cor*-tication the hand points toward the heart (*cor*), whereas in decerebration the hand points away from the heart. Finally, if the thalamus is entirely dysfunctional, there is no response to a painful stimuli or simply a bending of the knees, which is usually a simple spinal reflex. (See figure at top of facing page.)

10. What is the second layer in the brainstem?

The midbrain.

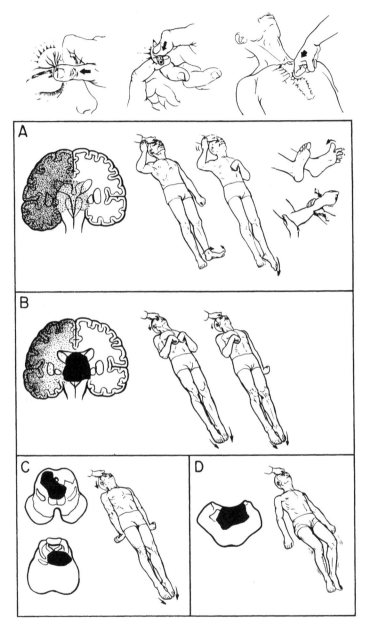

Motor responses to noxious stimulation in patients with acute cerebral dysfunction. Noxious stimuli can be delivered with minimal trauma to the supraorbital ridge, the nail bed, or the sternum as illustrated at top. Levels of associated brain dysfunction are roughly indicated at left. The text provides details. (From Plum F, Posner JB: The Diagnosis of Stupor and Coma, 3rd ed. Philadelphia, F.A. Davis, 1980, with permission.)

11. Which reflex tests the function of the midbrain?

The pupillary reflex, which consists of shining a light into the patient's eye and looking for a closing of the pupil (both ipsilaterally and contralaterally). Paralysis of the pupil (i.e., inability to constrict in response to light) indicates an ipsilateral dysfunction of the midbrain (**midbrain pupils** = midposition or slightly widened and fixed pupils unreactive to light). **Pontine pupils** are bilateral small pupils that still react to light, even though it may be necessary to use a magnifying glass. They reflect anatomic lesions in the tegmentum. **Pinpoint pupils** are small and constricted but reactive; they often are seen in patients with metabolic encephalopathy and may be due to opiates. **Bilaterally dilated pupils**, on the other hand, may be encountered in patients with atropine and scopolamine toxicity.

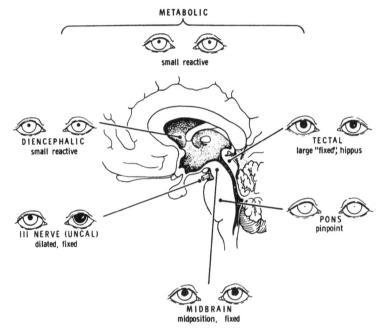

Pupils in comatose patients. (From Plum F, Posner JB: The Diagnosis of Stupor and Coma, 3rd ed. Philadelphia, F.A. Davis, 1980, with permission.)

12. What is anisocoria?

Anisocoria (from the Greek *aniso* = unequal and *kore* = pupil) indicates a pupillary asymmetry that is often congenital (in as much as 5% of the population).

13. How can one distinguish congenital anisocoria from pathologic anisocoria?

In congenital anisocoria pupils are reactive to light but asymmetric in size.

14. What is the third level in the brainstem?

The pons.

15. Which reflex tests the function of the pons?

The doll's eye reflex.

16. What is the doll's eye reflex?

This confusing term was used in the heyday of physical diagnosis, when Victorian dolls were much more popular than now. The neurologic term *oculocephalic reflex* is preferable because it conveys an anatomic sense of the reflex pathway.

17. What is the pathway of the oculocephalic reflex?

1. The stimulus is given either mechanically (by rotating the head of the patient along the horizontal plane) or calorically (by injecting a syringeful of liquid in the external canal of the ear—after ascertaining, of course, that the eardrum is intact).

2. As a result of this stimulus, the receptors contained in the inner ear (more specifically, in the semicircular canals and utriculus) are set into motion.

3. The afferent signals are carried to the central nervous system via the eighth cranial nerve, which enters the brainstem at the cerebellar-pontine angle.

4. The efferent pathway is carried to the eye muscles, eliciting movement of the eyes across the horizontal plane. This movement is controlled by the third and sixth cranial nerves. Because the third cranial nerve resides in the midbrain and the sixth cranial nerve in the upper pons, it is necessary to use a connecting wire to lead the electric impulse from the lower pons to the upper pons and midbrain. This connecting wire is the **medial longitudinal fasciculus** (MLF).

Therefore, when we test the oculocephalic reflex, we basically test the integrity of the MLF. The reflex is important not because of the MLF per se, but because the MLF is totally surrounded by the **reticularis activating system** (RAS), which is responsible for preserving the cortical function and awake state. Thus, the MLF acts as a sort of innocent bystander, like the canary that was used to identify leakage of gas in coal mines. Dysfunction of the MLF signals dysfunction of the surrounding RAS. Therefore, the absence of an oculocephalic reflex means the absence of RAS function in the pons and indicates a brainstem coma.

18. What is a normal oculocephalic response?

It depends on whether the patient is awake or comatose and whether coma is due to a primary (cortical) dysfunction or a cortical dysfunction secondary to a pontine insult. In a comatose patient with preserved brainstem function, application of the stimulus (rotation of the head) generates a combined movement of the eyes toward the opposite side. In other words, the eyes do not stay fixed in the midline, as they would in a patient with brainstem dysfunction. Death closely resembles brainstem dysfunction: the eyes remain fixed in the midline, as if they were painted. In an awake patient, on the other hand, eye movement is suppressed in response to head rotation because the cortex of an awake patient is active and thus suppresses the oculocephalic reflex to allow the eyes the see where the head is pointing. (See figure on following page.)

19. Does any other reflex test the function of the pons?

Yes. The corneal reflex is similar to the oculocephalic reflex. The input, however, is a delicate painful stimulus to the cornea with a cotton whisk. This stimulus triggers sensory input across the trigeminal (fifth) nerve, which enters the brainstem at multiple levels, including the pons and medulla. The efferent pathway is carried to orbicularis muscle, along the seventh nerve, and elicits blinking of the eye. Thus, the corneal reflex consists of a long loop that relies on several connecting wires, such as the MLF, all imbedded in the RAS. Like the oculocephalic reflex, the corneal reflex assesses the function and integrity of the RAS.

20. What is the fourth and lowermost layer of the brainstem?

The medulla.

21. Which reflex tests the function of the medulla?

The most basic and primitive of all reflexes—the integrity of cardiorespiratory function. The medulla houses the major cardiac and respiratory centers. Therefore, dysfunction of these centers manifests with cardiorespiratory instability, such as major irregularities of heart rate and rhythm, unstable blood pressure, and apnea.

22. What is an apnea test?

Inability of the patient to take a spontaneous breath after maximal carbon dioxide stimulation (60 mmHg) indicates major medullary dysfunction. Because of the hazards of hypoxemia,

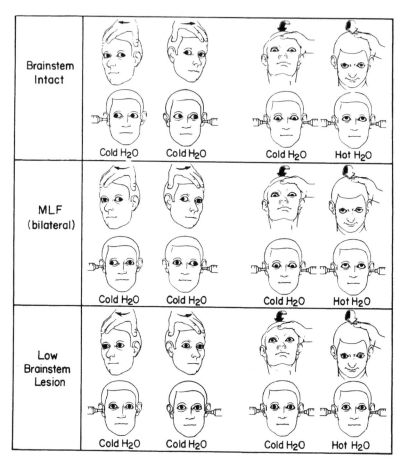

Ocular reflexes in unconscious patients. The upper section illustrates the oculocephalic (above) and oculo-vestibular (below) reflexes in an unconscious patient whose brainstem ocular pathways are intact. Horizontal eye movements are illustrated on the left and vertical eye movements on the right: lateral conjugate eye movements (upper left) to head turning are full and opposite in direction to the movement of the face. A stronger stimulus to lateral deviation is achieved by douching cold water against the tympanic membrane(s). There is tonic conjugate deviation of both eyes toward the stimulus; the eyes usually remain tonically deviated for 1 or more minutes before slowly returning to the midline. Because the patient is unconscious, there is no nystagmus. Extension of the neck in a patient with an intact brainstem produces conjugate deviation of the eyes in the downward direction, and flexion of the neck produces deviation of the eyes upward. Bilateral cold water against the tympanic membrane likewise produces conjugate downward deviation of the eyes, whereas hot water (no warmer than 44° C) causes conjugate upward deviation of the eyes.

In the middle portion of the drawing, the effects of bilateral medial longitudinal fasciculus lesions on oculocephalic and oculovestibular reflexes are shown. The left portion of the drawing illustrates that oculocephalic and oculovestibular stimulation deviates the appropriate eye laterally and brings the eye, which normally would deviate medially, only to the midline, since the medial longitudinal fasciculus (MLF), with its connections between the abducens and oculomotor nuclei, is interrupted. Vertical eye movements often remain intact. The lower portion of the drawing illustrates the effects of a low brainstem lesion. On the left, neither oculovestibular nor oculocephalic movements cause lateral deviation of the eyes because the pathways are interrupted between the vestibular nucleus and the abducens area. Likewise, in the right portion of the drawing, neither oculovestibular nor oculocephalic stimulation causes vertical deviation of the eyes. On rare occasions, particularly with low lateral brainstem lesions, oculocephalic responses may be intact even when oculovestibular reflexes are abolished. (From Plum F, Posner JB: The Diagnosis of Stupor and Coma, 3rd ed. Philadelphia, F.A. Davis, 1980, with permission.)

this test is performed under 100% oxygen. The patient will not become hypoxic, although he or she may become apneic.

23. What is the implication of the global absence of brainstem function?

Global absence of brainstem function means death. Given the implications of this diagnosis, a repeat neurologic exam usually is required at a 12-hour interval. Other, possibly reversible conditions that may lead to global dysfunction of the central nervous system need to be excluded (i.e., toxic-metabolic coma).

24. What is meant by toxic-metabolic coma?

Toxic-metabolic coma is a wastebasket term associated with both exogenous and endogenous toxins. Although such toxins may affect both cortical and brainstem function, they usually affect the cortex first. Thus, comatose patients with an intact brainstem should be considered to have a toxic-metabolic process until proved otherwise.

25. What is the differential diagnosis of a toxic-metabolic coma?

Toxic-metabolic comas may be due to either exogenous or endogenous toxins. By definition, such toxins should affect the cortex bilaterally and diffusely. Thus, a localized cortical process, such as an ischemic or hemorrhagic stroke, may lead to some disturbance in consciousness, such as lethargy or stupor, but it should *not* cause coma.

Exogenous toxins include poisons. A toxic screen should be part of the work-up of all comatose patients, even when the diagnosis of overdose is not clear-cut. **Endogenous toxins** also may act as poisons and induce a toxic-metabolic coma. Endogenous toxins usually are generated through dysfunction of the major detoxifying parenchymas: liver, kidneys, and lungs (in which case the toxin is carbon dioxide). Hepatic, renal, and hypercapnic encephalopathies are common examples of metabolic coma.

Failure of the major endocrine systems also may cause coma. Examples include hypothyroidism (myxedema coma) and global dysfunction of either the hypophysis (panhypopituitarism) or adrenal glands (Addisonian crisis). In addition, **defects in glucose metabolism**, either in excess (such as diabetic ketoacidosis or hyperosmolar nonketotic coma) or in deficiency (hypoglycemic encephalopathy) may lead to coma. **Electrolyte disturbances** (either in excess or deficiency) also may lead to disturbances in consciousness. Examples include hypo- and hypernatremia, hypercalcemia, and hypermagnesemia.

Another major cause of toxic-metabolic coma is direct, **generalized poisoning of the cerebral cortex**. Poisons of this sort usually are spread along the subarachnoid space; the two most common are blood (subarachnoid hemorrhage) and pus (purulent meningitis). Therefore, a lumbar puncture should be part of the standard work-up of comatose patients whenever there is a high index of clinical suspicion for this condition.

A **generalized electrical disturbance** (such as a seizure) also may lead to coma. Coma may occur during or after the crisis (postictal coma). Seizures may not present with classic tonic-clonic contractions. In subclinical seizures, patients may either be immobile or exhibit a fine fluttering of the eyelids. Such cases must be investigated aggressively, and electroencephalography (EEG) should be a standard component of coma work-up.

Finally, a common cause of metabolic coma is **hypoxic encephalopathy**. This term is actually incorrect because the bilateral cortical dysfunction characterizing such patients is caused more by reperfusion injury than by true hypoxia. Because of the resiliency of the brainstem, its function usually is preserved, and such patients are not dead. After going through the initial state of shock and coma (i.e., sleep-like state), patients with hypoxic encephalopathy emerge into a persistent vegetative state. As a result, the brainstem restarts its regular function, sending impulses to the cortex, even though the cortex is unable to process them. Patients in persistent vegetative state (vigil coma) open their eyes, which rove around the room. They send ambivalent messages to family and friends, leading them to believe that they have emerged from coma when in reality they have entered the much more prolonged and unfortunate state of persistent vegetation.

26. What is asterixis?

Asterixis (from the Greek *a* = lack of and *sterixis* = fixed position) is the flapping tremor that can be observed and elicited in patients with metabolic encephalopathy, particularly impending hepatic coma. It is due to the inability to maintain a voluntary muscular contraction. Thus, by definition, it requires patient cooperation and cannot be elicited in either stuporous or comatose patients. Asterixis consists of involuntary jerking movements, characterized by a sequence of flexions and extensions. Although it involves all muscles that are required to maintain posture (such as fingers, toes, eyelids, and even tongue), it is typically described in the hands.

Asterixis is best elicited by having patients extend their arms, dorsiflex their wrists, and spread their fingers (as if they were to stop traffic). Given the frequent association with severe hepatic failure, it is commonly referred to as liver flap. But it also may be encountered in other forms of metabolic encephalopathy, such as uremia, hypercapnia, poisoning, or electrolyte imbalances. It may even be seen (albeit more rarely) in patients with severe congestive heart failure or sepsis and usually indicates a severe condition. Indeed, patients with hepatic failure presenting only with asterixis have a mortality rate that is twice as high as in patients without asterixis.

Flapping tremor was first described in 1949 by Foley and Adams. Foley, a notorious wit, coined the word "asterixis" while drinking at a Greek bar across from Boston City Hospital. He then used the term semiseriously in a paper without expecting much of it. To his amazement, however, the word became the official academic term for flapping tremor.

27. What is the definition of death?

The definition of death is based on the results of a presidential commission appointed in the mid 1980s by Ronald Reagan. In this case, death is defined as brainstem death. The diagnosis of death, therefore, requires full and global dysfunction of the brainstem at each of its levels. There is no need to obtain an EEG; the diagnosis requires only two neurologic examinations, 12 hours apart, and exclusion of toxic-metabolic causes.

28. What conditions may look like coma but are not coma?

The differential diagnosis of coma should include a series of conditions that may be commonly encountered:

1. **Locked-in state** is a condition characterized by discrete and localized damage of the brainstem, usually involving the junction between the upper third and the lower two-thirds of the pons. Given the high location of the lesion, patients have enough activity of the reticularis to be awake even though there is no function below the pons. Patients, therefore, have control only of the cranial nerves above the lesion, which are primarily the third and the sixth. As a result, patients are able to move their eyes and keep their eyes open but cannot move their extremities and have no sensation in them. The patient can see and hear the examiner but cannot feel any touch or respond to stimuli by moving the extremities. A warning sign of the locked-in state is the fact that the eyes are open, whereas in true coma, which is a sleep-like state, the eyes are closed. Moreover, the patient's eyes often track the examiner around the room. If tracking is detected, the examiner should instruct the patient, "If you hear me, blink your eyes." Usually the locked-in state is a fatal condition that leads to death within a matter of days. In some cases, however, the patient has lived for many years. A famous case involves a World War I British soldier who lived for many years in this state, eventually learning to communicate by blinking his eyes in a Morse code fashion.

2. Patients with **hysteric coma** are not in coma but in a coma-like state as a result of major psychological disorders. Hysteric coma at times can be identified by raising the patient's hand over his or her head and letting it drop. Patients in hysteric coma rarely let the hand fall heavily on their head and usually slide it gently on the side.

3. **Catatonic coma** (from the Greek *katatonas* = depressed) is similar to hysteric coma, although different in pathogenesis. Patients with catatonic coma usually have a history of preexisting depression and develop catatonia as a result of a major intercurrent medical illness. The eyes tend to be open, and patients are indeed awake but immobile. The mechanism is hyperactivity of

some cortical centers that suppress the rest of the cortex. The hyperactive centers usually can be inhibited by a benzodiazepine or a short-acting barbiturate. The patient is restored to an awake state and is able to respond to verbal commands.

29. What is uncus herniation?

A rostral-caudal herniation of the uncus of the temporal lobe with secondary compression of the brainstem. Patients lose brainstem function in a layer-by-layer fashion (first the thalamus, then the midbrain, then the pons, and finally the medulla). Neurologically patients first exhibit ipsilateral cerebral posturing (decortication and then decerebration), eventually followed by no response to painful stimuli. They then develop unilateral paralysis of the pupil and lose the oculocephalic reflex on the ipsilateral side. Finally, because of compression of the medullary respiratory center, they develop respiratory arrest. Prompt intervention with hyperventilation and antiedema therapy is crucial to avoid death.

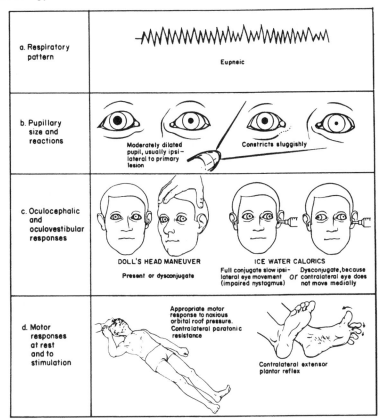

Signs of uncus herniation, early third nerve stage. (From Plum F, Posner JB: The Diagnosis of Stupor and Coma, 3rd ed. Philadelphia, F.A. Davis, 1980, with permission.)

30. What are the most common causes of uncus herniation?

The most common causes are intracranial space-occupying processes, such as an ischemic or hemorrhagic stroke, brain abscess, or tumor. Because brain edema peaks at 48–72 hours after an acute injury, patients who suffer a stroke over time may become stuporous, then comatose, and finally, immediately before respiratory arrest, exhibit progressive signs of uncal herniation.

31. Is the pattern of breathing helpful in identifying the site of a brainstem lesion?

Yes and no. Some patterns can help to identify which section of the brainstem has been damaged. Other breathing patterns, despite conventional teaching, are much less helpful. One pattern that probably belongs more to the folklore than to the science of bedside diagnosis is **Cheyne-Stokes respiration**. This periodic breathing is a regularly irregular pattern characterized by a progressive increase in the depth and at times frequency of respiration with a crescendo-decrescendo shape that eventually culminates in an apneic phase. This pattern is important to recognize because the associated apnea may be quite frightening to an untrained staff; indeed a few patients have even been "resuscitated." Cheyne-Stokes respiration, however, may be encountered in normal people as a result of aging or obesity. It is, nonetheless, a feature of congestive heart failure or various neurologic disorders that make the respiratory centers of the brain a bit too sluggish to respond promptly to variations in carbon dioxide. As a result, there is a need for major swings in carbon dioxide levels, which lead the patient either to hyperventilate or to become apneic. Cheyne-Stokes respiration, therefore, may be encountered in patients with meningitis, bilateral or unilateral cerebral infarctions, and pontine damage.

32. Who were Cheyne and Stokes?

John Cheyne (1777–1836) was a Scottish physician, the son of a surgeon. As a young boy, Cheyne often helped his father to care for patients by bleeding and dressing them. After graduating at age 18 from the University of Edinburgh, he served in the army for four years. During this time he took part in the battle of Vinegar Hill, which in 1798 broke Irish resistance to British rule. In 1809 the went to Dublin, where he was eventually appointed physician-in-general for Ireland, becoming the founder of modern Irish medicine.

William Stokes (1804–1878) was an Irish physician and the son of the anatomy professor who succeeded John Cheyne at the College of Surgeons School in Ireland. Although he received no formal education (his father wanted to protect him from a society that did not abide by the scriptures), Stokes eventually went to Edinburgh, where he graduated with an M.D. in 1825. In Scotland he learned about Laennec and his recent invention, the stethoscope. He became so enamored of this tool that he wrote an introductory book on the subject, the first of its kind in the English language. Stokes' interest in stethoscopy was so great that he became a vocal advocate for its use in medical practice, a habit that provoked quite a few reactions and even some sarcasm among his colleagues. A well-liked physician, he worked among the poor during the Dublin typhus epidemic in 1826 (he even contracted the disease and survived) and also during the subsequent cholera epidemic. William Stokes' name is linked not only to the pattern of respiration but also to Stokes-Adams syncope, which the Irish surgeon Robert Adams described in 1827 and which Stokes included in his 1854 book "Diseases of the Heart and Aorta."

33. What other respiratory patterns are important and worthy of recognition?

1. **Biot's breathing** is a variant of Cheyne-Stokes respiration in the sense that it is a succession of hyperpneas/hyperventilations and apneas. However, it lacks the typical crescendo-decrescendo pattern, abrupt beginning, and regularity of Cheyne-Stokes breathing. It is less common than the Cheyne-Stokes pattern and usually is encountered in patients with either meningitis or medullary compression; it therefore carries a much worse prognosis, usually resulting in complete apnea and cardiac arrest.

2. **Apneustic breathing** is a peculiar pattern characterized by a deep inspiratory phase followed by a breath-holding period, then rapid exhalation. This respiratory pattern is usually indicative of brainstem lesions (usually in the pons).

3. **Central hyperventilation** is often encountered in patients with midbrain/upper pons lesions. This ongoing pattern of hyperpnea and tachypnea (i.e., deep and rapid respirations) is quite different from Kussmaul's respiration.

4. **Kussmaul's breathing** was described by the German physician Adolf Kussmaul (1822–1902) in patients with diabetic ketoacidosis. It is, however, encountered in other forms of metabolic acidosis (such as lactic acidosis or uremia). Patients attempt to maintain pH balance by

respiratory compensation. To achieve this goal, hyperpnea is usually more effective than tachypnea. Thus, Kussmaul's respiration tends to be not as fast as central hyperventilation but often deeper. Kussmaul also linked his name to Kussmaul's sign (the paradoxical inspiratory increase in jugular venous pressure encountered in patients with constrictive pericarditis or tricuspid stenosis) and to the clinical description of pericarditis.

5. Patients with damage to the medullary respiratory centers have **ataxic ventilation** (from the Greek a = lack of and *taxis* = order). This totally anarchic respiratory pattern, a sort of fibrillation of the respiratory centers, is characterized by continuous shifts from hyperventilation to hypoventilation and even apnea. It is often called agonal respiration and usually precedes death.

BIBLIOGRAPHY

1. Hardison WG, Lee FI: Prognosis in acute liver disease of the alcoholic patient. N Engl J Med 275:61–66, 1966.
2. Plum F, Posner JB: The Diagnosis of Stupor and Coma, 3rd ed. Philadelphia, F.A. Davis, 1980.
3. Sapira J: The Art and Science of Bedside Diagnosis. Baltimore, Urban & Schwarzenberg, 1990.

21. THE PEDIATRIC EXAM

Ira Strassman, M.D.

Children are the spice of life. The only problem is that they keep turning into grown-ups.
Gemma Mangione
All children are artists. The problem is how to remain artists once they grow up.
Pablo Picasso

TOPICS COVERED IN THIS CHAPTER

Vital Signs
Normal respiratory rate
Normal heart rate
Normal blood pressure
Normal urine output
Apgar score
Assessment of toxicity
General Approach
Assessment for dehydration/hypovolemia
Skin turgor
Capillary refill time
Compensated and uncompensated shock
Head, Ears, Eyes, Nose, and Throat
Fontanels
  Bulging/sunken
  Closure
Epicanthal fold
Palpebral fissure slant
Chlamydial and gonococcal conjunctivitis
Nasolacrimal duct obstruction
Strabismus
  Alternate cover test
  Corneal light reflex
Leukocoria
Aniridia
Low-set ears
Otitis media
Preauricular ducts and skin tags
Choanal atresia
Asymmetric crying facies syndrome
Teeth eruption
"Strep" throat
Neck
Normal and abnormal lymph nodes
Torticollis
Neck webbing
Heart
Cyanosis
Point of maximal intensity and its
  displacement
Separate right ventricular impulse

Heart *(continued)*
Signs of congestive heart failure
Innocent murmurs
  Peripheral pulmonic stenosis
  Still's murmur
  Venous hum
  Carotid bruit
  Pulmonary flow murmur
Findings of congenital heart disease
Ventricular septal defect
Atrial septal defect
Patent ductus arteriosus
Delayed and diminished femoral pulses
Lungs
Signs of respiratory distress
Chlamydial pneumonia
Pertussis
Causes of crackles
Causes of wheezes
Causes of stridor
Abdomen
Palpable "olive"
Bilious vomiting
Pancreatitis
Appendicitis
Genitalia
Galactorrhea
Inguinal hernias
  Direct
  Indirect
Hydrocele
Hypospadias and epispadias
Chordee
Cryptorchidism
Phimosis and paraphimosis
Tanner stages for sexual maturation
Extremities
Ortolani and Barlow manuevers
Angle of gait
Polydactyly and syndactyly
Continued on following page

CONVENTIONAL TEACHING WATCH

The pediatric exam is an important and unique area of physical diagnosis. Examination of younger patients is in fact different and varies remarkably, depending on the child's age. This chapter presents only a selection of issues that may be encountered in pediatric physical examination and reviews them system by system. We present not only major abnormal findings but also pertinent normal findings, giving preference as much as possible to the most common and important signs and maneuvers.

FINDING		CONVENTIONAL TEACHING REVISITED
Vital signs	⇑	Quite different, depending on age; familiarity with normalcy is key.
Apgar score	⇑	Time-honored assessment of newborns.
Assessment for dehydration/ hypovolemia	⇑	Quite important in children and different from adults.
Eye exam	⇔	Few items to remember, limited to pediatric population.
Ear exam	⇔	Otitis media is key item.
Mouth exam	⇑	Beware of "strep" throat and its differences from viral pharyngitis.
Neck exam	⇔	Lymph nodes and torticollis should be kept in mind.
Innocent murmurs	⇑	Important and common finding.
Congenital heart disease	⇑	As above.
Congestive heart failure	⇑	Different findings in children.
Respiratory distress	⇑	As above.
Lung auscultation	⇔	Differential diagnosis of various findings is bit different from adult auscultation.
Abdominal exam	⇔	In infants and young children, beware of pyloric stenosis and intussusception.
Genitalia	⇔	Congenital malformations and hernias are most important topics.
Extremities	⇔	Need to know about hip dysplasia and scoliosis.
Skin	⇔	Series of infantile rashes and congenital lesions with which one should be familiar.
Neurology	⇔	Neurologic exam of infants focuses on series of motor automatisms that disappear over time.

VITAL SIGNS

1. What is a normal respiratory rate for a child?

Like other pediatric vital signs, it is age-dependent:

1. The normal respiratory rate for an **infant** several hours old may vary between 20–80 breaths per minute, with an average of 30–40.
2. During **childhood** the normal respiratory rate falls to 20–30 breaths per minute.
3. In **adolescence** it falls even further to the normal adult rate of 12–20 breaths per minute.

The normal breathing pattern of newborn infants is almost entirely diaphragmatic, and neonates commonly present with irregular and shallow respirations. Indeed, **periodic breathing** (crescendo-decrescendo respirations followed by periods of apnea as long as 10–15 seconds) may be quite common in premature infants. It is less common in full-term newborns, yet still relatively normal. On the other hand, apneic pauses of 20 seconds or more or pauses accompanied by pallor, cyanosis, or bradycardia should always be considered pathologic (**apnea of infancy**).

2. What is a normal heart rate for a child?

Each age group has a different upper and lower limit of normal heart rate:

- 0–3 months   80–205 beats per minute
- 3–24 months   75–190 beats per minute
- 2–10 years   60–140 beats per minute
- Older than 10 years   50–100 beats per minute

Persistent unexplained tachycardia should be a clue to the presence of congestive heart failure (see below). In an infant the heart rate may be determined by counting the visible pulsations through the anterior fontanel.

3. What is a normal systolic blood pressure for a child?

As a rule of thumb, the lower limit of normal systolic blood pressure for a pediatric patient is calculated as follows:

$$70 \text{ mmHg} + (2 \times \text{age in years})$$

Blood pressure is determined by cardiac output and systemic vascular resistance. When cardiac output falls, children can maintain normal blood pressure simply by vasoconstriction and an increase in heart rate. When these compensatory mechanisms fail, however, hypotension occurs. A fall in blood pressure, therefore, is a late finding in pediatric cardiovascular decompensation.

4. When can blood pressure be assessed by by auscultation?

Blood pressure can be assessed successfully by auscultation in children more than 3–4 years old.

5. What is the normal urine output of a child?

Normal urine output depends on the size of the child. In adults normal urinary output is 400–600 cc/day; anuria is defined as less than 50 cc/day and oliguria as 50–400 cc/day. In children, on the other hand, anuria is defined as 0–0.5 cc/kg/day and oliguria as 0.5–1 cc/kg/day. Normal urine output in children, therefore, is any value greater than 1 cc/kg/day.

6. What is the Apgar score?

The Apgar score is a clinical assessment of the newborn infant developed by Virginia Apgar, a New Jersey anesthesiologist. It is often remembered as the acronym:

A = **Appearance** (skin color)
P = **Pulse**
G = **Grimace** (reflex irritability)
A = **Activity**
R = **Respiration**

The Apgar score is measured at 1 minute after birth and then repeated 5 minutes later. If the neonate is doing poorly, the Apgar score should be measured again after 10 minutes. The maximal score is 10. Most infants do not get a perfect 10 because they lose a point for skin color. Thus, a score equal to or greater than 8 usually indicates normal cardiopulmonary function and successful transition to postnatal life. Conversely, a score of 3–4 at 1 minute indicates severe cardiopulmonary depression and need for resuscitation, whereas a score of 5 or 6 indicates mild central nervous system depression.

The Apgar Test

SIGN	SCORE		
	0	1	2
Color	Blue, pale	Pink body with blue extremities	Completely pink
Heart rate	Absent	Below 100	Over 100
Reflex irritability*	No response	Grimace	Sneeze or cough
Muscle tone	Flaccid	Some flexion of the extremities	Good flexion of the extremities
Respiratory effort	Absent	Weak, irregular	Good crying

* Determined by placing a soft catheter into the external nares.

7. How do you assess acute illness in an infant?

Assessing the degree of toxicity of an infant or toddler during a febrile illness is important and usually is accomplished by the *Acute Illness Observation Scales* (AIOS). The AIOS is composed of six items, each with a 3-point scale (1 = normal, 3 = moderate impairment, 5 = severe impairment). The AIOS scores range from 6 (optimal) to 30 (most toxic). A score greater than 10 usually indicates an ill-appearing child.

Acute Illness Observation Scales

OBSERVATION ITEM	1 NORMAL	3 MODERATE IMPAIRMENT	5 SEVERE IMPAIRMENT
Quality of cry	Strong with normal tone or content and not crying	Whimpering or sobbing	Weak, moaning, or high-pitched
Reaction to parent stimulation	Cries briefly then stops or content and not crying	Cries off and on	Continual cry or hardly responds
State variation	If awake, stays awake; if asleep and stimulated, wakes up quickly	Eyes close briefly, or awakes with prolonged stimulation	Falls to sleep or will not rouse
Color	Pink	Pale extremities or acrocyanosis	Pale, cyanotic, mottled, or ashen
Hydration	Skin and eyes normal, mucous membranes moist	Skin and eyes normal and mouth slightly dry	Skin doughy or tented and dry mucous membranes and/or sunken eyes
Response to social overtures	Smiles or alerts (≤ 2 mo)	Brief smile or alerts briefly (≤ 2 mo)	No smile Face anxious, dull, expressionless or no alerting (≤ 2 mo)

Adapted from Willms JL, Schneiderman H, Algranati PS: Physical Diagnosis. Baltimore, Williams & Wilkins, 1994.

GENERAL APPROACH

8. What is the significance of dry mucous membranes?

Dry mucous membranes signify early dehydration. Several physical findings suggest dehydration in children. The number of findings increases with the severity of the condition:

1. **Mild dehydration** leads to tachycardia and dry mucous membranes.

2. **Moderate dehydration** is also associated with sunken eyes, a sunken fontanel, and disappearance of tears.

3. **Severe dehydration** is usually manifested by cold, dry, and mottled skin; decreased skin turgor; prolonged refill time; and, eventually, hypotension.

9. How do you assess skin turgor in a child?

By pinching the abdominal skin of the child, pulling it upward over the abdominal plane, and suddenly releasing it. Skin turgor is expressed by the degree of skin elasticity and by its ability to spring back into place. Tenting of the skin (i.e., persistence of the skin in a crease located above the abdominal plane) is therefore a useful sign of significant dehydration. Tenting, however, may be absent in cases of obesity or dehydration associated with hypernatremia because skin turgor reflects not only hydration (including electrolyte status) but also nutrition. More specifically, skin turgor is related to the amount of subcutaneous fat.

Pearl. Assessment of skin turgor is valuable to determine not only the degree of hydration of a child but also the degree of nutrition.

10. What does poor subcutaneous tissue suggest?

Malnutrition. A well-nourished child has a good store of subcutaneous fat that is easily palpated on examination of the extremities and abdomen. A child who is malnourished, on the other hand, feels like "skin and bones." This finding reflects the presence of diminished subcutaneous tissue.

11. What is the general appearance of a child in shock?

General appearance depends on end-organ damage. Three main organ systems can be easily assessed to help determine if a patient is in shock: (1) the skin, (2) the kidneys, and (3) the brain:

1. A mottled appearance or poor capillary refill (> 2 seconds) is a sign of shock.

2. Poor urine output is also a sign of shock. Because the kidneys are not adequately perfused, they cannot produce urine.

3. Lethargy, another sign of shock, indicates insufficient brain perfusion.

12. How do you assess capillary refill time?

By squeezing the infant's fingertip between your thumb and index finger until it blanches and then suddenly releasing it. The number of seconds that it takes for the fingertip to regain its color is the capillary refill time.

13. What is the difference between compensated and uncompensated shock?

Shock is defined as the inability of the blood supply to meet the metabolic requirements of the various organs. In **compensated shock**, therefore, the child is still able to maintain normal blood pressure. If this hemodynamic imbalance is not promptly corrected, the child progresses to **uncompensated shock**, the stage of cardiovascular instability in which blood pressure no longer can be maintained. Uncompensated shock is ominous and leads to cardiorespiratory failure if not treated quickly.

HEAD, EYES, EARS, NOSE, AND THROAT

14. When does the anterior fontanel close?

The anterior fontanel (in French *fontanel* = fountain) may actually enlarge after birth. But by age 6 months the fontanel should begin to decrease in size, and by 9–18 months it should be fully closed.

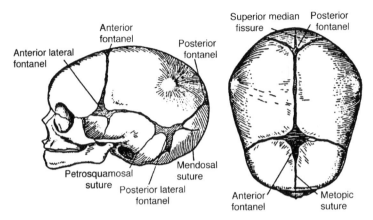

The cranium at birth, showing major sutures and fontanels. No attempt is made to show molding or overlapping of bones, which sometimes occurs at birth. (From Silverman FN, Kuhn JP (eds): Caffey's Pediatric X-Ray Diagnosis, 9th ed. St. Louis, Mosby, 1993, p 5, with permission.)

15. When does the posterior fontanel close?

The posterior fontanel is often closed at birth; it usually is closed by 2–4 months of age.

16. When do cranial sutures fuse?

Not until early adulthood. Until that time, they are composed of relatively pliable fibrous tissue. If one or more of these sutures closes prematurely (craniosynostosis), deformity of the head and damage to the brain may result.

17. What is the significance of a bulging or sunken fontanel?

The normal fontanel of a sitting baby is soft and slightly sunken. Bulging indicates an increase in intracranial pressure, whereas a sunken fontanel is an important sign of dehydration.

18. What is an epicanthal fold?

It is a small fold of skin that covers the medial corner of the eye. If associated with other abnormalities (see below), an abnormal epicanthal fold should raise the suspicion of Down syndrome.

19. How does one determine the palpebral fissure slant?

By drawing an imaginary line through the medial and lateral canthus of each eye (the canthus is the corner of the eye). If this line slants upward while going from medial to lateral, the palpebral fissure has a **mongoloid slant**. Conversely, if the line slants downward, the palpebral fissure has an **antimongoloid slant**. These findings may be related to the patient's ethnic background or may be clues to the presence of Down syndrome.

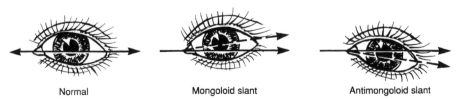

| Normal | Mongoloid slant | Antimongoloid slant |

Adapted from Willms JL, Schneidermann H, Algranati PS: Physical Diagnosis. Baltimore, Williams & Wilkins, 1994.

20. Where is the conjunctiva located?

Over the sclera (bulbar conjunctiva) and, through back reflection, over the inside of the eyelid (palpebral conjunctiva). Both bulbar and palpebral conjunctivae should be inspected carefully. This goal is easily accomplished by everting the upper and lower eyelid. This maneuver is essential to identify lesions of the conjunctiva and to locate (and remove) foreign bodies.

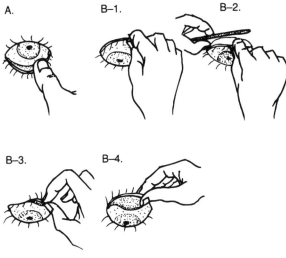

A, Eversion of the lower lid is easily accomplished with the thumb or index finger pressing on the soft tissue below the lid and pulling it downward. B, Eversion of the upper lid. Tell the patient to look downward and *(1)* with the right thumb and forefinger grasp a few cilia of the upper eyelid and pull the lid away from the globe; *(2)* lay an applicator along the crease made by the superior edge of the tarsal plate and the soft adjacent tissue; *(3)* quickly fold the lid over the applicator so the tarsal plate turns over and its upper edge faces downward; *(4)* replace the right thumb and finger by the corresponding left ones to hold the lid. (From DeGowin R: DeGowin and DeGowin's Diagnostic Examination, 6th ed. New York, McGraw-Hill, 1994, with permission.)

21. What is the mechanism for chlamydial conjunctivitis?

In the United States conjunctivitis due to *Chlamydia trachomatis* (from the Greek *trachoma* = rough, harsh) is primarily a sexually transmitted disease. Newborns acquire the organism while passing through an infected birth canal. Chlamydial conjunctivitis (trachoma) is present at 5–14 days of life with the typical findings of an injected bulbar and palpebral conjunctiva as well as a nonpurulent discharge. In most parts of the world, however, trachoma is an endemic disease affecting not only children but also adults. This form of chlamydial conjunctivitis (often called contagious granular conjunctivitis or Egyptian ophthalmia) remains the most common cause of preventable blindness in several parts of North Africa, sub-Saharan Africa, the Middle East, and Asia. In these countries transmission of the disease is not venereal but from eye to eye via mechanisms such as hands, towels, or flies. The clinical presentation is characterized initially by hypertrophy of the conjunctiva with formation of minute grayish or yellowish translucent granules that represent small lymphoid follicles and usually are located on the upper tarsal conjunctiva. As the inflammation progresses, scarring of the conjunctiva occurs and, in turn, causes retraction and distortion of the eyelids with inward movement of the eyelashes (entropion). This inversion of the eyelashes (with its resulting brushing against the cornea) eventually causes corneal abrasion and blindness.

22. How is gonococcal conjunctivitis acquired?

During delivery. It usually presents at 2–5 days of life with injected bulbar and palpebral conjunctivitis, thick and purulent discharge, and swollen eyelids. Gonococcal conjunctivitis may lead to erosion of the cornea and even perforation of the globe. Therefore, prompt and aggressive treatment is imperative.

23. What treatment is used in the delivery room to prevent gonococcal conjunctivitis?

Instillation of 1% silver nitrate into the eyes of the newborn. This procedure, however, may cause chemical conjunctivitis. Because of this side effect, many hospitals use antibiotic ointment (such as 0.5% erythromycin), which is as effective as silver nitrate without the irritant side effects. Because antibiotic ointment also can prevent trachoma, it has become the standard eye prophylaxis in newborns.

24. What is the significance of a mucus discharge from an infant's eye without associated evidence of conjunctivitis?

It indicates an obstructed nasolacrimal duct (blocked tear duct). This finding is quite common during infancy and usually becomes symptomatic after the first few weeks of life because of the time discrepancy between production of tears (which begins at about 2–3 months) and patency of the nasolacrimal duct (which is not complete until 5–7 months). Usually this blockage resolves spontaneously before 1 year of age. Thus, the typical treatment for tearing or crusting of eye secretions in one or both eyes of a child less than 1 year of age should be simply to wipe away the discharge with a clean moist cloth. On the other hand, if tearing persists after 1 year of age, the child should be referred to an ophthalmologist to probe the duct and rule out obstruction. Massage over the nasolacrimal sac (which consists of stroking the side of the nose in a repeated downward motion) is also clinically valuable. A purulent or mucoid discharge in response to massage further supports a diagnosis of nasolacrimal obstruction.

Pearl. *Obstruction of the nasolacrimal ducts is not associated with reddened conjunctivae. Therefore, reddening of the eye suggests a diagnosis of conjunctivitis.*

25. What is the alternate cover test?

It is a bedside maneuver for determining whether a child has useful vision in each eye and, therefore, is a good tool for assessment of strabismus. The maneuver is carried out by having the patient fixate on a distant object while the examiner covers the eyes alternately and watches closely for fixation movement by the uncovered eye. In older infants, the covering can be obtained by using the thumb and rapidly swinging it over the child's eyes. Movement of the uncovered eye indicates that it is returning from a convergent or divergent position and that the patient therefore has strabismus. Conversely, if the eye does not move when it is uncovered, no strabismus is present. Intermittent misalignment of the eyes is not uncommon in newborns and young infants but usually disappears by 3 months of age. Conversely, a fixed misalignment of the eyes is always abnormal.

26. What is the corneal light reflex?

It is another maneuver often used to screen children for strabismus and may be carried out in infants over 3–4 months of age. The maneuver consists of testing for asymmetric reflection of a light shined over the corneas. The corneal light reflex is normal in pseudostrabismus (see chapter 4).

27. What does leukocoria suggest?

Loss of the normal red reflex. The term *leukocoria* means white pupil or, more specifically, a white pupillary reflex (see chapter 4). When looking at an infant's eye from a distance of 10–12 inches with an ophthalmoscope with zero diopters, one should be able to see a normal red reflex, which indicates no serious obstruction to light between the cornea and retina. Absence of the red reflex (with a pupil that looks white) is, therefore, a sign of leukocoria and in a child may suggest one of the following abnormalities: retinoblastoma, cataract, retinopathy of prematurity, or retinal detachment. All patients with leukocoria should be referred to an ophthalmologist.

28. What is aniridia? With what neoplasm is it associated?

Congenital aniridia (absence of the iris) and hypoplasia of the iris are associated with an increased incidence of Wilms' tumor (nephroblastoma of children described in 1899 by the German surgeon Max Wilms). Serial examinations of the abdomen, along with periodic abdominal ultrasounds, are therefore required. The condition is autosomal dominant and associated with a specific deletion of chromosome 11.

29. How do you determine the presence of low-set ears?

By drawing an imaginary horizontal line between the medial corners of the eyes and the ears. Normally at least one-tenth to one-fifth of the total height of the ear should be above this line. If not, the ears are considered low-set. This important finding often is associated with renal and auditory abnormalities. The method of determining the setting of the ears, therefore, is quite valuable and can be used in any age group.

If $\frac{a}{b} \times 100 \leq 10$,
the ears are low set.

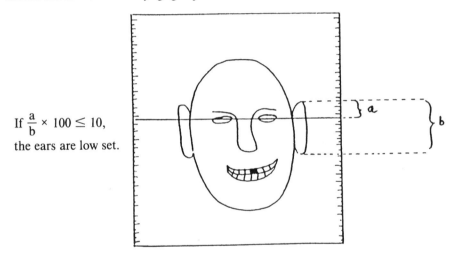

From Markel H, Oski J, Oski F, McMillan J: The Portable Pediatrician. Philadelphia, Hanley & Belfus, 1992, with permission.

30. What are the typical physical findings in otitis media?

Otitis media is an infection of the middle ear. Otoscopic examination is key to its diagnosis. Children with otitis media, in fact, may appear entirely well. The typical abnormalities found by visualizing the tympanic membrane (TM) are listed below in temporal sequence:

1. An **increase in blood flow to the TM** is revealed as membrane redness or injection.

2. **Thickening of the TM** is recognized by loss of the cone of light that normally is seen on an intact membrane. Because of this loss, the light reflecting off the TM becomes diffuse.

3. **Inability to visualize the middle ear ossicles**. Thickening of the membrane and loss of translucency, combined with the presence of fluid, make it impossible to visualize the ossicles. Inability to see the ossicles is called loss of landmarks.

4. Because the middle ear is frequently filled with serous fluid or purulent material, insufflation of air against the TM results in **poor or no mobility of the membrane**. An air-fluid level also may be seen behind the eardrum, along with bubbles. This finding is particularly common in serous otitis media, which is characterized by the presence of fluid in the middle ear without the presence of acute inflammation.

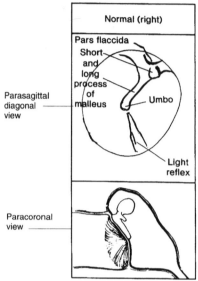
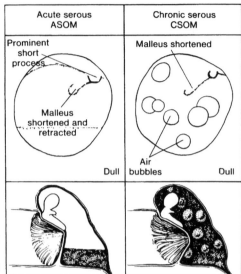

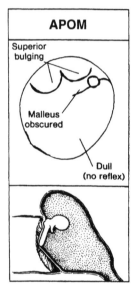

ASOM = acute serous otitis media, CSOM = chronic serous otitis, APOM = acute purulent otitis media. (Adapted from Willms JL, Schneidermann H, Algranati PS: Physical Diagnosis. Baltimore, Williams & Wilkins, 1994).

31. What is the embryogenesis of preauricular ducts and skin tags?

The pinna and tragus are formed from fusion of the first and second branchial arches. Abnormal fusion of these arches leads to preauricular ducts and skin tags. Such anomalies may be an isolated finding or associated with other face and ear abnormalities. Tags on or near the ears also may be found in normal children.

32. Why does nasal obstruction cause a respiratory emergency in infants?

Because infants are obligate nose breathers, normal respiration requires a patent nasal airway. Therefore, nasal obstruction causes respiratory distress. Bilateral choanal atresia, for example, presents early in life with respiratory distress. If no air appears to be flowing through a nostril, obstruction can be confirmed by trying to pass a number 5 or 8 French catheter through each external naris into the posterior nasopharynx.

33. What is the asymmetric crying facies syndrome?

It is a syndrome characterized by the inability of one side of the infant's mouth to turn down upon crying and indicates absence of the depressor anguli oris muscle. Usually cardiac and other abnormalities are associated findings.

34. At what age do infants' teeth emerge?

Normal eruption of teeth varies widely. Typically, the first teeth to erupt are the two lower central incisors (at 5–12 months of age). All deciduous or baby teeth should have erupted by the end of the third year; they should have fallen by 12–13 years of age.

35. At what age are children at risk for "strep throat"?

At 2 years of age or older; the highest incidence is at 6–8 years. The diagnosis of streptococcal pharyngitis at an age younger than 2 years is quite uncommon, accounting for only a few percent of cases. Most cases of strep throat occur from December to May with the peak in March.

36. How do you assess a patient for sinusitis?

Much as you assess sinusitis in an adult. In younger children, however, the paranasal sinuses develop at different rates and therefore may not yet be fully formed. If formed, they are susceptible to infection like the sinuses of older children and adults and therefore should be examined accordingly.

The exam of an older child or adolescent should begin with the nostrils. The examiner should use a short, wide speculum mounted on a handheld otoscope. The nasal mucosa should be inspected for color, edema, presence of nasal secretions and/or polyps, and characteristics of the septum. Septal deviation and nasal polyps in fact may contribute to nasal obstruction and recurrent sinusitis. Purulent secretion from the middle meatus is highly predictive of maxillary sinusitis.

Palpation for sinus tenderness should be carried out over the maxillary and frontal sinuses (ethmoid and sphenoid sinuses cannot be adequately assessed during physical exam). Tapping of the maxillary teeth also should be carried out, because 5–10% of all cases of maxillary sinusitis are secondary to dental root infection (in this case, tapping of the molars elicits pain). Finally, transillumination of the maxillary sinuses should be considered, but the test requires a completely darkened room, a proper instrument, and good technique. Interobserver agreement has been found to be low in examination of the sinuses; the only exception is assessment for the presence of sinus tenderness. Compared with roentgenologic standards, the accuracy of physical exam maneuvers, including transillumination, is quite wanting. Sinus tenderness, for example, has been found to have poor sensitivity and specificity in adults (48–50% and 62–65%, respectively, in two different studies in adults). In children sinusitis may be quite insidious, although concurrent otitis media is usually quite common. Indeed, the presence of tympanic membrane changes has a sensitivity of 68% in children and is the most common physical finding associated with sinusitis. Conversely, a fever higher than 101° is uncommon in children, with a sensitivity of only 12–21%.

37. What are the classic physical findings of strep throat?

Acute onset of fever, throat pain, and dysphagia after a 2–5-day incubation period. Physical findings include an erythematous pharynx with exudate on the tonsils and tender cervical lymphadenopathy. Patients also may have palatal petechiae and a "strawberry tongue" (reddened tongue with accentuation of papillae). Certain streptococcal strains also release a toxin, resulting in the red, sandpaper-like rash of scarlet fever.

NECK

38. At what size is a lymph node considered enlarged?

It depends on the area. In fact, normal infants and children may have small, pea-sized, soft, nontender, and palpable lymph nodes in the cervical, occipital, inguinal, and axillary areas. Such nodes are commonly referred to as "shotty" (they resemble buckshots) and are entirely normal. They usually represent the sequelae of a preceding viral infection and tend to resolve over time.

Anterior cervical adenopathy usually reflects upper airway infections and infection of the anterior portion of the mouth. Conversely, posterior cervical adenopathy usually reflects otitis media and scalp irritations. Shotty nodes should be smaller than 1 cm. In the cervical area, however, normal shotty lymph nodes may be smaller than 2 cm.

39. Are supraclavicular nodes normally palpable in infancy?
No. Palpable supraclavicular nodes are always pathologic. In fact, a palpable right supraclavicular node often is associated with lymphomas of the mediastinum, whereas a palpable left supraclavicular node suggests an abdominal malignancy (see chapter 18). The presence of an epitrochlear node in the absence of an arm infection also should be considered abnormal.

40. What are the features of an infected lymph node?
Enlargement, tenderness, warmth, and erythema of the overlying skin. The patient also may develop fever. Infected lymph nodes should be freely movable.

41. What are the features of a cancerous lymph node?
Firmness, rubbery quality, lack of tenderness, and fixation to surrounding structures. These features characterize the lymph nodes in Hodgkin's disease and lymphosarcoma.

42. What is torticollis?
It is an abnormal posture of head and neck in which the head is tilted to one side and the chin to the opposite side. This condition may have different causes, which usually are grouped as either congenital or acquired.
Congenital muscular torticollis, the most common form of torticollis in the neonatal period, is caused by a fibrotic contracture and shortening of the sternocleidomastoid muscle. On physical exam, the muscle is firm, nontender, and contracted to the point that it almost resembles a mass. Other forms of congenital torticollis usually involve abnormalities of the cervical vertebrae.
Acquired torticollis is often due to gastroesophageal reflux. Other causes include (1) strabismus (with tilting of the head to prevent double vision); (2) posterior fossa tumors (with tilting of the head to the affected side); (3) retropharyngeal abscess; (4) cervical lymphadenitis; (5) osteoid osteoma of the cervical vertebra; (6) eosinophilic granuloma involving the cervical vertebra; and (7) subluxation of the atlantoaxial joint.

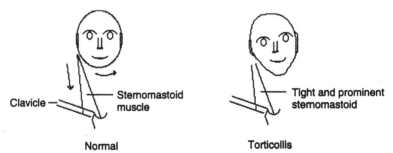

From Mehta AJ: Common Musculoskeletal Problems. Philadelphia, Hanley & Belfus, 1997, with permission.

43. What is paroxysmal torticollis?
It is a recurrent form of torticollis, which usually presents for no underlying reason. It may occur in infants and usually has a benign course.

44. What is neck webbing?
A very broad neck due to the presence of lateral folds of skin that extend from the clavicle to the head (pterygium colli). It typically occurs in Turner's syndrome but also may be present in other congenital conditions (see chapter 7).

HEART

45. What is the significance of cyanosis in a child?

Cyanosis may be the hallmark of congenital heart disease with a right-to-left shunt. Right-to-left shunts may result from an obstruction to right ventricular outflow in the setting of congenital atrial or ventricular septal defect (such as pulmonic stenosis) or from pulmonary hypertension in patients with septal defects or patent ductus arteriosus (Eisenmenger's syndrome).

46. How is the point of maximal intensity (PMI) different in infants and adults?

The PMI is in different positions in infants and adults. In palpating the chest of a normal adult, the PMI of the heart is usually in the fifth intercostal space along the anterior axillary line. In a normal infant, on the other hand, the PMI is in the fourth intercostal space along the midclavicular line. Hence, detecting a PMI in the anterior axillary line of the fifth intercostal space/anterior axillary line of an infant indicates a laterally displaced and clinically abnormal apical impulse.

47. What does a laterally displaced PMI suggest?

Left ventricular enlargement.

48. Where should you palpate a right ventricular (RV) impulse in an infant?

Nowhere. In fact, palpating just below the xiphoid process of the sternum (the area of chest projection of the right ventricle) should yield no impulse in a normal infant. Detection of a cardiac impulse in this region indicates a separate right ventricular impulse, which is a sign of disease.

49. What does a separate RV impulse suggest?

Right ventricular enlargement.

50. What are the four cardinal signs of congestive heart failure in small children?

1. Tachycardia
2. Tachypnea with shallow respirations and retractions
3. Cardiomegaly
4. Hepatomegaly

Conversely, findings such as peripheral edema, crackles, or wheezes (which may be common in the diagnosis of congestive heart failure in adults) tend to present much later in children. Similarly, distention of the neck veins is difficult to detect in infants. In fact, infants with congestive heart failure often are recognized because of tachycardia, irritability, profuse sweating (especially when feeding), and failure to thrive.

Pearl. *Persistent tachycardia (with a heart rate > 200 beats/min) in newborns or tachycardia > 150 beats/min in children up to 1 year of age should cause great concern.*

51. What is an innocent murmur?

An innocent murmur is not related to anatomic abnormality or significant heart disease. All innocent murmurs are systolic. The only exception is the venous hum, which is continuous. An exclusively diastolic murmur, therefore, should be considered pathologic until proved otherwise.

52. What does a murmur of peripheral pulmonic stenosis (PPS) sound like?

PPS causes a benign, short, and blowing midsystolic murmur that is flow-related, always less than grade 2/6, and not due to anatomic obstruction. In fact, the murmur is due to the oblique orientation of the pulmonary arteries in young infants, which causes turbulence in the flow. The PPS murmur is the most common innocent murmur in the newborn and usually is heard best over the distribution of the pulmonary arteries (left and right sternal border with transmission to the back and axilla). Indeed, a clue to the diagnosis is its audibility over both the right and left side of the chest (due to its origin in the peripheral pulmonary arteries). The PPS murmur usually resolves by 3 months of age.

53. Which innocent murmurs can be heard in preschool children?

Many. In fact, the preschool years are the most common age for detecting innocent murmurs (see chapter 12). The most common examples are listed below:

1. **Still's murmur:** a low-pitched, early systolic ejection murmur, best heard midway between the left lower sternal border and the apex. It is classically louder in the supine position. Indeed, the hallmark of this murmur is that it softens and even disappears upon standing. Still's murmur has a musical or vibratory quality (as opposed to the harsh quality of pathologic murmurs) and is rare before 2 years of age.

2. **Venous hum:** a continuous murmur (and therefore audible both in systole and diastole) that typically is heard over the right clavicular area (and at times even over the left infraclavicular area). It is produced by blood flowing through the great veins of the neck and therefore can be silenced by having the patient turn his or her head away from the side of the murmur or by simply compressing the ipsilateral internal jugular vein.

3. **Carotid bruit:** a systolic ejection murmur heard over the carotids. It classically softens when the stethoscope is moved downward toward the aortic and pulmonary areas.

54. Which innocent murmur can be heard in school-aged children?

The pulmonary flow murmur.

55. What findings in a newborn should raise the suspicion of congenital heart disease?

A persistent murmur (that is not the murmur of peripheral pulmonic stenosis), central cyanosis, pallor, diminished or absent peripheral pulses, respiratory distress, and poor feeding with failure to thrive. Any of the above should raise the suspicion of congenital heart disease.

56. What is the most common congenital heart disease?

Ventricular septal defect (VSD).

57. When does the murmur of VSD become audible?

Sometimes at birth but more often after several weeks of age, when pulmonic resistances have fallen and the left-to-right shunt has increased.

58. What does a VSD murmur sound like?

It is a harsh systolic murmur, often holosystolic in duration with more of a regurgitant than an ejection quality. In fact, the murmur often begins with S1 and ends with S2, covering them to the point of making both inaudible. The VSD murmur is best heard at the left lower or midsternal border. Its intensity is inversely related to the size of the defect (smaller defects sound louder and vice versa). Larger defects may be associated with a diastolic rumble produced by the large amount of shunted blood flowing from the left atrium into the left ventricle.

59. What does a murmur of atrial septal defect (ASD) sound like?

It does not sound. Flow through the ASD is silent because the interatrial pressure gradients are usually too low to generate enough turbulence to cause a murmur (this, of course, is not the case with VSDs). Thus, the murmur heard in patients with ASD (which is a soft systolic murmur over the left upper sternal border) is produced by increased flow over the pulmonary artery, caused by the left-to-right shunt seen in the early phases of ASD. The distinguishing auscultatory finding is the fixed splitting of the second heart sound, which persists in the standing position.

60. What does a murmur of patent ductus arteriosus sound like?

It sounds like a kite-shaped, to-and-fro, continuous, machinery-like murmur, also described as a "train-in-tunnel" murmur. It is heard not only in systole but also beyond S2 and well into diastole. The term *machinery-like* refers to the mechanical quality, and *continuous* refers to its duration throughout systole and diastole without pause. The murmur of patent ductus arteriosus is best heard anteriorly over the left upper sternal border and posteriorly over the left interscapular area.

61. What is the significance of femoral pulses that are diminished or delayed compared with brachial or radial pulses?

This finding suggests coarctation of the aorta, which is constriction of the aorta at any point from its ascending portion downward (but usually before or after the arch origin of the great vessels). Further evaluation usually is carried out by four-extremity blood pressure measurement, which should reveal higher pressures in the upper than in the lower extremities. This finding usually is diagnostic. In fact, the systolic blood pressure in the arms normally should be lower (usually by 10–20 mmHg), not higher, than in the legs.

LUNGS

62. What are the signs of respiratory distress in a child?

Much the same as in an adult: tachypnea, audible expiratory grunting, and nasal flaring as well as supraclavicular, intercostal, and subcostal retractions.

63. What is the classic cough in chlamydial pneumonia?

Because of its peculiar quality, this persistent and dry cough is often called a staccato cough (in Italian *staccato* = detached). In musical expression staccato refers to a sound composed of abrupt and disconnected parts, much like the cough of patients with chlamydial pneumonia.

64. How do newborns acquire chlamydial infection?

Usually they acquire it at birth by passing through an infected birth canal. Infection may lead to conjunctivitis and nasopharyngeal carriage of the organism with subsequent infection of the lower respiratory system. Conjunctivitis usually presents at 5–14 days, whereas the pneumonia presents at 1–4 months.

65. What is the classic cough of pertussis in an infant?

The classic "whooping" cough of pertussis is characterized by coughing spasms interspersed with deep, noisy inspirations. Only toddlers actually produce the typical "whoops"; infants with pertussis do not have enough intrathoracic pressure to generate the typical gasping noise. Thus, the classic cough of pertussis infants is usually a cluster of coughs closely grouped together without interspersed inspirations. It commonly is called a paroxysmal cough.

66. What causes crackles in children?

Much the same conditions that cause crackles in adults, with the exception of bronchiolitis, which is much more common in pediatric than adult medicine. Other conditions that cause crackles in children are pneumonia, pulmonary edema, tuberculosis, and bronchiectasis. Crackles also may be heard in a normal and healthy patient but should clear after a series of deep inspirations (see chapter 14).

67. What causes wheezing in children?

Usually asthma, but as the old saying goes, "Not all that wheezes is asthma." Causes of wheezing in children may include foreign bodies (particularly if localized), viral pneumonia, bronchiolitis, cystic fibrosis, gastroesophageal reflux with or without aspiration, vascular rings and slings, congestive heart failure, a mediastinal mass compressing lower airways, bronchopulmonary dysplasia, and tracheoesophageal fistula. Wheezes can be heard on both inspiration and expiration but usually are louder on expiration when the airways are narrower. Wheezes are never inspiratory only (an inspiratory wheeze is, by definition, a stridor).

68. What causes stridor in children?

Usually foreign bodies (children love to put stuff in their mouth), but any other cause of upper airway airflow obstruction may result in stridor. Examples include inflammatory, infectious, congenital, and even neoplastic processes. A common condition is croup (in Scottish *kropan* = to cry aloud), an inflammatory process of the upper airways that is common among children. It is characterized by varying degrees of epiglottitis, laryngitis, and tracheobronchitis, which may present with difficult and noisy respiration and a hoarse cough. A viral infection is responsible for 85% of cases and is the most common cause before the age of 3 years; *Hemophilus influenzae* type B has essentially disappeared with the greater availability of immunizations. Other causes of stridor in children include tracheobronchitis with laryngeal edema and spasm, sleep apnea as a result of hypertrophied tonsils, and, in the olden days, diphtheria. In infants developmental problems are not uncommon. Examples include vascular abnormalities of the aortic arch and its branches and glottic or subglottic webs.

69. What are the distinguishing characteristics of stridor?

Stridor is a harsh, high-pitched sound, generated by extrathoracic airflow obstruction and therefore best heard on inspiration. In a child, stridor usually has a distinctive clinical presentation due to its association with marked retraction of the supraclavicular, suprasternal, and subcostal spaces. Stridor is more common in children than in adults because the upper airways of infants and children are much smaller. Therefore, a small amount of inflammation that would cause minimal difficulty in an adult may lead to respiratory obstruction and stridor in a great number of infants.

Pearl.   Forced pharyngeal examination may precipitate acute airway obstruction in children with epiglottitis and should not be attempted in children who appear ill and have stridor.

ABDOMEN

70. Why do you auscultate before you palpate the abdomen?

Because deep palpation may cause transient ileus and therefore compromise the effectiveness of auscultation. The routine order of examination is to inspect, palpate, percuss, and then auscultate, but in examining the abdomen one should auscultate before palpating.

71. In what disease do you palpate an "olive"?

In pyloric stenosis a mass (described as having the shape of an olive) often can be palpated in the epigastric area just to the right of the midline. In the appropriate clinical setting of a 2-week to 3-month old infant with nonbilious projectile vomiting who wants to feed immediately after vomiting, the palpation of an olive is sufficient to establish a diagnosis of pyloric stenosis without further studies. If confirmatory testing is required, an abdominal ultrasound usually reveals the hypertrophic pylorus. Patients usually present to the physician after the first week or two of life because of projectile vomiting; they also may show signs of profound dehydration.

72. What does bilious vomiting suggest?

Bile-stained emesis is not an uncommon finding in children and suggests an intestinal obstruction because the biliary and the pancreatic ducts come together at the ampulla of Vater, where they empty into the small intestine. Thus, bile-stained emesis usually indicates an obstruction that is distal to the ampulla of Vater.

73. In what disease do you find intermittent fussiness with a sausage-shaped mass and eventually "currant jelly" stools and lethargy?

In intussusception, which consists of the telescoping of an intestinal segment into the segment just below it. The condition typically presents with intermittent episodes of pain and crying. Eventually, the child becomes lethargic and develops symptoms of shock. Abdominal exam frequently reveals a sausage-shaped mass in the right upper quadrant. Children with intussusception also frequently pass stools with blood and mucus known as "currant jelly stools." The diagnosis usually is established by history and physical exam. An abdominal roentgenogram may reveal a density in the area of the intussusception. Barium or air-contrast enema may be not only diagnostic but also therapeutic; the intussusception is reduced by the pressure of the enema.

74. Where does a patient with pancreatitis have pain?

Over the epigastrium. This constant pain usually radiates to the back. As a result, patients with pancreatitis tend to lie on the side and to stay as still as possible. Nausea and vomiting are often present. Examination of the abdomen reveals few bowel sounds and exquisite tenderness.

75. Where does a patient with appendicitis have pain?

It depends on the stage of the process. Initially, when the inflammatory process is limited to the visceral peritoneum, the pain of appendicitis is vague and localized in the umbilical area. As the overlying parietal peritoneum becomes inflamed, the pain becomes localized to the right lower quadrant. In older children the pain is usually well localized to McBurney's point (one-third of the way down the line connecting the anterior superior iliac spine and umbilicus). Atypical location of the appendix (such as retrocecal) may make the diagnosis of appendicitis even more difficult.

GENITALIA

76. What is physiologic galactorrhea?

Discharge of a milky substance from the breast. It may occur by the end of the first week of life in both sexes and is due to the presence of circulating maternal hormones. Neonates, therefore, have palpable breast tissue. Physiologic galactorrhea usually resolves within several weeks.

77. What are the two different types of inguinal hernias?

1. **Direct hernias** can be palpated as a swelling in the inguinal area and may be more pronounced when the patient is straining or crying.

2. **Indirect hernias** usually present as a swelling of the scrotum. This type of hernia is more common in children than adults.

78. How can you differentiate between a hydrocele and an indirect hernia?

Both indirect hernias and hydroceles may present as swelling of the scrotum. A hydrocele, however, is not due to viscus migration but to accumulation of fluid in the tunica vaginalis. Therefore, it does not increase in size with straining or crying. Other diagnostic features of a hydrocele include the following:

1. The mass easily transilluminates.
2. The mass cannot be reduced.
3. There are no bowel sounds over the mass.

Small hydroceles are quite common during early infancy, do *not* communicate with the peritoneal cavity, and usually resolve completely by 4–6 months of age. Conversely, hydroceles that vary in size over time are usually larger, communicating, and rarely resolving. Hydroceles of this type and, in general, hydroceles that persist over 6 months of age must be referred to surgery for repair. In fact, many such hydroceles reflect the presence of an indirect inguinal hernia. Rubbing a finger over the skin of the hydrocele often yields a peculiar sensation, commonly called the velvet-glove or silk-glove sign. This sensation feels as if two pieces of velvet or silk were rubbed together.

79. What is hypospadias?

It is a congenital malformation in which the urethral meatus opens on the ventral surface of the penis instead of on its tip (see chapter 16). This abnormality may be mild and occur on the glans (coronal hypospadias); it also may occur near the glans or anywhere else along the shaft. Five percent of patients with hypospadias also have either unilateral or bilateral cryptorchidism. Circumcision should *not* be performed on patients with hypospadias because the foreskin may be needed for repair of the lesion.

80. What is epispadias?

It is a congenital malformation in which the urethral meatus opens on the dorsal side of the penis (see chapter 16). This abnormality is less common than hypospadias. Early urologic consultation is required; circumcision should not be performed.

81. What is a chordee?

Chordee (pronounced kor-day), which is French for corded, also is referred to as penis lunatus (crescent-like penis). This downward curvature of the penis frequently is seen in hypospadias as a result of the congenital shortness of the ventral skin. On more rare occasions, chordee also in encountered in children with a normally situated meatus; ventral fibrous bands result from lack of distensibility. In adults a penis lunatus usually indicates a painful erection with an abnormal curvature of the corpus cavernosum urethrae. This condition usually results from either gonorrhea or Peyronie's disease (see chapter 16).

82. What is the meaning of a unilaterally empty scrotum in an infant?

It indicates an undescended testis (cryptorchidism). This condition should be promptly recognized and corrected in order to avoid testicular atrophy.

83. What is phimosis?

Phimosis is characterized by the inability to retract the foreskin over the glans and usually results from scarring of the foreskin. Almost all uncircumcised male neonates have unretractable foreskins but do not have phimosis. In fact, they simply have adhesions between foreskin and glans with no evidence of scarring. By 4 years of age, adhesions have resolved sufficiently to allow retraction of the foreskin in 80% of such children. Conversely, premature lysis of the adhesions by forceful retraction of the foreskin may cause scarring and therefore lead to true phimosis.

84. What is paraphimosis?

It is the trapping of the retracted foreskin behind the glans. Paraphimosis is a urologic emergency because the trapped foreskin may cause decreased venous flow, which, in turn, may lead to worsening edema and further ischemia. If uncorrected, this condition eventually may cause necrosis of the tip of the penis.

85. What are Tanner's stages for sexual maturation?

They are a valuable method for assessing sexual maturation by observation of (1) breast and pubic hair growth in girls and (2) growth of pubic hair and development of penis, testes, and scrotum in boys. The examiner should record two ratings, one for the pubic hair and the other for the genitalia in boys or the breasts in girls. For Tanner's stages in girls, refer to chapter 17.

EXTREMITIES

86. What are the Ortolani and Barlow maneuvers?

Two bedside maneuvers often carried out in newborns to determine joint stability and to rule out developmental dysplasia of the hip. Because the Ortolani maneuver may become falsely negative after the neonatal period, it should be limited to the examination of newborns. The **Ortolani maneuver** is carried out in the following sequence:

1. The infant lies supine. The examiner flexes the legs at the hips by holding the knees between thumb and first finger. The examiner's thumbs are placed over the infant's lesser trochanters while the first fingers are placed over the greater trochanters.

2. The examiner then applies a downward pressure to the infant's thighs, pushing them toward the examination table. This part of the test represents the **Barlow variation** of the Ortolani maneuver and evaluates dislocatability of the hip. If the examiner feels or hears a clunk while applying the downward pressure, the hip has slid out of the acetabulum and is now dislocated. A hip that is dislocated as a result of the Barlow maneuver is, by definition, dysplastic. A normal hip should not dislocate.

3. Finally, the examiner abducts the hips to almost 90°. If while carrying out this abduction the examiner feels or hears a clunk, the patient's hip probably was initially out of the acetabulum and was put back into the acetabulum as a result of the maneuver. Thus, the Ortolani maneuver tests reducibility of the hip.

Feeling the clunk is even more important than hearing it. A clunk is quite different from a click, a sound that may be produced by the knees and therefore may be present in normal infants. Both the Ortolani and the Barlow maneuvers can be carried out on one hip at a time or on both hips simultaneously. If either of these maneuvers is positive, congenital dysplasia of the hip is likely and can be confirmed by an ultrasound of the hips.

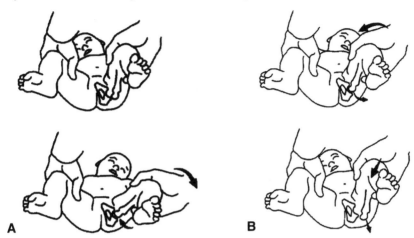

A, The Ortolani test. This maneuver reduces a posteriorly dislocated hip. The affected hip is gently abducted while the femoral head is reduced with an anteriorly directed force provided by the fingers placed over the greater trochanter. *B,* The Barlow test. This maneuver tests for dislocation or subluxation of a reduced hip. This is done by gently adducting the examined hip while directing a posterior force across the hip. (From Staheli LT: Pediatric Orthopedic Secrets. Philadelphia, Hanley & Belfus, 1998, with permission.)

87. What is the angle of gait?

It is the angle between the line of progression and the long axis of the child's foot. In-toeing or out-toeing gaits may be helpful clues to excessive rotational forces to hips, tibias, and feet with resulting torsional deformities.

From Staheli LT: Pediatric Orthopedic Secrets. Philadelphia, Hanley & Belfus, 1998, with permission.

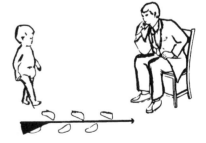

88. What is polydactyly?

It is the presence of an extra digit (literally, *multiple fingers* in Greek). This abnormality may be associated with various syndromes but commonly presents as an isolated finding, usually as a little skin tag on the ulnar side of the hand.

89. What is syndactyly?

It is the fusion or webbing of the digits. Like polydactyly, this finding may be either isolated or associated with other abnormalities.

90. What is Osgood-Schlatter disease?

Osteochondritis of the tibial tuberosity with a resulting partial avulsion. It is typically seen in adolescents (apophysitis tibialis adolescentium), in whom it presents with localized painful swelling of the tibial tuberosity. Usually it is self-limited.

91. Who were Osgood and Schlatter?

Robert B. Osgood (1873–1956) was an American orthopedic surgeon. A Harvard graduate and later the chief of orthopedics at the same school, Osgood was well published in his field, including even a book about the history of orthopedics. He described Osgood-Schlatter disease in 1903.

Carl Schlatter (1865–1934) was a Swiss surgeon who graduated, practiced, and taught in Zurich. Interested in trauma and its management, he even volunteered during World War I to work in a German prisoner-of-war camp and military hospital. He described Osgood-Schlatter disease in 1908.

92. How do you test for scoliosis?

By inspecting the back of a child stripped to the waist. The occiput should be aligned with the intergluteal cleft, and shoulders and scapulas should be at the same height. Once inspection is completed, ask the child to bend down and touch the toes with both arms. Children with scoliosis have a unilateral elevation of the lower ribs. This elevation can be detected even better by previously marking the patient's spinous processes with a felt-tip pen. A deviation of the marks on assuming a bent-forward position confirms the presence of scoliosis.

Pearl. Despite being the most important part of the musculoskeletal examination of children between 6 and 12 years of age, the common methods to detect scoliosis have neither good sensitivity nor good specificity.

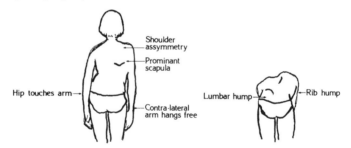

Scoliosis screening test showing the most important diagnostic features. (From Staheli LT: Pediatric Orthopedic Secrets. Philadelphia, Hanley & Belfus, 1998, with permission.)

93. What is a clubfoot?

A foot that points downward and medially, like the foot of a horse. This congenital abnormality should be recognized in the newborn and referred for early surgical correction.

SKIN

94. What is erythema toxicum?

It is a red, blotchy rash characterized by erythematous macules over the trunk, face, and limbs of newborns. At times lesions also may be papules with white centers, but the palms and soles are always spared. Eyrthema toxicum may be seen intermittently during the first 2 weeks of life, requires no treatment, and resolves spontaneously. Despite the name, there is nothing toxic about it. The cause of the rash is unknown, but eosinophils usually can be seen on material obtained by scraping the central white papules.

95. What is transient neonatal pustular melanosis (TNPM)?

TNPM is another benign rash of newborns. In contrast to erythema toxicum, however, TNPM is usually more common in darkly pigmented infants. It presents with vesicles and pustules that are scattered throughout the trunk, face, and limbs of neonates. The rash, however, also may affect palms and soles. Within a few days the lesions rupture and eventually heal with a pigmented macule surrounded by a fine scale, which, ultimately, leaves no sequelae.

Pearl. *Pustules in the newborn should raise the suspicion of infection by* Staphylococcus aureus. *Conversely, vesicles should raise concern for infection by* herpes simplex.

96. What is "cradle cap"?

Cradle cap is a form of seborrhea (see chapter 3) that appears during the first few months of life. It presents as a nonpruritic, greasy, yellow, and scaly rash usually involving the scalp, face, and eyebrows. The retroauricular skin, neck folds, axillae, groin, and umbilicus also may be involved but usually appear erythematous and scaly. Cradle cap presents slightly before eczema (see below) and usually resolves spontaneously after a few months of life.

97. What skin disease involves erythema and scaling of the flexor surfaces?

Atopic dermatitis (eczema). In infants, however, this disease presents a little differently, with dryness of the skin, erythema, scaling and crusting of face (especially the cheeks), scalp, trunk, and extensor surfaces of the extremities. The rash is highly pruritic, and excoriations are quite common. The distribution changes during childhood to involve the flexor surfaces of the extremities and eventually becomes localized to hands, feet, and flexor surfaces in adolescence and adulthood.

98. What is a strawberry hemangioma?

It is a red, well-demarcated vascular birthmark that is strawberry in color. It usually appears after a few weeks, growing in size throughout the first year of life and then beginning a slower period of involution with resolution by middle childhood. At birth it may be invisible, although more often it is heralded by a localized hypovascular lesion covered by telangiectasias.

99. What is a port-wine stain hemangioma?

This congenital vascular lesion is usually present at birth as a unilateral, pinkish/reddish, flat, and well-demarcated hemangioma. It may be found anywhere but tends to prefer the face and neck. Port-wine stain hemangiomas darken with age and match the child's growth. As a result, they may acquire a large, often disfiguring size. If located over the area of distribution of the ophthalmic branch of the trigeminus, a port-wine hemangioma may be an important clue to diagnosis of Sturge-Weber syndrome (cerebral vascular and neurologic abnormalities, mental retardation, and seizures).

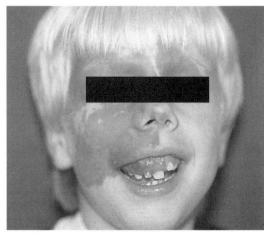

The port-wine stain of Sturge-Weber syndrome. (From Fitzpatrick JE, Aeling JL: Dermatology Secrets. Philadelphia, Hanley & Belfus, 1996, with permission.)

100. How can you differentiate between a mongolian spot and a bruise?

A **mongolian spot** is a bluish macular patch commonly seen on the back and extremities of Asian and African-American babies. It is due to pigment located deeply within the dermis. A **bruise** or **ecchymosis** is caused by extravasation of blood or blood pigments into the skin. Clinically, a mongolian spot is quite homogeneous in appearance, whereas an ecchymosis is usually heterogeneous (because of the variable rate of metabolism of the blood pigments). If the ecchymosis is due to trauma, it is tender on palpation. The mongolian spot, on the other hand, is painless. Whereas a mongolian spot on the sacrum of an infant is a normal variant, central bruising carries a different meaning. It is, in fact, an important sign of child abuse.

101. What is the importance of a hypopigmented ash leaf macule?

It can be an early sign of Bourneville-Pringle disease, also called tuberous sclerosis. These white spots are shaped like an ash leaf and located over the trunk and limbs. They are best seen under ultraviolet light and often are the first manifestation of disease. Other cutaneous findings in tuberous sclerosis include the following:

1. **Shagreen patch** refers to an oval-shaped, thick, rough, and yellowish patch of skin appearing in early childhood on the trunk or lower back. The name derives from the resemblance of the lesion to sharkskin or pigskin.

2. **Angiofibromas of the face**, often referred to as adenoma sebaceous, present as fine, wartlike lesions distributed in a butterfly pattern over cheeks and forehead.

3. **Periungual fibromas.**

Tuberous sclerosis is an important disease because of the associated involvement of internal organs by a series of neoplastic malformations. Sites commonly affected include the heart (rhabdomyomas), brain (cortical astrogliosis, often with calcification), kidneys, liver, pancreas, and adrenal glands. Patients, therefore, may present with seizure, arrhythmia, mental retardation, and various other clinical manifestations.

102. Who were Bourneville and Pringle?

Desiré M. Bourneville (1840–1909) was a French neurologist who worked as a surgeon during the Franco-Prussian War of 1870–1871 and subsequently took part in the Commune of Paris, where he saved a great number of lives.

John James Pringle (1855–1922) was an English dermatologist. A bon vivant and a fine singer with an attractive personality, a handsome figure, and a good sense of humor, Pringle was also a kind and gentle person who treated both charity and private patients with the same degree of compassion. Adored by his many students (who used to refer to him affectionately as "Jimmy"), he had a passion for music and theater. He was famous for having learned his impeccable French while attending performances of the Comédie Française. In his later years he was plagued by tuberculosis and eventually traveled to New Zealand, hoping to regain his health. He died there at age 67.

103. What is the significance of multiple café-au-lait spots?

Café-au-lait spots are oval, tan macules with distinct borders. Many normal people have one or two small spots. A diagnosis of neurofibromatosis, therefore, is suggested only by the presence of (1) six or more café-au-lait spots greater than 5 mm in diameter in a prepubertal child and (2) five or more café-au-lait spots greater than 15 mm in diameter in a postpubertal child.

104. Describe the classic skin rash of chickenpox.

It is a rash characterized by skin lesions that come in crops. They start as erythematous macules that rapidly progress to papules and within 48 hours become vesicles. In turn, the vesicles eventually evolve into pustules, umbilicate, ulcerate, and crust. Successive crops of lesions appear over 2–5 days so that at any one time lesions of all different stages can be seen. Lesions commonly involve mucosal surfaces, and a low-grade fever is common.

105. Which skin disease has erythematous plaques with adherent silvery scales on the extensor surfaces?

Psoriasis. Another form of psoriasis, called guttate psoriasis, presents with discrete papules with adherent silvery scales. Common sites of involvement include scalp, eyebrows, ears, extensor surfaces of upper and lower extremities, gluteal folds, genitalia, and nails.

106. What rash forms a Christmas-tree pattern on the neck?

Pityriasis rosea, which presents as a skin rash with oval, scaly papules on the trunk that follow the lines of skin stress. As a result, they create a Christmas-tree pattern on the back. Most patients with pityriasis have a herald patch that precedes the generalized rash. The herald patch is usually located on the trunk and can be confused with tinea corporis before the appearance of the generalized rash typical of pityriasis rosea.

NEUROLOGIC EXAM

107. When does an infant's Babinski reflex become downgoing?

After 6–9 months of age, by which time the patient's corticospinal tracts become fully myelinated and the Babinski reflex finally changes from upgoing to downgoing. Lack of myelination of the corticospinal tracts also explains why most infants cannot walk until they are at least 9 months of age. They may in fact have the strength to walk before that time, but without corticospinal myelination they do not have the required coordination.

108. Can you test an uncooperative infant's cranial nerves (CNs)?

Yes, but only to a certain point:
- CN II can be tested as the afferent limb of the pupillary light reflex.
- CNs III, IV, and VI can be tested as the nerves responsible for intact extraocular movements.
- CN V can be tested as the afferent limb of the corneal reflex.
- CN VII can be tested as the efferent limb of the corneal reflex.
- CN VIII can be tested as a response to a loud noise.
- CN IX can be tested as the afferent limb of the gag reflex (supplying the posterior one-third of the tongue)
- CN X can be tested as the efferent limb of the gag reflex.
- CNs XI and XII are much more difficult to assess in an uncooperative patient.

109. What is the Moro reflex?

It is one of the many reflexes and motor automatisms that are found exclusively in neonates. It was first described by the Austrian pediatrician Ernst Moro (1874–1951) and is often called the startle reflex. It consists of the symmetric abduction of the upper extremities with extension of the fingers followed by adduction and flexion. It is often associated with a loud cry. Moro's reflex normally is seen during the first 3–6 months of life. Its absence suggests generalized depression of the central or peripheral nervous system. An asymmetric response suggests a focal lesion of the central or peripheral nervous system (as may be seen in various forms of palsies). Finally, its persistence after 6 months of age suggests a cortical disturbance. The reflex can be elicited by a loud noise but more commonly is elicited by passive movement of the child's head. This maneuver usually is carried out by supporting the infant's body in the right hand and the head in the left hand. The head then is allowed suddenly to drop 10–15° (see figure at top of following page).

110. What other motor automatisms can be elicited in an infant?

Based on the infant's position, they are grouped as follows:
1. **Reflexes triggered in an infant turned over and held prone.** The two most common reflexes of this type are Galant's and Perez's reflexes (from the names of the physicians who

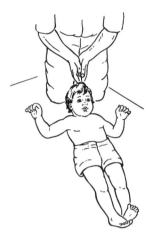

Moro reflex. (From Staheli LT: Pediatric Orthopedic Secrets. Philadelphia, Hanley & Belfus, 1998, with permission.)

described them in the 19th century: the Russian Nikolay Fedorovich Galant and the French Bernard Perez). Both reflexes are normally present in infants, and both should disappear after 2–3 months of age:

- **Galant's reflex** is characterized by an ipsilateral curvature of the spine in response to gentle stroking of one side of the infant's back. The maneuver is carried out along a paravertebral line, 2–3 cm from the midline and from shoulder to buttocks. The normal response is a lateral curvature of the trunk (including shoulder and hip) toward the side of stimulation.
- **Perez's reflex** is characterized by an extension of the whole body triggered by running a finger along the spine from the sacrum to the head. In response to this maneuver, there may even be urination, particularly in newborn infants. As with Galant's reflex, the infant should be held in a prone position.

  2. **Reflexes triggered in an infant lying supine**
- **Rooting response** is elicited by gently touching the corner of the mouth in an infant who is lying on the back with hands held against the chest. The normal response is a turning of the head toward the side of the stimulation and opening the mouth to grasp the finger. This reflex should disappear after 3–4 months of age.
- **Plantar grasp** is elicited by flexing the leg at hip and knee and dorsiflexing the infant's foot. The normal response is plantarflexion of the toes. This reflex should disappear after 9–12 months of age.
- **Palmar grasp** is elicited by placing the examiner's index finger in the neonate's palm. The normal response is to grasp the finger. This reflex should disappear after 3–5 months of age.

  3. **Reflexes triggered in an infant laid down on the examination table and picked up by the examiner**
- The **placing response** is elicited by having the dorsum of one of infant's feet touch the underside of the table. The normal response is to flex the knee and hip of the stimulated foot and to place it over the table.
- The **stepping response** is elicited by putting both soles of the infant over a table. The normal response is an alternating movement of both legs. Both the placing and the stepping response should disappear after 2–5 months of age.

111. What is Gowers' sign?

Gowers' sign is the typical way in which a child with Duchenne muscular dystrophy rises from the floor. It is due to weakness in the muscles of the lower back and pelvic girdle. As a result, the child "walks" the hands in front of the legs, pushing up against them until he or she is upright.

112. Who was Gowers?

Sir William Gowers (1845–1915) was a British neurologist with a penchant for pathophysiology and a love for synthesis (he used to quip that "words have a strong tendency to cause opacity if too numerous"). This love eventually led to an obsession with shorthand writing, which he used for all his patients and for which he founded the Society of Medical Stenography. Interested in botany, archeology, and architecture, he personally studied and wrote about the remains of some of the old churches in Suffolk and their history. His contribution to neurology was related primarily to his skills in classifying diseases and relating them to anatomopathologic changes.

113. Who was Duchenne?

Guillaume B.A. Duchenne (1807–1875) was a French neurologist and quite a character. Trained by giants of the caliber of Laennec and Dupuytren, Duchenne studied medicine despite his father's hopes for a seafaring career, which was much more in accordance with family traditions. Perhaps because of this background, Duchenne remained throughout his life a nonconformist free spirit who neither held nor pursued an academic appointment and had no official position in Parisian teaching hospitals. Instead he had plenty of time and will to roam the wards, particularly early in the morning, actively looking for new patients to examine and study. This gave him opportunity to become an excellent clinician, highly esteemed by the great Trousseau and nicknamed "the master" by Charcot. His major contribution to medicine was probably the introduction of biopsy as a diagnostic tool, a move that created a lot of controversies in the lay press. Estranged from his son, he had a moving reunion when the son eventually took up neurology in 1862. This reunion was brief, however, because the son died from typhoid fever in 1871. Duchenne never recovered.

BIBLIOGRAPHY

1. Behrman RE, Kleigman RM, Arvin AM (eds): Nelson Textbook of Pediatrics, 15th ed. Philadelphia, W.B. Saunders, 1996.
2. Chameides L: Pediatric Advanced Life Support. American Heart Association, 1997.
3. Delp MH, Manning RT (eds): Major's Physical Diagnosis. Philadelphia, W.B. Saunders, 1981.
4. Green M (ed): Pediatric Diagnosis, 6th ed. Philadelphia, W.B. Saunders, 1998.
5. Hoekelman RA (ed): Primary Pediatric Care, 3rd ed. St. Louis, Mosby, 1997.
6. Weston WL, Lane TL (eds): Textbook of Pediatric Dermatology, 2nd ed. St. Louis, Mosby, 1996.
7. Williams JV, Simel DL: Does this patient have sinusitis? JAMA 270:1242–1246, 1993.
8. Willms JL, Schneidermann H, Algranati PS (eds): Physical Diagnosis. Baltimore, Williams & Wilkins, 1994.

22. THE MUSCULOSKELETAL SYSTEM

Bruce I. Hoffman, M.D.

The Rheumatism is a common name for many aches and pains, which have yet got no peculiar appellation, though owing to very different causes.
William Heberden (1710–1801), *Commentaries on the History and Cure of Disease*

As to my health, thanks be to God, as long as I sit still I am without any pain, but if I do but walk a little I have pains in my legs, but that is, I suppose, caused by former colds and because my legs have carried my body for so long.
Anton Van Leeuwenhoek (1632–1723), Letter to J. Chamberlayne, 1707

Appearances are deceptive. I knew a man who acquired a reputation for dignity because he had muscular rheumatism in the neck and back.
J. Chalmers Da Costa (1863–1933), *The Trials and Triumphs of the Surgeon*

TOPICS COVERED IN THIS CHAPTER

Generalities
Significance of joint swelling, tenderness, and warmth
Crepitus and cracking and their significance
Pattern of joint involvement in arthritis
Tendinitis, ligamentous injury, and differentiation from arthritis
Bursitis

The Hand
Findings of osteoarthritis
Findings of rheumatoid arthritis
Nerve supply to the hand
Triggering of the fingers
Telescoped fingers
Mallet deformity
Bunnel-Littler test
Diabetic stiff-hand syndrome

The Wrist
Carpal tunnel syndrome
de Quervain tenosynovitis
Rheumatoid arthritis
Ulnar neuropathy

The Elbow
Normal range of motion of the elbow
Varus elbow
Tennis elbow
Golfer's elbow
Olecranon bursitis
Ulnar nerve entrapment
Rheumatoid nodules vs. gouty tophi

The Shoulder
Normal range of motion of the shoulder
Important areas to palpate in the shoulder
Shoulder effusion and its assessment
Painful arc sign
Impingement sign
Complete rotator cuff tear
Supraspinatus tendinitis
Bicipital tendinitis
Acromioclavicular arthritis
Referred shoulder pain
Shoulder pad sign

The Head and Neck
Examination of the temporomandibular joints
Motor innervation, sensory distribution, and reflexes of the cervical spinal roots
Torticollis
Occipital neuralgia

The Thoracic Spine
Scoliosis and kyphosis
Sprengel's deformity
Tenderness of vertebral spines
Winging of the scapula

The Lumbar Spine
Relative leg length
Spinal stenosis
Schober's maneuver
Straight leg-raising test
Crossed straight leg-raising test

Continued on next page

The Lumbar Spine (*continued*)
    Reversed straight leg-raising test
    Sacroiliac joint tenderness
    Trendelenburg sign and symptoms
    Hoover's test
The Hip
    Log rolling of the hip
    FABER maneuver
    Trochanteric bursitis
    Gait abnormality in hip disease
    Psoas pain
The Knee
    Assessment of quadriceps atrophy
    Flexion contracture and extension lag
    Ligamentous integrity
    Effusions of the knee

The Knee (*continued*)
    Meniscal tear
    Patellar tracking
    Patellofemoral disease
    Popliteal cyst
    Pseudothrombophlebitis
The Ankle and Foot
    Pes cavus and pes planus
    Hallux valgus
    Cock-up deformity of the toes
    Corns and bunions
    Rheumatoid foot
    Morton's neuroma
    Achilles tendinitis
    Plantar fasciitis
    Tarsal tunnel syndrome

CONVENTIONAL TEACHING WATCH

A sometimes difficult area of physical exam, but often necessary and rewarding in ambulatory medicine.

FINDING/MANEUVER		CONVENTIONAL TEACHING REVISITED
Examination of hand	⇑	Important site of involvement in both degenerative and inflammatory disorders; may reflect systemic diseases (gout)
Examination of wrist	⇑	Common site of injury, especially with increased use of computer keyboards (carpal tunnel syndrome)
Examination of elbow	⇑	Important site to examine, not only in golfers or tennis players.
Examination of the shoulder	⇑	Frequent site of injury. Be familiar with its maneuvers.
Examination of head and neck	⇑	Important to be aware of motor innervation, sensory distribution, and reflexes of cervical spinal roots.
Examination of thoracic spine	⇑	Common site of abnormality, which may affect lung function.
Examination of lumbar spine	⇑	Common site of injury and degenerative disease.
Examination of knee	⇑	As above.
Examination of hip	⇑	As above.
Examination of ankle and foot	⇑	Common site of deformities and inflammatory arthritis.

1. Describe the types of joint swelling.

Joints are swollen either from osteophytes or from synovial swelling and effusion. Osteophytes occur in osteoarthritis and have a bony feel on palpation. With synovial swelling palpation reveals a range of findings from indistinctness of joint margins to sponginess.

2. What is the significance of joint tenderness?

Normal joints can be palpated with significant force without eliciting pain. Tenderness in joints, which ranges from mild discomfort to severe pain on touch, is a sign of joint pathology.

3. What is the significance of joint warmth?

Normal joints are cooler than the surrounding areas. A joint that is warmer than the surrounding extremity is abnormal.

4. Explain crepitus.

Crepitus is the sensation of grinding felt with palpation of joints during motion. It may originate from irregularities in the cartilage, bone-on-bone articulation, or tendon abnormalities.

5. What is the significance of joint cracking?

Most people describe the sensation of cracking or popping in some joints. This symptom is not significant unless accompanied by pain. It is probably caused by tendon or ligament slippage over a bony prominence.

6. List the patterns of joint involvement in arthritis.
- Monoarthritis—one joint
- Pauciarthritis—four or fewer joints
- Polyarthritis—more than 4 joints
- Asymmetric—different joints involved in different extremities
- Symmetric—same joints or rows of joints on the extremities

7. What is the function of tendons and what is tendinitis?

Tendons attach muscle to bone and transmit the force of muscle across joints. Tendons are often covered in a sheath of synovium and connective tissue called the tenosynovium. Tendinitis is the general term to describe disorders of the tendon and includes tears in the body of the tendon or at the bone attachment (the enthesis) and inflammation of the tenosynovium.

8. How are disorders of tendons differentiated from joint problems?

With tendon disorders pain occurs with joint motion that requires muscle contraction, or it occurs when the tendon is stretched passively at its extreme range of motion. Passive motion of the joint produces no pain.

9. What is a bursa? How do you identify bursitis?

Bursae are sacs of synovium that are found over bony prominences and between adjoining muscle bundles with different directions of contraction. Bursitis is identified by point tenderness over the bursae. In superficial bursae an effusion can be appreciated.

10. How is joint hypermobility demonstrated?

Findings in patients with joint hypermobility, either of the common benign type or in association with Ehlers-Danlos syndrome, include (1) ability to oppose the thumb passively to the forearm, (2) hyperextension of the fingers, (3) > 10° of hyperextension of the elbows and knees, and (4) ability to touch the palms to the floor with flexion at the waist.

11. What are the findings in liagamentous injury?

The findings depend on the degree of injury. Tenderness is present over the ligament, and stretch of the ligament produces pain. Significant disruption of the ligament results in abnormal motion of the joint and gapping with stretching of the ligament. Ecchymosis may be seen over the site of injury.

THE HAND

12. What are the findings of osteoarthritis in the hand?

Bony swelling typically affects the distal interphalangeal (DIP) and proximal interphalangeal (PIP) joints. These findings may be associated with lateral deviation of the joint. (See chapter 23.)

13. Describe the typical deformities of rheumatoid arthritis.

At the PIP joints one may see boutonnière deformities (fixed flexion at the PIP and extension at the DIP) or swan-neck deformities (extension at the PIP and extension at the DIP). The fingers may deviate to the ulnar side at the metacarpal phalangeal joints (ulnar deviation).

14. Explain the significance of triggering of the fingers.

Triggering (or trigger finger) is the sensation that the fingers are stuck in flexion. The patient has to straighten the digit forcibly, sometimes using the other hand. Triggering results from catching of the flexor tendon as it runs through the fibrous flexor sheath, which is called the A1 pulley. This process is called flexor tendinitis.

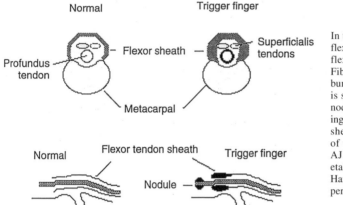

In trigger finger, the fibrous flexor sheath surrounding the flexor tendon is thickened. Fibers of the flexor tendon bunch up into a nodule that is sometimes palpable. This nodule has difficulty in sliding through the fibrous flexor sheath during movements of the finger. (From Mehta AJ: Common Musculoskeletal Problems. Philadelphia, Hanley & Belfus, 1997, with permission.)

15. What are the physical findings of triggering?

The tendon often is tender at the volar side of the metacarpal. When the finger is flexed and extended, a click can be palpated. Pain is elicited when the tendon is stretched by extension of the finger at the metacarpal.

16. What is the nerve supply of the hand?

The median nerve supplies sensation to the palmar side of the first, second, and third fingers and the radial half of the fourth finger. It also supplies sensory fibers for the distal fingers on the dorsal side to the DIP of the first to third fingers and motor fibers to the thenar muscles. The ulnar nerve supplies sensation to the ulnar fourth finger and the fifth finger on both the dorsal and volar side and to the contiguous portion of the hand. It also supplies motor innervation to the interosseous muscles. The radial nerve supplies the sensory innervation to the dorsal portion of the hand not supplied by the median and ulnar nerves.

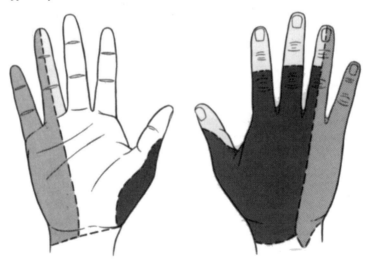

Cutaneous innervation from the median nerve *(white area)*, ulnar nerve *(light shading)*, and radial nerve *(dark shading)*. (From Concannon MJ: Common Hand Problems in Primary Care. Philadelphia, Hanley & Belfus, 1999, with permission.)

17. What is the significance of a swollen finger?

Diffuse swelling of a finger or toe, when not associated with trauma, is seen with psoriatic arthritis and sarcoidosis. The swollen digit is called a sausage digit.

18. What are telescoped digits?

Patients with extreme joint destruction may lose the entire joint. On examination the joint, usually the PIP, can be moved in and out by the examiner.

19. Describe a mallet deformity.

A mallet deformity (or mallet finger) is the inability to extend the DIP joint fully, with some degree of flexion of the DIP at rest. It results from injury to the long extensor tendon with lengthening of the tendon during healing.

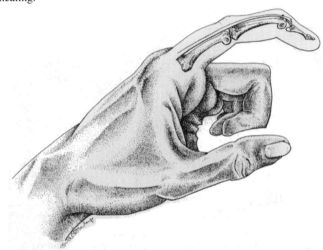

Mallet finger. The extensor tendon is usually torn near its insertion. Occasionally a small fragment of the distal phalanx is avulsed by the tendon. The DIP joint cannot be actively extended. (From Mellion MB: Office Sports Medicine, 2nd ed. Philadelphia, Hanley & Belfus, 1996, with permission.)

20. What are the findings of a paronychia? A felon?

A paronychia is an infection at the nail margin accompanied by swelling, erythema, and tenderness in the area adjacent to the nail. As it progresses, the infection points to the margin of the finger. A felon is an infection of the pulp space of the finger and causes swelling, erythema, and tenderness over the finger pad.

21. Describe the Bunnel-Littler test.

The Bunnel-Littler test (see figure at top of following page) differentiates between interosseous tightness and capsular contraction in patients who have difficulty with flexion of the PIP joint. The metacarpophalangeal (MCP) is held in a few degrees of extension. If the patient is unable to flex the PIP joint, the MCP is placed in flexion, and a second attempt is made to flex the PIP. With interosseous tightness the PIP is able to flex with the second maneuver. With capsular contraction flexion of the PIP is limited with both maneuvers.

22. What are the findings of diabetic stiff hand syndrome?

Stiff hand syndrome develops in patients with long-term type I diabetes and often parallels microvascular injury. The patient develops limitation of movement of the fingers with varying degrees of flexion contracture and limitation of flexion of the PIP joints. The syndrome is demonstrated by asking the patient to place the palms together. Patients with diabetic stiff hand syndrome are unable to oppose the flexor surfaces of the PIPs (prayer sign). The syndrome often is associated with thickening of the flexor tendon sheaths and waxy thickening of the skin over the fingers.

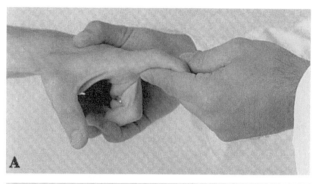

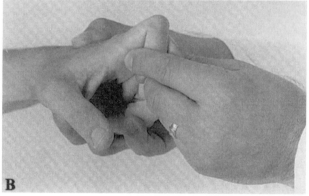

Bunnel-Littler test. *A,* To distinguish between intrinsic muscle tightness and joint contracture, the metacar-pophalangeal joint is extended. *B,* The proximal interphalangeal joint is then moved into flexion. (From Shankar K, Nayak NN, Dowdell BC: Commonly used clinical tests and gait abnormalities. Phys Med Rehabil State Art Rev 10:631–652, 1996, with permission.)

23. Describe the findings of osteoarthritis of the first carpometacarpal (CMC) joint.
Osteoarthritis of the CMC joint leads to pain at the base of the thumb with tenderness on pal-pation and crepitus on rotation of the joint. The proximal part of the first metacarpal protrudes, producing a change in contour at the base of the thumb called a mushroom deformity.

THE WRIST

24. What are the physical findings of carpal tunnel syndrome?
The symptoms may be reproduced with a tap over the median nerve at the wrist (Tinel's sign) or with holding the wrists fully flexed with the dorsal sides held together for 1 minute (Phalen's sign). Later findings include sensory loss in the distribution of the median nerve and at-rophy of the thenar muscles. (See figure at top of following page.)

25. What is the usual cause of pain on the radial side of the wrist? What physical finding is used to identify this disorder?
De Quervain tenosynovitis is a common cause of pain along the radial side of the wrist and forearm. It involves the tendons of the thumb as they travel over the radius. The diagnostic maneuver is Finkelstein's test, in which the thumb is placed in the palm and the fingers are wrapped around the thumb. The wrist is ulnar-deviated, and the pain should be reproduced.

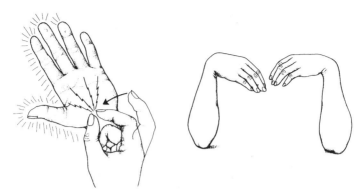

Tinel's sign *(left)* and Phalen's sign *(right)*. (From the American Society for Surgery of the Hand: The Hand: Examination and Diagnosis, 3rd ed. New York, Churchill Livingstone, 1990, with permission.)

26. What are the typical findings in the wrist of rheumatoid arthritis?

Early findings include swelling of the extensor carpi ulnaris tendon. Later findings include protrusion and instability of the distal ulna due to laxity of the radial ulnar ligaments. In advanced disease the carpal rows may sublux toward the dorsal side, causing the bayonet deformity.

27. How is a ganglion identified over the wrist?

Ganglia are fluid-filled cystic spaces within tendon sheaths. The swelling is fluctuant and moves with the involved tendon.

28. What are the findings of ulnar neuropathy?

The ulnar nerve can be compressed at the elbow or at the wrist in Guyon's canal. Findings include paresthesias in the ulnar side of the hand, the fifth finger, and the ulnar half of the fourth finger. Later findings include atrophy and weakness of the interosseous muscles.

THE ELBOW

29. What is the range of motion of the elbow?

The elbow should extend to 0° and flex to 150°. The patient should be able to touch the thumb to the shoulder. The forearm should supinate and pronate 80°; the motion occurs primarily at the elbow.

30. What is a varus elbow?

The normal angle of the elbow is in valgus with the elbow fully extended. After fractures in children the elbow may develop a varus angle (gunstock deformity). Remember that valgus means bent or twisted away, and varus bent or twisted toward, the midline of the limb or body.

31. Where is swelling of the elbow joint palpated?

Swelling of the elbow joint is appreciated in the groove between the olecranon and lateral epicondyle. Mild swelling is appreciated as a filling in of the groove. Greater degrees of swelling cause loss of the bony margins on palpation.

32. What is the most common finding with an abnormal elbow joint?

With any abnormality of the elbow joint a flexion contracture develops and may persist permanently. It is common to see residual contractures from previous fractures. Elbow flexion contractures also are seen in people whose occupation requires them to keep the elbow flexed for long periods, such as long-distance truck drivers.

33. Describe the physical findings of tennis elbow.

Tennis elbow or lateral epicondylitis is caused by an injury to the proximal attachment of the extensor muscles of the forearm. The patient notes pain at the lateral epicondyle, which refers down the forearm. Point tenderness of the lateral epicondyle corresponds to the site of injury. The pain may be elicited by grasp and/or with resisted wrist extension (see figure).

34. What are the findings of golfer's elbow?

Golfer's elbow is the common name given to injury at the medial epicondyle of the elbow. Palpation reveals tenderness of the medial epicondyle, and pain is elicited by resisted wrist flexion. The mechanism of injury is similar to lateral epicondylitis but is less common because the flexor muscles are stronger and less likely to be overstressed.

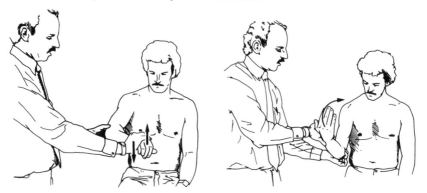

Testing for lateral epicondylitis *(left)* and medial epicondylitis *(right)*. (From Mellion MB: Office Sports Medcine, 2nd ed. Philadelphia, Hanley & Belfus, 1996, with permission.)

35. What is olecranon bursitis? How is it identified?

Olecranon bursitis is inflammation of the bursae lying over the olecranon. Of the many causes, trauma, infection, and gout are the most common. The condition is identified by finding a fluctuant swelling over the olecranon. It may dissect down the ulna. Usually elbow motion is normal.

36. What finding differentiates infectious from other causes of olecranon bursitis?

Definitive differentiation depends on aspiration of fluid from the bursae, but if erythema extends past the margins of the bursae, infection is the most likely cause.

37. What are the findings of ulnar nerve entrapment?

Most ulnar nerve entrapment occurs in the cubital tunnel at the medial side of the elbow. Tinel's sign can be elicited over the nerve. The patient may experience sensory loss in the ulnar distribution of the hand and, in later stages, interosseous atrophy and weakness.

38. How can a rheumatoid nodule and gouty tophus be differentiated?

Both produce nodules at the extensor surface of the elbow and other sites at which pressure occurs. No findings definitively differentiate the two entities. Aspiration for monosodium urate crystals or biopsy must be done. Occasionally tophi drain to the surface, and urate is recovered from an ulcer over the nodule.

THE SHOULDER

39. What is the range of motion of the shoulder?

The shoulder abducts to 180°, of which 90° is glenohumeral motion; the remainder is scapular rotation. It has 180° of forward flexion and 90° of external and internal rotation.

40. What are the important areas to palpate in the shoulder girdle?

The rotator cuff posterior to the acromion, subacromial areas, long head of the biceps tendon in the bicipital groove, and acromioclavicular joint.

41. Where are shoulder effusions appreciated?

The shoulder should be observed in comparison with the opposite shoulder to appreciate effusion. Fluid is palpated over the anterior surface of the joint.

42. What is the painful arc sign?

The painful arc is the physical maneuver used to evaluate the cause of a painful shoulder. The shoulder is abducted from the side to 180°. Supraspinatus tendinitis and partial rotator cuff tear produce pain between 40° and 120°. Patients with glenohumeral arthritis feel pain throughout the arc.

43. Describe the impingement sign.

The arm is forcibly elevated, and pain is elicited with compression of the rotator cuff under the acromion.

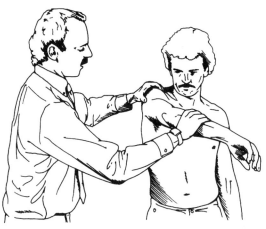

Impingement test. (From Mellion MB: Office Sports Medicine, 2nd ed. Philadelphia, Hanley & Belfus, 1996, with permission.)

44. What are the findings of a complete rotator cuff tear?

The arm cannot be actively abducted from 0°. If the arm is abducted passively above 90°, it can be held and actively moved to 180°. If the arm is lowered below 90°, it falls to the side. In addition, with the elbow held against the side, the arm cannot be actively placed in external rotation.

45. How can pain of supraspinatus tendinitis be elicited?

With the shoulder abducted to 90° and internally rotated to 90°, the arm is held against resistance. Pain is elicited. Pain also can be elicited when the elbow is held against the side and forced into external rotation against resistance.

46. What are the signs of bicipital tendinitis?

Pain is elicited in the anterior shoulder when the arm is forcibly supinated with the elbow at 90° and the hand pronated (Yergason's maneuver). The elbow is flexed against resistance.

47. What are the findings of acromioclavicular arthritis?

Tenderness is present over the acromioclavicular joint, and pain is elicited in the joint by touching the hand of the involved arm to the opposite shoulder.

48. How is shoulder instability demonstrated?

The apprehension test is used to demonstrate shoulder instability. The arm is abducted to 90° and externally rotated 90°. The examiner pushes forward on the arm. Pain, motion, and, at times, a click are signs of instability. (See figure at top of next page.)

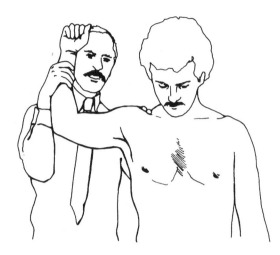

Apprehension test. (From Mellion MB: Office Sports Medicine, 2nd ed. Philadelphia, Hanley & Belfus, 1996, with permission.)

49. What physical findings suggests that shoulder pain is referred from a remote site?
The pain cannot be reproduced on physical examination of the shoulder.

50. What is the shoulder pad sign?
The shoulder pad sign is bilateral shoulder effusions. It is most characteristic of amyloidosis.

THE HEAD AND NECK

51. How are the temporomandibular joints examined?
The examiner places his or her fingers in the tragus of the ear, and the patient opens and closes the mouth. With abnormalities of the joints, either a crepitus or a click in the joint can be appreciated. The examiner also should watch the tract of the mandible with opening of the mouth; it should be directed down. An abnormal joint often produces asymmetry of jaw motion; the jaw deviates to one side during opening.

52. What is torticollis?
Torticollis is rotation of the head due to spasm of the cervical musculature. The head is held to one side or turns involuntarily.

53. What are the findings of occipital neuralgia?
Occipital neuralgia results from impingement of the occipital nerve as it exits from the skull at the occipital notch. Pressure by the examiner over this area reproduces the pain, which radiates from the occiput to the vertex of the head.

54. List the motor innervation, sensory distribution, and reflexes of the cervical spinal roots.

ROOT	MUSCLES	SENSATION	REFLEX
C5	Deltoid, biceps	Lateral arm	Biceps
C6	Wrist extension, biceps	Lateral forearm	Brachioradialis
C7	Wrist flexors, finger extension, triceps	Middle finger	Triceps
C8	Finger flexion, hand intrinsics	Medial forearm	—
T1	Hand intrinsics	Medial arm	—

THE THORACIC SPINE

55. How is scoliosis appreciated?

The examiner runs a finger down the vertebral spine. If scoliosis is present, the finger moves with the spine toward the side of the curve.

56. Describe the causes of accentuated kyphosis of the thoracic spine.

The thoracic spine normally has a kyphotic curvature, which may be accentuated in several circumstances. In younger patients accentuated kyphosis results from Scheuermann's disease, which produces juvenile kyphosis. In older patients it generally results from osteoporotic compression fractures, which produce increased kyphosis referred to as dowager's hump. Any cause of multiple thoracic compression fractures, such as trauma, accentuates thoracic kyphosis.

57. What is Sprengel's deformity?

Sprengel's deformity results from partial descent of the scapula, which produces an asymmetric appearance of the shoulders and upper back.

58. What is the significance of tenderness of the vertebral segments?

Tenderness of the vertebral segments, as demonstrated by striking the fist at each spinal level or firmly palpating over each vertebra, is highly suggestive of underlying bony abnormalities, such as fractures, infection, or tumor.

59. How is chest expansion measured?

A tape measure is placed around the chest at the nipple line. The patient is asked to inhale to forced maximal inspiration and then to do a forceful exhalation. The difference in chest circumference between maximal expiration and maximal inspiration is the chest expansions. The normal value is approximately 5 cm.

60. What is winging of the scapula? How is it demonstrated?

Winging refers to the protrusion of the scapula from the chest wall and suggests weakness of the serratus anterior muscle. It can be elicited by having the patient place both hands on a wall and push outward. This maneuver accentuates the protrusion of the scapula.

THE LUMBAR SPINE

61. What are the planes of motion of the lumbar spine?

The lumbar spine flexes forward and laterally and extends.

62. How can relative leg length be assessed?

The examiner stands behind the patient, who stands with feet together and both knees extended. The examiner places his or her hand on the iliac crests. The relative height of each hand gives an assessment of relative leg length. This test also is influenced by scoliosis and relative pelvic tilt.

63. How are radicular symptoms reproduced in patients with spinal stenosis?

The patient is asked to extend maximally or to flex laterally the lumbar spine. Either maneuver reproduces the radicular symptoms in patients with spinal stenosis.

64. What is the Schober test?

With the patient standing straight, a line is drawn 10 cm above the dimples of Venus. A mark is placed on the skin at each end, and the patient is asked to flex forward to the maximal extent.

This maneuver should result in distraction of the lumbar spine of 5 cm so that the distance between the marks is 15 cm. This measurement is reduced in ankylosing spondylitis and other settings that involve fusion of the lumbar spine.

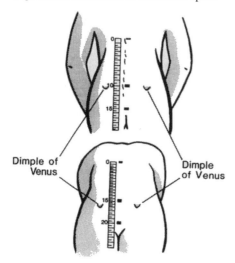

Dimple of Venus

Dimple of Venus

Schober test. (From Mellion MB, Walsh WM, Shelton GL: The Team Physician's Handbook, 2nd ed. Philadelphia, Hanley & Belfus, 1997, with permission.)

65. What is the straight leg-raising test? How is it performed?

The straight leg-raising test is indicative of nerve root compression. With the patient supine, the symptomatic leg is flexed with the knee fully extended. A positive test reproduces radicular symptoms with pain referred from the buttock down the leg.

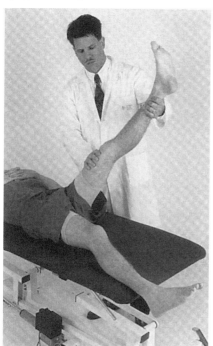

Straight leg raise. (From Shankar K, Nayak NN, Dowdell BC: Commonly used clinical tests and gait abnormalities. Phys Med Rehabil State Art Rev 10:631–652, 1996, with permission.)

66. Describe another way to perform the test.

With the patient sitting, the knee is fully extended, producing the same angle as the standard leg-raising test. This maneuver should reproduce symptoms. It is often done to check for malingering.

67. What is the crossed straight leg-raising test?

When the straight leg-raising test is performed, the patient experiences symptoms in the opposite leg. This finding also indicates nerve root compression.

68. What is the reverse straight leg-raising test?

With the patient lying on the abdomen, the leg is extended with the knee flexed. Reproduction of pain in the anterior thigh is seen with high nerve root lesions. A positive test also is seen with lesions of the psoas, such as an abscess.

69. How is sacroiliac joint tenderness assessed?

There are several tests of sacroiliac joint (SIJ) tenderness. With the patient lying on the side, the pelvis is compressed and pressure is applied over the lateral pelvis. This maneuver may cause pain in the areas of the SIJ. In Gaensler's maneuver, the patient is supine and lies with one side of the pelvis off the examination table; the contralateral leg is flexed at the hip and knee and held by the patient. The hip on the examined side is extended with the leg below the edge of the table. This maneuver elicits pain on the examined side.

70. What is Trendelenburg's sign?

It is a sign of weakness of the gluteus medius muscle. When a normal person stands on only one leg, the contralateral side of the pelvis is elevated by the effort of the gluteal muscles. Elevation does not occur with weakness of the gluteus medius muscle, which usually results from congenital dislocation of the hip, trochanteric fracture, poliomyelitis, or spinal nerve root lesions with muscular atrophy.

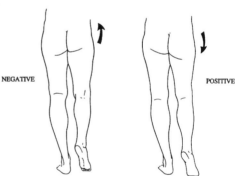

Trendelenburg's sign. (From Goldstein B, Chavez F: Applied anatomy of the lower extremities. Phys Med Rehabil State Art Rev 10:601–630, 1996, with permission.)

71. How is Trendelenburg's sign elicited?

By standing behind the patient and looking at the dimples over the posterior superior iliac vertebrae (dimples of Venus). In a patient who is standing upright, with feet together and weight evenly distributed between the legs, the two superior iliac vertebrae and the two buttocks should be symmetric and at the same level. If the patient then flexes one leg and stands only on the opposite leg, there should be a normal elevation of the hemipelvis and buttock on the unsupported side. Lack of elevation (or even more, a sagging of the buttock) indicates weakness of the ipsilateral gluteus medius muscle and represents a positive Trendelenburg's sign.

72. What is Trendelenburg's gait?

It a waddling gait seen in patients with weakness or paresis of the gluteal muscles. It often is observed in progressive muscular dystrophy.

73. Describe the neurologic examination of the lumbar roots.

DISC	ROOT	MUSCLES	SENSATION	REFLEX
L3–L4	L4	Anterior tibialis	Medial leg and medial foot	Patellar reflex
L4–L5	L5	Extensor hallucis longus	Lateral leg and dorsum of foot	None
L5–S1	S1	Peroneus longus and brevis	Lateral foot	Achilles

74. What is Hoover's test?

It is a maneuver used during examination of lower extremity strength designed to assess the patient's effort. The maneuver is based on the fact that when a person lying supine on a couch is asked to raise one leg, he or she involuntarily exerts counterpressure with the heel of the other leg. This response occurs even if the contralateral leg is paralyzed: the patient marshals whatever muscular power is left in the leg and involuntarily applies pressure on its heel. Of course, if the patient attempts to lift a paralyzed leg, counterpressure is exerted with the contralateral (healthy) heel, regardless of whether movement occurs in the paralyzed limb. This sign is absent in hysteria or malingering but is present in hemiplegia. It is, therefore, particularly helpful in evaluating weak patients who exhibit poor effort.

75. How is Hoover's test carried out?

1. The examiner's hands are placed below the heels of a supine patient. The patient is then asked to press down on the examiner's hands with both feet. If the patient has hemiplegia, pressure is less on the paralyzed side.

2. The examiner then places one hand above the patient's nonparalyzed leg and asks the patient to raise the leg. If the patient is making a maximal effort, the opposite (paralyzed) leg still exerts downward pressure, even if the patient is hemiplegic. Failure to do so suggests lack of effort and malingering.

3. Finally, one hand is placed under the heel of the patient's healthy leg, while the patient is asked to raise the other (paralyzed) leg. Even in this case, pressure is exerted by the patient's heel against the examiner's hand. This pressure, however, is greater than the pressure exerted by the paralyzed leg.

THE HIP

76. What is log-rolling of the hip?

With the leg fully extended, the leg is rolled side to side. Pain elicited by this maneuver comes only from the hip joint and helps to differentiate hip joint pain from pain caused by other structures.

77. Describe the FABER maneuver.

The **FABER** maneuver is a screening test for hip disease. The hip is **f**lexed, **ab**ducted, and **e**xternally **r**otated. Normally, the lateral leg should be able to lay on or near the examination table with the foot against the opposite knee.

78. How is a flexion contracture of the hip demonstrated?

The opposite hip is flexed, the patient holds the knee, and the thigh is extended until it lies on the table. If the thigh cannot touch the table, a flexion contracture is present.

79. Describe how trochanteric bursitis is localized.

There are several bursae around the greater trochanter. Bursitis leads to pain in the lateral thigh that may be referred laterally down the leg. Palpation over the bursae reveals tenderness, and the pain may be reproduced with internal rotation of the hip.

80. What are the characteristics of the gait abnormality in patients with hip disease?

Patients walk by shifting their weight over the involved side, giving a characteristic pattern to their limp. The involuntary shifting of weight reduces the pressure on the joint by reducing the multiplying effect of the femoral neck, which acts as a lever arm.

81. What structure can cause swelling over the hip?

The iliopectineal bursa lies anterior to the hip. It often is in communication with the joint. Fluid in the bursa produces a fluctuant mass in the inguinal region.

82. How is pain referred from the psoas identified?

Lesions of the psoas (i.e., abscess or hematoma) may cause pain referred to the inguinal area. The origin at the psoas is suggested by pain elicited with extension of the hip.

THE KNEE

83. How is quadriceps atrophy appreciated and measured?

Atrophy of the quadriceps muscle is appreciated by comparing the muscle bulk of the two sides. In more subtle atrophy, asking the patient to contract the quadriceps muscle accentuates the anatomy and allows appreciation of unilateral muscle loss. The quadriceps can be measured by drawing a line from the midpoint of the patella to a point 15 cm up the thigh and measuring the circumference at that point.

84. Describe the deformities of the knee.

Malalignment commonly is observed in the knee. Angulation of the distal leg toward the midline is **genu varum** deformity or bowlegs. Angulation of the distal leg away from the midline is **genu valgum** or knock-knee deformity. Both may be congenital or acquired. In an unusual condition called windswept knees, one knee is in varum and one knee in valgum.

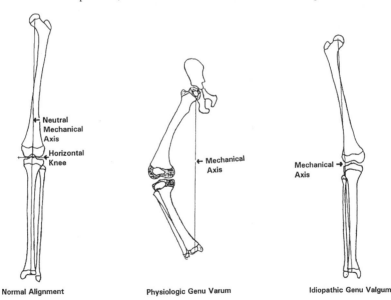

Normal alignment and malalignment of the knee. (From Staheli LT: Pediatric Orthopedic Secrets. Philadelphia, Hanley & Belfus, 1998, with permission.)

85. Define a flexion contracture and extension lag of the knee.

A flexion contracture is the inability of the examiner to extend the knee to 0°. This is a common finding in knee pathology. An extension lag is the inability of the patient to extend actively the knee that can be passively extended by the examiner. It is due to problems with the patellofemoral mechanism.

86. How is ligamentous integrity of the knee tested?

The medial and lateral collateral ligaments are tested by the examiner, who cradles the lower leg and applies force to the lateral side of the knee (to test the medial collateral ligament) and to the medial knee (to test the lateral collateral ligament). Instability is shown by the opening of the joint space. The cruciate ligaments are tested by having the patient lie supine and flex the knee to approximately 60°. The examiner fixes the foot and pulls forward on the tibia to test the anterior cruciate ligament and then pulls the tibia back to test the posterior cruciate ligament. Movement of the tibia in relation to the femur indicates instability.

87. How are effusions of the knee demonstrated?

The demonstration of knee effusions depends on the volume of fluid. Small effusions are demonstrated with the bulge sign. The medial side of the knee is stroked, pushing fluid into the suprapatellar pouch. The examiner runs his or her hand down the lateral side of the knee from proximal to distal. The fluid is pushed medially, and a bulge of the fluid wave is appreciated. Larger effusions can be appreciated by ballottement of the patella or the fluid wave test. The patellar ballottement is performed by grasping the knee at the level of the suprapatellar pouch. The examiner uses the other hand to push down on the patella. If significant effusion is present, the patella can be felt to move up and down. To perform the fluid wave test, the examiner places one hand around the suprapatellar pouch and uses the other hand to squeeze the knee. If fluid is present, a fluid wave is felt in the suprapatellar area.

88. Describe the palpation of the knee and possible findings.

The knee should be palpated with the patient in a seated position, starting at the tibial tuberosity and moving along each side of the tibial plateau and then up each femoral condyle. Tenderness localized to the joint line is seen with meniscal tears. Tenderness along the medial side of the knee extending above and below the joint line is seen with collateral ligament injury and in some substantially obese people. Tenderness over the medial femoral condyle is seen with osteonecrosis. Tenderness over the medial tibial plateau is seen in anserine bursitis, stress fractures of the plateau, and osteonecrosis.

89. What are the physical findings of meniscal tear?

The knee is tender over the joint line. Several tests can demonstrate meniscal tear. The McMurry test is performed with the patient supine. The knee is fully flexed, and the examiner places his or her hand over the medial and lateral joint line. The knee is extended. Then the knee is again flexed and extended, first with internal and then with external rotation applied to the lower leg. A positive test is indicated by increased pain with extension of the knee and rotation of the leg and by palpation of a click over the meniscus.

90. How is patellar tracking demonstrated?

With the patient seated, the knee is extended while the examiner places his or her finger over the midpoint of the patella. The patella should remain midline in the femoral groove. Abnormalities are indicated if the patella moves medially or laterally.

91. What are the findings of patellofemoral disease?

With the patient supine, the patella is moved laterally across the femur. Crepitus or pain is a sign of disease of the patellofemoral joint. Abnormal findings can be elicited if the maneuver is performed with the quadriceps tightened (patellar inhibition sign).

92. What is a popliteal cyst? Where is it palpated?
A popliteal cyst is fluid from the knee that has dissected through the popliteal space. The cyst can be felt as a fluctuant swelling in the popliteal space or dissected into the calf.

93. What is pseudothrombophlebitis?
When a cyst ruptures, fluid drains down the facial plane of the calf and causes swelling and erythema of the calf. This phenomenon is called pseudothrombophlebitis. The fluid causes a crescent-shaped ecchymosis at the medial or lateral malleolus (crescent sign).

THE ANKLE AND FOOT

94. Describe the deformities of the foot.
There are two abnormalities of the longitudinal arch. An abnormally high arch is called **pes cavus**, whereas loss of the arch is called **pes planus**, which may be flexible or fixed. Flexible flat feet have some discernible arch at rest, but it is lost with weight-bearing. Fixed flat feet have no arch at rest.

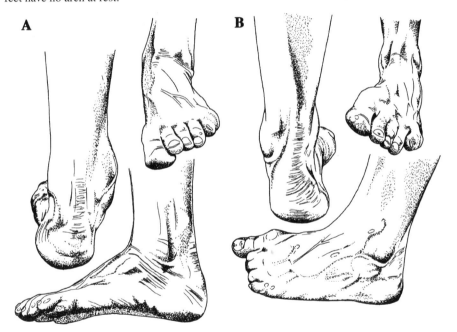

A, Pes planus (flat foot). *B,* Pes cavus (high-arched foot). (From Mellion MB, Walsh WM, Shelton GL: The Team Physician's Handbook, 2nd ed. Philadelphia, Hanley & Belfus, 1997, with permission.)

95. What ankle deformity is associated with pes planus?
Valgus or pronation deformity of the ankle is commonly associated with pes planus. It is appreciated by observing the patient standing. There is a variable degree of inward rotation of the medial malleolus. From behind the heel points away from the midline.

96. Describe hallux valgus and bunions.
Hallux valgus is a common deformity of the great toe, characterized by deviation away from the midline toward the second toe. Osteophytes may be palpable at the joint line. The true bunion is a bursa that develops over the medial border of the first MTP and produces an effusion.

97. Describe cock-up deformity of the toes.

Cock-up deformities are due to ligamentous instability, which causes flexion at the interphalangeal joint of the toe. Often the toe no longer touches the floor when the patient stands.

98. What are corns?

Corns are areas of skin thickening that develop over the toe as a result of chronic mechanical irritation. Hard corns develop over interphalangeal joints of the toes when cock-up deformity causes pressure on the joint in shoes. Soft corns are areas of skin thickening between the toes from abnormal pressure as the toes move against each other.

99. Describe the findings with dropped metatarsal heads.

Subluxation of the metatarsal heads toward the plantar surface of the foot is a common occurrence and is typically part of the foot deformities of rheumatoid arthritis. The metatarsal heads can be palpated on the plantar surface of the foot. With more severe degrees of subluxation the protrusion of the bone can be seen. Thickening of the plantar skin (calluses) is seen over the bone.

100. How is the loss of the anterior arch of the foot demonstrated?

Loss of the anterior arch of the foot causes widening of the forefoot. The patient places the foot on a piece of paper, and the margins are traced. The patient then is asked to step on a pencil placed parallel to the foot. With loss of the arch the margins of the foot lie within the original borders on the paper.

101. What are the typical deformities of the rheumatoid foot?

Rheumatoid arthritis can lead to extensive foot deformity. Patients may develop pes planus with pronation deformities of the ankle. They may exhibit loss of the anterior arch with widening of the foot. They have hallux valgus, cock-up deformities of the toes, and dropped metatarsal heads.

102. How is Morton's neuroma demonstrated?

Morton's neuroma is a collection of nerve fibers developing in the web space of the toes. It causes pain in the forefoot and is demonstrated by applying pressure to the web space, which elicits pain.

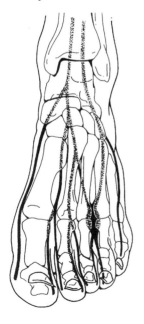

Morton's neuroma. (From Mellion MB, Walsh WM, Shelton GL: The Team Physician's Handbook, 2nd ed. Philadelphia, Hanley & Belfus, 1997, with permission.)

103. Describe the findings of Achilles tendinitis.

Several areas may be involved with Achilles tendinitis. Pain in the Achilles tendon can be elicited with passive dorsiflexion of the ankle or active plantarflexion (standing on the toes). Swelling may occur at the insertion to the calcaneous, in the midpoint of the tendon at the Achilles bursa, or along the length of the tendon. Tenderness may occur at the insertion to the calcaneous (retroachilles bursa).

104. What are the findings of Achilles tendon tear?

Active plantarflexion is absent, and a gap may be palpated in the tendon at the tear.

105. What are the findings of plantar fasciitis?

Plantar fasciitis causes pain on the plantar surface of the calcaneous. The patient complains of pain on standing. Examination reveals tenderness at the calcaneous at the midpoint of the plantar surface. Frequently a spur is seen on radiograph at the attachment of the plantar fascia, although it is not the cause of the pain.

106. What is tarsal tunnel syndrome? What are the findings?

Tarsal tunnel syndrome is entrapment of the tibial nerve as it winds under the medial malleolus. This entrapment leads to paresthesias and pain in the medial plantar surface of the foot from the first toe to the heel. The syndrome can be demonstrated by tapping over the area beneath the malleolus and eliciting the symptoms. This maneuver is called the tarsal tunnel tap and is analogous to Tinel's sign for carpal tunnel syndrome.

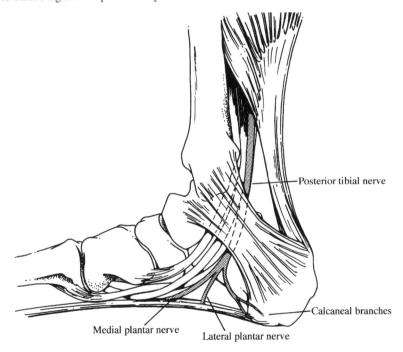

Tarsal tunnel syndrome. (From Mellion MB, Walsh WM, Shelton GL: The Team Physician's Handbook, 2nd ed. Philadelphia, Hanley & Belfus, 1997, with permission.)

BIBLIOGRAPHY

1. Ad Hoc Committee: Guidelines for the initial evaluation of the adult patient with acute musculoskeletal symptoms.Arthritis Rheum 39:1–8, 1996.
2. Doherty M, Hazelman BL, Hutton CW, et al: Rheumatology Examination and Injection Techniques. Philadelphia, W.B. Saunders, 1999.
3. Gomez JE, Landry GL, Bernhardt DT: Critical evaluation of the 2-minute orthopedic screening examination. Am J Dis Child 147:1109–1113, 1993.
4. Gredinger EL, Hellmann DB: Arthritis: What to emphasize on the rheumatologic exam. Consultant 35:1609–1617, 1995.

23. THE EXTREMITIES

Salvatore Mangione, M.D.

In Medicine it is always necessary to start with the observation of the sick and to always return to this as this is the paramount means of verification. Observe methodically and vigorously without neglecting any exploratory procedure, using all that can be provided by physical examination.

Antoine B.J. Marfan

TOPICS COVERED IN THIS CHAPTER

Hands and Feet
Heberden's nodes
Bouchard's nodes
Haygarth's nodes
Tophi
Janeway's lesions
Osler's nodes
Pachuco mark
Arachnodactyly
Hand changes in bulimia
Hand changes in acromegaly
Clubbing and hypertrophic osteoarthropathy
Raynaud's phenomenon
Dupuytren's contracture

Peripheral Arteries
Allen's test
Peripheral Veins
Trendelenburg's test
Evaluation of varicose veins of the saphenous system
Evaluation of deep vein thrombosis

CONVENTIONAL TEACHING WATCH

Often examined last, the extremities can provide important clues to the astute observer. This chapter also includes evaluation of peripheral arteries and veins.

FINDING/MANEUVER		CONVENTIONAL TEACHING REVISITED
Heberden's, Bouchard's, and Haygarth's nodes	⇑	Often difficult to tell apart, but still valuable diagnostic clues
Tophi	⇑	Pathognomonic of gout when located over the hands.
Osler's nodes and Janeway's lesions	⇓	Common in the heyday of endocarditis; much less frequent nowadays.
Clubbing and hypertrophic osteoarthropathy	⇑	Important finding with wide differential diagnosis.
Raynaud's phenomenon	⇑	As above.
Dupuytren's contracture	⇑	As above.
Allen's test	⇑	Essential to guide arterial puncture and cannulation.
Trendelenburg's test	⇑	Useful for evaluation of saphenous vein varicosities.
Assessment of patient with suspected deep vein thrombosis	⇔	Neither as overvalued as in remote past nor as undervalued in recent past.

HANDS AND FEET

1. What are Heberden's nodes?

They are painless nodules on the distal interphalangeal (DIP) joints. They may involve one or more fingers but typically spare the thumb. The overlying skin is normal. The nodules are hard, measure 2–3 mm in diameter, do not interfere with movement of the finger, have a twin presentation, and typically are located on the lateral and medial dorsal surface of the DIP. If the nodules affect the proximal interphalangeal (PIP) joint, they often are called Bouchard's nodes. Heberden's and Bouchard's nodes are signs of localized osteoarthritis. Therefore, they are encountered more commonly in elderly people. Involvement of a single joint is usually more common in men, whereas multiple-joint involvement is more common in women (in whom the condition is usually postmenopausal and hereditary).

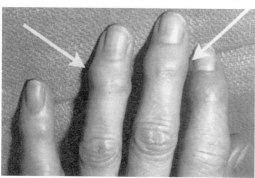

Patients with degenerative joint disease of the hands can present with Heberden's nodes *(arrows)*. These nodules represent osteophytes at the DIP joint. (From Concannon MJ: Common Hand Problems in Primary Care. Philadelphia, Hanley & Belfus, 1999, with permission.)

2. Who were Heberden and Bouchard?

William Heberden (1710–1801) was an English physician who studied in Cambridge and practiced in London at the local university. A devout Christian, he was a leading Latin and Hebrew scholar, referred to by Samuel Johnson as "the last of the Romans" ("Dr. Heberden ultimus Romanorum—the last of our learned physicians"). His contributions to medicine included the aforementioned nodules and classic descriptions of angina, chickenpox, and night blindness.

Charles J. Bouchard (1837–1915) was a French physician. He is also famous for the first description of spider nevi in chronic liver disease.

3. What are Haygarth's nodes?

They are quite different from Heberden's and Bouchard's nodes. In fact, Haygarth's nodes are inflammatory, not degenerative. Therefore, they are associated with signs of inflammation, such as flushing of the overlying skin, increased temperature, thickening of the joint capsule, fluid in the cavity (which is in part responsible for the fusiform swelling of the nodes), and limitation of movement. Unlike Heberden's lesions, Haygarth's nodes can be painful and tender. Haygarth's nodes are the typical lesions of rheumatoid arthritis (RA). They affect the middle and proximal PIP joints instead of the DIP joint (RA never involves the DIP) and therefore resemble Bouchard's nodes more closely than Heberden's nodes. Subcutaneous nodules are common in RA; they have been found on the extensor surfaces of upper extremities (primarily elbows, but also fingers), knees, ankles, and occiput. Subcutaneous nodes are not exclusive to RA. In fact, they may be encountered in other rheumatic disorders, such as lupus, rheumatic fever, sarcoidosis, syphilis, granuloma annulare, and tuberous xanthomatosis.

4. Who was Haygarth?

John Haygarth (1740–1827) was an English physician from the city of Bath. A graduate of Cambridge, Haygarth had a penchant for epidemiology, which led him to study the diseases that occurred in the ancient city of Chester (where he also investigated the value of isolation in infectious disease and the usefulness of smallpox as a method of immunization). Haygarth's work with rheumatism and rheumatic fever was published in 1798 upon his return to Bath.

5. What are tophi?

They are deposits of uric acid (in Latin *tophus* = calcareous deposit from springs, tufa). Tophi may be present over the ears, feet, and hands of patients with gout. In the hands they are pathognomonic of gout, although often they are confused with rheumatoid nodules.

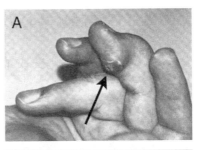

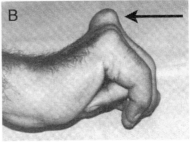

A, Gouty tophus deposition on the volar aspect of the long finger *(arrow)*. This patient has severe gouty arthritis with multiple tophaceous deposits. *B,* A large tophus over the metacarpophalangeal joint of the dorsal long finger *(arrow)*. (From Concannon MJ: Common Hand Problems in Primary Care. Philadelphia, Hanley & Belfus, 1999, with permission.)

6. What are Janeway lesions?

They are small, nontender, erythematous or hemorrhagic lesions of palms or soles. Like Osler's nodes (which are swollen, tender, raised, pea-sized lesions of fingerpads, palms, and soles), Janeway lesions usually are seen in bacterial endocarditis. The two lesions are often difficult to differentiate. Before the introduction of antibiotics they were seen in 40–90% of patients with endocarditis; now they are present in only 10–23% of cases. They also may be seen in lupus erythematosus, bacteremia without endocarditis, gonococcal sepsis, and marantic endocarditis. They result from septic emboli or sterile vasculitis.

7. Who was Janeway?

Edward G. Janeway (1841–1911) was an American physician. A student of Austin Flint, Janeway followed his mentor to Bellevue Hospital Medical College in New York, where he established himself as one of the first full-time consultants in American medicine. He had an interest in public service and later became health commissioner for New York and founder of the first infectious disease hospital in Manhattan.

8. What is the Pachuco mark?

It is a cross-like tattoo that during the 1970s used to be common over the anatomic snuffbox of intravenous drug abusers. The snuffbox is the hollow space on the radial aspect of the wrist and can be seen when the thumb is fully extended. The Pachuco mark was considered a sort of identification card in the drug-dealing world, easily visible upon handshake. Incidentally, Pachuco is an American-Spanish term, possibly an alteration of *payuco* (yokel, rustic in Spanish). The term also has been used to identify a Mexican-American youth or teenager, especially one who dresses in flamboyant clothes and belongs to a neighborhood gang.

9. What is the shape of the hand in acromegaly?

The hand has a spade-like shape because of enlargement of the distal portion of the body, which is, indeed, the defining feature of acromegaly.

10. What is arachnodactyly?

Arachnodactyly refers to the spider-like fingers of patients with Marfan syndrome. Although the condition was described in 1896 by the French pediatrician Antoine B. Marfan in a 5-year-old patient, the term arachnodactyly was actually coined six years later by Achard. The fingers are thin and long, resembling the bent legs of a spider. The test for arachnodactyly is **Marfan's thumb sign.** The patient is asked to open both hands and extend each thumb as far as possible across the palm. The patient then should fold the fingers across the thumb and make a fist. The test is considered positive if any part of the tip of the thumb protrudes beyond the ulnar surface of the fist. The sign is typical of Marfan syndrome and its various forms but also may be seen in other conditions of hypermobility of the joints, such as Ehlers-Danlos syndrome.

11. Who was Marfan?

Antoine B. Marfan (1858–1942) was a French pediatrician, the son of a provincial medical practitioner. He contributed to several areas of medicine, including the astute observation that tuberculosis acquired before the age of 15 seems to provide a unique resilience to patients. This observation inspired Calmette to develop the bacille Calmette-Guérin vaccine. Active in public health and public service, Marfan also had a passion for literature and the arts, enjoying concerts and trips to Italy. He was particularly fond of Venetian paintings. He befriended, among others, Emile Broca, of whom he wrote a biography. He left most of his fortune to the Society for the Preservation of Infants against Tuberculosis, which he had helped to create.

12. What is a short fourth metacarpophalangeal bone?

It is an unusually short and inwardly dimpled fourth knuckle. Although usually seen in patients with pseudohypoparathyroidism and Turner's syndrome, it occurs in as many as 10% of normal people.

13. What is the significance of calluses and abrasions on the dorsal aspect of the fingers?

They are an important clue to a diagnosis of bulimia. They are caused by interaction with the teeth during induction of vomiting.

14. What is clubbing?

Digital clubbing is focal enlargement of the connective tissue in the terminal phalanges of fingers and toes; it is especially prominent on the dorsal surface of the digits. The phenomenon has fascinated physicians since its original description by Hippocrates in a patient with empyema. Interest was rekindled in the nineteenth century by the German Eugen Bamberger and the French Pierre Marie and by their description of hypertrophic osteoarthropathy (HOA), a frequently concomitant disorder. By the end of World War I both clubbing and HOA were well known to physicians, usually as a sign of chronic infections. Today they are more commonly remembered for their association with cancer, usually bronchogenic carcinoma. In fact, this association is so strong that HOA is often referred to as hypertrophic pulmonary osteoarthropathy, even though it is not necessarily limited to pulmonary disorders. Despite increased awareness of both clubbing and HOA, the pathogenesis of the two conditions remains an unsolved and confusing mystery. In fact, a recent study showed that even the definition of clubbing varies tremendously among physicians. Still, given their frequent association with serious disorders, clubbing and HOA are too important to go unrecognized.

15. Is clubbing painful?

No. Although at times patients may complain of an aching discomfort in their fingertips, clubbing is usually painless.

16. Is clubbing limited to the fingers?

No. It usually involves both fingers and toes; however, it may involve only fingers or only toes. This selective distribution usually is seen with cyanotic forms of congenital heart disease, which selectively perfuse with oxygen-desaturated blood either the upper or lower half of the body. As a result, patients have differential cyanosis and clubbing in either the fingers or toes. Underlying disorders include (1) patent ductus arteriosus with pulmonary hypertension (in which the reversed shunt limits cyanosis to the feet and spares the hands) and (2) right ventricular origin of both great vessels. In this disorder both the aorta and pulmonary artery arise from the right ventricle; concomitant disorders include ventricular septal defect, patent ductus arteriosus, and pulmonary hypertension. As a result, oxygenated blood from the left ventricle enters the pulmonary trunk through the septum, shunts through the patent ductus into the descending aorta, and eventually flows to the lower extremities. Conversely, oxygen-desaturated blood from the right ventricle enters the ascending aorta and brachiocephalic vessels, thereby reaching the upper extremities. Hence, hands are cyanotic and clubbed, but feet are normal (reversed differential cyanosis). Identical and symmetric cyanosis and clubbing of both fingers and toes indicate the presence of right-to-left intracardiac shunt.

17. What is the cause of unilateral clubbing?

Most often an aneurysm of either the aorta or the innominate/subclavian arteries. Pancoast's tumor and lymphangitis also may cause unilateral clubbing. Another unusual cause of unilateral clubbing is placement of an arteriovenous fistula for dialysis.

18. Is increased nail convexity a special form of clubbing?

No. Clubbing requires accumulation of soft tissue with elevation of the base of the nail and loss of the subungual angle (see below).

19. What is the significance of increased nail convexity?

It is a separate sign, often present in the absence of clubbing. Clubbing is not defined by increased nail convexity but by (1) loss of subungual angle, (2) ballottability of the nail, and (3) abnormal phalangeal depth ratio (see below). Ironically, increased nail convexity may be a more frequent hallmark of chronic debilitating conditions than clubbing. In fact, it is quite common in hospitalized patients with chronic disorders, such as carcinoma of the lung, pulmonary tuberculosis, and rheumatoid arthritis. Increased nail convexity usually takes longer to develop than true clubbing. In fact, it requires the formation of an entirely new nailplate ridge. This transverse ridge appears 1 month after the causative event and reaches full formation over 6 months. By completion, an entirely new nail has been created, characterized by an abnormal and more convex profile (watchglass nail).

20. What are the diagnostic features of digital clubbing?

It depends on whether clubbing is present alone or in association with periostosis (see below). **Clubbing without periostosis**, the time-honored Hippocratic nail, has three main diagnostic features:

1. **Loss of Lovibond's angle,** which is the angle between the base of the nail and its surrounding skin (hyponychial or unguophalangeal angle). In a normal person this angle is less than 180°. In a person with clubbing, the angle is either obliterated (straight line) or greater than 180°. The loss of Lovibond's angle can be easily visualized by resting a pencil over the nail. In normal people there is a clear window below the pencil and above the nail. In patients with clubbing, on the other hand, there is no clear window; the pencil rests fully over the nail.

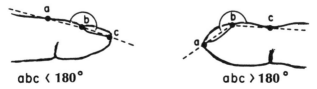

Measurement of Lovibond's angle. (Adapted from Hansen-Flaschen J, Nordberg J: Clubbing and hypertrophic osteoarthropathy. Clin Chest Med 8:287–298, 1987.)

2. **Floating nails (ballottability of the nail bed)** is increased sponginess of the soft tissue at the base of the nail. As a result, the nailplate acquires a peculiar "springy" feeling. When the skin just proximal to the nail is compressed, the nail sinks deep toward the bone; when released, it springs backward and outward (floating fingernail base). This feeling can be effectively simulated by the following maneuver:

(1) Press your right index finger over the skin just proximal to the nail of your left middle finger. In a normal person the nailplate feels solidly attached to the underlying bone.

(2) Repeat the maneuver, but this time apply some tension to the nail by pulling downward the nail's free edge with your left thumb, thereby increasing the natural convexity of the nailplate. After doing so, the nailplate feels detached from the underlying bone, capable of sinking down during pressure and springing back upon release, almost as if the nail were floating on a spongy pad.

3. **Abnormal phalangeal depth ratio** consists of a greater depth of the fingertip when measured at the cuticle (distal phalangeal depth [DPD]) vs. the interphalangeal joint (interphalangeal depth [IPD]). The DPD/IPD ratio of normal people is, on average, 0.895. Patients with clubbing have a DPD/IPD ratio equal to or greater than 1.0 (i.e., in excess of the norm by approximately 2.5 standard deviations). The DPD/IPD ratio is an excellent marker for clubbing with good sensitivity and specificity. For example, a ratio greater than 1.0 is found in 85% of children with cystic fibrosis and less than 5% of children with chronic asthma.

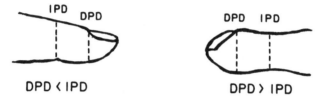

Phalangeal depth ratio. (Adapted from Hansen-Flaschen J, Nordberg J: Clubbing and hypertrophic osteoarthropathy. Clin Chest Med 8:287–298, 1987.)

21. What is a drumstick finger?

It is one of several terms used to describe the more advanced stages of digital clubbing. The accumulation of connective tissue extends well beyond the base of the nail and involves the entire digit. Depending on where the accumulation of connective tissue predominates, a few colorful terms have been created. For example, in parrot's beak clubbing, the swelling is primarily localized to the proximal portion of the distal digit; in the drumstick type, it is circumferential; and in the watchglass form, swelling is mainly localized to the base of the nail.

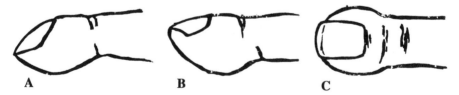

Types of digital clubbing: parrot's beak *(A)*, watchglass *(B)*, and drumstick *(C)*. (Adapted from Hansen-Flaschen J, Nordberg J: Clubbing and hypertrophic osteoarthropathy. Clin Chest Med 8:287–298, 1987.)

22. How quickly can such changes occur?

Very quickly. In the setting of a lung abscess, for example, loss of the unguophalangeal angle and ballottability of the nail bed have occurred within 10 days after aspiration.

23. Is ballottability of the nail always an indication of clubbing?

No. It also may be found in older patients without clubbing. Nonetheless, ballottability remains an important and valuable sign for the diagnosis of clubbing.

24. What is Schamroth's sign?

It is another bedside maneuver that can confirm the loss of the subungual angle. It consists of the disappearance of the diamond-shaped window normally present when the terminal phalanges of paired digits are juxtaposed. Schamroth actually noticed this sign on himself during recurrent episodes of clubbing caused by bouts of endocarditis.

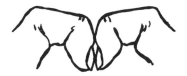 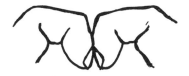

Schamroth's sign. (Adapted from Hansen-Flaschen J, Nordberg J: Clubbing and hypertrophic osteoarthropathy. Clin Chest Med 8:287–298, 1987.)

25. What is digital clubbing with periostosis?

Hypertrophic pulmonary osteoarthropathy (also called Marie-Bamberger syndrome from the names of its two discoverers), a systemic disorder of bones, joints, and soft tissues most commonly associated with an intrathoracic neoplasm (usually bronchogenic carcinoma but also lymphomas and metastatic cancers). The hallmark of HOA is periosteal new-bone proliferation that accompanies digital clubbing. This periostosis is especially prominent in the long bones of the extremities. Other features of HOA include (1) symmetric arthritis-like changes in one or more joints (ankles, knees, wrists, and elbows); (2) coarsening of the subcutaneous tissue in the distal portions of arms and legs (and occasionally the face); and (3) neurovascular changes in hands and feet (with chronic erythema, paresthesias, and increased sweating). HOA may occur in some disorders that commonly present with clubbing, but this is not always the case. For example, HOA may be seen in cystic fibrosis, bronchiectasis, chronic empyema, and lung abscesses (all typically associated with clubbing) but is rare in pulmonary interstitial fibrosis (also frequently associated with clubbing). Thus, HOA is in a league of its own.

26. Is HOA symptomatic?

Yes. In contrast to pure clubbing (which is painless), HOA is associated with aching and sometimes frank bony pain and tenderness. In addition, the pretibial skin looks shiny and is often thickened and warm to touch. Often autonomic manifestations also are present, such as increased sweating, warmth, or paresthesias. Of interest, all of these changes resolve with ablation or cure of the associated condition.

27. How is the diagnosis of HOA established?

Diagnosis is made not by physical exam but by bone radiography or scintigraphy. Both studies show periostosis. Physical exam may suggest the diagnosis, particularly in a patient presenting with clubbing and pretibial discomfort. Clubbing, on the other hand, is diagnosed exclusively by physical exam.

28. What is pachydermoperiostosis?

Pachydermoperiostosis (from the Greek *pachys* = thick, *derma* = skin, *peri* = around, *osteon* = bone, *osis* = condition) is a congenital and hereditary form of HOA characterized by digital clubbing and periosteal new bone formation (especially over the distal ends of the long bones). Other features include coarsening of facial features with thickening, furrowing, and oiliness of the facial and forehead skin (cutis verticis gyrata) as well as seborrheic hyperplasia with open sebaceous pores filled with plugs of sebum. In contrast to simple HOA, pachydermoperiostosis is characterized by less bony pain and greater skin changes. The syndrome is autosomal dominant and more severe in males; it becomes clinically evident during adolescence.

29. What is thyroid acropachy?

It is a disorder characterized by thickening of peripheral tissues (from the Greek *acro* = distal and *pachys* = thick). It occurs in 1% of patients with Graves' disease and often is associated with exophthalmos and myxedema of hands and feet. Thyroid acropachy resembles HOA in the sense that it is associated with digital clubbing and periosteal new bone formation. Yet it preferentially involves hands and feet instead of the long bones of the lower extremities. Moreover, thyroid acropachy spares the joints and is usually painless.

30. What are the causes of clubbing?

Disorders Commonly Associated with Digital Clubbing

Intrathoracic	Cardiovascular
Bronchogenic carcinoma*	Congenital cyanotic heart disease
Metastatic lung cancer*	Subacute bacterial endocarditis
Hodgkin's disease	Infected aortic bypass graft*
Mesothelioma*	**Hepatic and gastrointestinal**
Bronchiectasis*	Hepatic cirrhosis*
Lung abscess	Inflammatory bowel disease
Empyema	Carcinoma of esophagus or colon
Cystic fibrosis	
Pulmonary interstitial fibrosis	
Pneumoconiosis	
Arteriovenous malformations	

* Commonly associated with hypertrophic osteoarthropathy.
From Hansen-Flaschen J, Nordberg J: Clubbing and hypertrophic osteoarthropathy. Clin Chest Med 8:287–298, 1987, with permission.

Clubbing often presents as a familial congenital form (particularly in African-Americans). Congenital clubbing is extremely important to recognize and should be well documented in the patient's records to avoid future misunderstandings. Many patients are unaware of this abnormality and may not remember if asked about it. According to Sapira, congenital clubbing may be characterized more by loss of the subungual angle than by presence of ballottement.

31. What are the causes of a weaker and delayed pulse in the left arm compared with the right arm?

It depends on the age of the patient. In elderly people the most common cause is probably either atherosclerotic obstruction or dissection of the aorta. In younger patients it is usually coarctation. Depending on the level of the obstruction, asymmetry and delay in pulses may affect only the arteries of the lower extremities. Hence the importance of examining *all* peripheral pulses, particularly in symptomatic or hypertensive patients. Asymmetry of the pulse may be confirmed by measuring systolic blood pressure in the two arms or in the lower extremities for comparison with the upper extremities.

32. What is Raynaud's phenomenon?

It is a particular sensitivity of the hands and fingers to cold, resulting in spasm of the digital arteries and transient ischemia of the digits. Upon exposure to cold, the fingers exhibit a typical triple response. This response, appropriately for Raynaud, follows the colors of the French flag: pallor and blanching first (white), cyanosis later (blue), and finally rubor (red). Eventually the fingers return to their baseline pink color. This white-blue-red response at times may be out of sequence. In fact, some patients may have a blue-white-red response or even a single-color response (only blue or only white). Many also have finger numbness or pain.

33. What causes Raynaud's phenomenon?

Spasm of the digital arteries causes ischemia of the fingers, with pallor at first and cyanosis later (due to increased oxygen extraction from the trapped and noncirculating erythrocytes). The final stage of redness coincides with reperfusion, following release of the arterial spasm. This is also the phase mostly characterized by finger numbness or pain (a bit like the numbness and pain experienced in legs that have "fallen asleep").

34. How can Raynaud's phenomenon be triggered?

By immersing the patient's hand in a bucket of ice water.

35. What is the clinical significance of Raynaud's phenomenon?

Raynaud's phenomenon usually precedes several important disorders:

1. Connective tissue diseases (systemic lupus erythematosus, mixed connective tissue disease, rheumatoid arthritis, dermatomyositis, polymyositis, and especially progressive systemic sclerosis, which is present in 17–28% of patients with Raynaud's phenomenon)

2. Various blood disorders (including cryoglobulinemia, polycythemia, monoclonal gammopathy)

3. Disorders characterized by arterial compression (such as thoracic outlet and carpal tunnel syndromes)

4. Vasculitis and atherosclerotic arterial disease

5. Various drugs and toxins

6. Miscellaneous disorders, including hypothyroidism, reflex sympathetic dystrophy, primary pulmonary hypertension, Prinzmetal angina, acromegaly, Addison's disease, and use of percussion or vibratory tools.

Approximately 20% of patients with Raynaud's phenomenon seem to have no other underlying disorder. They are labeled as having Raynaud's disease.

36. Who was Raynaud?

Maurice Raynaud (1834–1881) was one of the great nineteenth century French physicians. The son of a university professor, he graduated in Paris at age 28 with a thesis in which he described his famous syndrome. The thesis made him an instant celebrity. Raynaud was an excellent clinician and a beloved teacher. He was also passionately interested in literature, history, and the arts. In fact, throughout his life he sought the chair of medical history at the University of Paris but died before his dream was fulfilled. His contributions to medical knowledge include a book entitled *Medicine in Molière's Time* and an article about the Greek physician, Asclepiades of Bithynia (an opponent of Hippocratic medicine and the unrivaled authority of his times. Among his patients were Cicero, Crassus, and Marc Anthony). In 1881 Raynaud wrote an address to the International Medical Congress of London entitled "Scepticism in Medicine, Past and Present" but died shortly before he was scheduled to deliver it.

37. What is Dupuytren's contracture?

It is a condition characterized by thickening and eventually contracture of the palmar tendons on the ulnar side of the hand. It results in flexure of the fingers, predominantly the fourth and fifth (the thumb is always spared). The hand of patients with Dupuytren's contracture is so typical that it has been dubbed "the hand of papal benediction." Dupuytren's contracture is seen in several clinical settings:

1. 18–66% of patients with alcoholic liver disease (either cirrhotic or noncirrhotic)

2. 13–42% of patients with chronic pulmonary tuberculosis

3. 8–56% of treated epileptics

4. 35% of men over the age of 60, usually smokers

Contrary to conventional teaching, however, Dupuytren's contracture does *not* occur in manual laborers or brewery workers. In addition, 31–48% of patients with Dupuytren's contracture are alcoholic (with or without liver disease); 10–35% have either peptic ulcer disease or cholecystitis, 6–25% have diabetes mellitus (strongly correlated with retinopathy); 93% have glucose intolerance; and 2.5% have Peyronie's disease.

In Dupuytren's contracture, fibrous bands of diseased palmar fascia can contract to pull the finger into flexion. *A,* The fibrous band can be seen at the level of the proximal palmar crease of the ring finger. *B,* Early Dupuytren's contracture producing flexion of the fifth finger. (From Concannon MJ: Common Hand Problems in Primary Care. Philadelphia, Hanley & Belfus, 1999, with permission.)

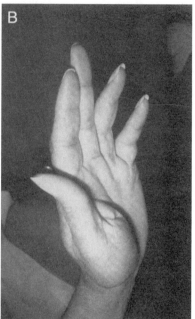

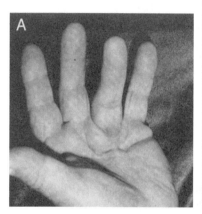

38. Who was Dupuytren?

A very weird character. Guillaume Dupuytren (1777–1835) was born just one year after the American Revolution, but some of the ideas of his time must have rubbed off on him. In fact, throughout his life he remained quite an eccentric and flamboyant character. For example, he was famous for operating in a cloth cap and carpet slippers and infamous for his arrogance, cynicism, and vindictiveness. Of humble origins, he was nonetheless an attractive and intelligent child—to the point of being kidnapped at age four by a rich lady from Toulouse (she later returned him to his family). As a teenager he moved to Paris, where at age 24 he became a prosector at the local school of health. This position gave him the opportunity to work directly with two of the medical giants of his time, Laennec and Bayle. Soon, however, Laennec realized that Dupuytren was trying to gain credit for Bayle's work, and the collaboration immediately ceased. Dupuytren eventually joined the Paris Hôtel Dieu (House of God), where he made a name for himself as a skilled surgeon and gifted speaker. He remained, however, as obnoxious as ever, to the point of being called "first of surgeons and last of men." Still he *was* a great surgeon: he not only described his eponymous contracture but even devised an operation to cure it. He was also the first to create a classification system for burns and one of the first great promoters of plastic surgery. A workaholic rumored to see an average of 10,000 patients per year, Dupuytren was also cheap. These two traits helped to make him a rich but unpopular man. His motto was "Fear nothing but mediocrity." This motto won him few friends in Paris but helped to make him famous well beyond the borders of France.

PERIPHERAL ARTERIES

39. What is Allen's test? What is its significance?

Allen's test is a bedside maneuver to assess patency of the arterial circulation of the hand. More specifically, it evaluates the patency of the radial and ulnar arteries and deep palmar arch. It is, therefore, a good test to learn about the risks of a radial artery puncture or cannulation. The test is conducted as follows:

1. The examiner compresses the patient's radial artery until blood flow is stopped.

2. The patient clenches and unclenches the hand several times in sequence until the hand visibly blanches.

3. When the patient finally relaxes the hand, the capillary bed from the ulnar side visibly refills, with return of the normal pink color within 5 seconds.

4. Absence of refilling (i.e, pallor persists despite the hand's relaxation) or delay in refilling (i.e., return of color takes longer than 5 seconds) indicates a positive test, which reflects decreased flow of either the ulnar artery or the deep palmar arch.

5. The maneuver is then repeated on the contralateral hand, comparing size of the refill area and length of refill time.

6. The entire sequence is finally repeated, but this time the ulnar arteries are compressed, first on the right and then on the left.

40. Can Allen's test be conducted by compressing the ulnar and radial arteries simultaneously?

This approach is, in fact, a variant of Allen's test. The maneuver is performed as follows:

1. Compress both the radial and ulnar arteries (see *A* in figure).

2. Ask the patient to clench and unclench the hand sequentially and vigorously to squeeze all blood out of it. When the palm finally blanches, ask the patient to relax the hand.

3. Release pressure only on the ulnar artery, and measure the time it takes for the palm to regain its color. This is the refill time for the ulnar artery (see *C* in figure).

4. If refill is delayed or absent (see below), do not attempt a radial puncture, but consider either a brachial stick or an arterial puncture on the contralateral hand (after similarly checking the arterial supply, of course).

5. The test can be repeated, but this time by releasing pressure on the radial artery only, thereby measuring refill time for the radial artery (see *B* in figure).

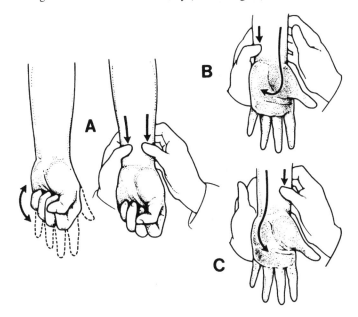

Allen's test. (From James EC, Corry RJ, Perry JF: Principles of Basic Surgical Practice. Philadelphia, Hanley & Belfus, 1987, with permission.)

41. How do you report the results of Allen's test?

By indicating (1) the name and side of the artery compressed (for example, RR for right radial) and (2) the refill time expressed in seconds. Thus, RR5/RU3 means that it took 5 seconds to refill the capillary bed of the right palm after releasing the right radial artery and 3 seconds after releasing the right ulnar artery. If refill takes longer than 15 seconds, the artery being tested should not be cannulated; ideally, cannulation should be conducted on the contralateral hand.

42. Who was Allen?

Edgar V. Allen (1900–1961) was an American physician. A native of Nebraska and a graduate of the state university, Allen eventually moved to the Mayo Clinic, where in 1947 he became professor of medicine. His contributions to medical knowledge include the introduction of coumarin anticoagulants in clinical practice and a landmark textbook about peripheral vascular diseases.

PERIPHERAL VEINS

43. What is Trendelenburg's test?

It is a test of the functionality of the valves of the leg veins. It is carried out as follows:

1. Raise the leg of a supine patient above the level of the heart until the veins are completely empty and collapsed.

2. Apply a tourniquet to the mid-thigh, thereby compressing the greater saphenous vein and preventing it from draining blood.

3. Ask the patient to stand and closely observe the leg veins. In a normal patient, the greater saphenous vein refills *slowly* from below the obstruction. Refill takes less than 1 minute because of unimpeded arterial flow in the face of obstructed venous drainage.

4. Release the tourniquet 60 seconds after standing.

5. Closely observe the leg veins for engorgement.

44. How are the results of Trendelenburg's test interpreted?

• Rapid refilling of the greater saphenous vein *before* the tourniquet is released indicates *backfilling* from incompetent valves of the communicating veins.

• Rapid refilling of the greater saphenous vein *after* the tourniquet is released indicates *backfilling* from incompetent valves of the greater saphenous vein itself.

• Patients with arterial insufficiency may have a false-negative test.

If the saphenous vein has incompetent valves, it also functions as a manometer of intraabdominal pressure. In other words, the saphenous vein is to the abdomen what the internal jugular is to the right atrium. This monitoring function can be carried out by raising the leg at various angles and studying the level of the column of blood in the saphenous vein both at baseline and after maneuvers that increase abdominal pressure (such as coughing or straining).

45. Who first described Trendelenburg's test?

The test was first described by Sir Benjamin Brodie in 1846, almost 50 years before Trendelenburg's report. For this reason the maneuver is still called the Trendelenburg-Brodie test.

46. How do you check for the presence of communicating veins?

By using another maneuver devised by Trendelenburg. It consists of applying a tourniquet on the saphenous vein while the patient is still supine and varicose veins are engorged. The leg is then raised high above the level of the heart, and varicosities are monitored closely. Their gradual disappearance indicates that there is a communication between the saphenous and deep veins, that the valves of the communicating veins are competent, and that the deep venous system is patent. Conversely, veins that remain engorged indicate either occlusion of the deep venous system or absence of the communicating veins.

47. What is the Trendelenburg position?

Originally it was a supine position on the operating table with the bed inclined at such an angle that the pelvis was always higher than the head. Trendelenburg's position is still used during and after pelvic operations. It is also used for patients in shock to redirect blood from the legs and abdomen into the chest and brain. In such acutely ill patients, Trendelenburg's position is sometimes called "the Titanic position."

48. Who was Trendelenburg?

Friedrich Trendelenburg (1844–1924) was a professor of surgery at the University of Leipzig. An innovator in his field, Trendelenburg developed the position that still carries his name. He experimented, however, in many other areas. For example, he devised an operation for the treatment of varicose veins; hence the aforementioned Trendelenburg's tests. He even attempted a pulmonary embolectomy in 1908. The first successful embolectomy, however, was performed in 1924, the year of Trendelenburg's death, by Kirsher, one of his students. Fortunately, Trendelenburg lived to see the success of the procedure. His interests included a passion for medical history, which led him to write a book about ancient Indian surgery. Trendelenburg's name is linked not only to eponymous tests and position but also to Trendelenburg's sign and symptom (see chapter 22).

49. What is Perthes' test?

Another bedside test of varicose veins, devised by the German surgeon Georg C. Perthes of Calvé-Legg-Perthes disease fame. Perthes' test is aimed at determining patency of the deep venous system and competence of the valves of the saphenous and communicating veins. It is carried out by placing a tourniquet around the mid-thigh of a standing patient whose leg veins are fully engorged. The patient is then asked to walk for 5 minutes, and the veins are reexamined.

50. How are the results of Perthes' test interpreted?

- If the veins below the tourniquet *collapse* as a result of walking, the deep venous system is patent and the valves of the communicating veins are competent.
- If the veins below the tourniquet *remain unchanged*, the valves of both saphenous and communicating veins are incompetent.
- If the veins below the tourniquet *become more engorged* and the patient experiences leg pain, the deep venous system is occluded and the communicating veins are incompetent.

Perthes' test is based on the "milking" effect that muscle compression exerts on the greater saphenous vein. As a result, walking squeezes blood from the saphenous veins into the communicating system and from there into the deep veins.

51. What is the role of palpation in examining the varicose veins of the saphenous system?

Palpation can confirm the presence of incompetent valves. The maneuver is carried out by placing the fingers of one hand over the engorged saphenous vein (below the knee) while at the same time flicking the same vein 1 foot cephalad (above the knee) by using the other hand. Incompetence of the valves results in transmission of the impulse downward and backward.

52. What is the role of physical examination for the diagnosis of deep venous thrombosis (DVT)?

Physical examination is part of a comprehensive approach, including review of risk factors, symptoms, and physical signs.

53. What are the risk factors for DVT?

Major risk factors
- Active cancer (treatment ongoing or within previous 6 months or palliative)
- Paralysis, bedridden > 3 days, and/or major surgery within 4 weeks

- Localized tenderness along the distribution of the deep venous system in calf or thigh
- Swollen thigh and calf (should be measured)
- Calf swelling by > 3 cm compared with asymptomatic leg (measured 10 cm below tibial tuberosity)
- Strong family history of DVT (> 2 first-degree relatives with history of DVT)

Minor risk factors
- History of recent trauma (≤ 60 days before development of symptoms)
- Pitting edema in symptomatic leg only
- Dilated superficial veins (nonvaricose) in symptomatic leg only
- Hospitalization within previous 6 months
- Erythema

Items excluded from the model are age, duration of symptoms, sex, obesity, presence of varicose veins, a palpable cord, and Homans' sign.

54. How are the risk factors for DVT interpreted?
High probability
≥ 3 major factors and no alternative diagnosis *or*
≥ 2 major factors and ≥ 2 minor factors and no alternative diagnosis
Low probability
1 major factor and ≥ 2 minor factors and an alternative diagnosis *or*
1 major factor and ≥ 1 minor factor and no alternative diagnosis *or*
0 major factors and ≥ 3 minor factors and an alternative diagnosis *or*
0 major factors and ≥ 2 minor factors and no alternative diagnosis
Moderate probability
all other combinations

55. What are the common symptoms of DVT?
Commonly reported symptoms in patients with suspected DVT include leg pain and swellling.

56. Describe the physical examination of patients with suspected DVT.
1. Careful inspection of the leg looking for pitting edema, warmth, dilated superficial veins, and erythema
2. Measurement of leg circumference
3. Elicitation of Homans' sign (development of calf pain after forceful and abrupt dorsiflexion of the ankle with the knee in a flexed position)

All of these signs, however, are quite inaccurate. Tenderness, swelling, redness, and the assessment of Homans' sign cannot adequately separate patients with or without DVT. The sensitivity of the clinical examination is 60–88% with a specificity of 30–72%. Findings such as pitting edema, increased temperature, erythema, and dilated superficial veins are, in fact, neither sensitive nor specific for DVT. They may be caused, for example, by leg trauma, cellulitis, obstructive lymphadenopathy, superficial venous thrombosis, postphlebitic syndrome, or Baker cysts. The same applies to the other maneuvers.

57. What, then, should be the approach to a patient with suspected DVT?
Because of the low sensitivity and specificity of clinical examination, many authors in the past recommended exclusive reliance on noninvasive objective tests. Yet five clinical findings still seem to be associated independently and significantly with the presence of proximal DVT: (1) swelling below the knee, (2) swelling above the knee, (3) recent immobility, (4) cancer, and (5) fever. Overall, the sensitivity of a positive clinical examination (associated with the presence of one or more independent predictors) is 96% (95% confidence interval = 92–100%), although the specificity is still low (20%). The absence of any of these findings is associated with a less than 5% chance of proximal DVT. Conversely, the presence of two or more of these clinical findings is associated with a 46% chance of proximal DVT.

Thus, although individual symptoms and signs of DVT by themselves are *not* very useful, a careful review of risk factors, symptoms, and signs may still help to determine the pretest probability of disease and guide interpretation of noninvasive diagnostic tests. This rekindled value of clinical evaluation recently has led to the hypothesis that when pretest probability of disease and noninvasive tests of lower extremity veins are concordant, DVT can effectively be ruled in or out, whereas when pretest probability of disease and noninvasive tests are discordant, further evaluation is necessary. This approach has led to the creation of a clinical prediction guide for the management of patients with suspected DVT.

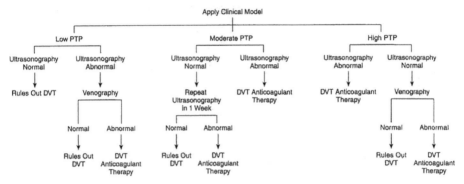

Prediction guide for management of patients with suspected deep vein thrombosis (DVT). PTP = pretest probability. (From Anand S, Wells P, Hunt D, et al: Does this patient have deep vein thrombosis? JAMA 279:1094–1099, 1998, with permission.)

58. Who was Homans?

John Homans (1877–1954) was an American surgeon who worked with Harvey Cushing at Johns Hopkins and eventually became professor of surgery at Peter Bent Brigham. His interest in peripheral vascular disease led to a monograph on the subject in 1939. He also wrote a successful textbook of surgery based on his Harvard course.

BIBLIOGRAPHY

1. Anand S, Wells P, Hunt D, et al: Does this patient have deep vein thrombosis? JAMA 279:1094–1099, 1998.
2. DeGowin RL: DeGowin and DeGowin's Diagnostic Examination, 6th ed. New York, McGraw-Hill, 1994.
3. Hansen-Flaschen J, Nordberg J: Clubbing and hypertrophic osteoarthropathy. Clin Chest Med 8:287–298, 1987.
4. Pyke DA: Finger clubbing: Validity as a physical sign. Lancet 2:352–354, 1954.
5. Sapira JD: The Art and Science of Bedside Diagnosis. Baltimore, Urban & Schwarzenberg, 1990.
6. Willms JL, Schneiderman H, Algranati PS: Physical Diagnosis. Baltimore, Williams & Wilkins, 1994.

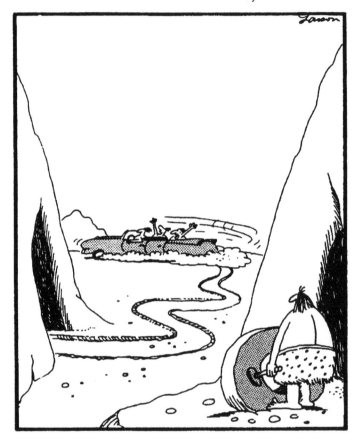

INDEX

Page numbers in **boldface type** indicate complete chapters.

Index